S0-BXN-333

Musculoskeletal Oncology
A Multidisciplinary Approach

Musculoskeletal Oncology
A Multidisciplinary Approach

MICHAEL M. LEWIS, MD, Editor

Robert K. Lippmann Professor of Orthopaedics,
Mt. Sinai School of Medicine, New York, New York

Chairman, Leni and Peter W. May Department of Orthopaedics,
Mt. Sinai Medical Center, New York, New York

Orthopaedic Surgeon-in-Chief,
Mt. Sinai Hospital, New York, New York

W. B. SAUNDERS COMPANY
Harcourt Brace Jovanovich, Inc.
Philadelphia ■ London ■ Toronto ■ Montreal ■ Sydney ■ Tokyo

W. B. SAUNDERS COMPANY
Harcourt Brace Jovanovich, Inc.

The Curtis Center
Independence Square West
Philadelphia, Pennsylvania 19106

Library of Congress Cataloging-in-Publication Data

Musculoskeletal oncology : a multidisciplinary approach /
Michael M. Lewis, editor.

p. cm.

ISBN 0–7216–5771–0

1. Musculoskeletal system—Cancer. I. Lewis, Michael M. (Michael Martin). [DNLM: 1. Bone Neoplasms. 2. Muscles—pathology. 3. Musculoskeletal System—pathology. 4. Soft Tissue Neoplasms. WE 140 M9858]

RC280.M83M87 1992

616.99′27—dc20

DNLM/DLC 91–35082

Editor: Jennifer Mitchell
Developmental Editor: W. B. Saunders Staff
Designer: Anne O'Donnell
Production Manager: Linda R. Garber
Manuscript Editors: Terry Russell and Amy Norwitz
Illustration Specialist: Peg Shaw
Indexer: Ellen Murray

Musculoskeletal Oncology: A Multidisciplinary Approach ISBN 0–7216–5771–0

Printed in the United States of America.

Last digit is the print number: 9 8 7 6 5 4 3 2 1

To my wife Betsy, my best colleague,
and our children.

Contributors

CARL BARBERA, MD
Assistant Professor of Orthopaedic Surgery, State University of New York, Health Science Center at Brooklyn, Brooklyn, New York
Surgical Considerations in Tumors About the Knee

NORMAN D. BLOOM, MD
Professor of Surgery, New York Medical College; Chief of Surgical Oncology and Head and Neck Surgery, Metropolitan Hospital Center; New York, New York
Tumors of the Thoracolumbar Spine; Tumors of the Thoracic Skeleton

WILLIAM D. BLOOMER, MD
Claude W. Benedum Professor of Radiation Oncology, Chairman, Department of Radiation Oncology, University of Pittsburgh School of Medicine, Pittsburgh, Pennsylvania
Radiation Therapy in the Treatment of Bone and Soft Tissue Sarcomas

RONALD H. BLUM, MD
Professor of Medicine, New York University School of Medicine; Director, Division of Medical Oncology, Associate Director, Kaplan Cancer Center, New York University Medical Center; New York, New York
Adult Oncology

MARK S. BROMSON, MD
Department of Orthopaedics, Mt. Sinai School of Medicine, New York, New York
Metabolic Mimickers of Tumor

ROBERT N. BUTLER, MD
Brookdale Professor and Chairman, Gerald and May Ellen Ritter Department of Geriatrics and Adult Development, Mt. Sinai School of Medicine, New York, New York
The Geriatric Patient

MARTIN B. CAMINS, MD
Associate Clinical Professor of Neurosurgery, Mt. Sinai School of Medicine; Associate Attending, Department of Neurosurgery, Mt. Sinai Hospital; Associate Neurosurgeon, Division of Neurosurgery, Lenox Hill Hospital; New York, New York
Osseous Lesions of the Vertebral Axis and Tumors of the Cervical Spine

FRANK P. CAMMISA, Jr., MD
Assistant Professor of Orthopaedic Surgery, Cornell University Medical College; Assistant Attending Surgeon, The Hospital for Special Surgery, New York Hospital; Consultant in Orthopaedic Surgery, Memorial Sloan–Kettering Cancer Center; New York, New York
Malignant and Benign Primary Tumors of the Proximal Femur

HOPE A. CASTORIA, RN, BSN
Clinical Nurse Specialist, Pediatric-Oncology, Hackensack Medical Center, Hackensack, New Jersey
Nursing Considerations

JACK CHOUEKA, MD
Department of Orthopaedic Surgery, Hospital for Joint Diseases Orthopaedic Institute, New York, New York
Hand Tumors

MICHAEL CLAIN, MD
Orthopedic Surgeon, Greenwich, Connecticut
Tumors of the Foot and Ankle

CARLENE CORD, RN, BSN
Clinical Nurse Specialist, Pediatric-Oncology, Hackensack Medical Center, Hackensack, New Jersey
Nursing Considerations

THOMAS A. EINHORN, MD
Associate Professor of Orthopaedics, Director, Orthopaedic Research, Mt. Sinai Medical Center; Associate Attending, Mt. Sinai Hospital; New York, New York
Metabolic Mimickers of Tumor

CHARLES FORSCHER, MD
Assistant Professor, Department of Neoplastic Diseases, Mt. Sinai School of Medicine, New York, New York
Adult Oncology

LORI STEIN FREUDMAN, RN, MSN
Nurse Clinician, Pediatric Hematology-Oncology, Mt. Sinai Hospital, New York, New York
Nursing Considerations

GARY E. FRIEDLAENDER, MD
Professor and Chairman, Department of Orthopaedics and Rehabilitation, Yale University School of Medicine; Chief of Orthopaedics and Rehabilitation, Yale-New Haven Hospital; New Haven, Connecticut
Osteochondral Allografts and Bone Banking

DALE B. GLASSER, MS, MPhil
Epidemiologist, Research Division, The Hospital for Special Surgery; Consultant, Memorial Sloan–Kettering Cancer Center; New York, New York
Malignant and Benign Primary Tumors of the Proximal Femur

ADAM GREENSPAN, MD
Professor of Radiology and Orthopaedic Surgery, University of California School of Medicine, Davis; Chief, Orthopaedic Radiology, Department of Diagnostic Radiology, University of California, Davis Medical Center; Sacramento, California
Radiology and Pathology of Bone Tumors

MICHAEL GROPPER, DSW
Assistant Professor, Bar Ilan University School of Social Work, Ramat Gan, Israel
Psychosocial Dimensions of Bone Cancer: Social Work Services and Human Resources

PAUL GUSMORINO, MD
Assistant Clinical Professor, Department of Psychiatry, Mt. Sinai School of Medicine; Attending, Department of Behavioral Medicine, Hospital for Joint Diseases Orthopaedic Institute; Assistant Attending, Department of Psychiatry, Beth Israel Medical Center; New York, New York
Behavioral Medicine and Cancer: A Clinical Guide

MICHAEL B. HARRIS, MD
Associate Professor of Clinical Pediatrics, University of Medicine and Dentistry, Newark, New Jersey; Director, Tomorrow's Children's Institute, Director, Pediatric Hematology-Oncology, Hackensack Medical Center; Hackensack, New Jersey
Pediatric Ewing's Sarcomas, Osteosarcomas, and Primitive Neuroectodermal Tumors

MICHAEL J. HARRISON, MD
Department of Neurosurgery, Mt. Sinai School of Medicine, New York, New York
Osseous Lesions of the Vertebral Axis and Tumors of the Cervical Spine

MICHAEL R. HAUSMAN, MD
Assistant Professor of Orthopaedics, Mt. Sinai School of Medicine; Chief, Upper Extremity Surgery, Mt. Sinai Hospital; Attending Orthopaedic Surgeon, Elmhurst Hospital; New York, New York
Hand Tumors; Reconstructive Techniques in Orthopedic Oncology

JAMES F. HOLLAND, MD
Jane B. and Jack R. Aron Professor of Neoplastic Diseases, Professor of Medicine, Mt. Sinai School of Medicine; Chairman, Department of Neoplastic Diseases, Mt. Sinai Hospital; Director, Derald H. Ruttenberg Cancer Center, Mt. Sinai Medical Center; New York, New York
Adult Oncology

HATIM HYDERALLY, MD
Associate Professor, Department of Anesthesiology, Mt. Sinai School of Medicine, Attending Anesthesiologist, Mt. Sinai Hospital; New York, New York
Anesthetic Considerations in Limb Preservation Surgery for Neoplastic Disease

SHALOM KALNICKI, MD
Associate Professor, Department of Radiation Oncology, University of Pittsburgh School of Medicine; Director of Radiation Oncology Services, Magee-Womens Hospital, Pittsburgh, Pennsylvania
Radiation Therapy in the Treatment of Bone and Soft Tissue Sarcomas

CONSTANTINE P. KARAKOUSIS, MD, PhD
Clinical Professor of Surgery, State University of New York at Buffalo; Associate Chief, Surgical Oncology Department, Chief, Soft Tissue–Melanoma and Bone Service, Roswell Park Cancer Institute, Buffalo, New York
Soft Tissue Sarcomas and Limb Sparing

SAMUEL KENAN, MD
Associate Professor of Orthopaedics, Mt. Sinai School of Medicine; Associate Director, Orthopaedic Oncology, Mt. Sinai Hospital; New York, New York
Tumors and Tumor-like Conditions of the Shoulder Girdle

MICHAEL J. KLEIN, MD
Associate Professor of Pathology and Orthopaedics, Mt. Sinai School of Medicine; Associate Attending, Mt. Sinai Hospital; Consultant in Orthopaedic Pathology, New York Veterans' Administration Medical Center; New York, New York
Radiology and Pathology of Bone Tumors

FREDRIC A. KLEINBART, MD
Clinical Instructor, Temple University School of Medicine; Attending, Department of Orthopaedic Surgery, Temple University Hospital; Philadelphia, Pennsylvania
Tumors and Tumor-like Conditions of the Shoulder Girdle

JOSEPH M. LANE, MD
Professor of Orthopaedic Surgery, Cornell University Medical College; Director, Research Operations, Chief, Metabolic Bone Disease; Orthopaedic Attending, The Hospital for Special Surgery; Orthopaedic Attending, Memorial Sloan–Kettering Cancer Center; New York, New York
Malignant and Benign Primary Tumors of the Proximal Femur

MICHAEL M. LEWIS, MD
Robert K. Lippmann Professor of Orthopaedics, Mt. Sinai School of Medicine; Chairman, Leni and Peter W. May Department of Orthopaedics, Mt. Sinai Medical Center; Orthopaedic Surgeon-in-Chief, Mt. Sinai Hospital; New York, New York
Tumors and Tumor-like Conditions of the Shoulder Girdle; Surgical Considerations in Tumors About the Knee

HENRY J. MANKIN, MD
Edith M. Ashley Professor of Orthopaedic Surgery, Harvard Medical School; Chief of Orthopaedic Services, Massachusetts General Hospital; Boston, Massachusetts
Osteochondral Allografts and Bone Banking

KATHRYN McLEAN, RN, MSN, CPN
Nurse Clinician, Pediatric Hematology-Oncology, Mt. Sinai Hospital, New York, New York
Nursing Considerations

ROBERT J. MEISLIN, MD
Department of Orthopaedics, Hospital for Joint Diseases Orthopaedic Institute, New York, New York
Tumors of the Thoracolumbar Spine

JAMES R. NEFF, MD
Professor and Chairman, Department of Orthopaedic Surgery and Rehabilitation, University of Nebraska College of Medicine, Omaha, Nebraska
Metastatic Disease to Bone

MICHAEL G. NEUWIRTH, MD
Assistant Clinical Professor, Mt. Sinai School of Medicine; Chief, Spine Services, Hospital for Joint Disease Orthopaedic Institute; New York, New York
Tumors of the Thoracolumbar Spine

MARY I. O'CONNOR, MD
Senior Associate Consultant and Instructor in Orthopaedics, Mayo Graduate School of Medicine, Jacksonville, Florida
Pelvic Tumors

ISAAC PINTER, PhD
Assistant Professor of Clinical Rehabilitation Medicine, Mt. Sinai School of Medicine; Director, Department of Behavioral Medicine, Administrative Director, Pain Center, Hospital for Joint Diseases Orthopaedic Institute; New York, New York
Behavioral Medicine and Cancer: A Clinical Guide

KRISTJAN T. RAGNARSSON, MD
Dr. Lucy G. Moses Professor of Rehabilitation Medicine, Chairman, Department of Rehabilitation Medicine, Mt. Sinai School of Medicine; Director, Department of Rehabilitation Medicine, Mt. Sinai Hospital; New York, New York
Rehabilitation of Patients with Physical Disabilities Caused by Tumors of the Musculoskeletal System

STEVEN G. ROBBINS, MD
Orthopaedic Surgeon, St. Barnabas Medical Center, Livingston, New Jersey
Malignant and Benign Primary Tumors of the Proximal Femur

GARY ROSENBERG, PhD
Edith J. Baerwald Professor of Community Medicine (Social Work), Mt. Sinai School of Medicine; Senior Vice President, Mt. Sinai Medical Center; New York, New York
Psychosocial Dimensions of Bone Cancer: Social Work Services and Human Resources

BRUCE ROSENBLUM, MD
Clinical Assistant Professor, Department of Neurosurgery, Mt. Sinai Medical Center, New York, New York
Osseous Lesions of the Vertebral Axis and Tumors of the Cervical Spine

BEVERLY R. RYAN, MD
Associate Professor of Clinical Pediatrics, University of Medicine and Dentistry, Newark, New Jersey; Attending, Pediatric Hematology-Oncology, Tomorrow's Children's Institute, Hackensack Medical Center, Hackensack, New Jersey
Principles of Pediatric Oncology

DONNA M. RYNIKER, RN, MA
Clinical Coordinator, Surgical Oncology, Orthopaedics, Mt. Sinai Hospital, New York, New York
Nursing Considerations

FRANKLIN H. SIM, MD
Professor of Orthopedic Surgery, Mayo Medical School; Consultant, Department of Orthopedics, Mayo Clinic and Mayo

Foundation; Consultant, Methodist Hospital; Rochester, Minnesota
Pelvic Tumors

BARRY R. SNOW, PhD
Adjunct Assistant Professor of Public Health, Columbia University School of Public Health; Clinical Psychologist, Department of Behavioral Medicine; Associate Director, Research and Training, Pain Center, Hospital for Joint Diseases Orthopaedic Institute; New York, New York
Behavioral Medicine and Cancer: A Clinical Guide

DEMPSEY S. SPRINGFIELD, MD
Associate Professor in Orthopaedic Surgery, Harvard Medical School; Visiting Orthopaedic Surgeon, Massachusetts General Hospital; Boston, Massachusetts
Evaluation of Bone and Soft Tissue Tumors

CARLIN B. VICKERY, MD
Assistant Professor of Clinical Surgery, Mt. Sinai School of Medicine; Assistant Attending, Mt. Sinai Hospital; New York, New York
Reconstructive Techniques in Orthopedic Oncology

JOHN F. WALLER, MD
Clinical Assistant Professor of Orthopaedics, Mt. Sinai School of Medicine; Associate Attending, Mt. Sinai Hospital; New York, New York
Tumors of the Foot and Ankle

HUBERT WEINBERG, MD
Associate Professor of Surgery, Mt. Sinai School of Medicine; Associate Attending, Mt. Sinai Hospital; New York, New York
Reconstructive Techniques in Orthopedic Oncology

DONNA M. WEINER, RN, MA, OCN
Clinical Nursing Supervisor—Oncology, Mt. Sinai Hospital, New York, New York
Nursing Considerations

MICHAEL A. WEINER, MD
Associate Professor of Clinical Pediatrics, University of Medicine and Dentistry, Newark, New Jersey; Associate Director, Pediatric Hematology-Oncology, Tomorrow's Children's Institute, Hackensack Medical Center, Hackensack, New Jersey
Childhood Tumors That May Result in Metastatic Bone Disease

DIANA WILLIAMSON, MD
Oncology Research Fellow, New York University Medical Center, New York, New York
Adult Oncology

Preface

Many aspects of contemporary medicine involve significant interaction among multiple disciplines. Often practitioners in one area of specialization seek further depth and delineation in allied fields. This maximizes professional interaction, enhances patient care, and may serve as a catalyst for future progress. The goal of this book is to focus on an integrated approach to the study of musculoskeletal oncology that is presented in a relevant, organized, and readable fashion. Primary and secondary neoplastic disease processes and treatment as well as selected tumor-like conditions are discussed.

Organizing a text can be challenging. One aspect of this book concerns the definition and overall evaluation of these lesions. This includes sections on staging and the important correlation of pathology and radiology. Another area is directed toward the current approach and experience in pediatric, adult, and radiation oncology. Part of the surgical concepts and techniques section is presented utilizing a regional anatomic orientation. Although this can lead to a certain amount of redundancy, it is hoped that this is minimal and offset by the cohesiveness of each of these chapters. Another important aspect of this surgical discussion includes sections on soft tissue neoplasm, wound coverage, and bone banking. Furthermore, the very significant areas of nursing, anesthesia, rehabilitation, social work, pain, and behavioral medicine are incorporated into this text. It is the hope, then, that this book will serve as a useful resource for students, professionals, and the allied health care members of the musculoskeletal oncologic team.

MICHAEL M. LEWIS, M.D.

Acknowledgments

Not that long ago Mr. Ed Wickland, then senior editor at W.B. Saunders, and I were having an informal discussion. Out of that talk came the idea and commitment for this book. I am grateful to Ed for his enthusiasm and endurance that made this text a reality. I am extremely indebted to all of the authors who have so graciously contributed their expertise as well as their valuable time in the preparation of this book. A very special thanks to Dr. Norman Bloom, Dr. Michael Harris, and Dr. Samuel Kenan, who not only contributed to the text but also served as contributing editors. I would like to acknowledge Dr. Andrew Casden, Dr. Raymond Miller, and Dr. Michael Wesson, who helped review selective aspects of the book, and Deborah Bachner and Marisa Mantineo for their administrative assistance. In addition, great effort has been expended in the production of the book by Kathleen McCullough and Jennifer Mitchell on behalf of the publisher. Furthermore, my office administrator, Mary Quarto, and procedure coordinator, Lucille Carrao, have helped to collate clinical information over many years.

Two individuals merit special appreciation. Dr. Michael Klein has participated, with distinction, as an outstanding associate editor. Donna Ryniker, R.N., predictably proved to be a tireless and exacting coordinator for this book.

Contents

CHAPTER 1

Evaluation of Bone and Soft Tissue Tumors

DEMPSEY S. SPRINGFIELD

Tumors of the musculoskeletal system are rare, and the practicing orthopedist sees only a few patients each year with a musculoskeletal tumor; malignant tumors are particularly uncommon. More often than not, bone lesions are caused by an infection, are the results of trauma, or are due to metastatic deposit from a previously diagnosed or occult carcinoma. Their rare occurrence makes the recognition of primary musculoskeletal tumors, especially malignant tumors, more difficult, and it is understandable that they are often not initially identified. Physicians must remain alert and remember that any musculoskeletal complaint may result from an underlying primary tumor.

The most important part of the initial examination of a patient with a musculoskeletal tumor is recognizing its presence. Musculoskeletal neoplasms should always be in the differential diagnosis of a patient with musculoskeletal symptoms until excluded by further evaluation. There are no specific patient complaints or physical examination findings associated with musculoskeletal neoplasms, and any musculoskeletal symptoms could be due to tumor of the bone or soft tissues.

Recognizing the Problem

All soft tissue masses, especially those in an adult, should be considered primary soft tissue sarcomas until proved otherwise. Although lipomas are common, many surgeons have been surprised to find a malignant soft tissue tumor when they had assumed that the mass was a lipoma. Bone lesions range from old benign, inactive, unimportant tumors to metastases from an untreatable carcinoma. The early recognition of a primary malignant bone tumor and the proper initial management can mean the difference between a limb salvage and an amputation or the difference between life and death.

Primary musculoskeletal tumors are missed not because they are occult on the physical examination or plain x-ray films but because the possibility of their existence is forgotten or they are thought to be too rare to be worth considering. An excellent example is the usual presentation of a patient with sacral chordoma. Chordoma, a malignant tumor most often in the sacrum, is most easily diagnosed by palpation on rectal examination. Unfortunately, the average length of time a patient with a chordoma complains of pain, usually low back pain, and is under the care of a physician before having a rectal examination is 1 year.[10] Patients with a lesion in the distal femur or the proximal tibia too often have a diagnostic knee arthroscopy before the bone tumor is seen on the plain x-ray film.[15] Sometimes an x-ray film is not obtained or is not reviewed, but more often an obvious lesion on the plain film is missed because the possibility of a bone tumor is not considered and the x-ray film is not examined specifically for a tumor.

Musculoskeletal tumors occur in both sexes and in all age groups. No part of the anatomy is exempt from the risk of harboring a tumor. Every bone, all muscles, every nerve, and all anatomic compartments have been sites of a primary musculoskeletal tumor. The patients, even those with malignant tumors, usually appear healthy and often present exactly like the patient with a sprained joint or a pulled muscle. The teenager who bumped her shoulder and later has a small mass or the 25-year-old businessman whose knee is sore after he plays tennis may have a bone tumor. After about age 60, metastatic bone deposits are the most common lesion of bone, but myeloma is the most common primary malignant bone tumor in adults, and malignant fibrous histiocytoma of bone and chondrosarcoma are not rare in this age group. The possibility of these tumors must be remembered by the clinician. Only by suspecting the unexpected, asking the right questions, and examining the patient carefully will the tumor be correctly diagnosed or excluded from the possible diagnoses.

Initial Evaluation

Most patients with a musculoskeletal tumor initially seek medical attention because of pain. Others are seen because they have an unexplained mass, and some patients are referred because an abnormality was found on an x-ray film for an unrelated complaint. When pain is present, the patient should be asked about the pain. What is it like? Is it sharp, dull, intermittent, or constant? Does it radiate? Is it related to activity? Is it worse at night? Does it awaken the patient at night? Exactly where is the pain located? What is done to make it better? What makes it worse? What medication is being used for the pain? When the patient has a mass, the physician should ask about its duration, its rate of growth, the presence of symptoms, and prior trauma. If the patient has only abnormal radiographic findings and no symptoms, the single most important determination is whether he or she had a prior x-ray film of the area. Occasionally, a patient remembers having had radiography in the past, and review of the previous x-ray film can provide invaluable information about the patient and the lesion.

PATIENT HISTORY

After questioning the patient about the presenting symptoms, the physician evaluating a patient with a musculoskeletal complaint takes a complete history, including the past medical history, the family history, and a review of systems. This can provide important diagnostic clues. Children's athletic activities have increased during the past decade, resulting in an increase in fatigue fractures in patients with open epiphyseal plates. The periosteal reaction and pain of a fatigue fracture may be mistaken for Ewing's sarcoma or osteosarcoma, but a careful review of the child's activities can suggest the true cause of the lesion. Another common traumatic lesion mistaken for a malignant neoplasm is an avulsion of bone at the origin of the hamstring muscles. The patient has an ache in the buttock and the sensation of a mass, and on the x-ray film there is a radiodense lesion adjacent to the ischium. When specifically asked about a traumatic event, the patient usually remembers the "hamstring pull" that occurred 6 to 9 months before the discovery of the ischial mass. (This history essentially confirms the suspected diagnosis.)

The history is particularly important when seeing a patient with a pathologic fracture. Most children with a pathologic fracture have an underlying benign tumor, and the patient is best managed by letting the fracture heal before treating the lesion. If the patient had no symptoms before the fracture and the lesion is well circumscribed, it is unlikely that the lesion is significant, and the patient's fracture can be safely treated with minimal concern about the underlying process. If the patient had symptoms (pain) before the fracture, the physician should be more concerned that the underlying process is an aggressive benign or malignant tumor and consider an early biopsy. Older patients with known carcinoma who have a pathologic fracture need a careful review of symptoms and physical examination; other lesions may be found and early treatment can be instituted.

The past medical history may also provide vital information. Adult patients with a history of breast cancer, prostate cancer, or lymphoma that has been in remission for a few years may not volunteer that they have had a malignancy, and the physician must specifically ask about these diagnoses when the possibility of a metastatic lesion is suggested by the clinical presentation. Children who have mastoiditis (manifested by recurrent otitis media), diabetes insipidus, and a bone lesion have Hand-Schüller-Christian disease, but the family may not offer the information about the ear problems and kidney problems to the orthopedist, because they think he or she is interested only in the bones. It is the responsibility of the physician to get all the necessary information from the patient or the family.

PHYSICAL EXAMINATION

The physical examination must be as thorough as the history taking. Most patients evaluated by an orthopedist have normal physical examination findings, except for the area of complaint. This is true for most patients with musculoskeletal tumors, but for those with a suspected neoplasm, the physical findings, separate from those directly related to the patient's complaints, may play a major role in helping the physician determine a proper differential diagnosis and plan an appropriate evaluation. The adult patient with a pathologic fracture who has a thyroid nodule, a breast mass, or decreased breath sounds probably has a metastatic carcinoma, and the evaluation should include a careful study of the other abnormal organ system. A patient with a soft tissue mass who has numerous café au lait spots should be suspected of having neurofibromatosis, and the mass should be considered to be a neurofibroma or neurofibrosarcoma until proved otherwise.

Initially, the physician should examine the site of the complaint. Is there a visible mass? How big is it? (The physician should take measurements.) Is it tender? Is there increased temperature? What is the range of motion, passive and active, of adjacent joints? Is there atrophy of the muscles in the limb? What is the neurovascular status of the extremity? The remainder of the physical examination should be done with specific attention to those anatomic areas that may provide clues to the diagnosis. Are there other musculoskeletal abnormalities? Are there enlarged lymph nodes? Does the patient have an abdominal or rectal mass? After a complete history and physical examination has been done, the plain x-ray film can be requested.

RADIOGRAPHY

Plain x-ray films are a necessary part of the initial work-up of almost every patient with a musculoskeletal complaint. The x-ray films must be of good quality. Underpenetrated x-ray films of a bone lesion or overpenetrated x-ray films of a soft tissue lesion are not acceptable. They must include the entire area of interest. This usually means that the entire bone should be seen. One should not forget to obtain x-ray films of an anatomic site that may refer pain to another location (e.g., a lesion in the hip presenting as pain in the knee). Two views taken at right angles to one another are a minimum. The x-rays films should be reviewed systemically, the examiner looking at specific areas and asking specific questions. The clinician should not forget to look at the soft tissues. Is there calcification in the soft tissue? If the x-ray film is not studied in a systematic fashion, it is easy to miss an otherwise obvious lesion. The findings on the plain x-ray films help determine what other radiographic evaluations, if any, are necessary.

Enneking teaches that four primary questions should be answered when evaluating a lesion on a plain x-ray film.[7]

The first question is "Where is the lesion?" Is it in a long bone, a flat bone, or a short bone of the hand or the foot? Is it in the epiphysis, the metaphysis, or the diaphysis? Is it in the medullary canal, in the cortex, on the cortex, or surrounding the cortex?

The second question is "What is the lesion doing to the bone?" Is there bone destruction? Is it geographic, permeative, or "moth eaten"?

The third question is "What is the bone doing to the lesion?" Is there an endosteal reaction, and if there is, how mature is it? Is there a periosteal reaction? What type? Is there a Codman's triangle, a sunburst pattern, or "onionskinning," or is it a well-formed periosteal reaction? Is there an overreaction to the lesion?

The fourth question is "Is there any characteristic within the lesion to suggest a specific diagnosis?" Is there bone formation? Is there calcification? Does the lesion have a ground-glass appearance?

Although often a lesion is recognized without asking and answering each question, the exercise is useful. The answers may suggest other lesions that should be considered, reducing the chance that a potential diagnosis will be overlooked. The answers often provide the clues that lead to a specific diagnosis, but if they do not, they indicate the additional studies that need to be done.

Observation of a lesion over time can provide important information. One should remember to ask if the patient has had a previous x-ray film taken or if the area has been examined by another physician. If these have not occurred, it still may be possible to take advantage of the diagnostic value of observation over time. Lesions that are inactive (i.e., the patient has no symptoms, the reaction is a mature rim of bone, and the lesion is cold on the bone scan) can be watched, and the tumors' nature can be assessed over a few months. Only if there is a change in the lesion would it be necessary to do a biopsy. The primary objections to performing a biopsy for every abnormality seen on an x-ray film are that many need no treatment and the biopsy makes observation of the lesion's natural history impossible.

Other Studies

After the initial evaluation, a decision is made regarding the next step in the patient's examination or treatment. Although often the diagnosis and a final treatment decision can be based on the initial evaluation, in other cases the information is not sufficient to make a diagnosis or even to differentiate between major categories of illnesses. Lesions that are obviously benign, inactive, and self-healing (e.g., fibrous cortical defect, enchondroma, fibrous dysplasia, and exostosis) need no other evaluation, and the patient can be told that only observation is necessary. For lesions that are benign, are active, and need treatment that can be done without additional information (e.g., unicameral bone cyst), treatment can be planned and scheduled.

In other cases, the diagnosis is made from the initial evaluation but additional radiologic testing is needed before planning the definitive treatment (e.g., giant cell tumor of bone, chondroblastoma, osteoid osteoma, osteosarcoma, and chondrosarcoma), and these tests can be requested. It is important to discuss with the radiologist the reasons for any additional examination. The surgeon is principally interested in the anatomic extent of the lesion so that surgery can be planned. The radiologist is not a surgeon and cannot know what information is sought. In other patients, the initial evaluation does not provide sufficient information from which to make diagnostic or therapeutic decisions. Often, it is not possible to make a diagnosis or even to know whether a lesion is traumatic, infectious, or neoplastic in origin from only the history, physical examination findings, and plain x-ray films. In these cases, additional diagnostic tests are necessary. Although knowing the anatomic extent of the lesion, determined by radiography, is valuable, the more important information is that which helps decide the nature of the lesion. Even if a definitive diagnosis cannot be made after all radiologic tests are obtained, the information gained assists both in planning a biopsy and in allowing the pathologist to make an accurate diagnosis. As a rule, lesions that are difficult to diagnose from the clinical information are difficult to diagnose from the histology examination, and the pathologist often depends on the data obtained from the additional examinations to make the final diagnostic decision.

An orthopedist who is evaluating the patient with a musculoskeletal lesion must remember that the radiologist and the pathologist are usually not familiar with the patient's history. To increase the value of the consultation, the orthopedist requesting a special radiologic examination from a radiologist or a biopsy interpretation from a pathologist should tell the radiologist and the pathologist what specific information is needed.

The patient with a suspected metastatic deposit should be evaluated differently from the patient with an apparent primary sarcoma, but a cautious approach is suggested, and one should not assume that every destructive bone lesion in an elderly patient is a metastatic carcinoma. Chondrosarcoma and malignant fibrous histiocytoma of bone often masquerade as metastatic bone lesions. A destructive lesion of bone in a patient with a history of a prior carcinoma can be assumed to be a metastasis but usually needs to have a confirmatory biopsy. These lesions do not need further evaluation, as the treatment can usually be planned with only the initial information. The evaluation is limited to assessing the patient's general status and looking for other sites of metastasis, particularly bone metastasis. Patients suspected of having metastasis from the appearance of the bone lesions but in whom no primary focus is known should be examined for a primary carcinoma.

The search for an unknown primary carcinoma metastatic to bone should not be exhaustive. There is little to be gained by performing every diagnostic study available. Carcinomas of the paired central organs (thyroid, breast, lungs, kidneys, and prostate) most frequently metastasize to bone. These organs should be evaluated by physical examination (thyroid, breast, and prostate), chest radiography (lung), mammography (breast), acid phosphatase determinations (prostate), urinalysis (kidney), and intravenous pyelography (kidney). Abdominal ultrasound is increasingly popular to evaluate for kidney and other abdominal masses. Multiple myeloma is a common primary tumor of bone (the single most common primary malignant bone tumor of adulthood), and a serum immunoelectrophoresis should be done. The history and a review of symptoms are also important in the work-up of a patient suspected of having a metastatic lesion. If either the patient's history or the review of symptoms suggests a primary carcinoma, the organ system implicated should be thoroughly evaluated. For example, patients with abdominal pain or gastrointestinal symptoms should have the abdomen examined with a computed tomography (CT) scan and/or an upper and lower gastrointestinal radiograph series. If the history, the review of symptoms, and an initial review of the paired central organs do not reveal a primary tumor, biopsy of the bone lesion should be performed. This biopsy should be done as if the tumor were a primary bone sarcoma.

Many lesions are so suggestive of a primary bone tumor that they can be recognized as such, and a search for a primary carcinoma is not justified. A destructive lesion with intralesional calcification, in an adult, particularly in the proximal femur or the periacetabular pelvis, is most likely a chondrosarcoma, and the evaluation should be planned as if it were. The same is true in a teenager with a distal femoral or the proximal tibial lesion that both destroys bone and is producing bone. This is an osteosarcoma until proved otherwise and should be evaluated as such.

The evaluation of a primary bone sarcoma should determine the anatomic extent of the lesion and search for possible metastatic foci. Occasionally, the diagnosis can be made from the prebiopsy staging studies, but their principal purpose is to provide sufficient information so that the tumor's stage can be established with only the addition of data about the histologic grade, which is determined by examination of the tissue removed at biopsy. Plain x-ray films, linear tomograms, CT scans, magnetic resonance imaging (MRI), arteriograms, and scintiscans all play roles in discovering the anatomic extent and searching for metastatic foci of a primary sarcoma. The primary lesion should be studied with the aid of those studies that show its anatomic extent. The lungs and bones should be evaluated as potential sites of metastatic foci because of the propensity of sarcoma to metastasize to these organs. Physical examination is sufficient to evaluate the regional lymph nodes, and the liver and spleen do not need to be evaluated unless other findings suggest metastasis to one of these organs.

Special Diagnostic Studies

RADIONUCLIDE SCANS

Technetium-99m bone and gallium-67 scans are efficient, safe, and readily available.[16, 23] Technetium scans are used both to determine the activity of the primary lesion and to search for other bone lesions. Occasionally, the technetium bone scan reveals the intraosseous anatomic extent of a bone lesion better than other studies, but usually the CT scan or the MRI image is more accurate. The value of the intrinsic activity of the lesion on the bone scan is limited. Lesions that do not have increased activity on the technetium bone scan are almost always benign, inactive lesions and usually need no treatment. Myeloma and histiocytosis X bone lesions are exceptions and often appear normal or have decreased uptake on the technetium bone scan. Lesions with increased activity may be benign or malignant, and the intensity of the uptake is not predictive of the risk of malignancy. The technetium scan is sensitive and reveals metastatic foci in bone before the plain x-ray film findings are abnormal and often before the patient has symptoms. The technetium bone scan is the best method to screen the entire skeleton of a patient suspected of having bone metastases.

Gallium scans are less useful in the evaluation of a patient with a suspected musculoskeletal tumor.[9] The examination takes longer to perform (24 to 48 hours) and is more sensitive to inflammatory cells than to activity in the bone. Most, if not all, tumors have an inflammatory component and therefore have an increase in gallium uptake (a hot scan), but gallium scans are most useful in determining whether a mass is neoplastic or infectious. Unsuspected metastases from soft tissue sarcomas are occasionally found on a gallium scan.

LINEAR TOMOGRAPHY

Linear tomography was once an important method to evaluate bone tumors. It was used to see the details of the lesions, particularly intralesional calcification or ossification, cortical destruction, periosteal reaction, intraosseous extension, and intraarticular extension. Whole-lung linear tomography was used as the standard method to evaluate the lungs for pulmonary metastasis. CT scans have made linear tomography almost obsolete in the evaluation of a suspected bone tumor, though it does remain a good method to determine if a lesion has extended across the subchondral bone into the articular cartilage and therefore into the joint. Linear tomography is also useful in the evaluation of a suspected fatigue fracture.

ARTERIOGRAPHY

Whereas arteriography was once the best method for judging the extent of a bone or a soft tissue tumor,[13] it has become almost obsolete for this purpose. CT and MRI are better methods to visualize the extraosseous extent of a bone tumor or anatomically to localize a soft tissue mass. If intravenous contrast material is administered during the CT scan, the major vessels can be seen, and on MRI no contrast media are necessary to see the arteries and veins. Arteriography is indicated when the major vascular bundle cannot be seen with CT or MRI, when the vessels appear to be intralesional, when preoperative embolization is planned, or when intraarterial infusion of chemotherapeutic agents is used.

COMPUTED TOMOGRAPHY

The development of CT has done more for the ability to localize tumors anatomically than any other study since the discovery of x-rays.[12, 14, 28] Before CT scans, the surgeon had to rely on physical examination, linear tomograms, and arteriograms to define the anatomic extent of a musculoskeletal tumor. Technetium-99m bone scans were reported to be more accurate in predicting bone involvement, but this study was done with early CT scanning equipment.[14] Tumors evaluated without the use of CT or MRI were not accurately defined, and as a result, surgical resections were usually more radical than was necessary to ensure complete resection of the tumor. The increase in the percentage of limb salvage operations done in the last decade is in part (probably principally) due to the CT scan, and more recently MRI, with the resultant better definition of the tumor's extent.

As mentioned above, the orthopedist must discuss the purpose of the CT scan with the radiologist before the examination is done. The orthopedist should have specific expectations of the CT examination and should not assume that the radiologist knows what information is sought. Sometimes the CT scan is done as an additional diagnostic test, sometimes it is done only to determine the anatomic extent, and often it is done for both reasons. The CT scan is performed differently depending on the suspected diagnosis and questions that need to be answered.[4, 5, 12, 28] The radiologist must select the window settings of the scanner, the anatomic extent of the examination, and whether to use intravenous or oral contrast agents. The position of the extremity, whether the patient is prone or supine, and whether to include both extremities are other important variables when doing a CT scan. It is more complicated than a plain radiography and must yield more detail than a plain x-ray film if it is to be used to its full potential.

As a rule of thumb, all lesions should be studied with and without intravenous contrast media, tumor and normal tissue densities should be measured, permanent records should be made of the appearance of the lesion with both bone window settings and soft tissue window settings, the contralateral extremity should be included in the study for comparison, and the entire compartments involved should be studied. If the lesion is deformed by the weight of the patient's body, the patient should lie on the opposite side to eliminate this artefact.

MAGNETIC RESONANCE IMAGING (MRI)

MRI is in its infancy and its role is not yet clear. In the future, it will be possible to select which patients are better studied with CT scanning and which with MRI, but currently there is not sufficient experience.[1–3, 18–20, 29] The author's impression is that MRI is superior to CT in evaluating a soft tissue mass, for determining the extent of the extraosseous component of a bone tumor, and for determining the medullary canal extent of a tumor.[19, 25] MRI is not as accurate as CT in determining the relationship of a tumor to the cortex of a bone or in evaluating a lesion composed of dense bone.[11, 23]

The patient is exposed to no radiation during MRI, and views in three planes can be obtained without added time or danger to the patient. An additional advantage of MRI is its ability to distinguish between histologically different tissues of identical densities whereas CT scans rely only on different densities to distinguish between tissues. Most solid soft tissue tumors have densities similar to those of muscle, and on CT scans they are distinguished from the surrounding normal muscle only by their size or the increased vascular pattern seen when intravenous contrast material is used. MRI, on the other hand, reveals a tumor because of the types of signals emitted compared with those from normal tissues.[26, 27] As with the CT scan, the purpose of the MRI examination should be discussed with the radiologist before it is done.

Staging

Staging of lesions is useful for two reasons. First, the prognosis is related to the stage of a patient's disease, and by establishing the stage, the physician has an idea of the prognosis. Knowing the prognosis is important when planning treatment as well as when advising the patient of the options. A patient with an early or less advanced stage of a tumor is managed differently from a patient with the same tumor at a later stage. Second, staging permits meaningful classification of lesions, so that treatments can be evaluated. Without staging it would be impossible to compare treatments of similar lesions. The staging system should be prognostic, it should be practical, and it should assist in categorizing patients into separate treatment groups.

In 1977, the American Joint Commission on Staging and End Result Studies (AJC) published their proposed staging system for soft tissue sarcomas.[21] This system is based on the TNM system used in previous staging systems. T indicates size. T1 lesions are 5 cm or less in diameter. T2 lesions are larger than 5 cm. T3 lesions are those with extension into a major nerve, artery, or bone (the T3 category was excluded in the revised 1988 AJC staging system). N refers to the involvement of lymph nodes. N0 means no lymph node involvement, and N1 indicates that lymph nodes are involved. M refers to the presence of distant metastasis. M0 means there are no distant metastases, and M1 indicates the presence of distant metastasis. The histologic grade of the tumor (G) was added to the TNM classification. A three-grade system was selected. Grade 1 (G1) tumors have the least risk of metastasizing; grade 2(G2), an intermediate risk; and grade 3(G3), the greatest risk.

This initial system was modified in 1988.[24] The resultant system has four stages, each with two subclassifications (Table 1–1). The risk of distant metastasis increases from stage IA through stage IVB. This staging system is for soft tissue sarcomas only. There is no AJC staging system for bone tumors.

TABLE 1–1

Staging System for Soft Tissue Sarcoma

Stage	Description
Stage I	
IA	(G1, T1, N0, M0) Grade 1 tumor <5 cm in diameter with no regional lymph node or distal metastasis
IB	(G1, T2, N0, M0) Grade 1 tumor ≥5 cm in diameter with no regional lymph node or distant metastasis
Stage II	
IIA	(G2, T1, N0, M0) Grade 2 tumor <5 cm in diameter with no regional lymph node or distant metastasis
IIB	(G2, T2, N0, M0) Grade 2 tumor ≥5 cm in diameter with no regional lymph node or distant metastasis
Stage III	
IIIA	(G3, T1, N0, M0) Grade 3 tumor <5 cm in diameter with no regional lymph node or distant metastasis
IIIB	(G3, T2, N0, M0) Grade 3 tumor ≥5 cm in diameter with no regional lymph node or distant metastasis
Stage IV	
IVA	(G1–3, T1–2, N1, M0) Tumor of any grade or size with histologically verified metastasis to regional lymph nodes, but no distant metastasis
IVB	(G1–3, T1–2, N0–1, M1) Clinically diagnosed distant metastasis

From Suit HD, Mankin HJ, Wood WC, Gebhardt MC, Harmon DC, Rosenberg A, Tepper JE, Rosenthal D: Treatment of the patient with stage M0 soft tissue sarcoma. J Clin Oncol 6:854–862, 1988.

Enneking and associates proposed a staging system used for both bone and soft tissue sarcomas.[8] This system is a "surgical" staging system and was designed to be "clear cut, straightforward, and clinically practical."[8] It has been adopted by the Musculoskeletal Tumor Society and is used frequently in the literature. The system uses the histologic grade and anatomic extent to separate tumors into different stages. Only two histologic grades are used: low grade (I) and high grade (II). Low-grade tumors are those that have less than a 25% risk of developing distant metastasis, are histologically well-differentiated, and have few mitoses. High-grade lesions have a greater risk of metastasizing and have a high cell/matrix ratio, a high mitotic rate, necrosis, and microvascular invasion.

Anatomic extent is defined as either intracompartmental (A) or extracompartmental (B) (Table 1–2). The compartments are anatomic areas bounded by barriers to tumor extension. The cortex, the periosteum, and the articular cartilage are barriers to tumor extension; thus each bone is an anatomic compartment. The major fascial septae and tendinous origins and insertions of muscles are barriers to tumor extension; therefore the extremities are separated into compartments by their fascial septae and the origin and insertion of the muscles within that compartment.

TABLE 1–2

Anatomic Compartments

Intracompartmental (A)	Extracompartmental (B)
Intraosseous	Soft tissue extension
Intraarticular	Soft tissue extension
Superficial to deep fascia	Deep fascial extension
Paraosseous	Intraosseous or extrafascial
Intrafascial compartments	Extrafascial planes or spaces
Ray of hand or foot	Midfoot and hindfoot
Posterior calf	Popliteal space
Anterolateral leg	Groin—femoral triangle
Anterior thigh	Intrapelvic
Medial thigh	Midhand
Posterior thigh	Antecubital fossae
Buttocks	Axilla
Volar forearm	Periclavicular
Dorsal forearm	Paraspinal
Anterior arm	Head and neck
Posterior arm	
Periscapular	

From Enneking WF, Spanier SS, Goodman MA: A system for the surgical staging of musculoskeletal sarcoma. Clin Orthop 153:106–120, 1980.

TABLE 1–3

Surgical Stages of Sarcomas

Stage	Grade	Site
1A	Low (G1)	Intracompartmental (T1)
IB	Low (G1)	Extracompartmental (T2)
IIA	High (G2)	Intracompartmental (T1)
IIB	High (G2)	Extracompartmental (T2)
III	Any (G) Regional or distant metastasis	Any (T)

From Enneking WF, Spanier SS, Goodman MA: A system for the surgical staging of musculoskeletal sarcomata. Clin Orthop 153:106–120, 1980.

The surgical staging system has five categories (Table 1–3). There is an intracompartmental and an extracompartmental class for both low- and high-grade tumors. The fifth classification (Stage III) is for the patient with a distant metastasis to lymph node, bone, visceral organ, or lung.

An additional contribution made by Enneking and associates was the definition of a common set of terms to be used to describe surgical procedures.[8] They proposed four characterizations of surgical margins: intralesional, marginal, wide, and radical. An intralesional margin is accomplished when the plane of the operation is within the tumor; macroscopic tumor is left in the patient. A marginal margin is achieved when the plane of the excision is through the pseudocapsule of the tumor; microscopic tumor is left in the patient, if the lesion is locally invasive. A wide margin is accomplished when the entire tumor is resected with a cuff of normal tissue surrounding it. This margin has also been called an *en bloc* resection. If there are nodules of tumor outside the reactive pseudocapsule (satellite lesions) they are left in the patient, but a wide surgical margin is most appropriate for the majority of malignant tumors of the musculoskeletal system. A radical margin involves removal of the tumor and the entire compartment involved by the tumor.

Biopsy

The biopsy should be the last step in the evaluation of a bone or soft tissue tumor and is done only after careful planning.[6, 17, 22] Often, a biopsy proves unnecessary after the patient has been thoroughly examined, the diagnosis having been made by the clinical setting and radiographic findings. When a biopsy is required, the prebiopsy evaluation improves the chance that adequate and representative tissue will be obtained, the least amount of normal tissue will be contaminated, and the pathologist will be able to make an accurate diagnosis. Biopsies done without an adequate prebiopsy evaluation are likely to produce an unsatisfactory result.[17]

The majority of complications of biopsy occur because the biopsy is done without adequate knowledge of the anatomic extent and exact location of the tumor. The biopsy should not be done until a thorough evaluation has been completed and should not be done to justify a thorough work-up or an orthopedic oncologist.[7] Referring patients before a biopsy has been done means an unnecessary trip for some patients, but the early referral is more than justified by the better management the other patients receive from the multidisciplinary approach offered by a center specializing in musculoskeletal tumor.

The purpose of the biopsy is to confirm the diagnosis suspected by the physician after the initial evaluation or to determine which one of a limited number of differential diagnoses is correct. The tissue obtained must be sufficient for histologic grading as well as for establishing a specific diagnosis. It must be representative of the tumor. Because many musculoskeletal tumors are heterogeneous, the specific site from which the tissue is taken is important. The surgeon who is willing to assume the surgical management of the patient, regardless of the diagnosis, should be the one to perform a biopsy of the tumor. The biopsy incision and the tissue exposed during the biopsy must be excised with the tumor if a definitive resection is necessary. If the surgeon who must do the resection has planned and done the biopsy, the patient will have a better chance of a limb salvage and less risk of a local recurrence than if the surgeon doing the resection did not do the biopsy. The surgeon should consult with the radiologist and the pathologist before the biopsy to get their suggestion of the best tissue to obtain. Another advantage of a prebiopsy discussion of the case with the pathologist is that it allows the pathologist to be better prepared, rather than being expected to make a diagnosis from a frozen section without considering the possibilities beforehand and reviewing reference texts.

NEEDLE BIOPSY

Needle biopsy or fine needle aspiration biopsy is often suggested. They can usually be done without general anesthesia or a hospital admission, saving the patient money and the risk of general anesthesia. Needle biopsies do contaminate the tissue penetrated by the needle. The needle track can be seeded with tumor and should be excised at the time of the definitive resection. Needle biopsies and fine needle aspiration biopsies must be planned in the same manner as an open biopsy, and the surgeon should decide how the biopsy is to be done. A needle biopsy or fine needle aspiration biopsy yields a minimal amount of tumor and may not provide a sufficient sample of a heterogeneous lesion. Needle biopsies and fine needle aspiration biopsies are most useful for lesions suspected of being lymphoma, metastatic carcinoma, or myeloma. Diagnosis of these lesions is usually easily accomplished with a limited amount of tissue and necessitates neither resection nor histologic grading. Although an experienced pathologist can usually make the correct diagnosis from a successful needle biopsy or fine needle aspiration biopsy specimen, more diagnostic mistakes are based on needle biopsy specimens compared with specimens obtained by open biopsy. Histologic grading can be difficult or impossible without an open biopsy. Open biopsy is recommended for most musculoskeletal lesions. A needle biopsy or fine needle aspiration biopsy is reserved for a limited number of specific clinical circumstances.

INCISIONAL BIOPSY

The biopsy should be carefully planned. The surgeon should think about possible future treatment, especially a limb salvage resection. The skin incision and deep dissection should be made so that the incision and the exposed tissue can be resected with the tumor at the time of a definitive limb salvage operation. Longitudinal skin incisions are better than transverse skin incisions; transverse incisions are difficult to incorporate into a limb salvage resection, and usually the dissection for a biopsy through a transverse incision contaminates more tissue than one done through a longitudinal incision. The dissection should be as limited as possible, no flaps should be raised, and major neurovascular bundles should not be exposed. The dissection should be through a muscle and not between muscles. The violated muscle needs to be resected with the tumor, but if the biopsy dissection is between two muscles, they must both be subsequently removed. The tissue obtained should be sharply cut from the tumor. The tumor's pseudocapsule and a portion of the tumor should be excised as a block and sent to the pathologist. A frozen section examination should be done even when there are no plans for immediate additional surgery, and the pathologist should be sure that adequate and diagnostic tissue is available. Only when biopsy of dense bone is performed is it impossible to do a frozen section examination. The pathologist should set aside tissue for subsequent examination with an electron microscope. Some tissues should be kept frozen in the event that immunohistochemistry study is necessary.

The author uses a tourniquet during the biopsy but deflates the tourniquet before wound closure. The use of the tourniquet is controversial. Some believe that the use of the tourniquet increases the risk of metastatic disease. Although not documented, the belief is that tumor cells released from the tumor during the biopsy collect in the vein just distal to the tourniquet and are released as a bolus when the tourniquet is deflated. This bolus of tumor cells is thought to present an increased risk to the patient. Surgeons who use a tourniquet do not think that a tourniquet increases the risk of metastasis and believe that the biopsy is safer and the dissection is less extensive when the operation is done in a bloodless field. All authors agree that the surgeon should not use a compressive bandage to exsanguinate the extremity but rather should elevate the extremity for 3 to 5 minutes before inflating the tourniquet.

Extra care should be taken to obtain hemostasis before closing the wound. The hematoma from the biopsy may contain tumor cells and should be resected if surgery is the treatment. The wound may be drained, but the exit site of the drain must be in line with the incision and close to it. The drain track will be resected with the tumor and the biopsy incision.

EXCISIONAL BIOPSY

An excisional biopsy rather than an incisional biopsy is occasionally indicated. An excisional biopsy is appropriate when the lesion is small, when it can be easily excised, and when a wide excision will not significantly affect the patient's function. An excisional biopsy may be appropriate even when a major resection to obtain the proper wide margin is required. If the preoperative evaluation strongly supports the diagnosis of a malignancy, particularly if a frozen section specimen will be difficult to interpret (e.g., parosteal osteosarcoma or low-grade chondrosarcoma) or when the incision will contaminate tissue that will be difficult to resect at a later date (e.g., pelvis tumors), an excisional biopsy should be considered.

The choice between an incisional biopsy and an excisional biopsy is usually easy to make. A clinically obvious exostosis on the proximal tibia should have an excisional biopsy, if biopsy is performed at all. A large aggressive lesion in the distal femur invading the adjacent soft tissues should undergo incisional biopsy. It is more difficult to decide when the evaluation reveals a small "active," possibly low-grade malignancy. An incisional biopsy exposes uncontaminated tissues to the tumor, and if the tumor proves to be a malignancy, the definitive resection is more complicated. On the other hand, if the lesion can be treated with curettage or marginal excision, the incisional biopsy leads to the least functional loss. The final decision made for each individual patient is based on not only the tumor's characteristics but also the patient's desires. It is the surgeon's responsibility to discuss these issues with the patient so an informed decision can be made.

An added advantage of the excisional biopsy is that the pathologist is able to examine the entire lesion, improving the accuracy of the pathology examination results. Musculoskeletal tumors are often quite heterogeneous, and the amount of tissue obtained with an incisional biopsy is always limited. It is particularly difficult to distinguish active benign cartilage tumors from low-grade chondrosarcomas with limited histologic material. When the entire lesion, especially its interface with the adjacent bone and soft tissue, is seen the distinction is more easily made. Occasionally, even after studying the entire specimen, the pathologist is not able to differentiate between a benign cartilage tumor and a low-grade chondrosarcoma. In these cases, excisional biopsy with wide excision is particularly appropriate.

A final note of caution is offered regarding the biopsy. Osteomyelitis is more common than bone tumors, especially in children, and osteomyelitis often mimics neoplasia. The reverse is also true, so whenever doing a biopsy, even when the diagnosis seems obvious, the physician should "culture the tumor and biopsy the infection."

Summary

The initial examination of a patient with a suspected musculoskeletal tumor should be done with care. Specific information sought from the specialized diagnostic studies such as technetium bone scan, CT scan, and MRI before they are requested. The case should be discussed with the radiologist and the pathologist. The biopsy, be it open, needle, or fine needle aspiration, can be done as the final step in the evaluation of the musculoskeletal tumor.

References

1. Aisen AM, Martel W, Braunstein EM, McMillin KI, Philips WA, King TF: MRI and CT evaluation of primary bone and soft tissue tumors. AJR 146:749–756, 1986.
2. Bohndorf K, Reiser M, Locher B, de Lacroiz WF, Steinbrich W: Magnetic resonance imaging of primary tumors and tumor-like lesions of bone. Skeletal Radiol 15:511–517, 1986.
3. Brady TJ, Rosen BR, Pykett IL, McGuire MH, Mankin HJ, Rosenthal DI: NMR imaging of leg tumors. Radiology 149:181–187, 1983.
4. Chang AE, Schaner EG, Conkle DM, Flye MW, Doppman JL, Rosenberg SA: Evaluation of computed tomography in the detection of pulmonary metastases. Cancer 43:913–916, 1979.
5. Coffre E, Vanel D, Contesso G, Kalifia C, Dubousset J, Genin J, Masselot J: Problems and pitfalls in the use of computed tomography for the local evaluation of long bone osteosarcoma: Report on 30 cases. Skeletal Radiol 13:147–153, 1985.
6. Enneking WF: Editorial. The issue of the biopsy. J Bone Joint Surg 64A:1119–1120, 1982.
7. Enneking WF: Musculoskeletal Tumor Surgery. New York, Churchill Livingston, 1983, 137–138.
8. Enneking WF, Spanier SS, Goodman MA: A system for the surgical staging of musculoskeletal sarcomata. Clin Orthop 153:106–120, 1980.
9. Finn HA, Simon MA, Martin WB, Darakjian H: Scintigraphy with gallium-67 citrate in staging of soft-tissue sarcomas of the extremity. J Bone Joint Surg 69A:886–891, 1987.
10. Eriksson B, Gunterberg B, Kindblom LG: Chordoma. Acta Orthop Scand 52:49–58, 1981.
11. Gillespy T III, Manfrini M, Ruggieri P, Spanier SS, Petterson H, Springfield DS: Staging of intraosseous extent of osteosarcoma: Correlation of preoperative CT and MR imaging with pathologic macroslides. Radiology 167:765–767, 1988.
12. Heiken JP, Lee JKT, Swiathers RL, Totty WG, Murphy WA: CT of benign soft tissue masses of the extremities. AJR 142:575–580, 1984.
13. Hudson TM, Haas G, Enneking WF, Hawkins IF Jr: Angiography in the management of musculoskeletal tumors. Surg Gynecol Obstet 141:11–21, 1975.
14. Hudson TM, Schabel M II, Springfield DS, et al: The comparative value of bone scintigraphy and computed tomography in determining bone involvement by soft tissue sarcomas. J Bone Joint Surg 66A:1400–1407, 1984.
15. Joyce MJ, Mankin HJ: Caveat arthroscopos: Extra-articular lesions of bone simulating intra-articular pathology of the knee. J Bone Joint Surg 65A:289–292, 1983.
16. Kirchner PT, Simon MA: The clinical value of bone and gallium scintigraphy for soft tissue sarcomas of the extremities. J Bone Joint Surg 66A:319–327, 1984.
17. Mankin HJ, Lange TA, Spanier SA: The hazards of biopsy in patients with malignant primary bone and soft tissue tumors. J Bone Joint Surg 64A:1121–1127, 1982.
18. Moon KL, Genant HK, Helms CA, Chafetz WI, Crooks LE, Kaufman L: Musculoskeletal applications of nuclear magnetic resonance. Radiology 147:161–171, 1983.
19. Pettersson H, Gillespy T III, Hamlin DJ, Enneking WF, Springfield DS, Andrews ER, Spanier S, Slone R: Primary musculoskeletal tumors: Examination with MRI imaging compared with conventional modalities. Radiology 164:237–241, 1987.
20. Pettersson H, Hamlin DJ, Mancuso A, Scott KN: Magnetic resonance imaging of the musculoskeletal system. Acta Radiol (Diagn) (Stockh) 26:225–234, 1985.
21. Russell WO, Cohen J, Enzinger F, et al: A clinical and pathological staging system for soft tissue sarcomas. Cancer 40:1562–1570, 1977.
22. Simon MA: Biopsy of musculoskeletal tumors. J Bone Joint Surg 64A:1253–1257, 1982.
23. Simon MA, Kirchner PT: Scintigraphic evaluation of primary bone tumors. J Bone Joint Surg 62A:758–764, 1980.
24. Suit HD, Mankin HJ, Wood WC, Gebhardt MC, Harmon DC, Rosenberg A, Tepper JE, Rosenthal D: Treatment of the patient with stage M0 soft tissue sarcoma. J Clin Oncol 6:854–862, 1988.
25. Sundaram M, McGuire MH, Herbold DR, Wolverson MK, Heiberg E: Magnetic resonance imaging in planning limb-salvage surgery for primary malignant tumors of bone. J Bone Joint Surg 68A:809–819, 1986.
26. Totty WG, Murphy WA, Lee JKT: Soft-tissue tumors: MR imaging. Radiology 160:135–141, 1986.
27. Weekes RB, Bergquist TH, McLeod RA, Zimmer WD: Magnetic resonance imaging of soft-tissue tumors: Comparison with computed tomography. Magn Reson Imaging 3:345–352, 1985.
28. Weinberger G, Levinsohn EM: Computed tomography in the evaluation of sarcomatous tumors of the thigh. AJR 130:115–118, 1978.
29. Zimmer WD, Bergquist TH, McLeod RA, et al: Bone tumors: Magnetic resonance imaging versus computed tomography. Radiology 155:709–718, 1985.

CHAPTER 2

Radiology and Pathology of Bone Tumors

ADAM GREENSPAN
MICHAEL J. KLEIN

RADIOLOGIC EVALUATION

The radiologic evaluation of a tumor or a tumor-like lesion may necessitate a range of imaging modalities, including conventional radiography and tomography, arteriography, computed tomography (CT), magnetic resonance imaging (MRI), and radionuclide imaging (scintigraphy, bone scan). The most important among these for establishing the diagnosis is plain radiography. It provides the most useful diagnostic information—about calcifications, ossifications, and periosteal reaction—more readily than CT or MRI. Conventional tomography may help delineate the matrix composition, evaluate the cortex and periosteal reaction, and detect occult pathologic fracture. Arteriography is essential for mapping the tumor and its vascular supply, as well as for choosing the area suitable for open biopsy.

The radiologic features that help the radiologist reach a precise diagnosis of a tumor or a tumor-like lesion of bone include the site of the lesion (the location in the skeleton and in the individual bone), the borders of the lesion (the so-called zone of transition), the type of matrix of the lesion (the composition of the tumor tissue), the type of bone destruction, the type of periosteal response to the lesion (periosteal reaction), and the nature and extent of soft tissue involvement.[43, 77, 91, 92, 102, 104]

Acknowledgment: The authors wish to express their thanks to Ms. Mary Closson for her invaluable secretarial assistance and to Mr. Norman Katz and Mr. Daniel Benevento for their expert photographic work.

Site of the Lesion. The site of a bone lesion is important because some tumors have a predilection for specific bones or specific sites in bone. The sites of some lesions are so characteristic that a diagnosis can be suggested on this basis alone, as in the case of parosteal osteosarcoma or chondroblastoma.[31, 89] Similarly, certain entities can be readily excluded from the differential diagnosis on the basis of the lesion's location. For example, the diagnosis of a giant cell tumor should not be made for a lesion that does not reach the articular end of the bone, because few of these tumors are found in other locations.[64]

Borders of the Lesion. Evaluation of the borders, or margins, of a lesion is crucial to determining the growth rate. Slow-growing lesions, usually benign, have sharply outlined, sclerotic borders (a narrow zone of transition), whereas malignant or aggressive lesions typically have indistinct borders (a wide zone of transition).

Type of Matrix. Many tumors of bone are composed of characteristic extracellular tissue components, the tumor matrix. The identification of tumor bone (osteoid or bone produced by malignant cells) within or adjacent to the area of destruction should alert the radiologist to the possibility of osteosarcoma. However, the deposition of new bone may also be the result of a reparative process caused by bone destruction—so-called reactive sclerosis.

Cartilage is identified by the presence of typically punctate, annular, or comma-shaped calcifications. Because cartilage usually grows in lobules, a tumor of cartilaginous origin can often be suggested by lobulated growth.

Type of Bone Destruction. The type of bone destruction caused by a tumor is primarily related to the rate of growth of the tumor.[92] Although not pathognomonic of any specific neoplasm, the type of destruction, which can be described as geographic, moth eaten, or permeative, may suggest not only a benign or a malignant neoplastic process, but sometimes even the histologic type of the tumor, as in the permeative type of bone destruction characteristically produced by the so-called round cell tumors (Ewing's sarcoma, lymphoma, and myeloma).[91]

Periosteal Response. The periosteal reaction to a neoplastic process in bone is usually categorized as uninterrupted or interrupted. Uninterrupted reaction is characterized by solid layers of periosteal density, indicating a long-standing benign process. The interrupted type of periosteal reaction suggests malignancy or a highly aggressive nonmalignant process. It may appear as a sunburst pattern, an onionskin pattern, or Codman's triangle and is commonly seen in malignant primary tumors.[104]

Soft Tissue Extension. With few exceptions, benign tumors and tumor-like lesions of bone do not exhibit soft tissue extension; almost invariably, therefore, a soft tissue mass indicates an aggressive lesion and one that is in most instances malignant.

In the evaluation of intraosseous and extraosseous extension of a tumor, CT, MRI, and radionuclide imaging are crucial.[15, 45, 109, 112, 143] Both CT and MRI can determine with high accuracy the presence or absense of soft tissue invasion by a tumor.[15, 110] On occasion, particularly in the coronal plane, MRI may be superior to CT in delineating the intramedullary extent of the tumor and its relationship to surrounding structures.[3] Showing sharper demarcation between normal and abnormal bone tissue than CT does, MRI—particularly in evaluation of the extremities—reliably identifies the spatial boundaries of tumor masses, the encasement and displacement of major neurovascular bundles, and the extent of joint involvement.[15, 61] Axial images, together with coronal images, have been employed in determining the extent of soft tissue invasion in relation to important vascular structures.[3, 131] On the other hand, in comparison with CT scans, MRI images do not clearly depict or allow characterization of calcification in the tumor matrix; in fact, large amounts of calcification or ossification may be almost undetectable.[15, 109] Moreover, MRI was less satisfactory than CT and even plain films and tomography in the demonstration of cortical destruction.[3, 15, 112] The use of the inversion recovery mode to obtain strongly T1-weighted images and the application of the spin echo mode with variation of the pulse sequences may in time improve the evaluation of tumors by MRI.[45]

It must be stressed that, most of the time, neither CT nor MRI is suitable for establishing the precise nature of a bone tumor. In particular, too much faith has been placed in MRI for distinguishing benign from malignant lesions. Despite the utilization of various criteria, the application of MRI to tissue diagnosis has rarely brought satisfactory results.[135, 151] This is because, in general, the small number of protons in calcified structures renders MRI less useful in the evaluation of bone lesions. Valuable evidence concerning the production of the tumor matrix can be missed by MRI because of the unsatisfactory demonstration of small calcified structures. Moreover, as several investigations have shown, MRI was found to be an imaging modality of low specificity. T1 and T2 measurements are generally of limited value for histologic characterization of musculoskeletal tumors.[15] Quantitative determination of relaxation times has not proved clinically valuable in identifying various tumor types,[45] although it was demonstrated to be important in the staging of osteosarcoma or chondrosarcoma. In particular, T2-weighted images are a crucial factor in delineating extraosseous extension of tumor and peritumoral edema as well as in assessing the involvement of major neurovascular bundles. Necrotic areas change from a low-intensity signal in the

T1-weighted image to a very bright, intense signal in the T2-weighted images and could be differentiated from viable, solid tumor tissue.[13, 15, 61]

Scintigraphy may demonstrate the extent of intramedullary involvement by tumor better than plain film or conventional tomography. However, it cannot adequately evaluate the exact level of intramedullary spread because a radionuclide bone scan usually shows the extent of the lesion to be greater than it really is owing to the increased activity demonstrated in the areas of hyperemia and edema adjacent to the tumor.[132] Radionuclide imaging has, however, the advantage of being able to identify additional, remote skeletal lesions, so-called skipped lesions, and intraosseous metastases.

PATHOLOGIC EVALUATION

The task of categorizing an osseous lesion as benign or malignant is even more complex for the pathologist than for the radiologist. It is mandatory to consider all the radiologic criteria (see above), together with the data supplied by the clinician. Ideally, the pathologist should also consult with both the radiologist and the orthopedic surgeon. Although it may be obvious to a clinician that a teenager with a rock-hard, tender, 15-cm swelling of the femur almost undoubtedly has a tumor, a 4-mm sampling of tissue from the same lesion, unaccompanied by a history and radiologic studies, is fraught with diagnostic risk. Without consideration of all correlative measurements available before an attempt to interpret histologic sections, there is ultimately no assurance that a biopsy specimen is representative of the lesion or, indeed, that the actual abnormality has been sampled.

Several factors make the precise diagnosis of osseous tumors difficult. Although radiographic features have high correlation with malignancy, benignity, and sometimes even an exact histologic diagnosis, radiographic determination of these characteristics is based on statistical probabilities. Regardless of how persuasive a radiologist's clinical assessment of the biologic potential of a lesion may be to a pathologist colleague, any lesion, no matter how radiologically typical it appears, may represent an entirely different entity on histologic examination. A confident radiologic diagnosis may not outweigh the microscopic appearance of the lesion. To make matters more difficult for the practicing pathologist, the absolute number of bone tumors is small, and consequently few pathologists outside of large referral centers have sufficient diagnostic experience with them. For this reason, if any doubt exists as to the precise diagnosis of a bone tumor, consultation with a pathologist who has expertise in orthopedic pathology should be obtained.

After results of the necessary clinical correlation studies have been considered, the histologic diagnosis is rendered. The tumor cells and their arrangement and the intercellular matrix produced are compared with the appearance of radiographs and imaging studies to verify adequate and representative sampling. The histologic patterns are then compared and matched with similar or identical histologic patterns of known examples of bone neoplasms. In most instances, bone tumors are categorized in this manner. When pattern alone is insufficient for diagnosis, the application of special stains, immunohistochemical techniques, and even electron microscopy can help further in the categorization of bone tumors. For example, the application of leukocyte common antigen and neuron-specific stains, as well as the ultrastructural identification of neurosecretory granules, can assist in distinguishing malignant lymphoma and neuroblastoma from Ewing's sarcoma.

Despite the use of all the above studies, however, a small percentage of bone tumors are not easily categorized. The pathologist must then at least try to assess the biologic potential of the neoplasm, even if it cannot be given a specific name. In such cases, the classic signs of nuclear pleomorphism and hyperchromaticity, mitotic rate and the presence of atypical mitoses, and the identification of spontaneous necrosis are sought to help distinguish benign from malignant lesions. Observation of the interface area of the tumor with normal bone may reveal subtle infiltration of intertrabecular marrow spaces or haversian canals by tumor cells and point toward malignancy. Finally, more recent techniques such as flow cytometry to analyze nuclear DNA content are used increasingly in difficult diagnostic assessments.

In the final analysis, only close cooperation among the radiologist, the pathologist, and the orthopedic surgeon in the review of history, radiographic studies, and biopsy materials may lead to an accurate conclusion regarding the exact nature and character of a bone lesion. In most cases, careful analysis of all these variables makes it possible to identify the various benign and malignant tumors and tumor-like conditions.

Bone-Forming Tumors

BENIGN OSTEOBLASTIC LESIONS

Osteoma

Osteoma is an asymptomatic, slow-growing osteoblastic lesion, commonly encountered in the outer table of the calvarium and the frontal and ethmoid sinuses and, occasionally, in the long and short tubular bones. Growing on the surface of a bone, osteoma presents on plain film as a dense, ivory-like sclerotic mass attached to the bone, with sharply demarcated borders (Fig. 2–1*A*). Occasionally, it may resemble parosteal osteosarcoma. Its clinical importance lies in its common association with the complex of disorders known as Gardner's syndrome, characterized by epidermoid cysts, subcutaneous fibromas, and premalignant intestinal polyps.[52]

Histologically, osteomas are composed primarily of bone with a mature, lamellar architecture. This architecture may consist of concentric rings as in compact bone or, more usually, parallel plates as in cancellous bone.[64] The lesions are well circumscribed (Fig. 2–1*B*), and the stromal cells have the characteristics of osteocytes.

Osteoid Osteoma

Osteoid osteoma is a benign osteoblastic lesion that most commonly occurs between ages 10 and 35 years.[66] Its preferred sites are the long bones, particularly the femur and the tibia.[71] A typical history of pain can be elicited in about 75% of cases, and this serves as an important clue to the diagnosis. The pain is usually more severe at night and is dramatically relieved by salicylates (aspirin) in about 20 to 25 minutes.[51]

Four radiographically distinctive types of this lesion can be distinguished on the basis of its location in the bone: cortical, medullary, subperiosteal, and periarticular. Rarely, more than one nidus is encountered, in which case the lesion is called multicentric, or multifocal, osteoid osteoma.[53] The nidus characterizing osteoid osteoma manifests as either a purely radiolucent lesion or one with a sclerotic center. It usually measures less than 1 cm in diameter and usually is surrounded by a zone of reactive bone formation.

Plain radiographs may be sufficient to dem-

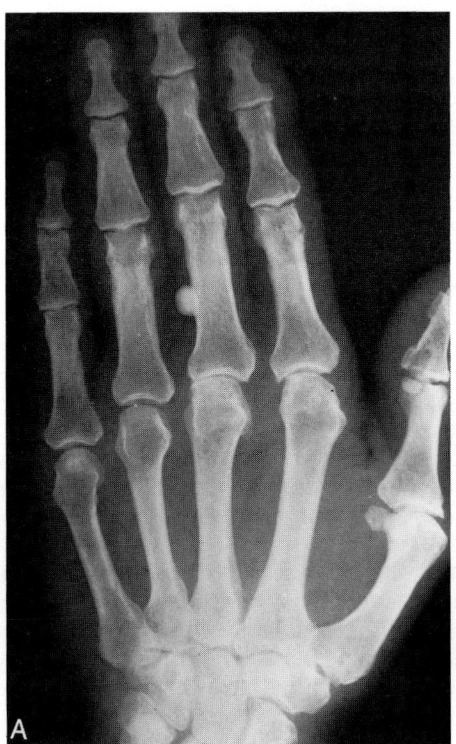

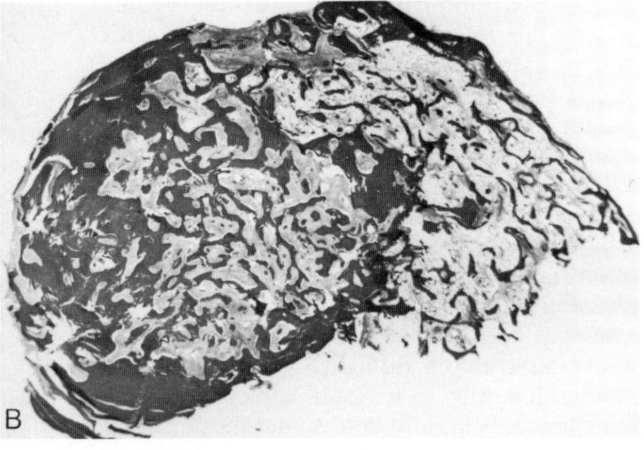

FIGURE 2–1. Osteoma. *A,* An ivory-like round mass is attached to the cortex of the proximal phalanx of the middle finger. (From Greenspan A: Orthopedic Radiology. Philadelphia, JB Lippincott, 1988.) *B,* Low-power micrograph demonstrates an admixture of compact bone (upper and lower left) and spongy bone (remaining areas), showing mature pattern (×3.6).

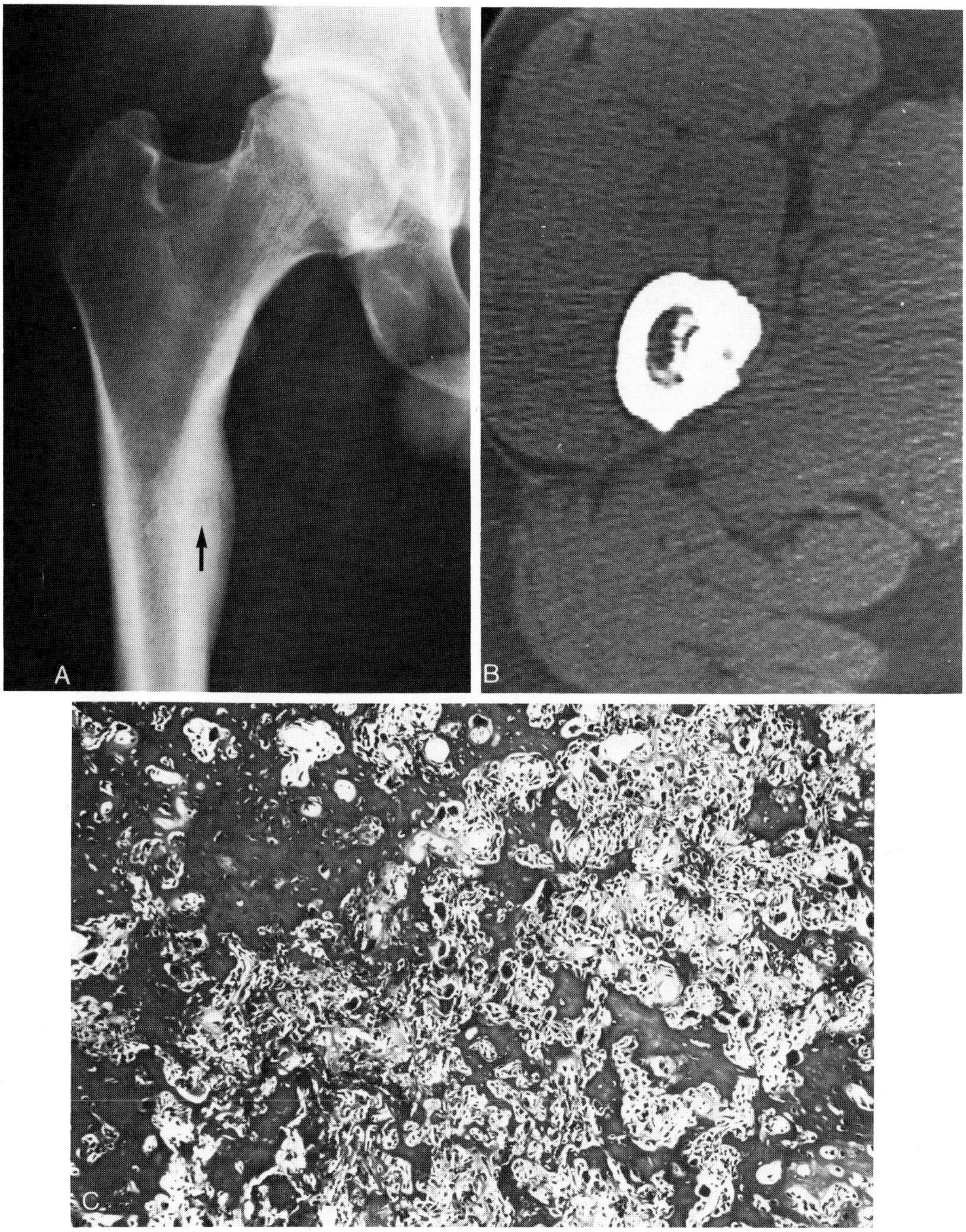

FIGURE 2–2. Osteoid osteoma. *A,* Cortical lesion is characterized by a radiolucent nidus (arrow) and extensive reactive sclerosis. (From Greenspan A: Orthopedic Radiology. Philadelphia, JB Lippincott, 1988.) *B,* Computed tomography (CT) section demonstrates the nidus to better advantage. Reactive sclerosis is seen to involve not only the cortex but also the medullary portion of the bone. *C,* Microtrabeculae produced in haphazard arrays are loosely arranged in a fibrovascular stroma. At this low power, remodeling is evidenced by numerous osteoclast giant cells. Perilesional osteosclerosis is seen at upper left (×22.4).

onstrate these features (Fig. 2–2 *A*), but usually conventional tomography or CT is necessary, particularly for precise localization of the nidus (Fig. 2–2 *B*). Radionuclide bone scan is also helpful because osteoid osteoma invariably shows a marked increase in uptake of radioisotope.[57]

With radiographic demonstration of the nidus, a diagnosis can usually be made with a great degree of assurance. Only an atypical presentation of the lesion may sometimes create diagnostic difficulty. It is important to keep in mind, however, that even when the classic radiographic appearance is exhibited, the differential diagnosis of osteoid osteoma should include stress fracture, bone abscess (Brodie's abscess), and bone island. In stress fracture, the radiolucent lesion is usually more linear and perpendicular or at an angle to the cortex, rather than parallel to the cortex as in osteoid osteoma. Bone abscesses may exhibit a radiographic appearance similar to osteoid osteoma's, but the presence of a serpiginous track extending from the radiolucent center of the lesion favors the diagnosis of an infectious process. In 90% of cases of bone island, radionuclide bone scan demonstrates no increase in isotope uptake, in contrast to the marked activity seen in osteoid osteoma.

Histologically, the nidus is composed of osteoid, or sometimes mineralized immature bone. It is a small, well-circumscribed, and self-limited lesion. Its microtrabeculae and irregular islets of osteoid matrix and bone are surrounded by a richly vascular fibrous stroma in which osteoblastic activity and osteoclastic activity are often prominent (Fig. 2–2 *C*). The perilesional sclerosis associated with osteoid osteoma is composed of dense bone in varying maturation patterns.[124] As the lesion gets closer to the periosteal surface, the sclerosis becomes more pronounced. The central portion of the lesion differs from bone island in that the latter lesion is structured like a spherical piece of cortical bone, including medullary haversian canals. Bone abscesses, although they may be associated with perilesional sclerosis, contain a combination of bland fibrous tissue and a polymorphous mixture of inflammatory cells of various types. On a strictly histologic basis, the differential diagnosis of osteoid osteoma includes various benign and malignant osteoblastic tumors. The best avenue to the correct diagnosis combines radiographic observations with low-power microscopic views of the arrangement of the lesion. High-power observation of active osteoblasts in this benign lesion, without consideration of the clinical findings, may lead to misconstruing osteoid osteoma as a more aggressive process.

Osteoid osteoma may be accompanied by a few complications. Accelerated growth of a bone may occur if the nidus is located near the growth plate, particularly in young children.[107] A vertebral lesion, particularly in the neural arch, may lead to painful scoliosis, with the concavity of the curvature directed toward the side where the lesion is. Moreover, an intracapsular lesion may result in precocious onset of arthritis. This complication serves as an important diagnostic clue when a typical history of osteoid osteoma is elicited from a patient and the nidus is not recognized radiographically.[106]

Treatment consists of complete resection of the nidus. Radiographs of the resected specimen and the involved bone should be obtained promptly to exclude the possibility of incomplete resection. The lesion recurs if it is not completely excised.[105]

Osteoblastoma

The patient's age at presentation of osteoblastoma is similar to that of osteoid osteoma: 75% of cases involve individuals in the first to third decades of life. Although the long bones are frequently involved, the vertebral column is a site of predilection.[70] In contrast to the clinical presentation of osteoid osteoma, that of osteoblastomas some may be asymptomatic; and if pain is present, it is not so readily relieved by salicylates.[34]

Osteoblastoma has three distinctive radiographic presentations:

1. A giant osteoid osteoma. The lesion is usually greater than 1.5 cm and often more than 2 cm in diameter, and it exhibits less reactive sclerosis and, possibly, more prominent periosteal response than osteoid osteoma does (Fig. 2–3 *A*).
2. A blown-out expansion, similar to that of an aneurysmal bone cyst, with small radiopacities in the center. This pattern is particularly common in lesions of the spine (Fig. 2–3 *B*).
3. An aggressive lesion, which may suggest malignancy.[93]

Plain film radiography and conventional tomography are often sufficient to demonstrate these features and suggest the diagnosis. One of the differential possibilities to be considered is bone abscess, which usually exhibits a serpiginous track or a lesion crossing the growth

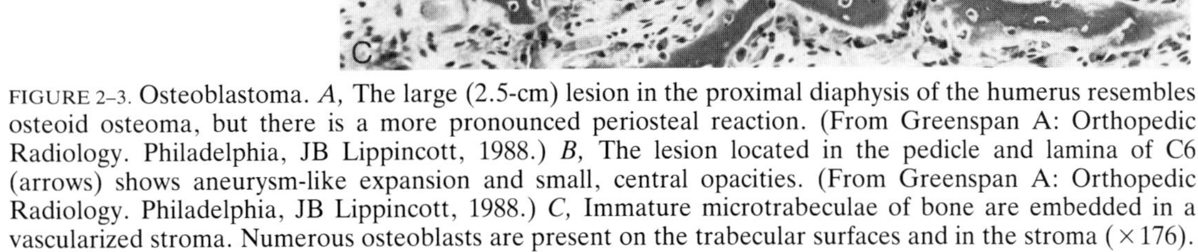

FIGURE 2–3. Osteoblastoma. *A,* The large (2.5-cm) lesion in the proximal diaphysis of the humerus resembles osteoid osteoma, but there is a more pronounced periosteal reaction. (From Greenspan A: Orthopedic Radiology. Philadelphia, JB Lippincott, 1988.) *B,* The lesion located in the pedicle and lamina of C6 (arrows) shows aneurysm-like expansion and small, central opacities. (From Greenspan A: Orthopedic Radiology. Philadelphia, JB Lippincott, 1988.) *C,* Immature microtrabeculae of bone are embedded in a vascularized stroma. Numerous osteoblasts are present on the trabecular surfaces and in the stroma (×176).

plate, phenomena almost never seen in osteoblastomas. Osteosarcoma must be considered when an aggressive osteoblastoma is encountered, and tomography may be helpful with the distinction. CT scan may be useful for evaluating lesions located in complex anatomic regions, such as the vertebrae. Occasionally, myelography or MRI may be needed to assess tumor extension into the thecal sac.

Osteoblastoma is histologically almost identical with osteoid osteoma (Fig. 2–3 *C*). Its osteoblastic stromal cells may vary from bland, differentiated osteoblastic morphologic features to large, sometimes even bizarre, variants that are difficult to distinguish from a malignant neoplasm. These bizarre stromal cells can pose a difficult diagnostic problem when the radiograph suggests an aggressive tumor.[124]

The most helpful features for resolving this problem are the pattern of matrix production and cellular proliferation. The lesion of osteoblastoma tends to mature at the periphery; in osteosarcoma, this pattern is usually reversed. Moreover, no matter how immature the matrix production may appear in osteoblastoma, it is never admixed with cartilage, which indicates the type of primitive multipotentiality seen in osteosarcoma.[100] Finally, the nuclear and cellular alterations in osteoblastoma are rarely as bizarre as they tend to be in osteosarcomas. Even the plump and prominent so-called epithelioid osteoblasts seen in aggressive osteoblastoma[41] seldom have the markedly increased nucleus-to-cytoplasm disproportion seen so regularly in osteosarcomas. The mitotic activity demonstrated in osteoblastoma is seldom as frequent and as bizarre as that seen in osteosarcoma.[41] Tumor necrosis, a hallmark of malignancy when it is combined with mitotic activity, is notably absent in osteoblastoma.

In addition to osteosarcoma and osteoid osteoma, the histologic differential diagnosis of osteoblastoma includes giant cell tumor of bone because of the large number of osteoclasts and osteoclast-like multinucleated giant cells that are typically found in osteoblastoma. Furthermore, the vascularity of the lesion and its giant cells may lead to confusion with aneurysmal bone cyst. This confusion is further complicated because a secondary aneurysmal bone cyst reaction is occasionally associated with osteoblastoma. Finding well-differentiated osteoblastic areas typical of osteoblastoma in histologic sections of such lesions can usually establish the diagnosis.

MALIGNANT OSTEOBLASTIC LESIONS

Osteosarcoma

Osteosarcoma comprises a family of tumors, with varying malignant potential, having in common the characteristic ability to produce bone or osteoid directly from connective tissue tumor cells. The collection of large series of osteosarcomas resulted in the identification of an increasing number of subtypes.[136] Although subclassification is essential for orthopedic pathologists and is of interest to bone radiologists, the variety of terms has become a source of confusion to the surgeons and the chemotherapists who need to know the degree of malignancy of a tumor and its likely response to therapy. The following discussion attempts to bring some order to the classification of osteosarcomas.

The vast majority of osteosarcomas are of unknown cause and can therefore be referred to as idiopathic, or primary, osteosarcomas. A smaller number of tumors can be related to known factors predisposing to malignancy, such as Paget's disease, fibrous dysplasia, external ionizing irradiation, or ingestion of radioactive substances. These lesions can be referred to as secondary osteosarcomas.[35]

All types of osteosarcoma may be further subdivided by anatomic site into lesions of the axial skeleton and lesions of the appendicular skeleton, with the exception of osteosarcomas of the jaw and multicentric osteosarcomas. Furthermore, they may be classified on the basis of their location with respect to the bone as central or juxtacortical.

Histopathologically, osteosarcomas can be graded on the basis of their cellularity, nuclear pleomorphism, and degree of mitotic activity. Generally speaking, central osteosarcomas are much more frequent than juxtacortical tumors, and they tend to have a higher histologic grade. Although pulmonary metastasis is the most common and most significant complication in most high-grade osteosarcomas, it is rare in osteosarcomas of the jaw and a late complication in multicentric osteosarcomas.

CONVENTIONAL OSTEOSARCOMA

Conventional osteosarcoma is the most frequently encountered type of osteosarcoma. It has its highest incidence in the second decade, with males affected slightly more often than females. The knee (the distal femur and the proximal tibia) is the most commonly affected site, followed by the proximal humerus.[30]

The lesion of conventional osteosarcoma exhibits distinctive radiologic features. Plain film often demonstrates medullary and cortical bone destruction, an aggressive periosteal reaction, a soft tissue mass, and the presence of tumor bone either within the destructive lesion or on its periphery, as well as in the soft tissue mass (Fig. 2–4*A*). If bone destruction is not so obvious, patchy densities, representing tumor bone, and an aggressive periosteal reaction are clues to the diagnosis. The sunburst and onionskin types of periosteal reaction and Codman's triangle are most commonly exhibited. CT examination is invaluable in the evaluation of these tumors, particularly in the determination of tumor extension in the bone marrow, an important factor if a limb salvage

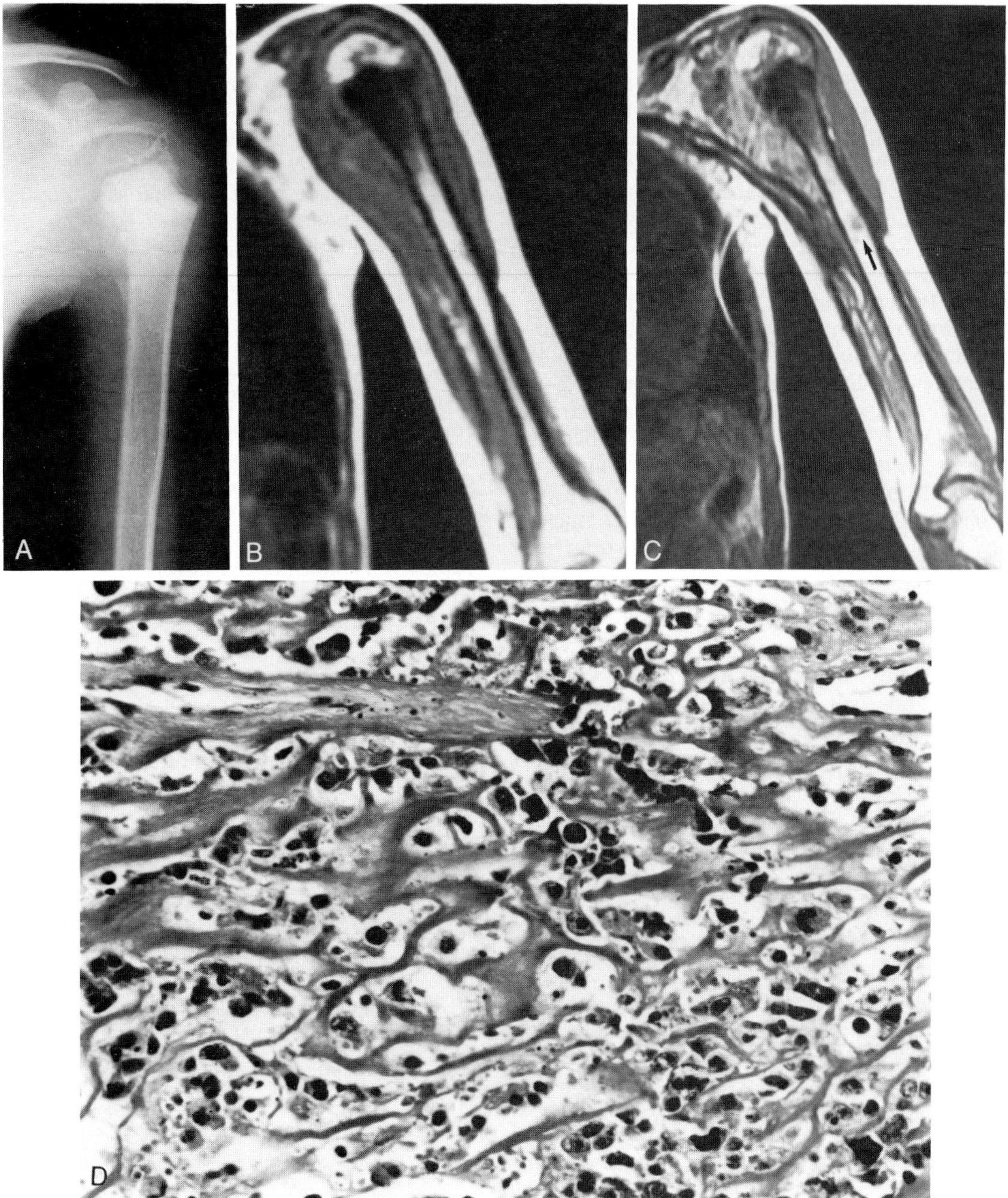

FIGURE 2–4. Conventional osteosarcoma. *A,* Sclerotic lesion in the metaphysis of the left humerus in a 6-year-old boy. There is an aggressive periosteal reaction and a soft tissue mass with tumor bone formation. *B,* Magnetic resonance imaging (MRI) section in coronal plane (T1-weighted image: TR 500 ms/TE 20 ms) of the same patient. Osteosarcoma demonstrates a low-intensity signal as compared with the high-intensity signal of normal bone marrow. *C,* MRI section in coronal plane (proton density–weighted image: TR 1800 ms/TE 20 ms). Sclerotic areas of a tumor closer to the growth plate display a low-intensity signal, whereas less sclerotic areas demonstrate an intermediate-intensity signal. Note a focus of lower-intensity signal representing a "skipped" lesion (arrow). *D,* Haphazardly connected microtrabeculae of osteoid form a lacelike filigree. A high degree of cellularity is present (×250).

procedure is contemplated.[82, 126] MRI is equally effective for evaluating soft tissue involvement and intraosseous tumor extension. In the T1-weighted images, the solid, nonmineralized parts of the osteosarcoma generally present as a dark area of low-intensity signal compared with bright-appearing normal bone marrow and fat. In the T2-weighted image, the tumor demonstrates a high-intensity signal. Osteosclerotic tumors demonstrate a low-intensity signal on T1- and T2-weighted images.

The formation of osteoid or bone by tumor cells is the criterion for histologic diagnosis.[28] The bone matrix appearance may be subtle, displaying sporadic wisps in a lacelike pattern resembling a doily or a lotus root (Fig. 2–4 *D*). The matrix may sometimes demonstrate bulky deposits, which have been described as "massive osteoid."[136] The tumor cells may be highly pleomorphic, but if osteoid deposition is plentiful, the tumor cells and their nuclei may become inconspicuous, a process referred to as "normalization" by Jaffe.[71]

LOW-GRADE CENTRAL OSTEOSARCOMA

Only recently identified, this rare form of osteosarcoma usually occurs in patients older than those in whom conventional osteosarcoma occurs; its sites of occurrence are similar.[141] Low-grade central osteosarcoma is radiographically indistinguishable from conventional osteosarcoma, but it is a slow-growing lesion, which consequently has a better prognosis.

Histologically, this tumor is extremely difficult to diagnose. It may resemble fibrous dysplasia, desmoplastic fibroma, and nonspecific reactive lesions. Even the usual histologic features of low-grade parosteal osteosarcoma (see below) have been reported. As a consequence, only with radiologic correlation is a diagnosis possible.

TELANGIECTATIC OSTEOSARCOMA

An aggressive type of osteosarcoma, the telangiectatic variant affects males twice as often as females and is seen predominantly in the second and third decades. Grossly, the tumor (resembling a "bag of blood") is characterized by blood-filled spaces, necrosis, and hemorrhage.[94] These features account for its radiographic presentation as a purely lytic, destructive, radiolucent lesion almost devoid of sclerotic changes. A soft tissue mass may be present. Pathologic fracture is not unusual if the lesion is sufficiently large (Fig. 2–5 *A*).

Histologically, the tissue generally consists of blood-filled spaces with few solid areas, a feature that it has in common with the major differential diagnostic possibility, aneurysmal

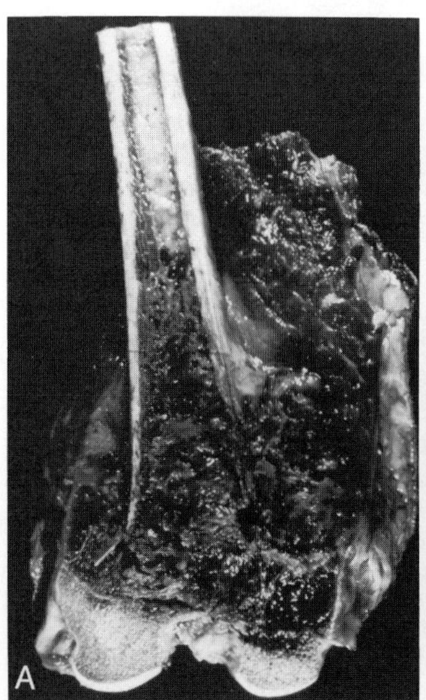

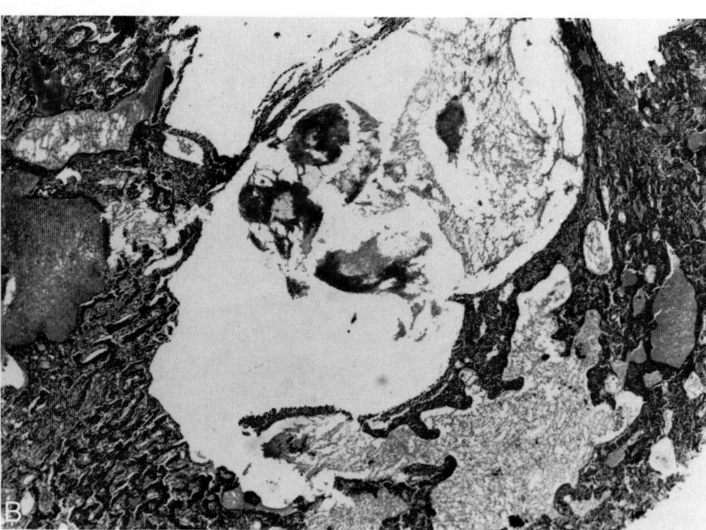

FIGURE 2–5. Telangiectatic osteosarcoma. *A,* The tumor extends from epiphysis to diaphysis and has caused a telescoped pathologic fracture associated with a hemorrhagic tumor mass laterally and medially. Note the lack of sclerosis and the resemblance to a "bag of blood." *B,* Photomicrograph of the specimen reveals large and small sinusoid spaces lined by osteoid and tumor cells (×20).

bone cyst. High-power examination of the cells lining the blood-filled spaces, however, shows significant pleomorphism, a high mitotic rate, and focal osteoid production (Fig. 2–5*B*).

MULTICENTRIC (MULTIFOCAL) OSTEOSARCOMA

This rare type of osteosarcoma, in which lesions develop simultaneously in multiple bones, is currently recognized as having two variants: synchronous and metachronous.[129] Whether this entity is truly separate or in fact represents multiple bone metastases from a primary conventional osteosarcoma remains a controversy.[5]

SMALL CELL OSTEOSARCOMA

Described by Sim and associates, small cell osteosarcoma usually occurs as a lucent lesion having permeative borders and a large soft tissue mass.[127] Its appearance thus mimics that of a round cell sarcoma of bone.

These lesions usually exhibit small round cells in many histologic fields, resembling Ewing's sarcoma to a great extent. To blur the distinction further, they may also show a positive staining for glycogen, as described for Ewing's sarcoma. However, the presence of definite spindling of the tumor cells in some areas and the often focal production of osteoid wisps or bone formation should direct the pathologist away from a consideration of Ewing's sarcoma and toward a confident diagnosis of small cell osteosarcoma.[44]

JUXTACORTICAL OSTEOSARCOMA

The term juxtacortical is a general designation for a group of osteosarcomas arising on the surface of a bone.[81] Usually, these lesions are much rarer and occur a decade later than their intraosseous counterparts. The great majority of juxtacortical osteosarcomas are low-grade tumors, although there are moderately and highly malignant variants.[142] Low-grade juxtacortical osteosarcoma is usually termed *parosteal* osteosarcoma. The lesion arises on the outside surface of the bone, virtually never elevating the periosteum.[140] Histologically, the proliferating portion of the neoplasm consists of a fibrous stroma, regarded as being derived from the outer fibrous periosteal layer. Intermediate grades of surface osteosarcomas are termed *periosteal.* These lesions may cause periosteal elevation and are usually composed mostly of cartilage. The lesions are thought to be derived from the inner, or cambium, layer of periosteum. *High-grade surface* osteosarcomas are located on the periphery of a bone. They have histologic features identical with those of intramedullary conventional osteosarcomas and have a similar metastatic potential.

Parosteal Osteosarcoma. This type of surface osteosarcoma, which is seen in patients in their third and fourth decades, has a characteristic site of predilection in the posterior aspect of the distal femur. Because the tumor is slow growing and usually involves only the surface of the bone, the prognosis is much better than for the other types of osteosarcoma.

Radiographically, the neoplasm appears as a dense oval or a spherical mass attached to the surface of the cortical bone; it is sharply outlined from the peripheral soft tissues. These features can be sufficiently demonstrated by conventional radiography (Fig. 2–6*A*), but CT or MRI is often necessary to determine cortical penetration and intramedullary invasion by tumor. The radiographic differential diagnosis of parosteal osteosarcoma includes juxtacortical myositis ossificans, soft tissue osteosarcoma, parosteal liposarcoma with ossifications, and sessile osteochondroma. The most frequent source of confusion arises in the differentiation of this tumor from myositis ossificans and osteochondroma. Unlike parosteal osteosarcoma, myositis ossificans exhibits the distinctive features of a zonal phenomenon and a cleft that completely separates the ossific mass from the cortex. Osteochondroma, on the other hand, demonstrates uninterrupted cortical continuity and medullary communication between the lesion and the host bone. These features are not present in parosteal osteosarcoma.

The histologic diagnosis of a low-grade malignant tumor is usually difficult to make without consideration of the radiographic features.[2] The bone is often trabeculated but at least partially immature, and even when the bone is mature, the intertrabecular spaces contain a fibrous tissue stroma in which it may be difficult to find frank atypicality (Fig. 2–6*B*). Osteochondromas, in contrast, usually exhibit fatty or even hematopoietic marrow in their intertrabecular spaces.

Occasionally, a cartilage cap is associated with a parosteal osteosarcoma, causing even more confusion with osteochondroma. The atypicality and disorderliness of the chondrocytes in this cap usually point to the correct diagnosis. The histologic distinction of parosteal osteosarcoma from myositis ossificans is

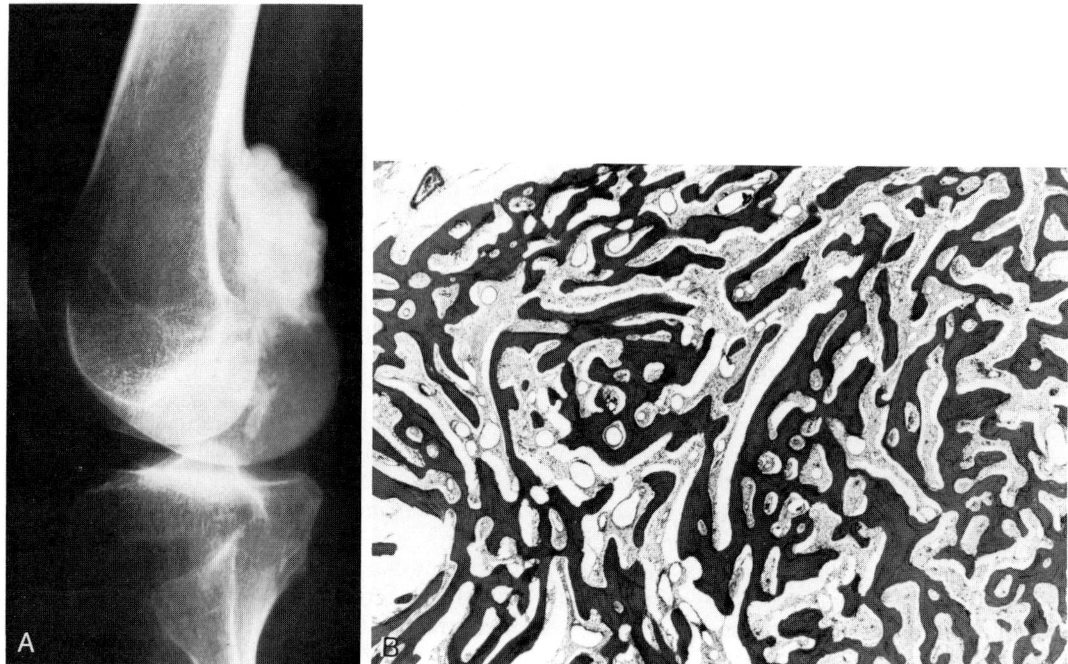

FIGURE 2–6. Parosteal osteosarcoma. *A,* Ossific mass with slightly lobulated borders is attached to the posterior cortex of the distal femur. *B,* Highly interconnected, immature and maturing bony trabeculae are haphazardly arranged in a loosely textured fibrous stroma (×24).

analogous to the radiographic zonal phenomenon. The heterotopic ossification of myositis ossificans matures in a centripetal fashion, the most mature portion of the lesion being the outermost. In parosteal osteosarcoma and higher-grade malignant tumors, the outer advancing portion of the lesion is usually the least mature.

Periosteal Osteosarcoma. This tumor, a rare type of osteosarcoma, grows on the surface of a bone, usually the midshaft of a long bone; it occurs most often in adolescence.[140] Because it is a surface lesion, it may resemble myositis ossificans, and the predominance of cartilage in the lesion may lead to confusion with periosteal chondrosarcoma. Together with the young age of the patient, the radiographic presence of ossification in the base of the lesion (Fig. 2–7*A, B*) and the histologic identification of at least some osteoid or bone formation by tumor cells (Fig. 2–7*C*) are helpful in differentiating this tumor from periosteal chondrosarcoma. The prognosis for periosteal osteosarcoma is somewhat better than for conventional osteosarcoma but worse than for parosteal osteosarcoma.[56, 125]

High-Grade Surface Osteosarcoma and Dedifferentiated Parosteal Osteosarcoma. The small percentage of juxtacortical osteosarcomas that are high-grade tumors carry the same prognosis as conventional osteosarcoma. The less common of these lesions, *high-grade surface* osteosarcoma, exhibits features like those of parosteal or periosteal osteosarcoma.[147] It is histologically indistinct from conventional osteosarcoma, and like the latter, it has a high potential for distant metastases. Intramedullary extension of the tumor is uncommon, but the cortex may be involved and pathologic fracture may occur (Fig. 2–8). *Dedifferentiated parosteal* osteosarcoma, the more common variant of the high-grade malignant surface osteosarcomas, usually initiates as a conventional low-grade parosteal osteosarcoma. Then either spontaneously (in which case both low- and high-grade components can be identified histologically) or secondarily in recurrences of inadequately resected low-grade parosteal tumors, the lesion undergoes transformation to a high-grade malignancy.[148] The latter situation is more common. Unni (1988) cites a dedifferentiation rate of 20% in such recurrences.[136]

SECONDARY OSTEOSARCOMA

The term *secondary* applied to osteosarcoma refers to a tumor arising in association with a preexisting alteration of the bone, which may

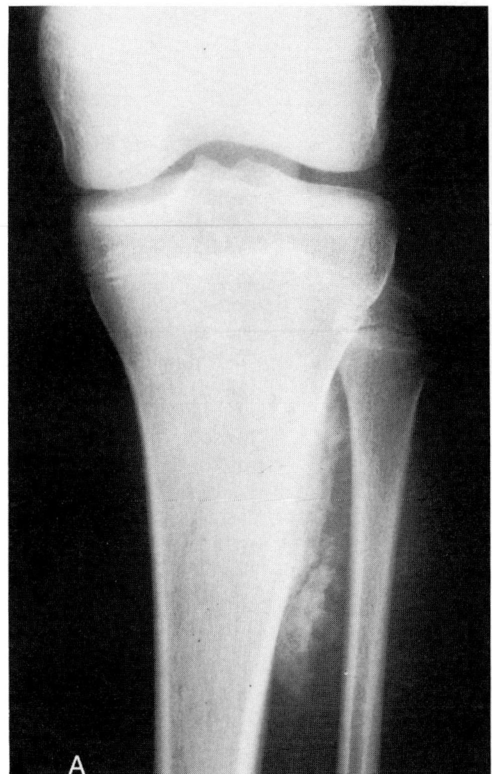

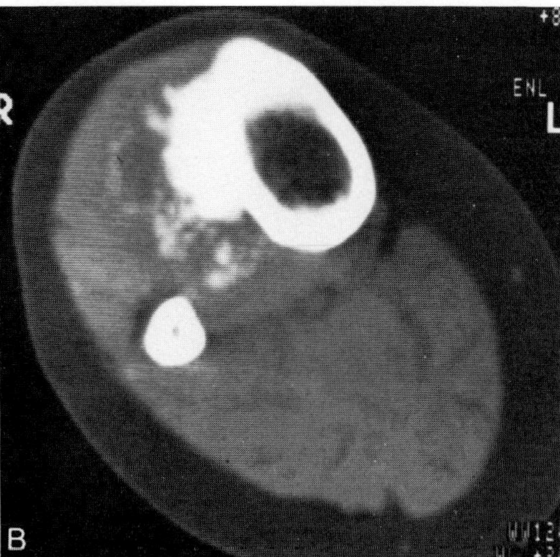

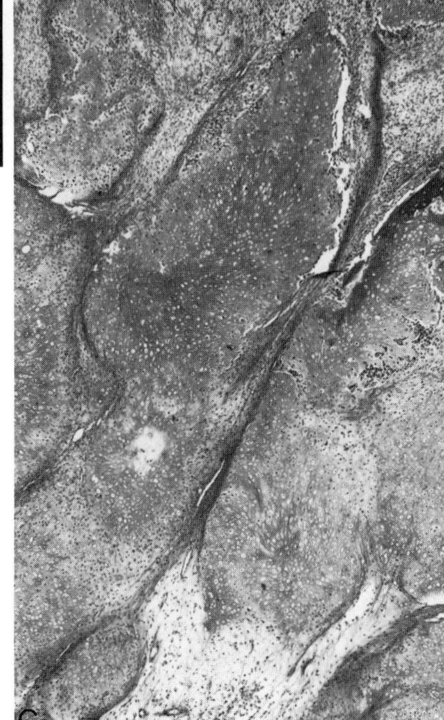

FIGURE 2–7. Periosteal osteosarcoma. *A,* Extensive calcifications and ossifications in the ill-defined mass attached to the lateral tibial cortex in a 12-year-old girl. (From Greenspan A: Orthopedic Radiology. Philadelphia, JB Lippincott, 1988.) *B,* CT section through the proximal tibial diaphysis of the same patient demonstrates bone and cartilage formation in the tumor situated on the surface of the bone. (From Greenspan A: Orthopedic Radiology. Philadelphia, JB Lippincott, 1988.) *C,* The field is dominated by highly cellular cartilage matrix interspersed with a cellular stroma and small amounts of bone (upper portion of photomicrograph) (×8).

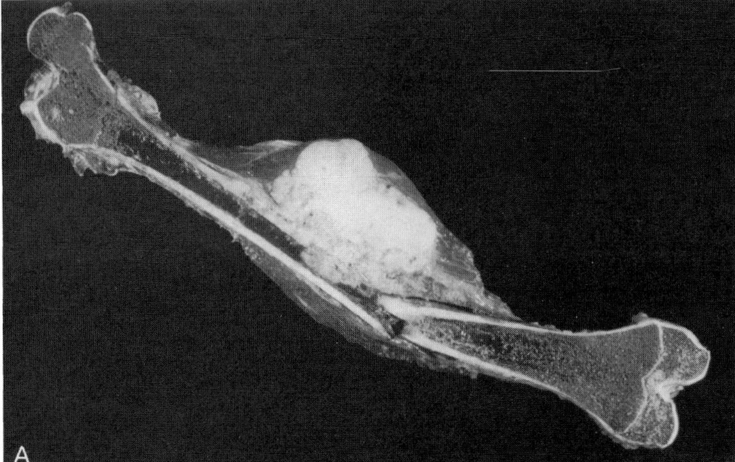

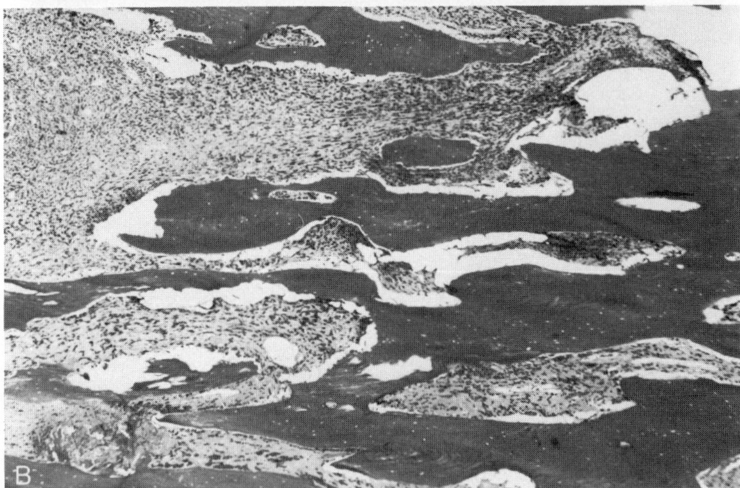

FIGURE 2–8. High-grade surface osteosarcoma. *A,* Secondary bone invasion and pathologic fracture. The radiograph of the specimen reveals a large tumor situated peripherally on the cortex of the middiaphysis with focal cortical and intramedullary extension. The periosteal reaction along the medial aspect is caused by fracture. *B,* Photomicrograph of the cortex reveals permeation of haversian systems by high-grade tumor with resorption of compact bone (×9).

or may not be neoplastic. Secondary lesions usually occur in an older population group than do primary tumors, a large percentage of secondary lesions arising as complications of Paget's disease.[96]

Typically, malignant transformation in pagetic bone can be recognized radiographically by the appearance of a destructive lesion, a soft tissue mass, and tumor bone production (Fig. 2–9). In older patients with Paget's disease, secondary osteosarcoma must be differentiated from metastatic carcinoma, especially from primary breast or prostate tumors, which are characteristically associated with osteosclerotic changes. However, metastases are uncommon in Paget's disease, despite the increased vascularity of pagetic bone.[145]

Radiation therapy for an unrelated previous condition may also give rise to secondary osteosarcoma. The criteria for diagnosis of postirradiation sarcoma are the following:

1. The initial disease and the postirradiation sarcoma must not be of the same histologic type.
2. The site of the new tumor must be within the field of irradiation.
3. At least 3 years must have elapsed since the previous radiation therapy.[129]

Postirradiation osteosarcoma may also develop after the ingestion and intraosseous accumulation of radioisotopes, as has been described in radium watch dial painters. The least commonly encountered instance, one in which secondary osteosarcoma arises, involves completely benign bone diseases, such as fibrous dysplasia, without prior irradiation.[138] Whatever its cause, the histopathologic features of secondary osteosarcomas are identical with those of primary osteosarcomas; the prognosis for these tumors is equally ominous.

Tumors of Cartilage Origin

To diagnose a lesion as originating from cartilage is rather simple for the radiologist. Its

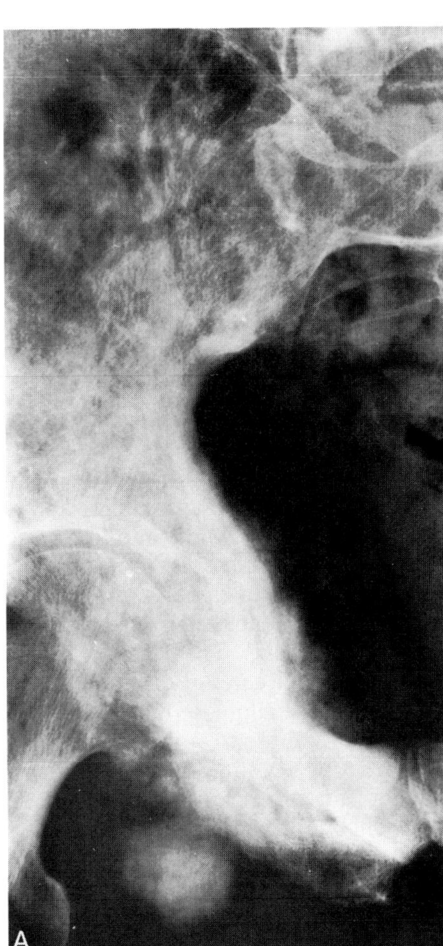

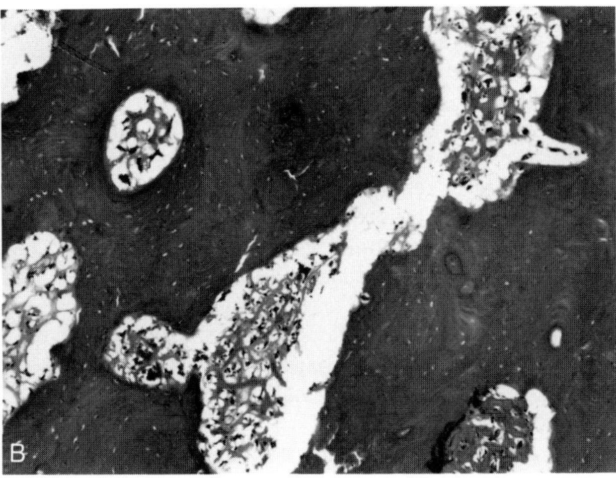

FIGURE 2–9. Osteosarcoma in Paget's disease. *A,* Destruction of the cortex of the right ischium and a soft tissue mass with tumor bone formation in a patient with extensive skeletal involvement by Paget's disease. (From Greenspan A: Orthopedic Radiology. Philadelphia, JB Lippincott, 1988.) *B,* The remodeled cortex shows tumor cells and osteoid matrix in the vascular canals (×63).

radiolucent matrix, scalloped margin, and annular, punctate, or comma-shaped calcifications usually suffice to establish its chondrogenic nature.[102, 103] On the other hand, determining whether a cartilaginous tumor is benign or malignant may at times be extremely difficult for the radiologist and the pathologist.[98, 99] Some slow-growing, low-grade chondrosarcomas can masquerade as enchondromas, and some aggressive-looking benign cartilaginous lesions may be mistakenly diagnosed as chondrosarcomas. Close cooperation among the radiologist, the pathologist, and the clinician in reviewing the history, the radiographic examination, and the biopsy specimens is crucial to reaching a conclusion about the exact nature of a cartilage lesion.

Clinically, the malignancy of a lesion is suggested by, among other signs, the development of pain in a previously asymptomatic lesion (e.g., malignant transformation of enchondroma to chondrosarcoma) or the development of swelling at the site of a lesion. Radiographically, the presence of a periosteal reaction, thickening or destruction of the cortex, and a soft tissue mass are highly suggestive of malignancy. Pathologic features of malignant cartilaginous tumors include the presence of hypercellular and pleomorphic tumor tissue, an appreciable number of plump cells with large or double nuclei, invasion (permeation) of bone trabeculae, and infiltration of the haversian systems and bone marrow.[27] In the pathologic evaluation, Dahlin states, "it is necessary to examine numerous fields in these tumors to be certain that these are not areas with sufficient evidence for a diagnosis of malignancy. . . .[27]" Evidence that a tumor is a chondrosarcoma rather than a benign enchondroma is frequently found in isolated areas within the mass. This is why biopsy specimens must be obtained from various areas of a tumor.[83]

BENIGN CARTILAGINOUS TUMORS

Chondroma (Enchondroma and Periosteal Chondroma)

Chondroma is a benign tumor characterized by the formation of mature hyaline cartilage. Several theories have been postulated regarding its etiology. One of these is that the lesion forms as a result of abnormal zones of dysplastic chondrocytes from the growth plate. These abnormal foci fail to undergo normal endochondral ossification; instead, they are deposited within the metaphysis and, as the bone grows, are displaced into the diaphysis.[98, 99]

Customarily, a lesion located centrally in the bone is called an *enchondroma,* whereas one located outside the cortex is called a *chondroma* (periosteal or juxtacortical).[84, 85] Although the tumor may occur throughout life, most cases are seen between the second and fourth decades;[64, 71] there is no sex predilection. The short tubular bones of the hand (the phalanges and the metacarpals) are sites of predilection, followed in frequency by the femur, the humerus, and the ribs. The lesion is often asymptomatic; a pathologic fracture through the tumor usually calls attention to the condition (Fig. 2–10*A*).

Plain film radiography and conventional tomography most often suffice to demonstrate the lesion and to establish its chondroid character. In short bones, the lesion is frequently purely radiolucent; but in long bones, it may display visible calcifications (Fig. 2–10*B*). If the calcifications are extensive, enchondromas are called calcifying. The lesion can also be recognized by scalloping of the inner cortical margins, reflecting the lobular growth pattern of cartilage. CT and MRI may further delineate the tumor and more precisely localize it in the bone (Fig. 2–10*C* to *E*). It must be stressed, however, that most of the time, neither CT nor MRI is suitable for establishing the precise nature of a cartilaginous lesion, nor can CT or MRI distinguish benign from malignant lesions. Despite the utilization of various criteria, the application of MRI to tissue diagnosis of cartilaginous lesions has not brought satisfactory results. This is because benign and malignant chondrogenic lesions have the same MRI characteristics: low-intensity signal compared with normal bone on T1-weighted images, and high-intensity signal on T2-weighted images.[13, 26]

The main differential diagnostic condition, particularly in long bones, is medullary bone infarct. At times, the two lesions may be difficult to distinguish from one another because of similar calcifications, particularly if enchondroma is small. The radiographic features helpful in the differential diagnosis are lobulation of the margins of an enchondroma, annular and punctate calcifications in the matrix, and the lack of a sclerotic outline (commonly seen in bone infarcts).[130]

Histologically, enchondroma consists of lobules of hyaline cartilage of varying cellularity and is recognized by the features of its intercellular matrix, which has a uniformly translucent appearance and contains relatively little collagen. The tissue is sparsely cellular and the cells contain small and darkly staining nuclei. The tumor cells are located in rounded spaces (lacunae). The nuclei of the chondrocytes are usually bland and single, although occasional double nuclei are found. The external borders of the lesion are well circumscribed and typically do not interdigitate with the intertrabecular spaces of the surrounding cancellous bone (Fig. 2–10*F*). Similarly, although the advancing border of enchondromas may thin the cortex, enchondromas do not penetrate its Volkmann canals or haversian systems. The punctate calcifications seen on plain radiographs correspond to the same type of calcification seen in the zone of provisional calcification in a growth plate or to actual endochondral ossification at the periphery of cartilage lobules (Fig. 2–10*G*).

The most important complication of the lesion is malignant transformation to chondrosarcoma.[108] In a solitary enchondroma, this occurs only in a long or flat bone, almost never in a short tubular bone. Malignant degeneration may be detected radiographically by thickening or destruction of the cortex and the presence of a soft tissue mass. An important clinical sign is the development of pain at the site of the lesion in a previously asymptomatic patient in the absence of a fracture.

Enchondromatosis (Ollier's Disease)

Enchondromatosis is a condition marked by multiple enchondromas generally about the metaphyses and the diaphyses. If the skeleton is extensively involved, the term Ollier's disease is applied.[71, 118] There is no hereditary or familial tendency in this disorder, which some investigators consider developmental rather than neoplastic, classifying it as a form of bone dysplasia. The condition has a strong preference for involvement of one side of the body. The clinical manifestations, like knobby swellings of the digits or gross limb length disparity, are frequently recognized in childhood and adolescence.

The radiographic appearance of enchondromatosis involving the hands and feet is characteristic. Radiolucent masses of cartilage with foci of calcifications markedly deform the bones (Fig. 2–11 *A*). Elsewhere, columns of radiolucent streaks extend from the growth plate into the diaphysis (Fig. 2–11*B*); interference with the growth plate causes foreshortening and deformity of the bones (Fig. 2–11*C*).

Histologically, the lesions in enchondromatosis are essentially indistinguishable from those of solitary enchondromas, although, on occasion, they tend to be more cellular.[71] The most frequent and severe complication of Ollier's disease is malignant transformation to chondrosarcoma. Unlike the solitary enchondroma, even lesions in the short tubular bones may undergo sarcomatous changes. This is particularly true in patients with so-called Maffucci's syndrome, a congenital, nonhereditary disorder, manifested by enchondromatosis and soft tissue hemangiomas. The skeletal lesions in Maffucci's syndrome have the same distribution as those in Ollier's disease, with a strong predilection for one side of the body.[64] The condition is recognized radiographically by multiple calcified phleboliths.

Osteochondroma (Osteocartilaginous Exostosis)

Osteochondroma, the most common benign bone lesion, is a cartilage-capped bony projection on the external surface of a bone.[130] Usually diagnosed in patients before the third decade, it most commonly involves the metaphyses of long bones, particularly around the knee and the proximal humerus. The lesion grows by endochondral ossification of its cartilage cap and usually stops growing at skeletal maturity.[71]

Its radiographic presentation depends on the type of lesion. The *pedunculated* osteochondroma manifests with a slender pedicle, which is usually directed away from the neighboring growth plate (Fig. 2–12 *A*); the *sessile* variant shows a broad base attached to the cortex (Fig. 2–12 *B*). In either type, the most important identifying feature is that the cortex of the host bone merges without interruption with the cortex of osteochondroma and the cancellous portion of the lesion is continuous with the medullary cavity of the adjacent diaphysis. These characteristics distinguish this lesion from the occasionally similar-appearing bone masses of juxtacortical osteosarcoma, soft tissue osteosarcoma, and juxtacortical myositis ossificans. Calcifications in the chondro-osseous portion of the stalk of the lesion are also typical features.

Histologically, the cap of the osteochondroma is composed of hyaline cartilage arranged similarly to that of a growth plate (Fig. 2–12*C*). A zone of provisional calcification corresponds to the areas of calcifications in the chondro-osseous portion of the stalk. Beneath this zone, there is vascular invasion and replacement of the calcified cartilage by new bone formation, which undergoes maturation and merges with the cancellous bone of the medullary cavity. The intertrabecular spaces between these maturing spicules contain fatty or sometimes hematopoietic marrow. In carefully prepared sections, a delicate fibrous membrane overlies the cartilage cap. This fibrous tissue, known as perichondrium, is the continuation of the periosteum of the adjacent bone cortex over the surface of the osteochondroma (Fig. 2–12*D*).

Osteochondroma may be complicated by pressure on adjacent nerves or blood vessels, as well as bone, occasionally with consequent fracture; by fracture of the lesion itself; and by inflammatory changes of the bursa exostotica covering the cartilage cap. Malignant transformation to chondrosarcoma is rare, occurring in fewer than 1% of solitary lesions.[68, 129, 130]

It is important to recognize the features suggesting malignant degeneration early.[76] Clinically, pain (in the absence of a fracture, bursitis, or pressure on nerves) and growth spurt or continued growth of the lesion after skeletal maturity are highly suggestive. The radiographic evaluation may reveal features suggesting this complication: development of a thick, bulky cartilage cap (usually more than 2 to 3 cm in thickness);[63] development of a soft tissue mass with or without calcifications; and dispersed calcifications within the cartilage cap, separate from those contained in the stalk, a new sign described by Norman and Sissons.[108] The most reliable imaging modalities for evaluating possible malignant transformation are plain radiography, conventional tomography, CT, and MRI. Plain films usually demonstrate

Text continued on page 34

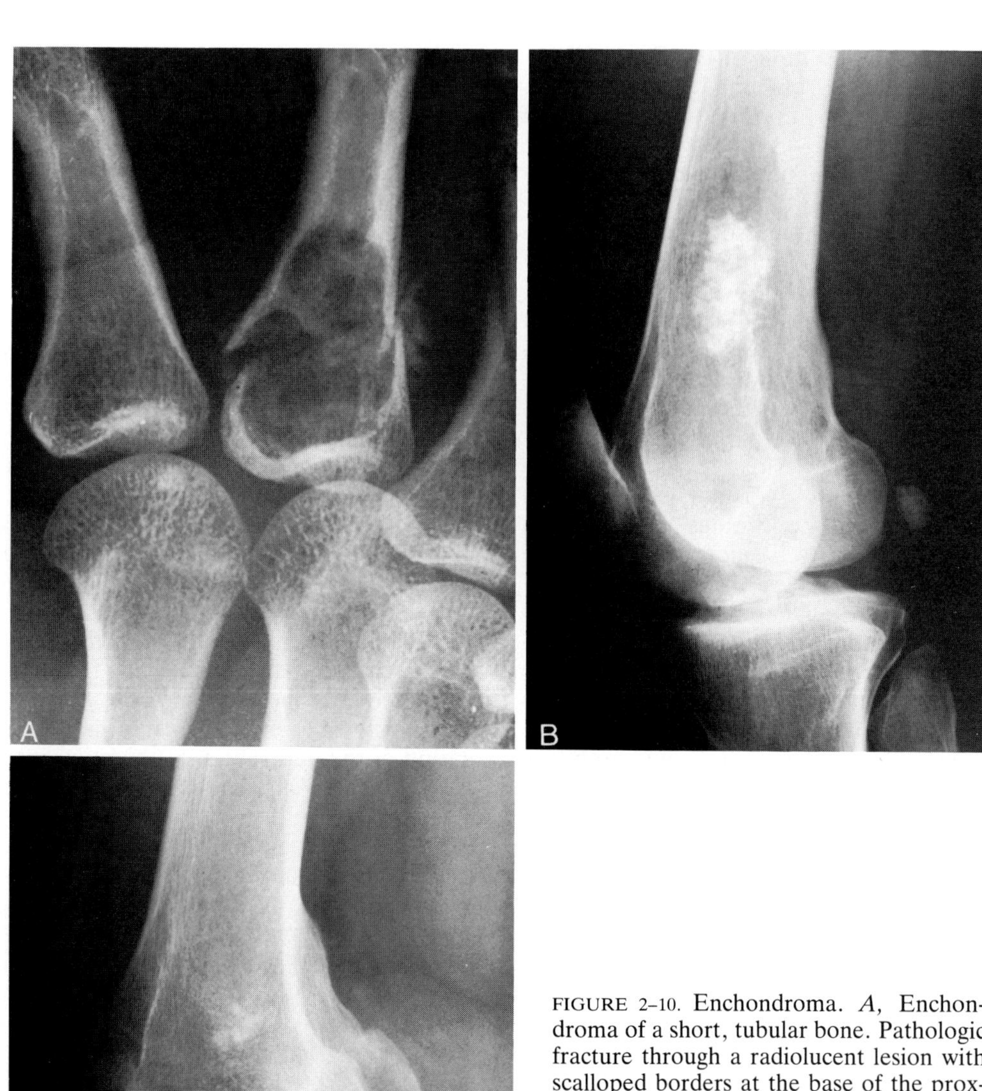

FIGURE 2–10. Enchondroma. *A,* Enchondroma of a short, tubular bone. Pathologic fracture through a radiolucent lesion with scalloped borders at the base of the proximal phalanx. *B,* Enchondroma of a long bone. Punctate and annular calcifications are present in the central portion of the lesion. *C,* Enchondroma in the distal femur. Lateral radiograph demonstrates only a small conglomerate of calcifications.

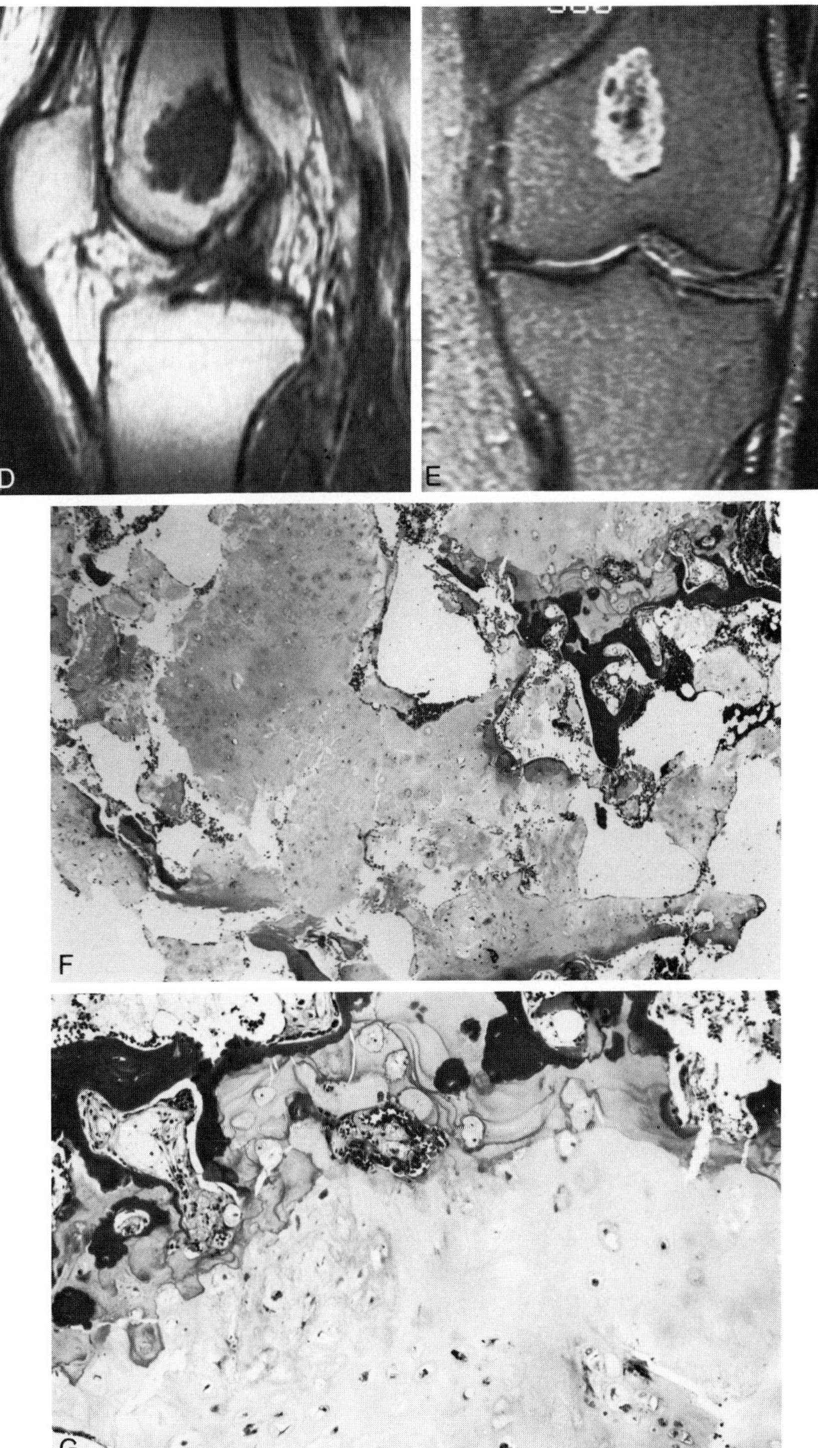

FIGURE 2–10 *Continued D,* MRI T1-weighted image in sagittal plane demonstrates the true extent of the lesion, which shows a low-intensity signal. *E,* T2-weighted image in coronal plane (TR 1800 MS/TE 70 MS). The enchondroma displays a high-intensity signal. The low-intensity foci in the central portion of the lesion represent calcifications. *F,* Multiple lobules of bland, hyaline cartilage of low cellularity (×24). *G,* Endochondral ossification at the periphery of a cartilage lobule (×115).

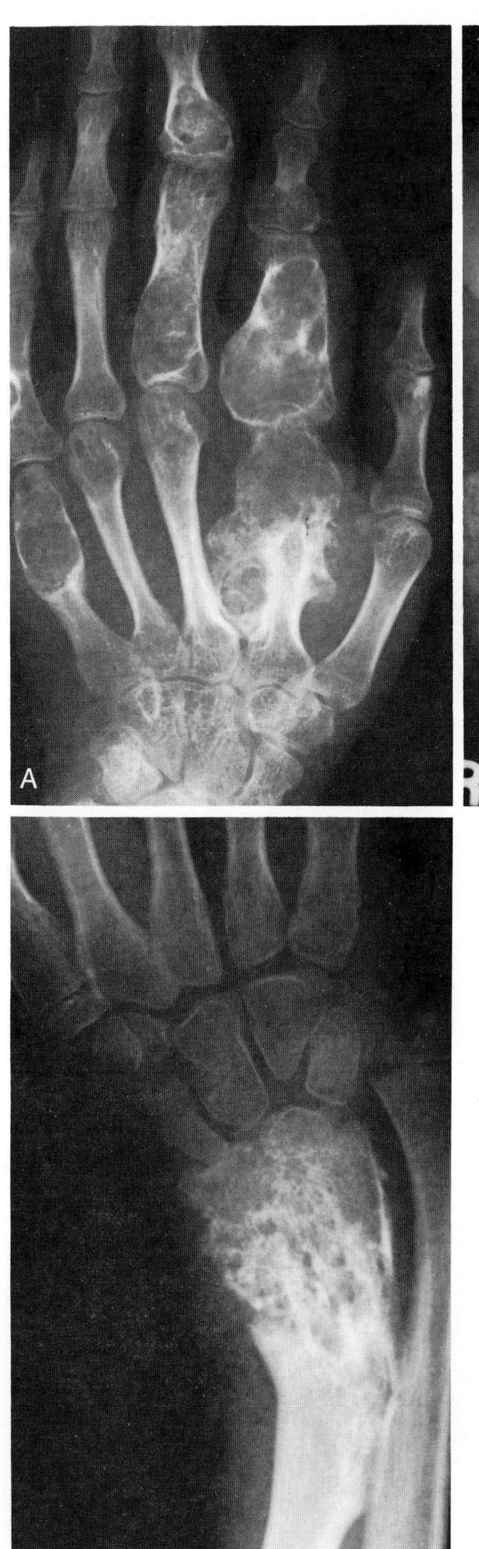

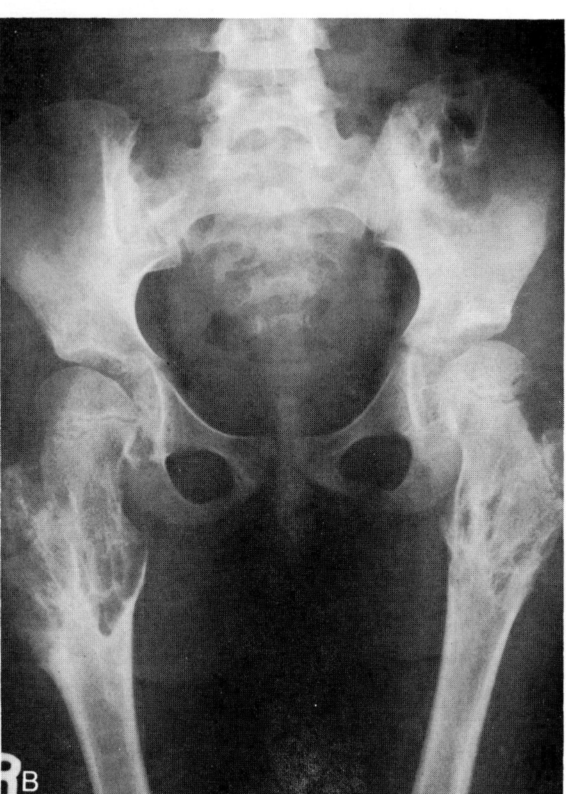

FIGURE 2–11. Enchondromatosis. *A,* Multiple expansile lesions are seen in the metacarpals and the phalanges, markedly deforming the bones. *B,* Tongues of cartilage extend from the growth plates of both femora into the diaphyses. Note the involvement of the iliac bones and the acetabula. *C,* Involvement of the metaphysis and the growth plate of the radius resulted in deformity of the distal forearm.

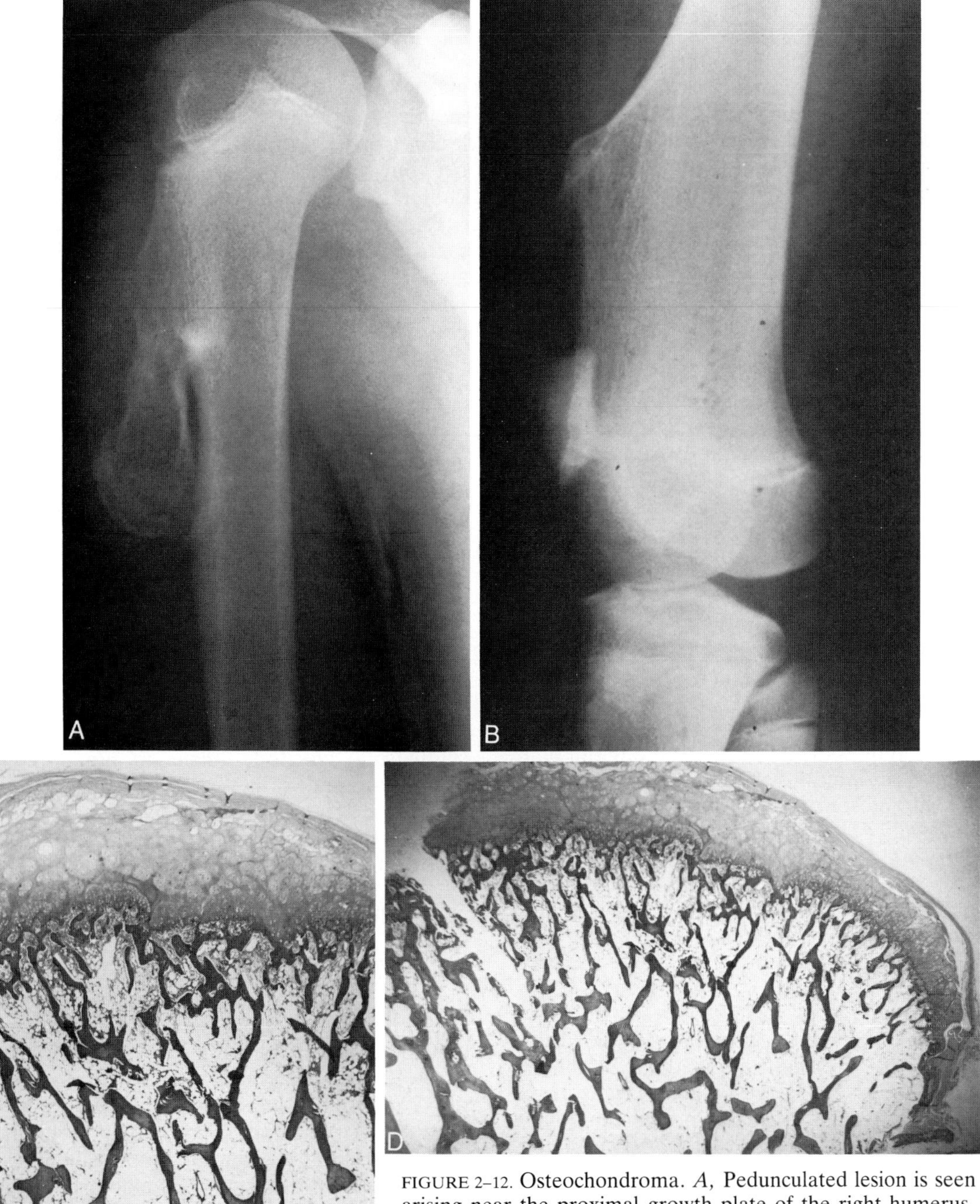

FIGURE 2–12. Osteochondroma. *A,* Pedunculated lesion is seen arising near the proximal growth plate of the right humerus. (From Greenspan A: Orthopedic Radiology. Philadelphia, JB Lippincott, 1988.) *B,* Sessile variant. The lesion is situated on the anteromedial aspect of the distal femoral diaphysis. Note that the cortex of the host bone merges without interruption with the cortex of the lesion. *C,* The hyaline cartilage cap transforms into bone and fatty marrow by endochondral ossification. A thin, fibrous membrane loosely overlies the cartilage (×4). *D,* The overlaying fibrous membrane perichondrium is in continuity with the periosteum (lower right field) (×2.5).

containment of the calcifications of osteochondroma within the stalk of the lesion, but occasionally conventional tomography can also be helpful in this regard. Dispersement of the calcifications in the cartilage cap and the increased thickness of the cap, the cardinal signs of malignant degeneration, can be demonstrated by any of the above-mentioned modalities.

Radionuclide bone scan may also be performed, and it may show increased uptake of radiopharmaceutical at the site of a lesion. Exostotic chondrosarcoma often exhibits greater intensity of uptake than a benign exostosis, but according to various investigators, this is not always a reliable distinguishing feature of malignant transformation. The increased activity of a benign exostosis on bone scan is related to endochondral ossification within the cartilage cap, whereas that of exostotic chondrosarcoma represents active ossification, osteoblastic activity, and hyperemia within the cartilage and bony stalk of the tumor.[60]

Multiple Osteocartilaginous Exostoses (Osteochondromatosis or Diaphyseal Aclasis)

Classified by some authorities among the bone dysplasias, multiple osteochondromas represent an autosomal dominant hereditary disorder.[27, 68, 71] The knees, the ankles, and the shoulders are the most frequently affected sites, and growth disturbances are often present, primarily in the forearms and the legs. The radiographic features are similar to those of a solitary osteochondroma; the sessile form of the lesion is more common (Fig. 2–13 *A*, *B*).

The pathologic features of multiple osteochondromas are the same as those of solitary lesions (Fig. 2–13*C*). Malignant transformation to chondrosarcoma is more common in osteochondromatosis (5 to 15%) than in solitary lesions. Lesions at the shoulder girdle and around the pelvis are usually at greater risk for this complication. Clinically and radiologically, the signs of malignant degeneration are identical with those of solitary osteochondroma. After skeletal maturity, any change in the size of the lesion or in the symptoms must be regarded as a possible indication of malignant change.

Chondroblastoma (Codman's Tumor)

Representing fewer than 1% of all primary bone tumors, this rare, benign lesion typically occurs in the epiphysis of long bones, such as the humerus, the tibia, and the femur.[14] Generally, the clinical symptoms are nonspecific; pain and swelling, usually lasting several months, are the most common complaints. The lesion is seen primarily before skeletal maturity, but some cases have been reported after obliteration of the growth plate.[32]

Radiographically, the lesion is usually located eccentrically. It is radiolucent, showing a sclerotic border and, in 25 to 50% of cases, popcorn-like calcifications (Fig. 2–14 *A*, *B*). Fewer than 10% of cases exhibit a periosteal reaction.[62, 97] If calcifications are not apparent on standard radiographs, conventional tomograms or CT scan can be helpful.[62]

Before the recognition of this entity by Jaffe and Lichtenstein (1942), examples were usually referred to as "epiphyseal chondromatous giant cell tumor."[25] Although the tumor contains giant cells (and it is still sometimes misdiagnosed as giant cell tumor), Jaffe and Lichtenstein argued that the giant cells were not part of the "primary pattern" of the tumor, stressing instead their relationship to cartilage.[73]

Histologically, chondroblastoma is composed of uniform large round cells with a large cytoplasmic envelope, clear to amphophilic cytoplasm, and rather defined cellular borders.[118, 122] The nuclei are ovoid and show occasional folding with prominent nuclear grooves (Fig. 2–14*C*). Although there are usually enough multinucleated osteoclast-like giant cells scattered about to make giant cell tumor a serious differential consideration, several features distinguish the two lesions histologically. First, in giant cell tumor, the giant cells are randomly and evenly distributed. Second, the stromal cells in giant cell tumor tend to be spindle shaped and polyhedral rather than round. Most importantly, giant cell tumor shows no true matrix production, whereas chondroblastoma produces an intercellular matrix resembling cartilage but seldom differentiating into true hyaline cartilage. The matrix shows variable amounts of calcification and even secondary necrosis, similar to what is found in epiphyseal growth plate but with an aberrant arrangement. Particularly characteristic are fine, lattice-like matrix calcifications surrounding apposing chondroblasts and having a spatial arrangement resembling the hexagonal configuration of chicken wire (Fig. 2–14*D*). The lesion is benign and a thorough curettage is usually adequate treatment. Occasionally, however, chondroblastoma can be

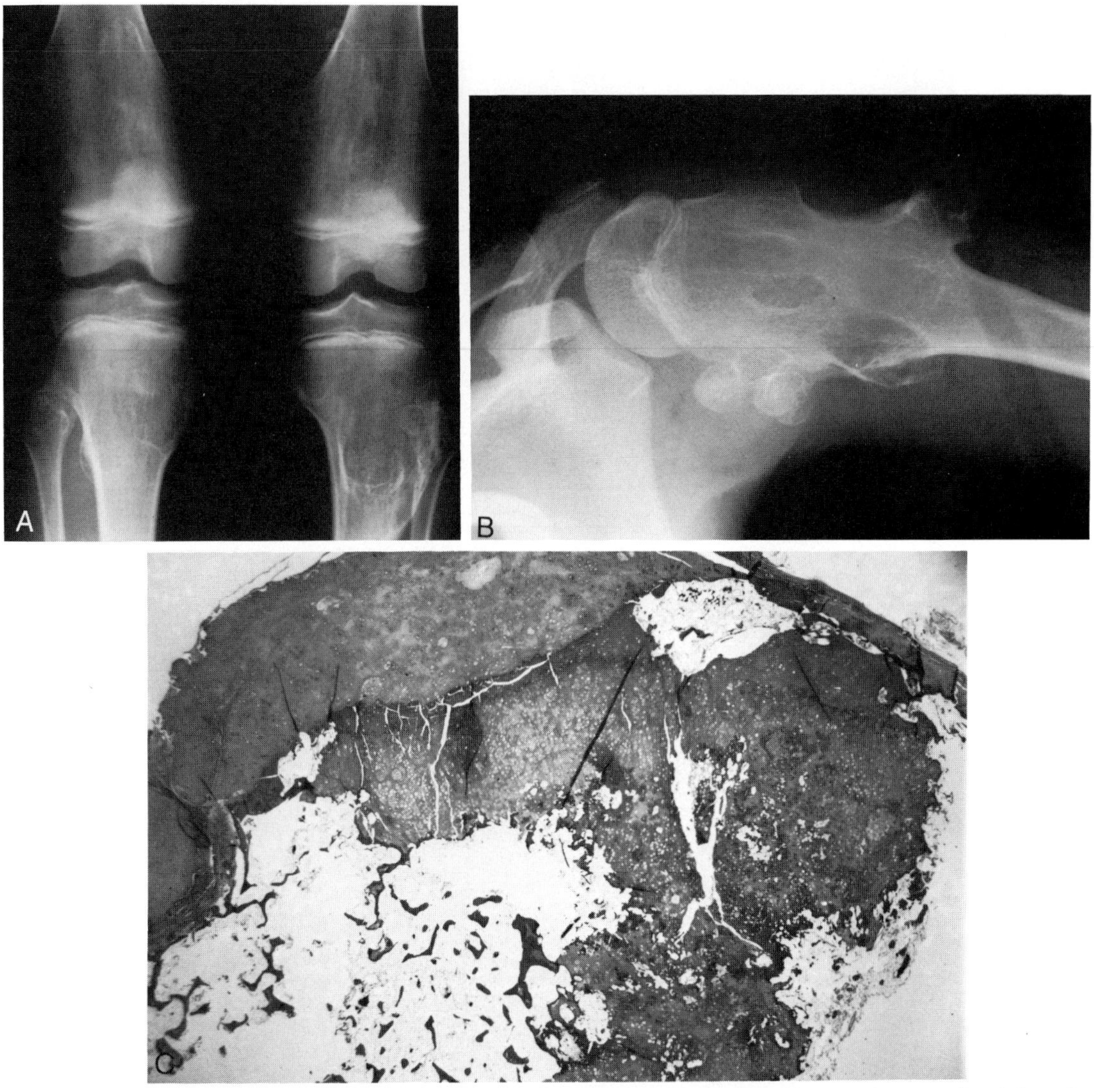

FIGURE 2–13. Multiple osteocartilaginous exostoses. *A,* Multiple osteochondromas are seen involving the distal femora and the proximal tibiae and fibulae. *B,* Multiple osteochondromas in the proximal diaphysis of the left humerus. Note the preponderance of sessile lesions. *C,* The cartilage cap is thicker and more irregular than that in Figure 2–12*C* and *D* but displays benign cellularity (×9).

a tenaciously recurrent local tumor. Pulmonary metastases have been reported in a minority of cases of chondroblastoma,[64, 79, 99] but no histologic evidence of malignancy has been reported in either the primary bone tumor or the pulmonary metastases.

Chondromyxoid Fibroma

This rare cartilage tumor, accounting for less than 1% of all primary bone tumors, occurs predominantly in adolescents and young adults and more commonly in males than in females (2:1).[27] It has a predilection for the bones of the lower extremities, usually the proximal tibia, and clinical symptoms include the presence of a peripherally located mass, together with local pain and swelling.[48]

Radiographically, the lesion may range from 1 to 10 cm in size, with an average of 3 to 4 cm.[27, 48] It is a lucent, eccentrically located lesion exhibiting a scalloped, sclerotic margin (Fig. 2–15*A*); it often erodes or balloons out from the cortex, and frequently a buttress of

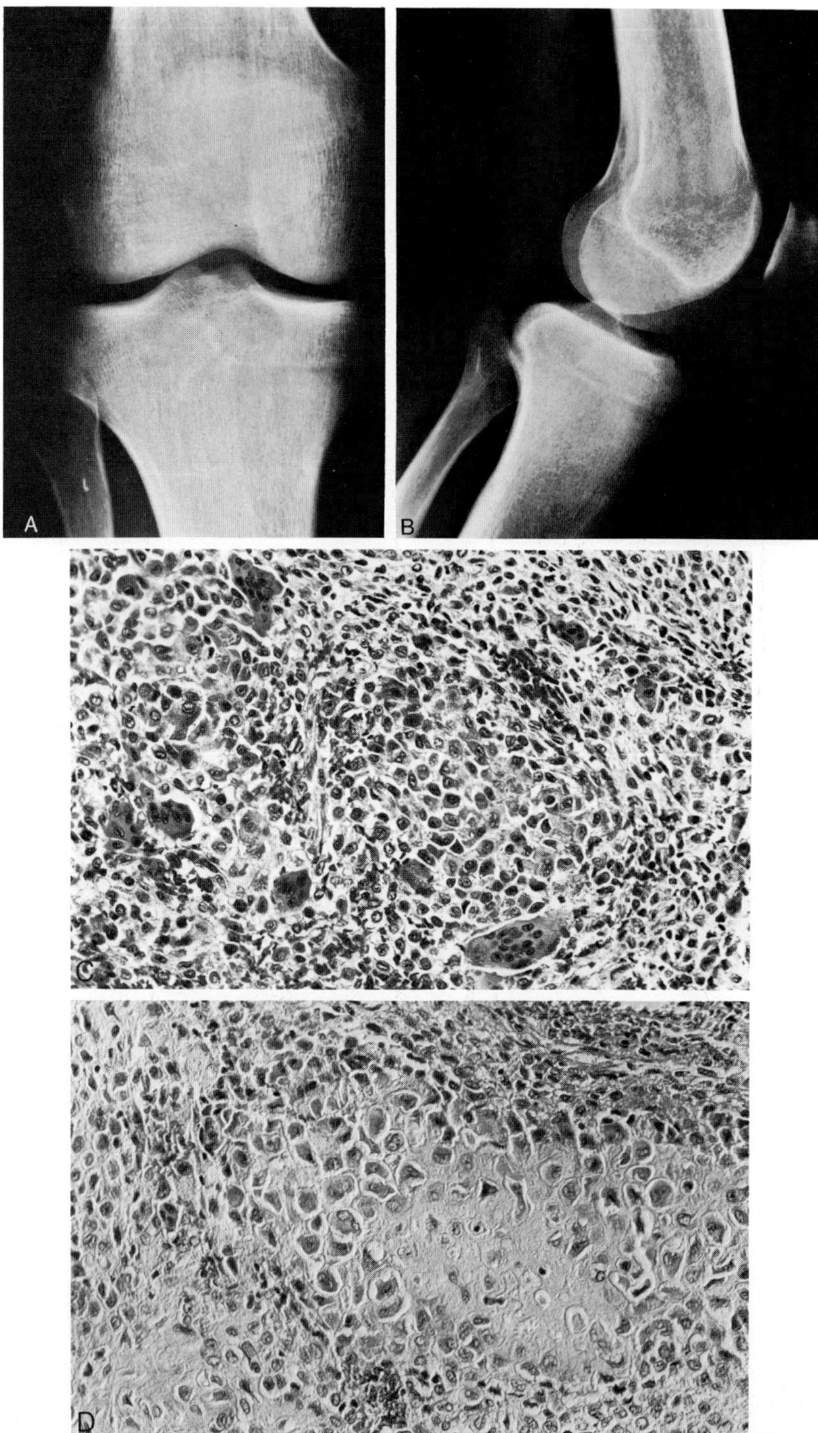

FIGURE 2–14. Chondroblastoma. *A, B,* Radiolucent, eccentrically located lesion in the proximal epiphysis of the tibia, with a thin, sclerotic margin and focal calcifications. (From Greenspan A: Orthopedic Radiology. Philadelphia, JB Lippincott, 1988.) *C,* Round chondroblasts and scattered multinucleated giant cells are characteristic of this tumor (×250). *D,* Chondroid matrix and "chicken wire" calcifications are histologic hallmarks of this lesion (×400).

periosteal new bone can be observed. Calcifications are not apparent radiologically. A few cases were reported with predominantly cortical involvement.[121] Occasionally, the lesion of chondromyxoid fibroma may be radiographically indistinguishable from an aneurysmal bone cyst.

Pathologically, curettage specimens from such a lesion are yellowish white, somewhat glistening and slippery, and devoid of blood, making their distinction from aneurysmal bone cyst simple. Histologically, the most important feature of the lesion is its lobular or pseudolobular arrangement into zones of varying cellularity (Fig. 2–15*B*). The center of the lobule is hypocellular and consists of a loosely arranged matrix rich in chondroitin sulfates and consequently showing positive staining with alcian blue at strongly acidic pH. Within this matrix are loosely arranged spindle-shaped and stellate cells with elongated processes. Occasionally, there are abortive spaces resembling chondrocyte lacunae surrounding some of the spindle-shaped and stellate cells, but the matrix almost never attains the completely rounded lacunar spaces surrounding true chondrocytes as seen in hyaline cartilage. The periphery of the lobules has a zone of dense cellularity containing an admixture of mononuclear spindle-shaped and polyhedral stromal cells with a variable number of multinucleated giant cells. Large pleomorphic cells may be present and can result in confusion with chondrosarcoma.[123] Mitotic figures and nuclear atypicality are sometimes observed in the densely cellular, narrow zone that serpiginously encircles the pseudolobules; however, the typical radiographic appearance usually permits recognition of the entity. Before the description of this entity by Jaffe and Lichtenstein in 1948,[74] many examples of chondromyxoid fibroma probably had been regarded as chondrosarcomas, but the tumor is now recognized as benign. Cases reported as myxomas or myxofibromas of long bones are also most likely chondromyxoid fibromas.[48]

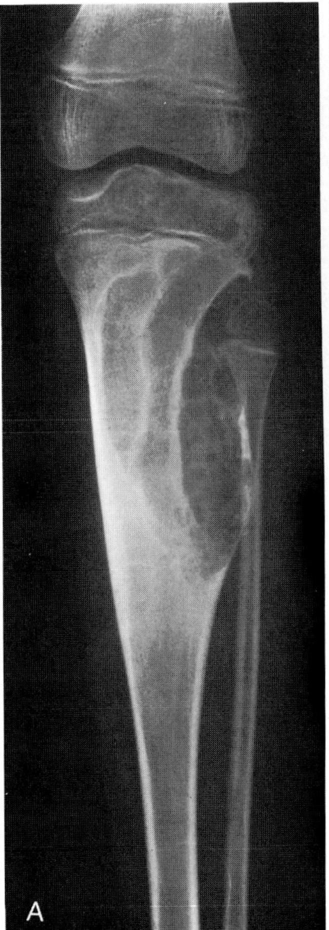

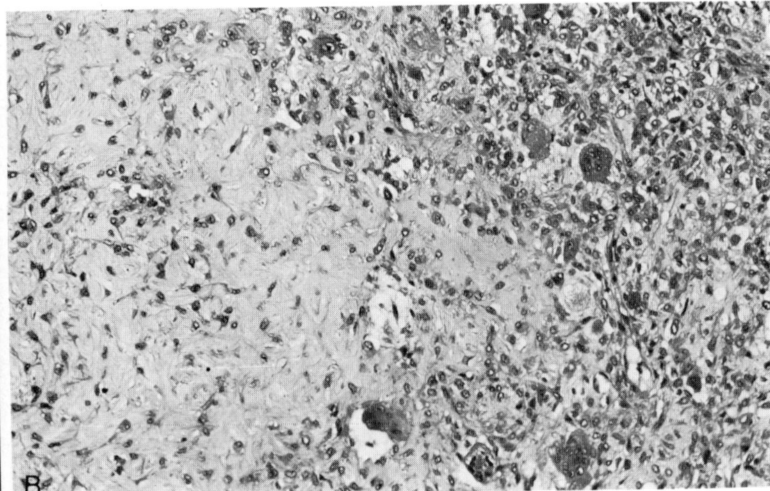

FIGURE 2–15. Chondromyxoid fibroma. *A,* Radiolucent lesion with sharply defined, sclerotic scalloped borders extends from the metaphysis into the diaphysis of the tibia. (From Greenspan A: Orthopedic Radiology. Philadelphia, JB Lippincott, 1988.) *B,* Myxochondroid lobule with stellate cells (left) bordered by hypercellular zone with multinucleated giant cells (right) (×125).

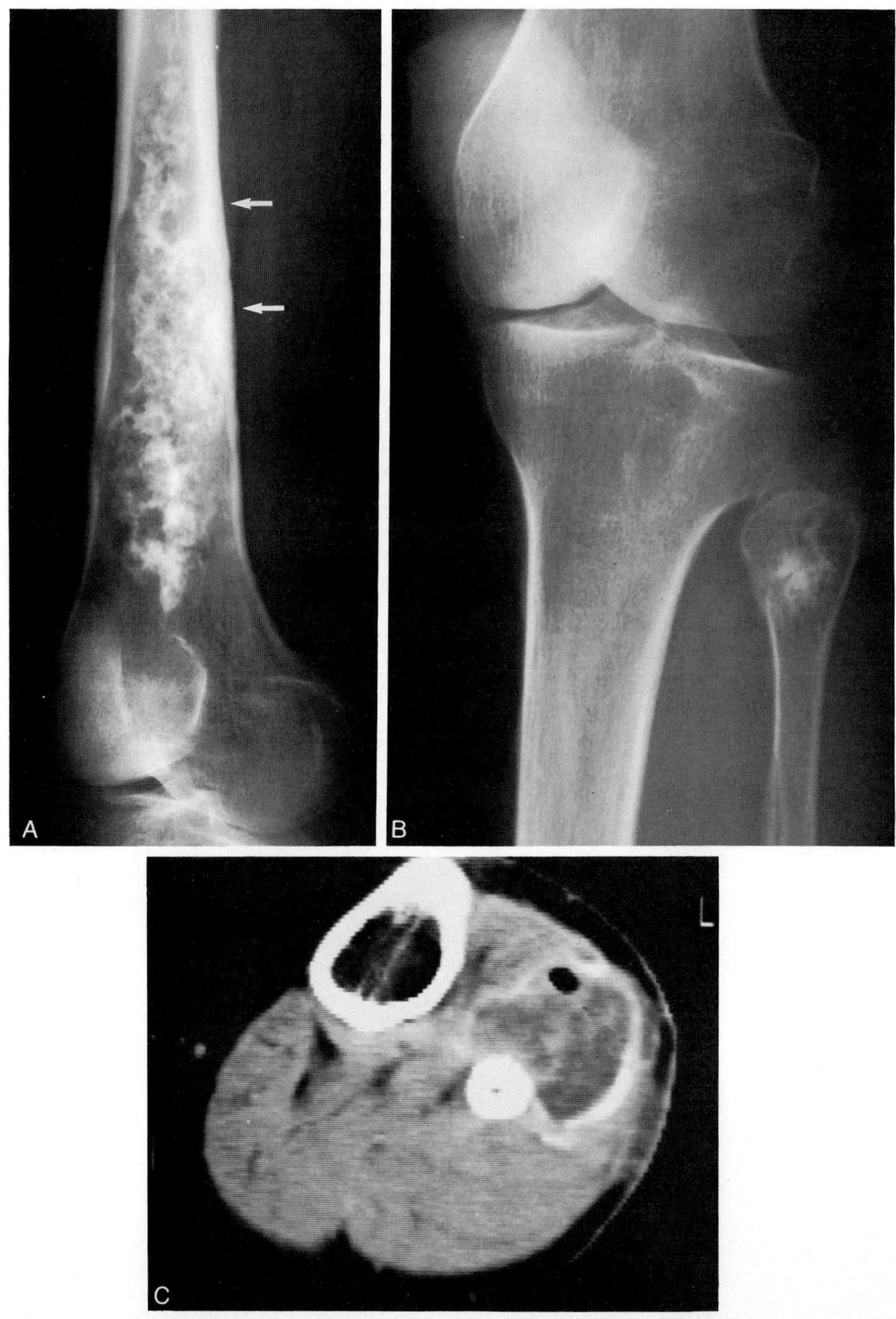

FIGURE 2–16. Chondrosarcoma. *A,* Expansile lesion in the distal femur demonstrates endosteal scalloping and typical chondroid calcifications. Note the thickening of the posteromedial cortex (arrows). (From Greenspan A: Orthopedic Radiology. Philadelphia, JB Lippincott, 1988.) *B,* Plain film shows a destructive lesion in the head of the fibula with central calcifications. The soft tissue mass is not appreciated. *C,* CT section of the lesion in *B* demonstrates involvement of the medullary cavity by the tumor and a large soft tissue mass.

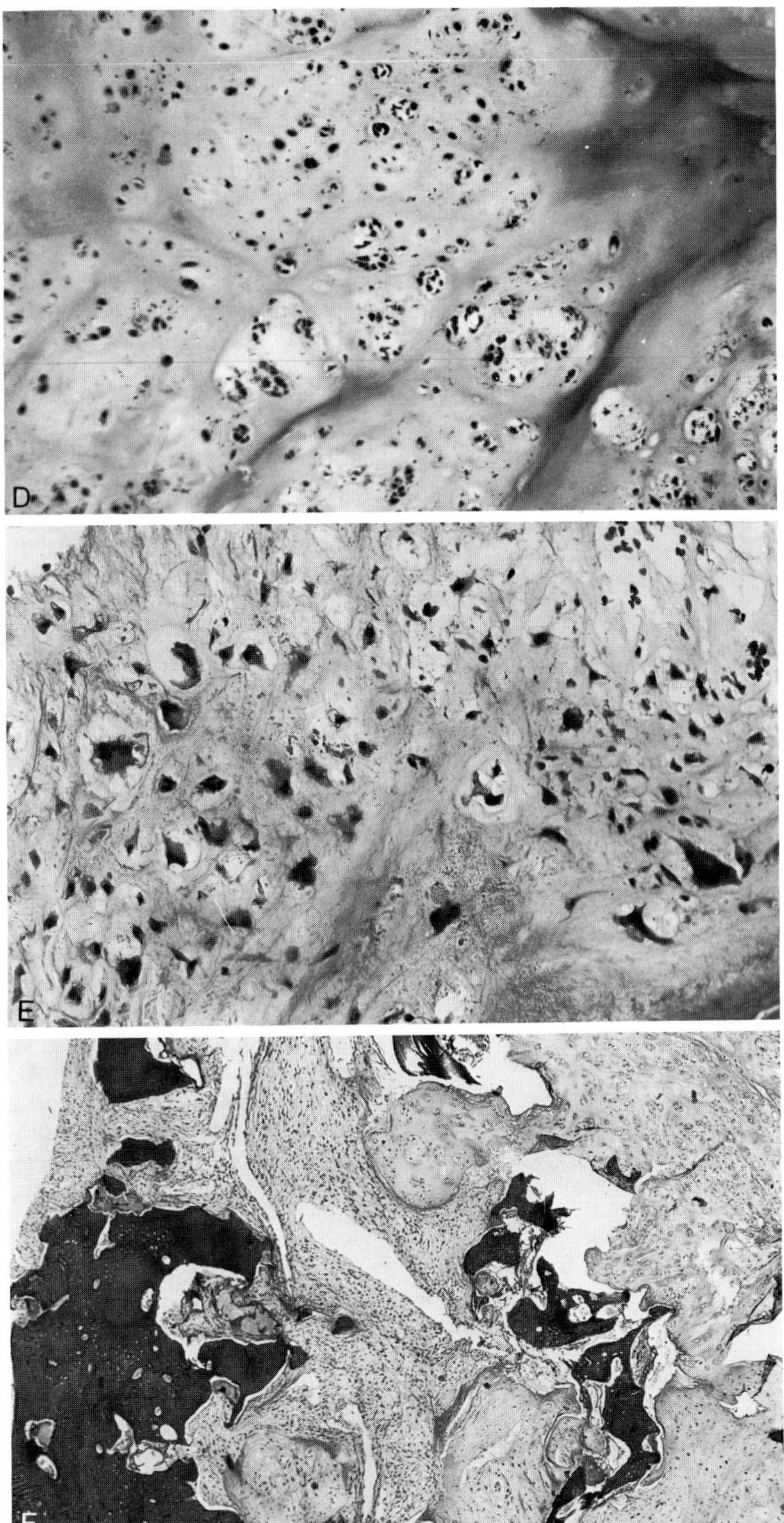

FIGURE 2–16 *Continued D,* Low-power magnification demonstrates a high degree of cellularity and multiple nuclei (×80). *E,* High-power view of grade 2 tumor reveals bizarre, hyperchromatic nuclei (×187). *F,* A low-grade tumor showing foci of trabecular permeation (×28).

MALIGNANT CARTILAGINOUS TUMORS

Chondrosarcoma

This malignant bone tumor is characterized by the formation of cartilage by tumor cells.[58, 87] Chondrosarcoma may be primary or secondary, depending on whether there was a preexisting lesion in which the chondrosarcoma took origin. In addition, these tumors are also referred to as *central* (or medullary) and *peripheral* (or surface) chondrosarcomas depending on their location. In general, most primary chondrosarcomas tend to be central and most secondary chondrosarcomas tend to be peripheral.

Several distinctive types of this tumor have been identified, each demonstrating characteristic clinical, radiographic, and histologic features.

CONVENTIONAL (MEDULLARY) CHONDROSARCOMA

Seen more commonly in adults, usually beyond the third decade of life, conventional chondrosarcoma affects men twice as often as women and is most often located in the pelvis and the long bones, particularly the femur and the humerus.[8, 36] It is a slow-growing tumor, and only in exceptional cases does it metastasize to distant organs.[116] Pathologic fractures through the tumor are rare.[21]

Radiographically, the lesion is characterized by expansion of the medullary portion of the bone, thickening of the cortex, and endosteal scalloping, as well as annular, punctate, or comma-shaped calcifications (Fig. 2–16*A*); occasionally, a soft tissue mass is present. The standard radiographic examination usually suffices to make a diagnosis, but CT and MRI may be helpful in delineating intraosseous extension of the lesion[109] and the extent of the soft tissue mass (Fig. 2–16*B, C*). In exceptional cases, the tumor can be indistinguishable from an enchondroma, particularly in the early stage.[58] For this reason, all central cartilaginous tumors in long bones, particularly in adult patients, should be regarded as malignant until proved to be benign.[111]

Histologically, chondrosarcoma is typified by the formation of cartilage by tumor cells.[129] Its more cellular and pleomorphic appearance and appreciable numbers of plump cells, with large or double nuclei, distinguish it from enchondroma (Fig. 2–16*D*). Mitotic cells are infrequent.[58]

Chondrosarcomas range in behavior from slow-growing, relatively benign lesions to highly malignant, metastasizing tumors. The histologic grade of these tumors is well correlated with their biologic behavior.[47, 116] The histologic distinction among low-grade, intermediate, and high-grade lesions is based on the cellularity of the tumor tissue, the degree of pleomorphism of the cells and nuclei, and the number of mitoses present.[47, 87] Microscopically, a well-differentiated (i.e., low-grade) chondrosarcoma differs only slightly from an enchondroma. The intercellular cartilage matrix is abundant in each, but the malignant tumor is more cellular, and the tumor cells are larger and more variable in appearance than those of a benign tumor. Cell nuclei, too, instead of being small and dark staining, are larger and have a more dispersed pattern of chromatin (Fig. 2–16*E*). Bizarre cells with pleomorphic nuclei are clear evidence of malignancy, but these may not always be present. A more subtle indication, according to some authorities, is the presence of appreciable numbers of binucleated cells.[71, 87] Mitoses are not always found in low-grade chondrosarcomas. Many of these tumors exhibit histologic evidence of malignancy in only part of the lesion; therefore, many sections may need to be examined before an unequivocal diagnosis can be made.

In both gross and microscopic appearance, high-grade chondrosarcomas resemble normal cartilage less closely than low-grade tumors do. Cellular and nuclear types of pleomorphism are more pronounced, and mitotic cells may be numerous. Intercellular cartilage matrix may be less abundant, and the tumor cells, which are not necessarily enclosed in lacunae, may be spindle shaped rather than rounded. The tissue of more malignant chondrosarcomas may show frank hypervascularity, a factor distinguishing them from an enchondroma or a low-grade malignancy.

Foci of calcification are frequently present in chondrosarcomas, and these may provide a reliable radiologic indication of the diagnosis. The areas of calcification may undergo replacement by endochondral bone, appearing radiographically as ringlike opacities, particularly in well-differentiated, slow-growing tumors.

Unlike benign cartilaginous tumors, chondrosarcomas show an invasive pattern of growth. The lesion's extension into the marrow spaces of cancellous bone and the vascular canals of cortical bone, whether it is apparent grossly or histologically, is an important diagnostic feature of chondrosarcoma (Fig. 2–16*F*). It may indicate the diagnosis when a limited sample of tissue fails to show definite cytologic evidence of malignancy.

CLEAR CELL CHONDROSARCOMA

This tumor, first described as a specific entity in 1976,[139] is a highly uncommon sarcoma, constituting less than 4% of all chondrosarcomas in the Mayo Clinic series.[27] Clear cell chondrosarcoma occurs twice as often in men as in women, usually in the third to fifth decades. The lesion often involves the proximal end of the humerus or the femur. It is considered a low-grade malignancy, and its clinical behavior is usually less aggressive than that of conventional chondrosarcoma.[78]

Radiologically, it presents most commonly as a lytic lesion with a sclerotic border; it may resemble a chondroblastoma (Fig. 2–17*A*).

Histologically, this clear cell variant exhibits larger and more rounded tumor cells than other chondrosarcomas, with fairly bland nuclei and clear or vacuolated cytoplasm, bearing a resemblance to chondroblasts (Fig. 2–17*B*). The clarity of the cells has been attributed to abundant intracellular glycogen and a paucity of cellular organelles and matrix.[6] A chondroid and osseous matrix is present, and trabeculae of reactive bone and the presence of numerous osteoclast-like giant cells are distinctive features of this tumor.[6, 12] These areas may contain foci of calcification, which are sufficiently pronounced to be apparent radiologically.

The histologic differential diagnosis includes metastatic epithelial neoplasms of clear cell type such as renal adenocarcinoma; however, the true diagnosis can usually be established by the finding of tumor cartilage and poor vascularity, both features of true chondrosarcoma. Clear cell chondrosarcomas are generally of low-grade malignancy, although metastatic lesions have been reported.[12]

MESENCHYMAL CHONDROSARCOMA

Mesenchymal chondrosarcoma is a rare lesion, representing less than 1% of all malignant bone tumors. It commonly occurs in the second and third decades of life. Its radiographic appearance is usually indistinguishable from that of a conventional chondrosarcoma; however, at times, this tumor may additionally exhibit a characteristic permeative growth pattern similar to that of round cell tumors (Fig. 2–18 *A*).

Histologically, mesenchymal chondrosarcoma is a highly malignant tumor, typified by the presence of areas of more or less differentiated cartilage, together with highly vascu-

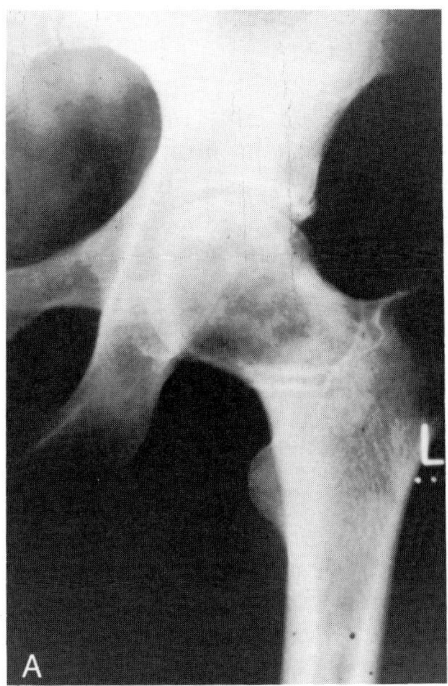

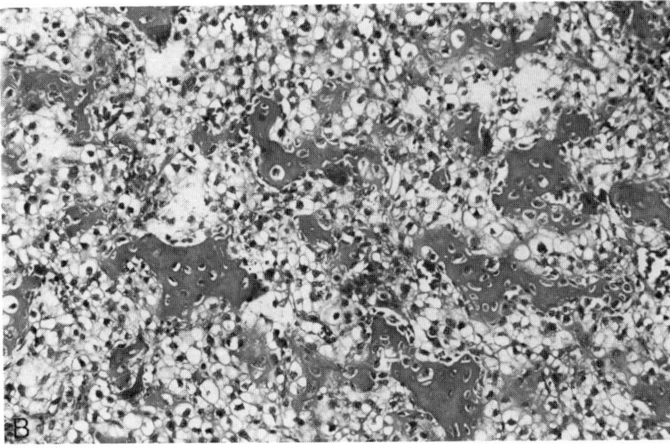

FIGURE 2–17. Clear cell chondrosarcoma. *A*, Radiolucent lesion with sclerotic border situated in the femoral head. Note the resemblance to chondroblastoma. (From Lewis MM, Sissons HA, Norman A, Greenspan A: Benign and malignant cartilage tumors. *In* Instructional Course Lectures, Vol 36. Chicago, American Academy of Orthopaedic Surgeons, 1987.) *B*, Hypovascular clear cell stroma with metaplastic bone. A few multinucleated giant cells are present (×125).

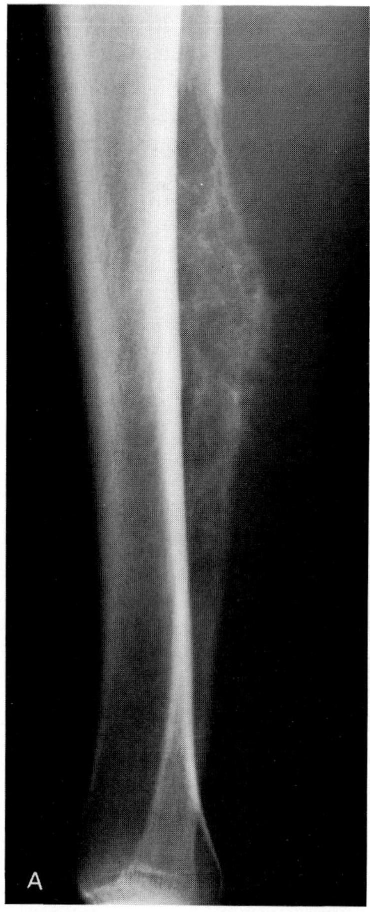

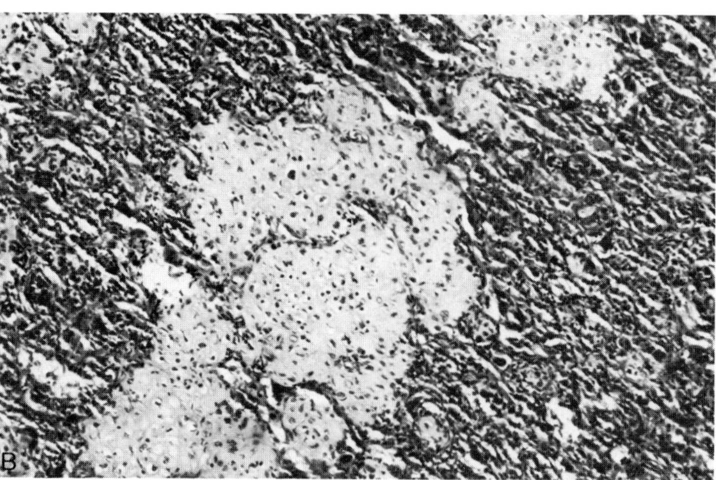

FIGURE 2–18. Mesenchymal chondrosarcoma. *A*, Highly destructive lesion in the middle portion of the fibula is associated with a large soft tissue mass. The cortex has been destroyed, and there are scattered, punctate calcifications in the medullary portion of the lesion. (From Lewis MM, Sissons HA, Norman A, Greenspan A: Benign and malignant cartilage tumors. *In* Instructional Course Lectures, Vol 36. Chicago, American Academy of Orthopaedic Surgeons, 1987.) *B*, Islands of hyaline cartilage with low-grade malignancy in a background of small round and spindle cells ($\times 100$).

lar spindle cell or round cell mesenchymal tissue.[31, 59] The microscopic appearances of these two components are strikingly different (Fig. 2–18*B*). When recognizable cartilage tissue is absent, the cellular mesenchymal component may be mistaken for Ewing's sarcoma or a malignant vascular tumor (hemangiopericytoma). The tumor has a high propensity for distant metastases but at unpredictable time intervals.[11]

PERIOSTEAL (JUXTACORTICAL) CHONDROSARCOMA

Although the great majority of primary chondrosarcomas are centrally located, in rare instances a tumor may arise in a periosteal (juxtacortical) location. These tumors have the same general radiologic and pathologic features as conventional (medullary) chondrosarcomas.[120] They may be confused radiographically with rare periosteal osteosarcoma, which also occurs on the external surface of long bones and consists largely of cartilage.[10]

DEDIFFERENTIATED CHONDROSARCOMA

The most malignant of all chondrosarcomas, the dedifferentiated variant, resembles conventional chondrosarcoma in its age group predilection and anatomic location. The patient typically has pain of long duration, followed by more recent onset of rapid swelling and local tenderness. The prolonged pain probably reflects a slow-growing lesion, and the swelling and tenderness may be related to the development of a rapidly growing, more malignant component. The tumor is associated with a poor prognosis, and the majority of patients die as a result of the disease within 2 years of diagnosis.

The radiographic presentation of dedifferentiated chondrosarcoma is variable.[38] It exhibits features of a conventional chondrosarcoma, as well as other characteristics such as an aggressive type of bone destruction and extension of the lesion into the soft tissues, producing a large mass (Fig. 2–19*A*). Focal calcifications in the tumor identify its cartilaginous nature. The hallmark of this lesion is the

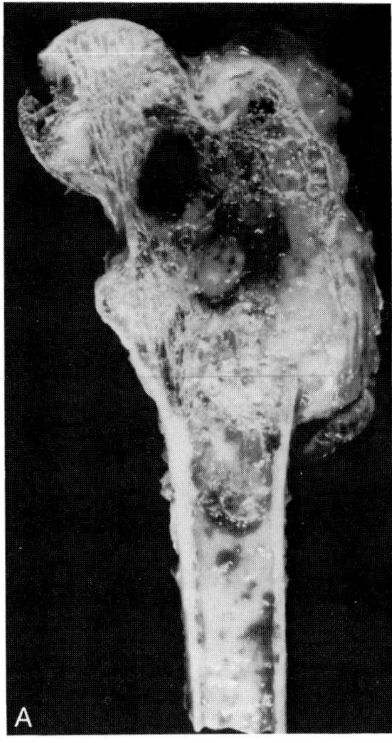

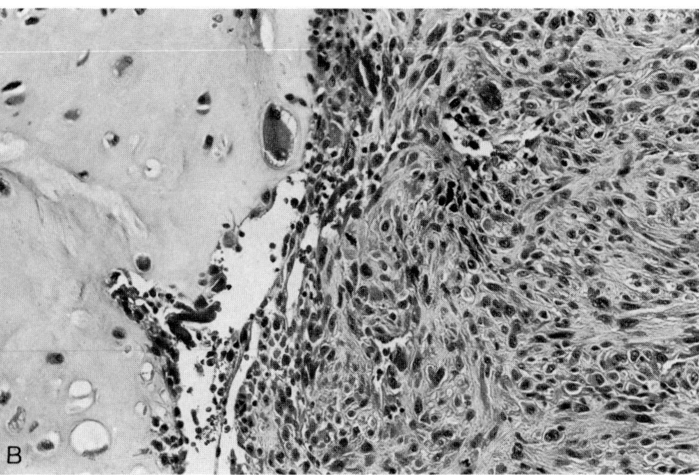

FIGURE 2–19. Dedifferentiated chondrosarcoma. *A*, Cartilaginous tumor with a fleshy component, producing a large soft tissue mass. The distal part of the lesion shows typical annular calcifications and scalloping of the endocortex, a less aggressive feature of cartilaginous tumor. *B*, The mixture of fleshy and cartilaginous tissues shows a high-grade spindle cell tumor and low-grade hyaline cartilage ($\times 158$).

appearance of an aggressive sarcoma engrafted on a benign-appearing chondrosarcoma.[29] The large size of the soft tissue mass and the presence of metastases are also helpful signs in the diagnosis.

Histologically, dedifferentiated chondrosarcoma often exhibits a cartilaginous component of low-grade malignancy combined with a highly cellular, sarcomatous tissue (Fig. 2–19*B*). Believed to develop from the cartilage by a process of dedifferentiation, this tissue may have the appearance of fibrosarcoma, osteosarcoma, or, as has more recently been reported, malignant fibrous histiocytoma.[29, 95, 117] The histologic diagnosis depends on the identification of two or more types of tissue, which are often distinct from one another.

Recently, the validity of the term dedifferentiation has been challenged. Studies using electron microscopy and immunohistochemistry support the concept that sarcomatous dedifferentiation in fact represents the synchronous differentiation of separate clones of cells from a primitive spindle cell sarcoma to various types of sarcoma.[50, 133]

SECONDARY CHONDROSARCOMA

The term secondary chondrosarcoma applies to any tumor arising as a result of malignant degeneration of a benign cartilaginous lesion, such as an osteochondroma or enchondroma. The incidence of malignant change in solitary lesions is very low, but it is greater in enchondromatosis and multiple osteochondromatosis. As many as 10% of cases of multiple osteocartilaginous exostoses have been reported to develop chondrosarcoma. Secondary chondrosarcomas develop at a somewhat earlier age than primary tumors do. They are usually of low-grade malignancy and follow a relatively benign course; they have a favorable prognosis. The features suggesting malignant transformation in enchondromatosis and multiple osteochondromatosis were discussed above.

Fibrous and Fibro-osseous Lesions

BENIGN FORMS

Fibrous Cortical Defect and Nonossifying Fibroma

Fibrous cortical defect and nonossifying fibroma are the most common fibrous lesions. Seen predominantly in childhood and adolescence and more commonly (2:1) in boys, they have a predilection for the long bones, particularly the femur and the tibia. *Fibrous cortical defect* (metaphyseal fibrous defect) is a small, asymptomatic lesion, found in 30% of the

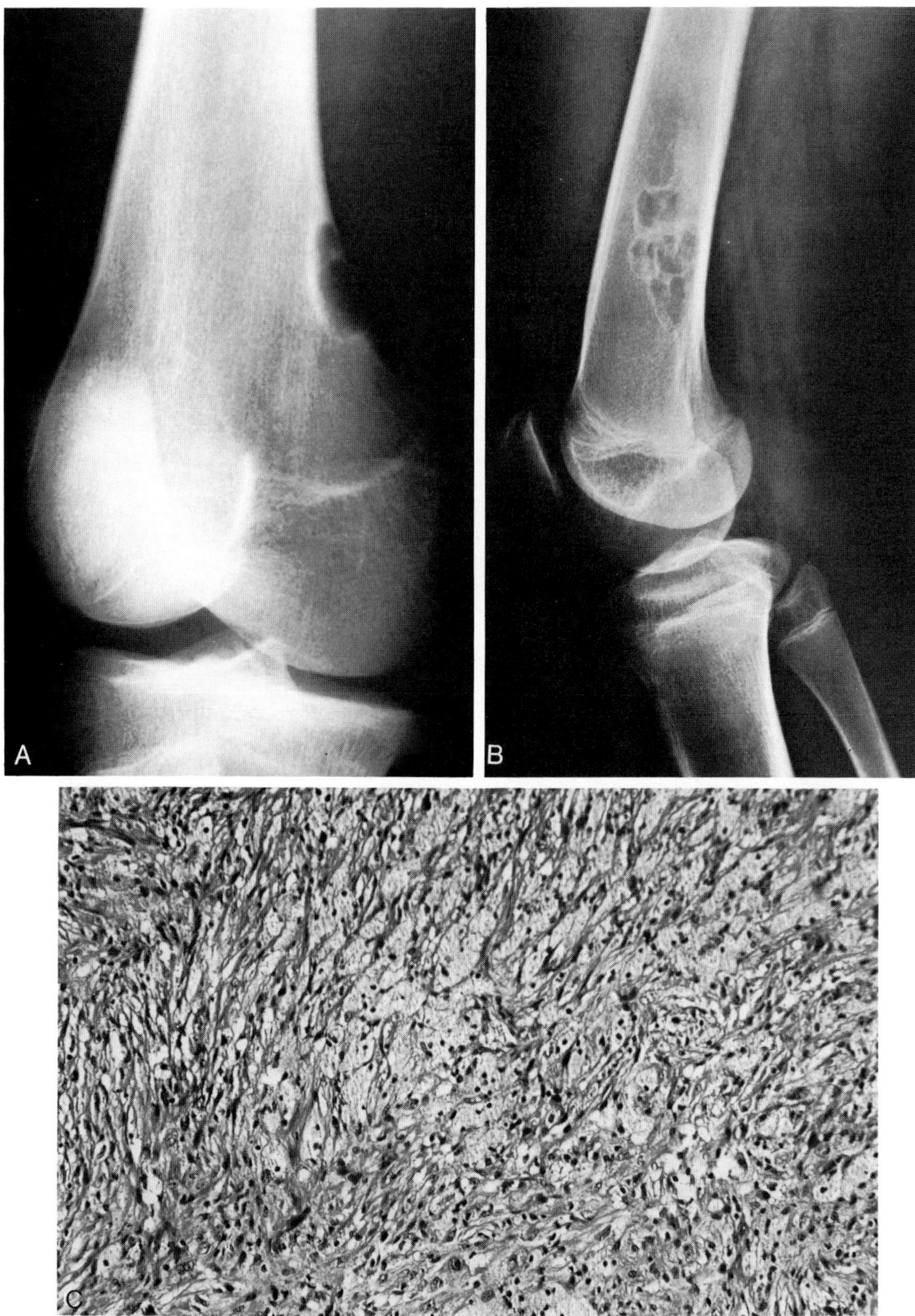

FIGURE 2–20. Fibrous cortical defect and nonossifying fibroma. *A,* Fibrous cortical defect. Radiolucent lesion in the medial metaphysis of the distal femur is demarcated by a thin zone of sclerosis. *B,* Nonossifying fibroma. Eccentrically located radiolucent lesion encroaches the medullary cavity of the distal femoral diaphysis and displays a scalloped, sclerotic border. (From Greenspan A: Orthopedic Radiology. Philadelphia, JB Lippincott, 1988.) *C,* Nonossifying fibroma. Foamy histiocytes admixed with spindle-shaped fibroblasts (×125).

normal population in the first and second decades of life. The term *nonossifying fibroma* is applied to this lesion if it enlarges and encroaches on the medullary portion of the bone.

Radiologically, the lesion is an elliptic, radiolucent defect confined to the cortex of a long bone near the growth plate and demarcated by a thin margin of sclerosis (Fig. 2–20*A*). Most foci undergo spontaneous involution (healing) by the remodeling process exhibited in osteosclerosis. A few lesions may continue to grow; and as they encroach on the medullary cavity, they characteristically display a scalloped, sclerotic border and are located eccentrically within the bone (Fig. 2–20*B*). Most such lesions are asymptomatic, but larger ones may undergo pathologic fracture.

Histologically identical regardless of size, fibrous cortical defect and nonossifying fibroma are composed of rather bland spindle cells admixed with histiocytic cells often having a clear, foamy cytoplasm. Usually, osteoclast-like multinucleated giant cells are present and, when numerous, may lead to confusion of the lesion with giant cell tumor of bone.[67] Typically, varying numbers of inflammatory cells, especially lymphocytes, and a few plasma cells are scattered in the background. The amount of collagen production may vary. No bone or cartilage formation should be present, unless a fracture or previous surgical disruption of the lesion has occurred. The cells are often arranged in a swirling storiform pattern typical of fibrohistiocytic lesions, but a fascicular arrangement may also be seen (Fig. 2–20*C*). A storiform architecture in a hypercellular lesion can lead to confusion with malignant fibrous histiocytoma, if the pathologist is unfamiliar with the clinicopathologic spectrum of fibrous cortical defect and nonossifying fibroma.

Benign Fibrous Histiocytoma

The term benign fibrous histiocytoma may be controversial,[146] but it provides a useful organizational term to subclassify lesions having similar histologic features to nonossifying fibroma but atypical clinical or radiographic patterns. The lesion, which is often symptomatic, is usually diagnosed in older patients. Radiographically, it may appear to be more aggressive than nonossifying fibroma (Fig. 2–21 *A*). The lesion is usually histologically quite similar to nonossifying fibroma (Fig. 2–21*B*); the background, however, may contain larger numbers of the histiocytic cells and Touton-type giant cells seen in xanthomatous tissue reactions.[24] Although frankly malignant histologic criteria are absent, mitotic activity may be in evidence.

Periosteal Desmoid

Periosteal desmoid is a tumor-like fibrous proliferation of the periosteum, which has a striking predilection for the posteromedial cortex of the medial femoral condyle.[7] It usually occurs between the ages of 12 and 20 years, and most lesions spontaneously disappear by the end of the second decade. Although many patients have a history of injury, trauma does not necessarily predispose to the development of this lesion. The radiographic features of periosteal desmoid are similar to those of fibrous cortical defect, except for the specificity of its location. Its hallmarks are a saucer-like radiolucent defect with sclerosis at its base; it may erode the cortex and appear as a cortical irregularity (Fig. 2–22 *A*). Occasionally, it may simulate an aggressive or even a malignant tumor. The histopathologic appearance of the lesion demonstrates fibroblastic spindle cells with a large amount of collagen production[17] (Fig. 2–22*B*).

Fibrous Dysplasia

Classified as a developmental abnormality by some authorities, fibrous dysplasia is a fibro-osseous lesion that may affect one bone (monostotic form) or several bones (polyostotic form).[86]

MONOSTOTIC FIBROUS DYSPLASIA

Most commonly affecting the femur (with a predilection for the femoral neck), the tibia, and the ribs, the lesion of monostotic fibrous dysplasia arises centrally in the bone; it usually spares the epiphysis in children and the articular end of the bone in adults.

The radiographic appearance of the lesion depends on the proportion of osseous-to-fibrous content. A lesion with greater ossification appears more dense and sclerotic; a more fibrous lesion exhibits greater radiolucency with a characteristic ground-glass appearance (Fig. 2–23*A*). When the lesion enlarges, it expands the medullary cavity. The cortex may be attenuated and even remodeled about the lesion; however, it is rarely directly involved by the lesion. Pathologic fracture through the structurally weakened bone is the most frequent complication of this disorder.

Histologically, fibrous dysplasia consists of

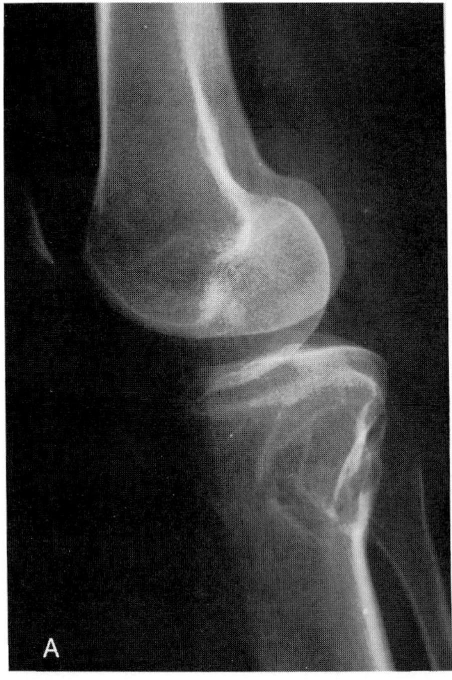

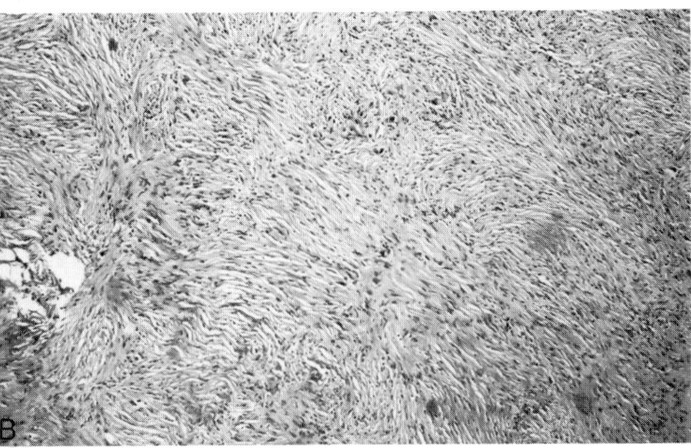

FIGURE 2–21. Benign fibrous histiocytoma. *A,* Radiolucent lesion with sharply defined, sclerotic borders in the posterior aspect of the proximal tibia has a radiographic appearance similar to that of a nonossifying fibroma. *B,* Spindle cells are arranged in a storiform pattern. These are occasional multinucleated giant cells (×63).

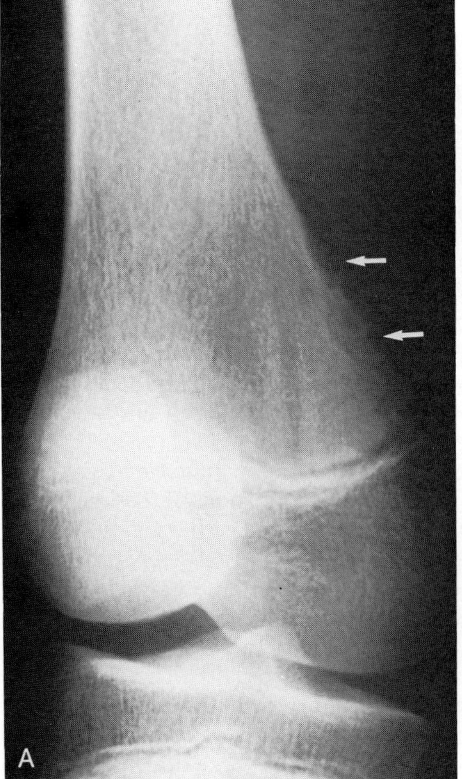

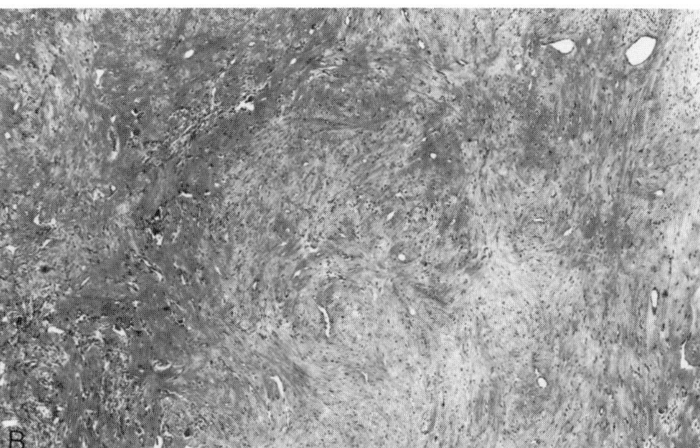

FIGURE 2–22. Periosteal desmoid. *A,* Radiolucent, saucer-like lesion resulted in a cortical irregularity at the medial aspect of the distal femoral metaphysis (arrows). *B,* Densely collagenized stroma and bland fibroblasts (×70).

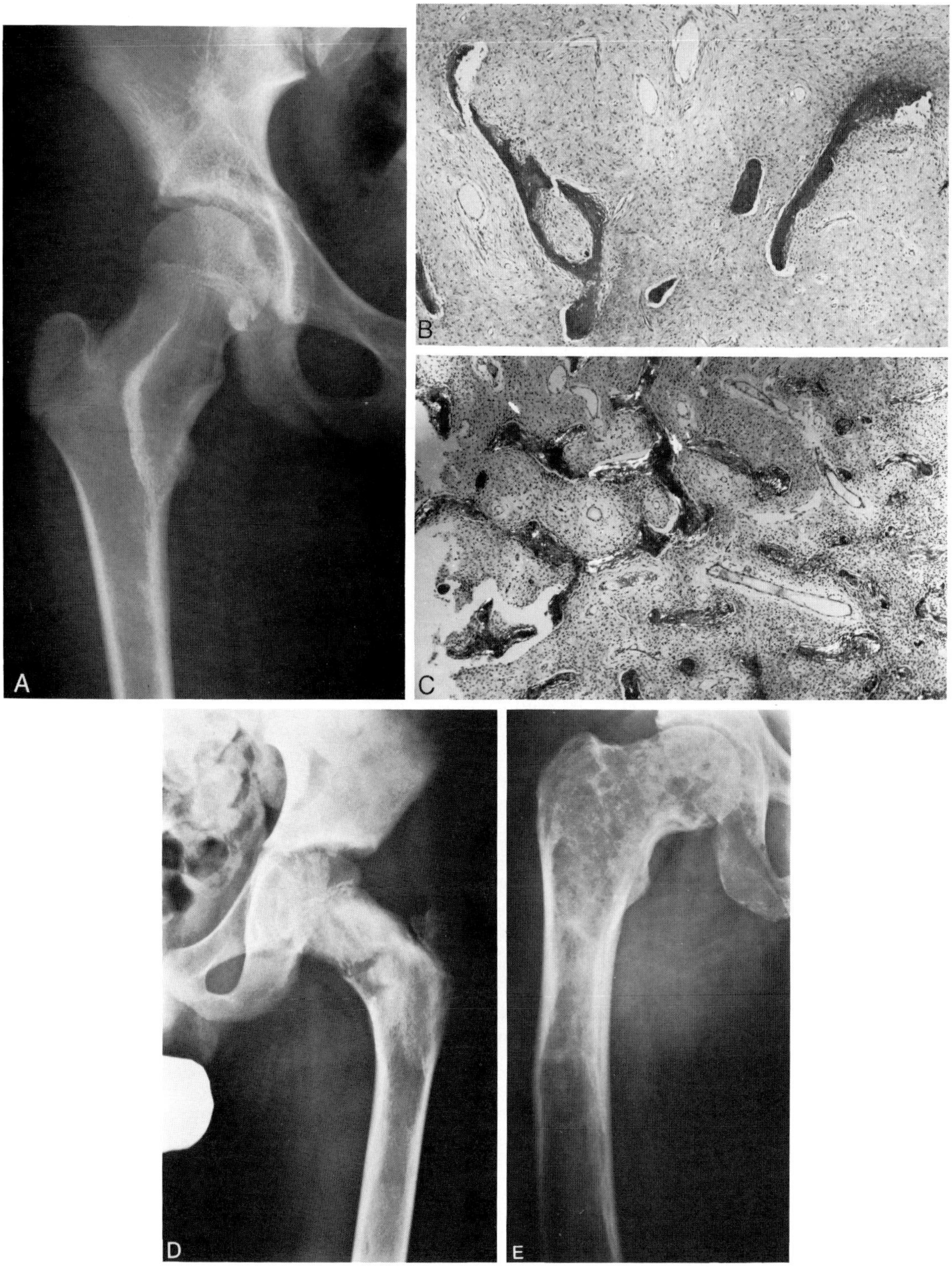

FIGURE 2–23. Fibrous dysplasia. *A,* Monostotic form. Radiolucent lesion in the femoral neck demonstrates sclerotic border and ground-glass appearance. (From Greenspan A: Orthopedic Radiology. Philadelphia, JB Lippincott, 1988.) *B,* Haphazard metaplastic trabeculae arranged in loose, fibrous stroma. Note the lack of osteoblastic activity ("naked trabeculae") (×50). *C,* Polarization of fibrous dysplasia reveals immature (woven) pattern in bone trabeculae (×50). *D,* Polyostotic fibrous dysplasia lesions involve the proximal femur and the acetabular portion of the ilium. Note that the proximal femoral epiphysis is not affected. (From Greenspan A: Orthopedic Radiology. Philadelphia, JB Lippincott, 1988.) *E,* Polyostotic type. Extensive involvement of the right femur resulted in the "shepherd's crook" deformity.

an aggregate of moderately dense fibrous connective tissue containing a haphazard distribution of bony trabeculae. Rather than being stress oriented, as in normal cancellous bone, these trabeculae tend to be curved and branching with sparse interconnections. Their low-power photomicrographic picture has been likened to Chinese characters or even alphabet soup. Under polarized light, the bony trabeculae are shown to be composed of woven, immature bone (Fig. 2–23*B, C*). Although they contain osteocytes, they exhibit no evidence of osteoblastic activity at any stage in their maturation ("naked trabeculae"); thus, the bone formed is viewed as metaplastic. The lesion of fibrous dysplasia may also contain areas of cartilage formation.

POLYOSTOTIC FIBROUS DYSPLASIA
Although radiographically similar to the monostotic form, polyostotic fibrous dysplasia often exhibits a somewhat more aggressive appearance. The lesions, moreover, are distributed differently in the skeleton, showing a striking predilection (more than 90% of cases) for one side of the body. They often involve the pelvis, followed in frequency by the long bones, the skull, and the ribs; the proximal end of the femur is a common site of occurrence. Generally, the lesions of polyostotic fibrous dysplasia progress in number and size until skeletal maturity is reached; they then become quiescent. Only 5% of lesions continue to enlarge.

Polyostotic fibrous dysplasia may also be associated with endocrine disturbances (premature sexual development, hyperparathyroidism, and other endocrinopathies) and skin pigmentation (café au lait spots), which together constitute the disorder called Albright-McCune syndrome.[4] This condition almost exclusively affects females, who exhibit true sexual precocity resulting from accelerated gonadotropin release by the anterior lobe of the pituitary. Typically, the café au lait spots of Albright-McCune syndrome show irregular, ragged ("coast of Maine") borders, in contrast to the smoothly marginated ("coast of California") café au lait markings seen in neurofibromatosis.

The characteristic radiographic changes of polyostotic fibrous dysplasia may occur in any portion of the long bones and involvement of the bone by the lesion may be limited or extensive. Moreover, as in the monostotic form, the articular ends of bones are usually unaffected. This latter phenomenon has given rise to speculation that a defect of the primary ossification center may lead to impairment of the production and maintenance of mature cancellous bone. The cortex, as in the solitary form, is usually intact but often thinned because of the expansile nature of the lesion. The borders of the lesion are well defined and the inner cortical margins may show scalloping. The variable amount of bone in the fibrous tissue that replaces the cancellous bone imparts a radiographic picture ranging from lucency to increased density (Fig. 2–23*D*). More fibrous lesions exhibit greater lucency, occasionally with a loss of the trabecular pattern and a ground-glass, milky, or smoky appearance. Massive formation of cartilage may be observed in the lesion, accompanied by secondary calcification and ossification patterns that can easily be confused radiographically with cartilaginous neoplasm. Radionuclide bone scan is the quickest method of determining the distribution of lesions in the skeleton. This examination may disclose unsuspected sites of involvement.

The most common complication of polyostotic fibrous dysplasia is pathologic fracture, which, occurring in the femoral neck, frequently leads to a "shepherd's crook" deformity (Fig. 2–23*E*). Occasionally, accelerated growth of a bone or hypertrophy of a digit may be observed. The development of a sarcoma in fibrous dysplasia is extremely rare, but it may occur either spontaneously[150] or, more commonly, following radiation therapy.

Osteofibrous Dysplasia

Osteofibrous dysplasia (ossifying fibroma, Kempson-Campanacci lesion) is a rare lesion with a decided preference for the tibia.[75] With rare exception, it is situated in the proximal third or midsegment of the bone and is often localized to the anterior cortex.[20, 22] In more than 80% of patients, some degree of anterior bowing is observed clinically. This lesion is seen predominantly in childhood, but occasionally it may first be discovered in adolescence.

Radiographically, the Kempson-Campanacci lesion bears a striking similarity to nonossifying fibroma and fibrous dysplasia. It is a radiolucent lesion with lobulated, sclerotic margins, usually confined to the cortex (Fig. 2–24*A*). Larger lesions may destroy the cortical bone and invade the medullary cavity.

Osteofibrous dysplasia and fibrous dysplasia, as the similarity in their names might suggest,

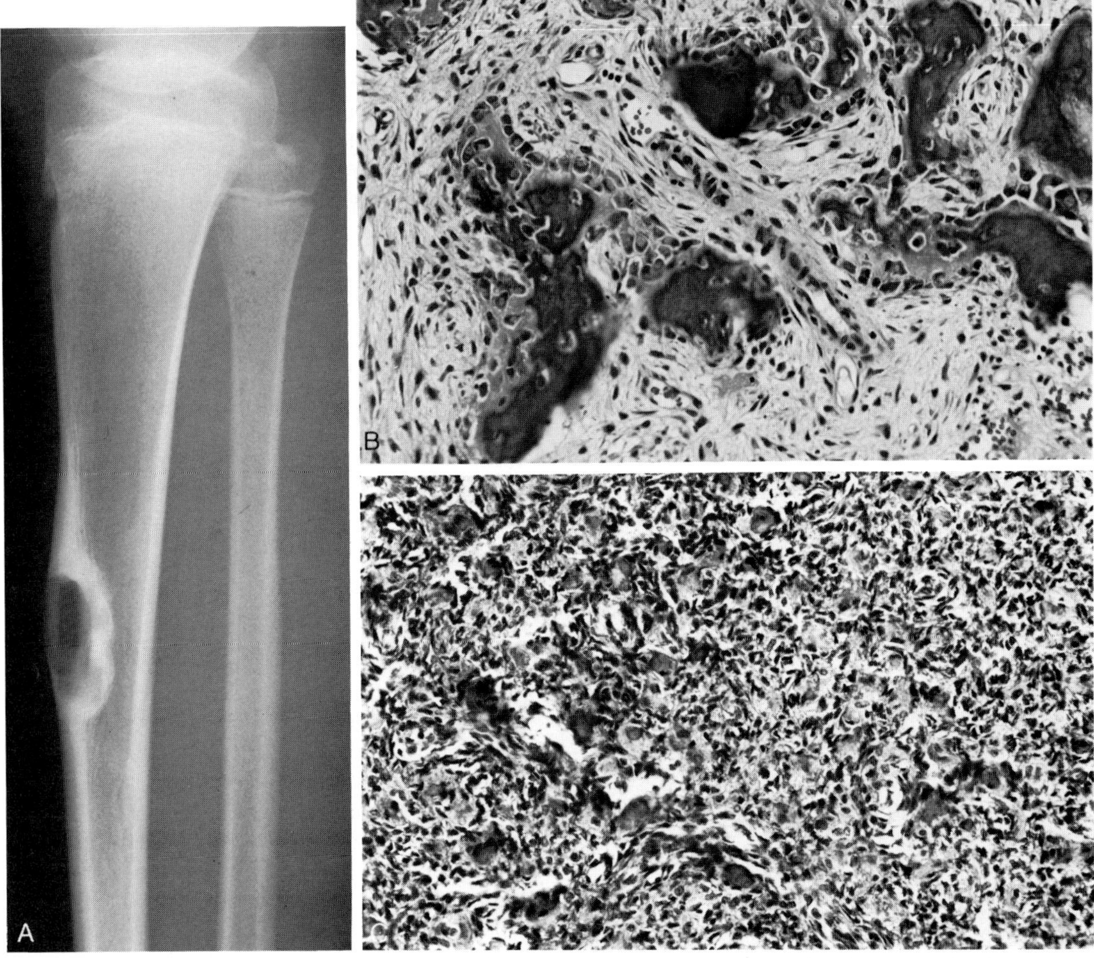

FIGURE 2–24. Osteofibrous dysplasia. *A,* A radiolucent lesion with sclerotic borders is present in the anterior aspect of the tibia. Note the similarity in radiographic appearance to that of a nonossifying fibroma. *B,* The bone trabeculae are rimmed by osteoblasts (×200). *C,* Ossifying fibroma. Section of type of lesion described by Sissons and colleagues[128] reveal plump spindle cells producing spherical bone fragments that resemble cementum (×200).

display a remarkable histopathologic similarity. Like fibrous dysplasia, osteofibrous dysplasia is composed of a fibrous background containing a rather haphazard arrangement of incomplete trabeculae. In osteofibrous dysplasia, however, these bony trabeculae often show appositional osteoblastic activity (Fig. 2–24*B*). Such activity, which may sometimes be seen at the earliest stages of bone development, is more often encountered surrounding larger trabeculae. Under polarized light, these trabeculae are seen to consist of an inner portion of woven bone surrounded by an outer zone of lamellar transformation. Because osteofibrous dysplasia and fibrous dysplasia exhibit nearly identical radiographic and histologic features, with the exception of the former lesion's predilection for the cortex of the tibia, it is possible that osteofibrous dysplasia represents a regional or localized presentation of fibrous dysplasia. The osteoblastic remodeling of trabeculae seen in osteofibrous dysplasia may represent a response to cortical stress trajectories rather than something inherent in the biologic character of the lesion itself.

Sissons and colleagues reported two cases of fibro-osseous lesions containing smaller aggregates of osseous material resembling cementum (Fig. 2–24*C*). They proposed the term *ossifying fibroma* for this lesion.[128] The term *osteofibrous dysplasia,* they suggested, should be reserved for the fibrous cortical lesions of the tibia and the fibula.

On occasion, osteofibrous dysplasia is

known to be a locally aggressive lesion. It frequently recurs after local excision and, according to some authors, may coexist with the malignant lesion adamantinoma.

Desmoplastic Fibroma

Desmoplastic fibroma is a rare tumor usually seen in individuals younger than 40 years; half of cases occur in the second decade of life.[27] There are no characteristic radiographic features of this tumor. The long bones and the pelvis are frequent sites of involvement. In the long bones, the lesion is diaphyseal, but it often extends into the metaphysis and may even extend into the articular end of the bone after closure of the growth plate. The epiphyses, however, are spared. Generally, it is an expansile, radiolucent lesion, usually with sharply defined borders (Fig. 2–25*A*). The cortex is thinned, but there is no significant periosteal response. Locally aggressive variants, which may simulate malignant bone tumors, are marked by bone destruction and invasion of the soft tissues.

Histologically, the lesion is composed of spindle-shaped and occasionally stellate fibroblasts associated with a densely collagenized matrix. It is variably cellular, but cells almost always constitute a smaller proportion of the lesion than does the collagenous matrix (Fig. 2–25*B*). For this reason, the biopsy specimen resembles scar tissue or a desmoid tumor of soft tissue. On purely histologic grounds, the lesion most resembles periosteal desmoid, but correlation with the radiographs clarifies its true nature. Moreover, a very cellular lesion may be confused with low-grade fibrosarcoma. In this case, the radiographs may be confusing, and the distinction can be made histologically on the basis of the quantity of collagen, the lack of nuclear atypia and hyperchromatism, and the paucity of mitotic activity.

MALIGNANT TYPES

Fibrosarcoma and Malignant Fibrous Histiocytoma

Fibrosarcoma and malignant fibrous histiocytoma are malignant fibrous tumors that have similar radiographic presentations and similar histologic features. Both usually occur in the third to sixth decades of life; their sites of predilection are the femur, the humerus, and the tibia.[65]

Radiographically, they are marked by an osteolytic area of destruction surrounded by a wide zone of transition. There is little or no reactive sclerosis and usually no periosteal reaction (Fig. 2–26 *A*). The lesions are often eccentrically located, close to or in the articular end of the bone. A soft tissue mass is frequently present.[49] They may resemble giant cell tumor of bone or telangiectatic osteosarcoma, and they may be mistaken for metastatic carcinoma because of the age group in which they usually occur. Some authorities believe that an almost pathognomonic sign of fibrosar-

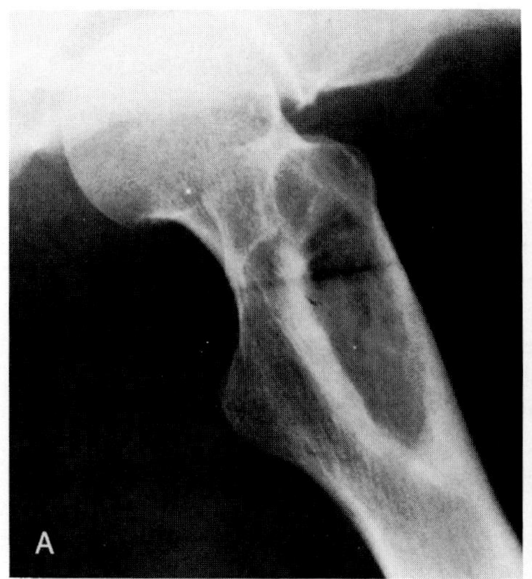

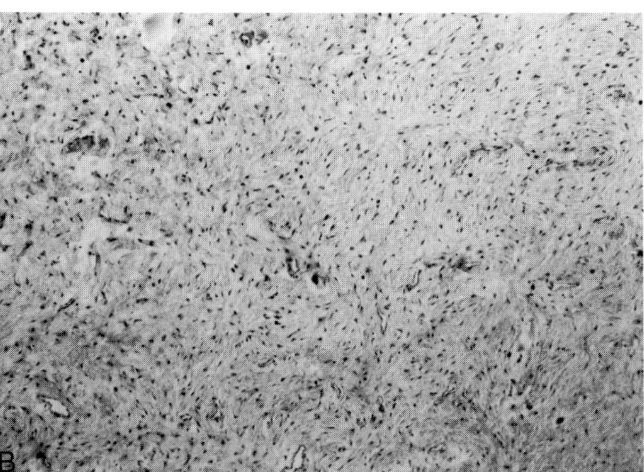

FIGURE 2–25. Desmoplastic fibroma. *A*, Osteolytic lesion with sparse central trabeculation and sclerotic rim is noted in the intertrochanteric region of the left femur. Note the thinning of the cortex but the lack of periosteal response. *B*, Moderately cellular fibroblastic stroma with extensive extracellular collagen (×70).

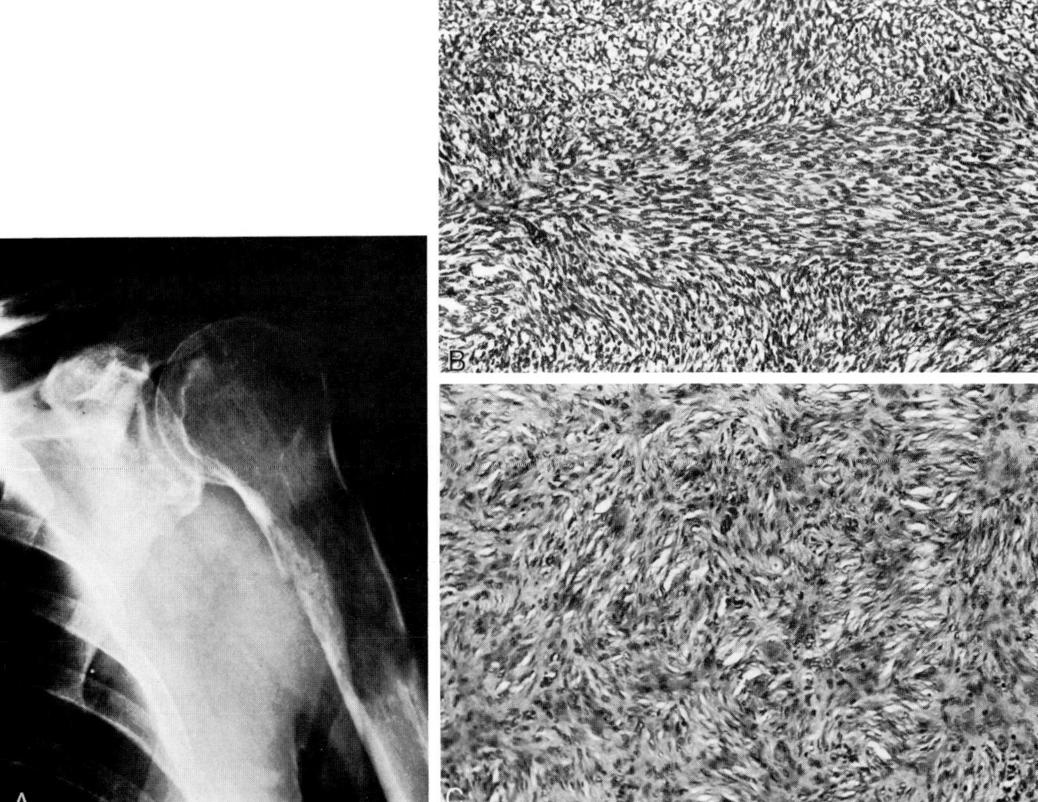

FIGURE 2–26. Fibrosarcoma and malignant fibrous histiocytoma. *A,* Fibrosarcoma. A destructive, purely osteolytic lesion in the proximal shaft of the left humerus with a pathologic fracture in a 62-year-old man. (From Greenspan A: Orthopedic Radiology. Philadelphia, JB Lippincott, 1988.) *B,* "Herringbone tweed" arrangement of malignant spindle cells in fibrosarcoma (×125). *C,* Malignant fibrous histiocytoma. Histologic section reveals malignant spindle cells arranged in a spiral nebular, or storiform, pattern (×200).

coma is its tendency to allow the preservation of small sequestrum-like fragments of cortical bone and spongy trabeculae, which may be demonstrated on conventional radiographs or CT examination.

Although both tumors are composed of sarcomatous spindle cells forming variable amounts of collagen, each tumor exhibits certain distinguishing features. The spindle-shaped cells of fibrosarcoma are largely arranged in long fascicles. These fascicles may run at right angles to one another, so that any plane of section shows some bundles of tumor cells running transversely and others running longitudinally. In some areas of sectioning, all bundles may be seen longitudinally, forming a "herringbone tweed" pattern in their spatial relationship to each other[33] (Fig. 2–26*B*). The spindle cells have hyperchromatic nuclei with an increased nucleus-to-cytoplasm ratio. Mitotic activity, including bizarre mitoses, may be present. Collagen production is usually evident in parts of the neoplasm, but it tends to be sparse in comparison with that of the benign fibroblastic tumors. It is important that there be no evidence of osteoblastic activity, a feature distinguishing fibrosarcoma from fibroblastic variants of osteosarcoma.

In contrast to the long fascicles of tumor cells in fibrosarcoma, the spindle cells of malignant fibrous histiocytoma tend to be arranged in sweeping, curved fascicles and expanding nodules. Their histologic appearance has been compared to pinwheels, spiral nebulae, or cut, matted straw (storiform pattern)[37] (Fig. 2–26*C*). Thought to be histiocytes acting as "facultative" fibroblasts, the cells of this tumor accordingly tend to show more pleomorphism than the simple fibroblasts of fibrosarcoma. Support for a histiocytic origin of this tumor may also be seen in phagocytic activity by occasional tumor cells and the usual presence of multinucleated giant cells, sometimes in large numbers. Predominantly spindle shaped, the tumor cells may also be round or polyhedral. In addition to the usual hyperchromatic nuclei, vesicular nuclei (as found in histiocytes) may be identified. Areas of necrosis are a frequent finding, and it is not unusual to observe a background with scattered chronic inflammatory cells. Occasionally, extracellular collagen production resembling osteoid may be found in malignant fibrous histiocytoma of bone, which may lead to diagnostic confusion. In such cases, experience is necessary to make the differentiation from true osteosarcomas.[146] Immunohistochemical studies have been helpful in the diagnosis of malignant fibrous histiocytoma by the demonstration of certain nonspecific markers of histiocytic enzymes (lysozyme, alpha$_1$-antitrypsin) in the tumor. On the other hand, studies of direct immunologic markers for monocyte-macrophage lineage yielded somewhat mixed results.[131, 149] The problem with many immunologic studies is that they have been performed on malignant fibrous histiocytomas of soft tissue; such tumors have not been subjected to the cellular alterations inherent in decalcification.

Both fibrosarcoma and malignant fibrous histiocytoma may complicate benign conditions such as fibrous dysplasia, Paget's disease, bone infarction, and chronic draining sinuses of osteomyelitis.[40] They may also arise in bones that were previously irradiated. The 5-year survival rates vary in different studies from 37 to 67%.

Tumors and Tumor-like Lesions of Hematopoietic, Reticuloendothelial, and Vascular Origin

Giant Cell Tumor

Giant cell tumor is a locally aggressive neoplasm characterized by proliferating mononuclear stromal cells containing numerous osteoclast-like multinucleated giant cells randomly but evenly distributed throughout.[27, 71] This tumor is seen almost exclusively after skeletal maturity, when the growth plates are obliterated, and affected patients are usually between ages 20 and 40 years. There is a female preponderance (2:1). At least 60% of cases occur in long bones, and nearly all extend to the articular end. The commonest skeletal sites are the distal femur, the proximal tibia, the distal radius, the proximal humerus, and the sacrum. The characteristic radiographic features are those of a purely destructive, radiolucent lesion without marginal sclerosis. There is usually no periosteal reaction (Fig. 2–27*A*). A soft tissue mass may be present, and in this respect, CT or MRI examination may be helpful. Although 5 to 10% of giant cell tumors undergo malignant degeneration, malignant giant cell tumor does not have any additional radiologic characteristics and therefore cannot be diagnosed radiographically. Recurrences after surgical curettage and bone grafting are often encountered. These may be recognized radiographically by resorption of the graft material and the reappearance of radiolucent areas similar to the original tumor.

The histologic features consist of a related dual population of mononuclear stromal cells and multinucleated giant cells (Fig. 2–27*B*). Morphologically, the giant cells bear some resemblance to osteoclasts and they display increased acid phosphatase activity. However, unlike the true osteoclasts, they are not apposed to trabecular surfaces and they do not possess a ruffled border. They never show mitotic activity; hence, the occasionally used term osteoclastoma for giant cell tumor is probably inappropriate. Because mitotic activity can be seen with regularity in the mononuclear stromal cells and the nuclei of the giant cells may resemble those of the stromal cells, it was thought for a long time that the giant cells represent a fusion product of the stromal cells. Studies by Burmester and colleagues and Ling and associates confirmed the monocytic nature of the stromal cells and the probable derivation of the giant cells from these mononuclear cells.[19, 90] The background of the tumor contains varying amounts of collagen. Bone or osteoid formation is seen where there has been a pathologic fracture or previous curettage or, occasionally, surrounding a focus of recurrent tumor in the soft tissue.

Although giant cell tumor is generally a benign lesion, malignant transformation may occur, either spontaneously or after radiation therapy. To diagnose malignant giant cell tumor, there must be either a frankly sarcomatous change occurring in the lesion or, alternatively, a sarcoma arising in the previous site of a treated giant cell tumor.[36] Histologic grading of giant cell tumors in an attempt to predict local recurrence has generally met with little success. Moreover, there are instances in which completely benign-appearing giant cell

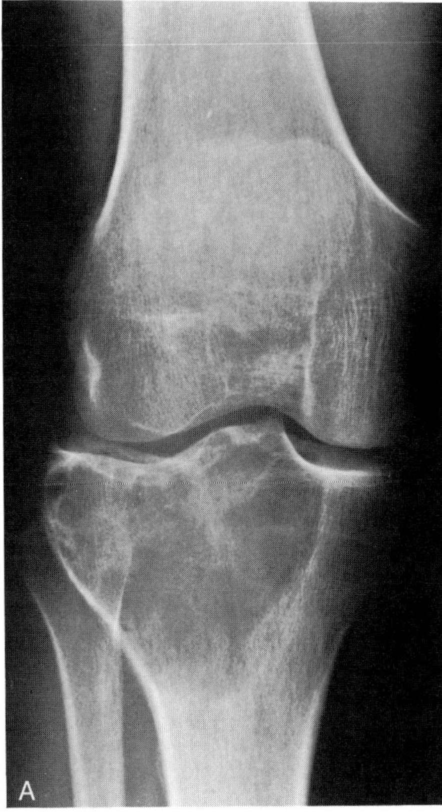

FIGURE 2–27. Giant cell tumor. *A,* A purely osteolytic lesion involves the articular end of the proximal tibia in a 30-year-old woman. (From Greenspan A: Orthopedic Radiology. Philadelphia, JB Lippincott, 1988.) *B,* Low-power micrograph demonstrates random and even distribution of multinucleated giant cells in a mononuclear stromal tumor (×20).

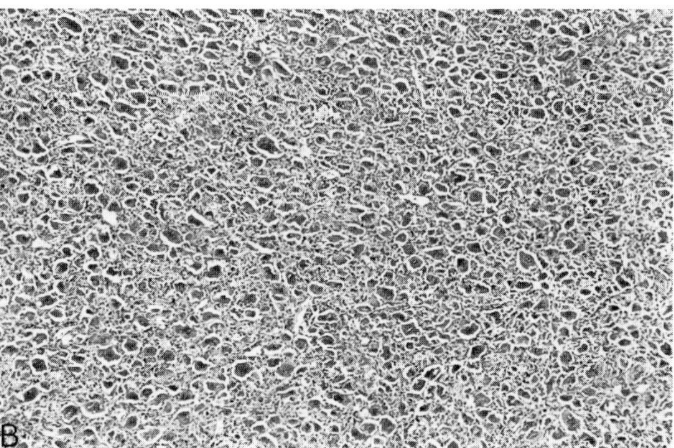

tumors have been followed, some months or years later, by distant metastases in the lungs, having the histologic characteristics of classic giant cell tumor.[36, 113]

Hemangioma, Hemangioendothelioma, and Angiosarcoma

These lesions constitute a spectrum of pathologic entities ranging from benign neoplasms (some of which may, in fact, represent congenital vascular malformations) to highly malignant tumors that metastasize widely and have low survival rates.[36] The malignant and locally aggressive varieties are quite uncommon.

Hemangioma is a benign lesion composed of blood vessels. Although its name suggests a neoplastic nature, the behavior of this lesion is that of a vascular malformation. Depending on its vascular composition, a hemangioma is subdivided into capillary, cavernous, venous, and mixed types. Women are affected twice as often as men. The incidence of discovery of these lesions increases with age, and most patients present after their fourth decade. The commonest sites are the spine (particularly the thoracic segment) and the skull; hemangiomas of the long and short tubular bones are less frequently encountered. In the spine, the lesion typically involves the vertebral body, although it may extend into the lamina and rarely into the spinous process. On occasion, multiple vertebrae may be affected. The majority of hemangiomas of the vertebral column are asymptomatic and are discovered incidentally. Symptoms occur when the affected vertebra expands in the direction of the spinal cord, causing compression. This neurologic complication is more commonly associated with lesions in the midthoracic spine. Another mechanism considered responsible for compression of the cord, although less frequently, is fracture of the involved vertebral body and the formation of a soft tissue mass or hematoma. On a plain roentgenogram, a hemangioma is characterized by the presence of coarse, vertical striations. This pattern in the vertebral body is referred to as honeycombing or corduroy cloth appearance (Fig. 2–28*A*) and is considered virtually pathognomonic of hemangioma.[80] On CT scan, it has the characteristic appearance of multiple dots, representing a cross section of reinforced trabeculae (Fig. 2–28*B*).

Histologically, most hemangiomas consist of simple endothelium-lined channels, morphologically identical with capillary endothelium

(Fig. 2–28*C*). Some or all of the vascular channels may be enlarged and have a sinusoidal appearance, in which case the lesion is referred to as cavernous type. Lesions in which the endothelium occurs as solid aggregates or in which the endothelial cells are plump and atypical are infrequent. If these areas predominate in a vascular tumor, the lesion is referred to as *hemangioendothelioma* (Fig. 2–28*D*). Hemangioendotheliomas are thought to be true neoplasms rather than malformations, because nuclear atypia is frequently seen, accompanied by occasional mitotic activity, and recurrence after inadequate local excision is not uncommon. It is also usual to find moderate to large numbers of eosinophilic leukocytes within these tumors. In general, such lesions behave in a benign fashion; however, there is always a small element of unpredictability in their outcome. Synonyms used for hemangioendothelioma, most notably hemangioendothelial sarcoma and low-grade angiosarcoma, reflect the uncertainty of pathologists in predicting their biologic behavior. Factors related to their grading include mitotic rate, degree of atypia, presence of necrosis, and the morphologic features of their vascular spaces. They may occur in any part of a bone, and it is not unusual to see multiple lesions in contiguous anatomic sites (i.e., in several carpal or tarsal bones) displaying a benign course. Hemangioendotheliomas are usually tumors of the mature skeleton, and there is no sex predilection. Radiographically, they are osteolytic and may either be well circumscribed or have a wide zone of transition. Unless a fracture is present, a soft tissue mass is unusual. That the cells composing these tumors are differentiated may be seen by their frequent positivity in immunohistochemical stains for Factor VIII and for the plant lectin *Ulex europaeus*.

Angiosarcomas of bone represent the most malignant end of the spectrum of vascular tumors. They have similar radiographic features to hemangioendotheliomas, except that they are usually single, almost invariably have a wide zone of transition, and frequently demonstrate a soft tissue mass. Histologically, they are composed of poorly formed blood vessels showing complicated infolding and irregular anastomoses. The endothelial cells lining these blood vessels display features of frank malignancy, including frequent and atypical mitoses, nuclear hyperchromatism, and the presence of often plump, interluminal cells resembling hobnails (Fig. 2–28*E*). Solid areas of the tumor may contain spindle cells and epithelioid cells. Spontaneous necrosis is frequently present. Staining for Factor VIII and *Ulex europaeus* has inconsistent and sometimes negative results, reflecting poor tumor differentiation. Metastasis to the lungs and other parenchymal organs is a frequent outcome.

Eosinophilic Granuloma

This is a tumor-like condition belonging to a group of disorders known as reticuloendothe-

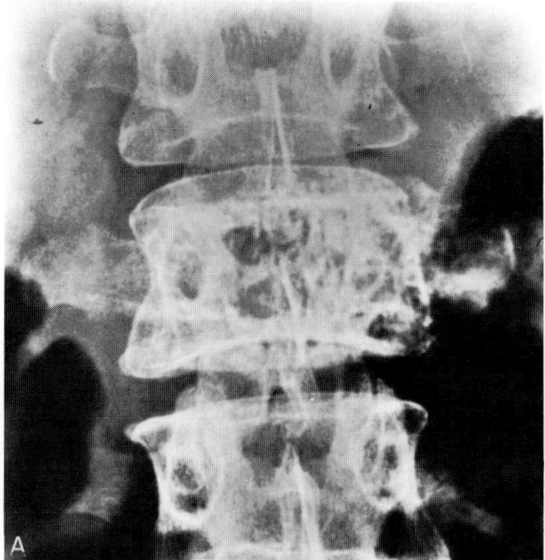

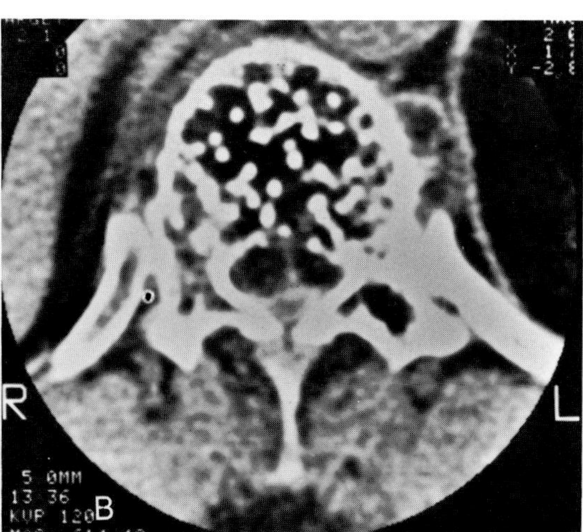

FIGURE 2–28. Hemangioma, hemangioendothelioma, and angiosarcoma. *A*, Hemangioma affecting the vertebral body of L2 displays a typical honeycomb appearance. *B*, CT section of hemangioma demonstrates coarse dots in the vertebral body of T8, representing reinforced vertical trabeculae of the cancellous bone.

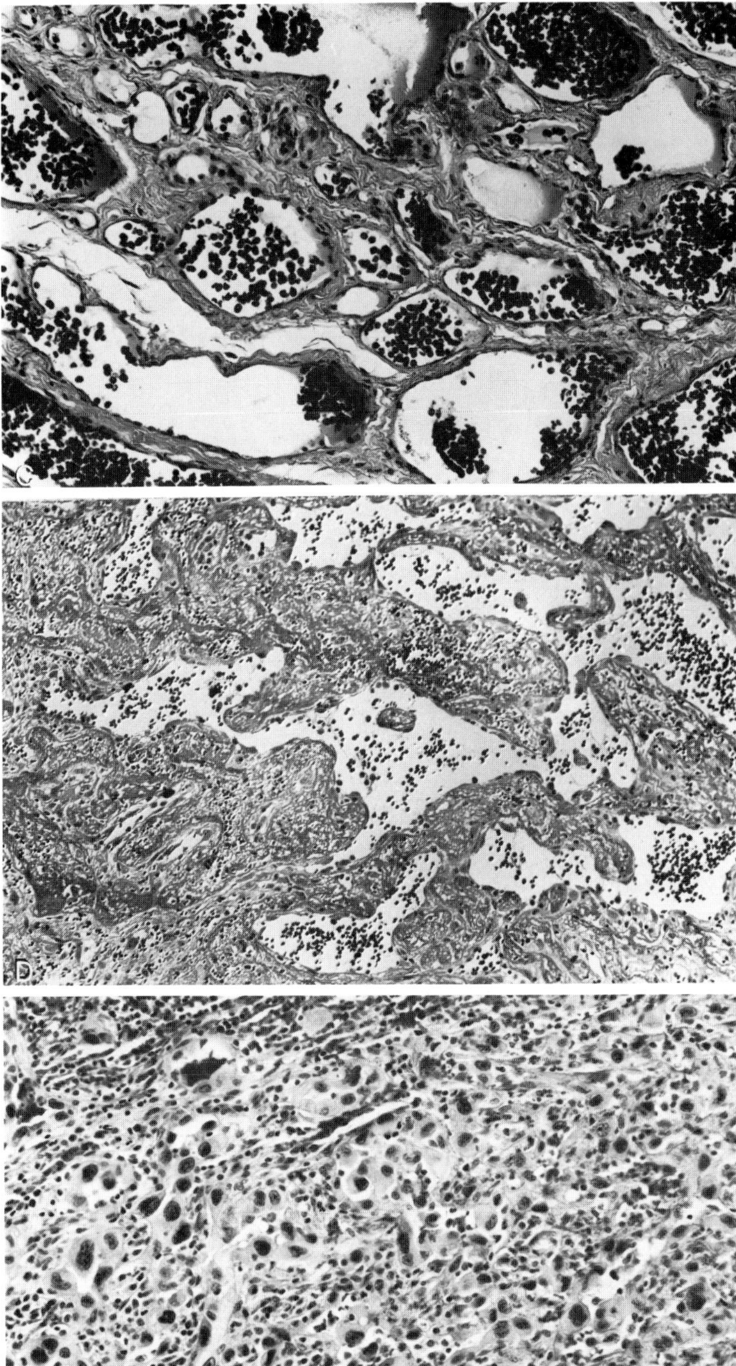

FIGURE 2–28 *Continued C,* Hemangioma. Endothelial-lined, simple vascular spaces supported by a fibrous stroma (×207). *D,* Hemangioendothelioma. Endothelium of vascular spaces is more prominent in some areas, and the vascular channels show infolding and complex interchannel anastomoses (×50). *E,* Angiosarcoma. Lumina of vascular spaces are largely obliterated by the proliferation of highly atypical endothelial cells and the proliferation of extravascular spindle cells infiltrated by a dense inflammatory component (×158).

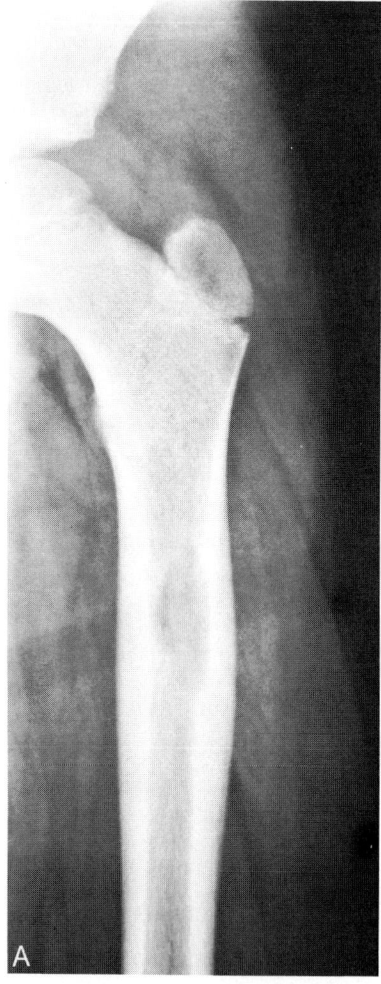

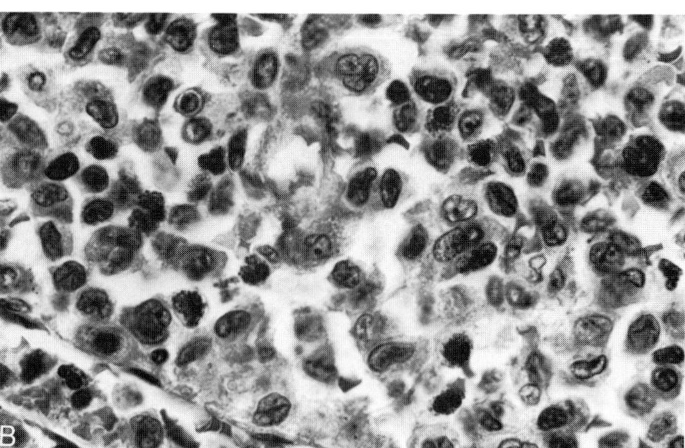

FIGURE 2–29. Eosinophilic granuloma. *A,* Osteolytic lesion in the femoral diaphysis is associated with fusiform thickening of the cortex and a solid periosteal reaction. (From Greenspan A: Orthopedic Radiology. Philadelphia, JB Lippincott, 1988.) *B,* Numerous histiocytes with vesicular, folded, and grooved nuclei, dotted with occasional, coarsely granular eosinophils (×440).

lioses. Lichtenstein proposed the name histiocytosis X for the three conditions—eosinophilic granuloma, Hand-Schüller-Christian disease (xanthomatosis), and Letterer-Siwe disease (nonlipid reticulosis)—because the lesions, being of unknown cause, seemed to represent an increasing spectrum of severity in which the common denominator was the presence of the histiocyte.[144] Although this concept gained a wide acceptance, the three diseases may, in fact, represent different entities.

Eosinophilic granuloma may manifest as a solitary lesion or as multiple lesions. It is most often seen in childhood, with a peak incidence between ages 5 and 10 years.[145] The most frequently affected sites are the skull, the ribs, the pelvis, the spine, and the long bones. In the mandible, radiolucent lesions and "floating teeth" are characteristic. In the spine, so-called vertebra plana is a typical manifestation and results from a collapsed vertebral body. The finding was for a long time mistakenly considered an osteochondrosis of the vertebra and named Calvé's disease after its proposer. In the long bones, eosinophilic granuloma presents as a radiolucent, destructive lesion, commonly associated with a lamellated periosteal reaction (Fig. 2–29*A*), and this appearance may mimic that of a round cell malignant tumor such as lymphoma or Ewing's sarcoma. In later stages, the lesion becomes more sclerotic, with dispersed radiolucencies. Distribution of the lesion is best ascertained by radionuclide bone scan. This may be helpful to detect silent lesions and to differentiate eosinophilic granuloma from Ewing's sarcoma, which rarely has multiple foci.

Histologically, eosinophilic granuloma is generally composed of a variable admixture of two types of cells (Fig. 2–29*B*). One type, the eosinophilic leukocyte, has a bilobated nucleus and coarse, eosinophilic cytoplasmic granules.

Although the eosinophil gives the lesion its name, the second cell type, a histiocyte, is the necessary histologic finding to make a diagnosis of eosinophilic granuloma. This pathognomonic cell was proved by electron microscopic observations to be identical with the Langerhans histiocyte seen in the skin.[144] These cells are plump and pink, displaying lightly granular cytoplasm. Their nuclei are translucent, ovoid or kidney bean shaped, have distinct nuclear membranes, and may possess longitudinal grooves. The eosinophils tend to be aggregated into small micronodules at various levels of the lesion and may not be appreciated in any given plane of section. The major histologic differential diagnostic condition is infection, because osteomyelitis is one of the diseases capable of producing a polymorphous infiltrate of several inflammatory cell types. Moreover, there is sometimes an inflammatory reaction simulating osteomyelitis at the periphery of eosinophilic granuloma, and so it is necessary to correlate histologic findings with the radiographic presentation before rendering a diagnosis.

Lymphoma of Bone

Primary lymphoma of bone is a rare tumor, having been termed reticulum cell sarcoma or lymphosarcoma in the past.[16] For the purpose of specific treatment, it must be distinguished from other small round cell malignant tumors of bone, as well as from secondary skeletal involvement by systemic lymphoma. Osseous lymphomas occur in the second to seventh decades of life, with peak incidence between ages 35 and 45 years. They are slightly more frequent in males. The sites of predilection are the long bones, the pelvis, and the ribs. Radiographically, lymphoma may exhibit a moth-eaten pattern of destruction or may be purely osteolytic (Fig. 2–30*A*), or it may occur as a mixed lesion with periosteal reaction (Fig. 2–30*B*). It may also have an ivory bone appearance, a picture commonly seen in vertebrae or flat bones. Lymphoma may resemble Ewing's sarcoma, particularly if it is present in younger patients, or Paget's disease, if it involves the articular end of the bone and displays a mixed sclerotic and osteolytic pattern (Fig. 2–30*C*, *D*).

Histologically, lymphomas may be subdivided into non-Hodgkin's lymphoma and Hodgkin's lymphoma. Although involvement of bones is relatively common in Hodgkin's lymphoma, primary Hodgkin's lymphoma of bone is extremely rare. Non-Hodgkin's lymphomas are considered primary in bone only if a complete systemic work-up reveals no evidence of extraosseous involvement. Moreover, some authorities consider that no evidence of extraosseous or nodal disease has to be present for at least 6 months after the discovery of the osseous focus in order that lymphoma be considered primary in the bone. Histologically, the tumor consists of aggregates of malignant lymphoid cells replacing marrow spaces and osseous trabeculae. Depending on the type of lymphoma, the infiltrate may be monomorphic or polymorphic, but even in the polymorphic variant, the cells have a malignant rather than inflammatory character (Fig. 2–30*E*). The mixed B cell lymphomas and especially the T cell lymphomas tend to show the largest admixture of cell types; in addition, the T cell lymphomas tend to be infiltrated by eosinophils.[36] The histologic differential diagnosis includes lymphoma, Ewing's sarcoma, metastatic neuroblastomas, and other small round cell tumors involving bone. Although the patient's age and overall tumor morphologic features usually are sufficient to categorize the tumor, the most important single procedure to distinguish lymphoma from all other major round cell tumors is the stain for leukocyte common antigen, because lymphoid cells are the only cells that stain positively. If lymphoma is a serious consideration at the time of biopsy, frozen sections may be prepared and stained for lymphoid markers to guide the patient's therapy and to determine the prognosis.[42]

Myeloma (Multiple Myeloma, Plasma Cell Myeloma, and Plasmacytoma)

Myeloma, a tumor originating in bone marrow, is the most common primary malignant tumor of bone. It is usually seen between the fifth and seventh decades and is found more frequently in men than in women. The axial skeleton is most commonly affected; however, no bone is exempt from involvement. Rarely, the lesion is solitary and is then termed plasmacytoma or solitary myeloma. More commonly, it is a widespread disease, in which case the name multiple myeloma is applied. Pain, mild and transient, enhanced by weight bearing and activity, may be the initial complaint and is present in about 75% of patients. Therefore, multiple myeloma may masquerade as sciatica or intercostal neuralgia in the stages before diagnosis is established. Rarely, a

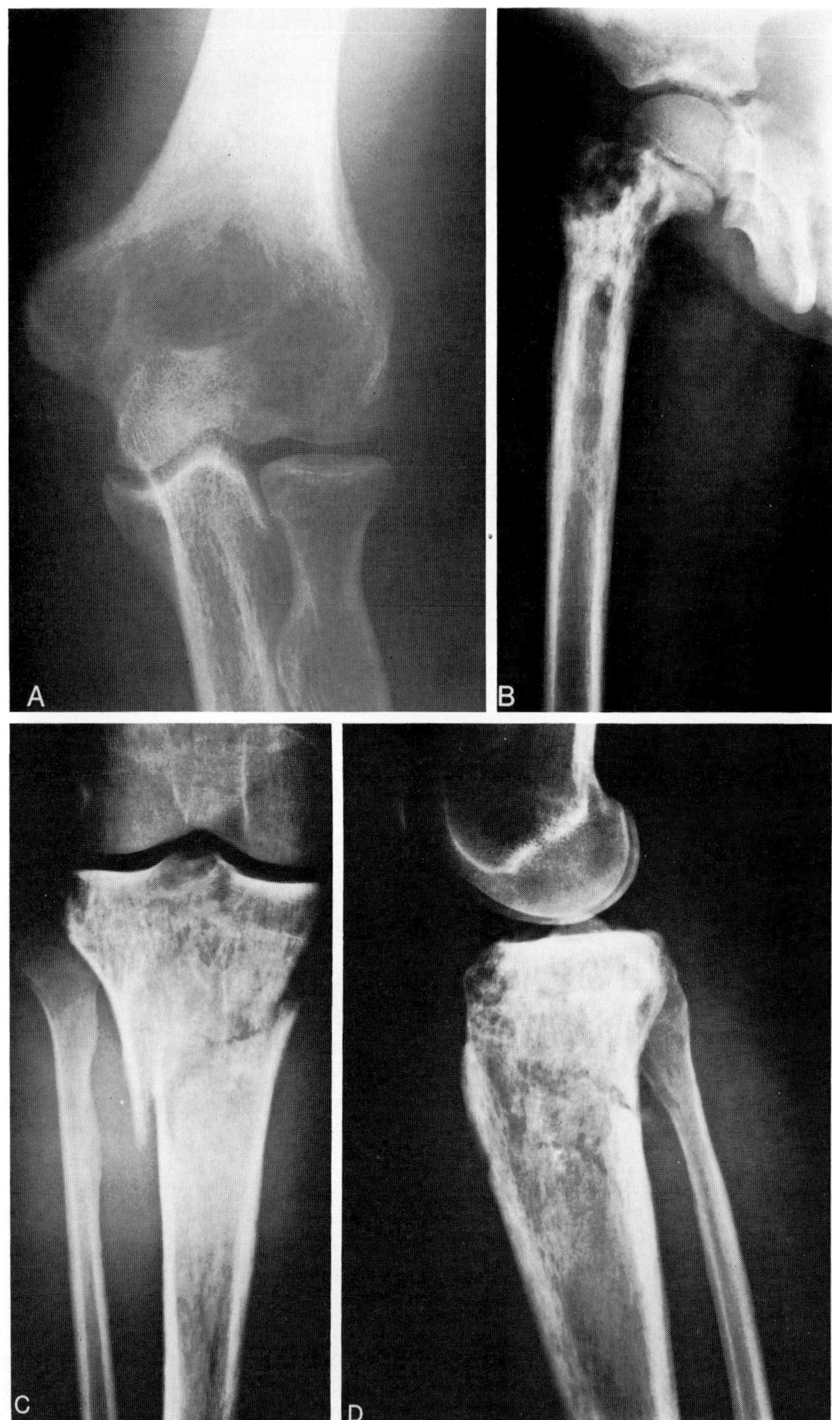

FIGURE 2–30. Lymphoma. *A,* An osteolytic lesion with ill-defined margins extends into the articular end of the distal humerus in a 43-year-old man. *B,* Destructive lesion with a mixed lytic and blastic pattern and an aggressive, lamellated periosteal reaction involves the metaphysis and the proximal diaphysis of the right femur in a 7-year-old girl. (From Greenspan A: Orthopedic Radiology. Philadelphia, JB Lippincott, 1988.) *C, D,* The mixed sclerotic and osteolytic character of the lesion affecting the proximal tibia and the thickening of the cortex resemble the coarse, trabecular pattern of Paget's disease. There is a pathologic fracture, but only minimal periosteal response is evident. (From Greenspan A: Orthopedic Radiology. Philadelphia, JB Lippincott, 1988.)

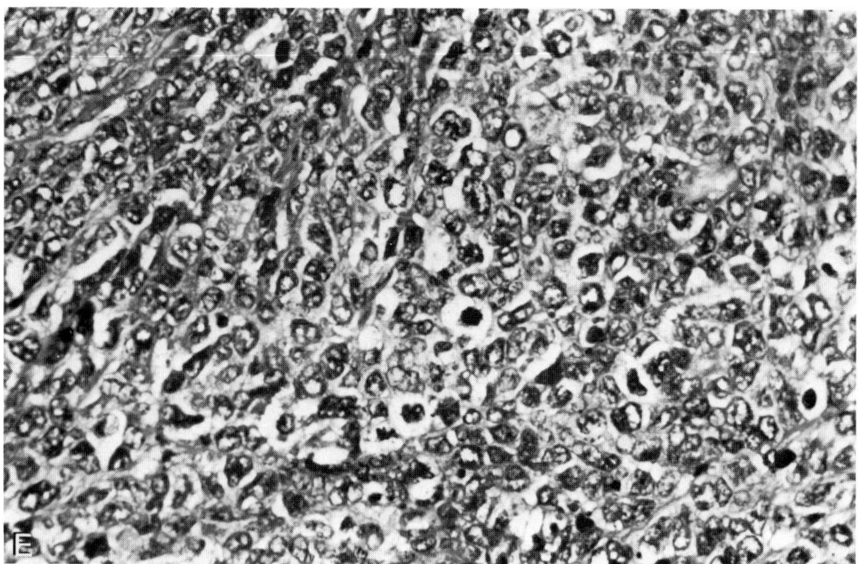

FIGURE 2–30 *Continued E,* Malignant lymphoma, large cell type. Sheets of malignant lymphocytes with large, noncleaved, vesicular nuclei and numerous mitoses. Immunohistochemistry study revealed B cell markers (×320).

pathologic fracture is the first sign of disease. Because the malignant cells represent a monoclonal proliferation of plasma cells, the tumor produces the specific immunoglobulin type associated with that particular neoplastic plasma cell. Characteristically, the ratio of serum albumin to globulins is reversed because of the high concentration of monoclonal immunoglobulin. Because the monoclonal immunoglobulin is of the same molecular weight and charge, during serum electrophoresis it moves to a single spot, and a concentrated narrow band, so-called M component, appears as a peak when densitometry is performed on the electrophoretic strip. Although the total immunoglobulin level is elevated because of the monoclonal protein, the normal serum immunoglobulin concentrations are markedly depressed, resulting in impaired humoral immunity. If light chains are produced in excess, these pass into the renal tubules and dimerize to form Bence Jones protein in the urine.[9]

Radiographically, particularly in the spine, multiple myeloma may present simply as osteoporosis with no definitely identifiable lesions. Multiple compression fractures of the vertebral bodies may be seen. A more common presentation than compression fractures, however, is the presence of multiple lytic lesions scattered throughout the skeleton. In the skull, characteristic punched-out areas of bone destruction, usually uniform in size, are noted (Fig. 2–31*A*). In the ribs, lacelike areas of bone destruction and small osteolytic lesions accompanied by soft tissue masses are occasionally seen.[103] In the flat and long bones, areas of medullary bone destruction are noted, and if these abut the cortex, endosteal scalloping of the inner cortical margin is seen (Fig. 2–31*B*). Characteristically, there is no evidence of sclerosis and no periosteal reaction. Fewer than 1% of myelomas may exhibit sclerosis (sclerosing myelomatosis).[18]

If the spine is involved, which occurs rather frequently, multiple myeloma must be differentiated from metastatic carcinoma. In this respect, the "vertebral-pedicle sign" identified by Murray and Jacobson, may be helpful.[103] They contend that, in the early stages of myeloma, the pedicle, which does not contain as much red marrow as the vertebral body, is not initially involved, whereas in metastatic carcinoma, the pedicle is affected to the same extent as the vertebral body, even in early stages. In the late stages of multiple myeloma, however, the pedicle and the vertebral body are both affected. A more reliable distinction between these two processes is achieved with the radionuclide bone scan. Although the bone scan is invariably abnormal in cases of metastatic carcinoma, myeloma seldom produces increased uptake of radiopharmaceutical.

A solitary myeloma may create even more diagnostic problems. As a purely radiolucent lesion, it may mimic other purely destructive processes such as giant cell tumor, brown tu-

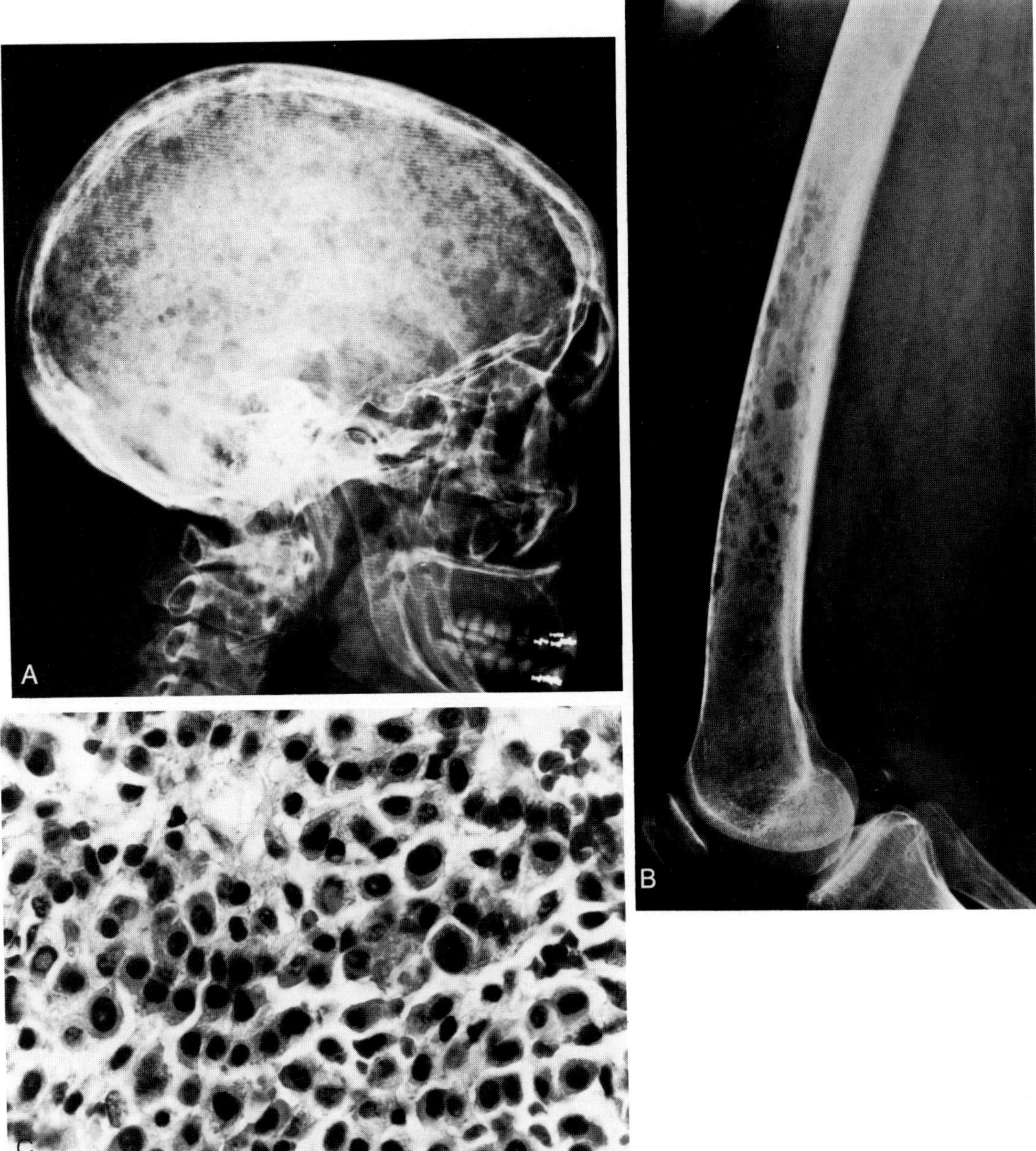

FIGURE 2–31. Myeloma. *A,* Multiple myeloma. Characteristic punched-out, lytic lesions, most of which are uniform in size and lack sclerotic borders. (From Greenspan A: Orthopedic Radiology. Philadelphia, JB Lippincott, 1988.) *B,* Multiple osteolytic lesions and endosteal scalloping of the cortex are typical of diffuse myelomatosis. (From Greenspan A: Orthopedic Radiology. Philadelphia, JB Lippincott, 1988.) *C,* Plasma cell myeloma. The tumor cells show eccentric nuclei, occasional paranuclear clear zones, and a few intranuclear aggregates of immunoglobulin (×780).

mor of hyperparathyroidism, fibrosarcoma, malignant fibrous histiocytoma, and a solitary metastatic focus from a carcinoma of the kidney, the lung, the thyroid, or the gastrointestinal tract. Moreover, only a small percentage of solitary myelomas are associated with the production of detectable monoclonal immunoglobulins.

Histologically, the diagnosis is made by finding sheets of atypical plasmacytoid cells replacing the normal marrow spaces. The neoplastic cells may contain double or even multiple nuclei. These nuclei are usually hyperchromatic and enlarged, and prominent nucleoli may be found. Despite the malignant cytologic features of the tumor cells, a spoke wheel chromatin distribution and a decided nuclear eccentricity usually seen in normal plasma cells help in their identification (Fig. 2–31*C*).

An interesting variant of sclerosing myeloma is the so-called POEMS syndrome, first described in 1968, but gaining wide acceptance only more recently. It consists of polyneuropathy (P); organomegaly (O), particularly of the liver and the spleen; endocrine disturbances (E), such as amenorrhea and gynecomastia; monoclonal gammopathy (M), and skin changes (S), such as hyperpigmentation and hirsutism. It is still debatable whether the sclerotic changes relate to plasma cells that fail to secrete osteoclast-activating factor or perhaps to the secretion of an osteoblast-stimulating factor. There are relatively few plasma cells in the marrow of patients with POEMS syndrome, and some investigators consider this entity to be a plasma cell dyscrasia rather than a true neoplasm.

Complications encountered with myeloma are pathologic fractures (of long bones, ribs, sternum, and vertebra), amyloidosis (in about 15% of patients), increased incidence of infection, anemia, and hyperviscosity syndrome. Most patients with solitary myeloma manifest the systemic form of myeloma within 5 to 20 years.[36]

Tumors and Tumor-like Lesions of Uncertain and Unknown Origin

Simple Bone Cyst

The simple bone cyst, sometimes called unicameral bone cyst, is a tumor-like lesion of unknown cause, attributed to a local disturbance of bone growth.[72] It is more common in males and is usually seen during the first two decades of life. The vast majority of bone cysts are located in the proximal diaphysis of the humerus and the femur, especially when they occur in patients younger than 17 years. In older patients, the incidence of involvement of atypical sites, such as calcaneus, talus, and ilium, rises significantly.

Radiographically, the appearance of a simple bone cyst is that of a centrally located, well-circumscribed, radiolucent lesion with sclerotic margins (Fig. 2–32*A*). Periosteal reaction is absent unless there has been a pathologic fracture, and this feature distinguishes it from aneurysmal bone cyst, in which there is almost invariably some degree of periosteal response. Diagnosis is best based on the plain film radiographs, and tomography is used only exceptionally in equivocal cases.

The commonest complication is pathologic fracture and this occurs in about 66% of cases. Occasionally, one can identify a characteristic "fallen fragment" sign. This represents a piece of fractured cortex that is in the interior of the lesion, indicating that it is either hollow or filled with fluid, as most simple bone cysts are. This sign permits differentiation of simple bone cysts from radiographically similar radiolucent lesions containing solid fibrous or cartilaginous tissue, such as fibrous dysplasia, nonossifying fibroma, or enchondroma. Bone abscess may occasionally mimic simple bone cyst, particularly if it is located in the sites of predilection for simple bone cyst. However, the presence of periosteal reaction and the frequent extension of the lesion beyond the boundaries of a growth plate are important features indicating bone abscess.

Histologically, simple bone cyst is a diagnosis of exclusion. A vigorous surgical curettage, if the lesion is not simply injected, yields almost no solid tissue, but the walls of the cavity may show remnants of fibrous tissue or, occasionally, a flattened single-cell lining (Fig. 2–32 *B*). If the fluid is examined chemically, it is usually found to contain elevated levels of alkaline phosphatase.

Aneurysmal Bone Cyst

Aneurysmal bone cyst is seen predominantly in childhood, and 90% of cases occur in patients younger than 20 years of age. The metaphysis of the long bones is the most frequent site of predilection, although the diaphysis, the flat bones, and even the spine may be involved.[69] When the spine is affected, the lesion is usually situated in the posterior elements. The radiographic hallmark of an aneurysmal bone cyst is a multicystic, eccentric expansion (blow out) of the bone with a buttress or thin shell of periosteal response (Fig. 2–33 *A*). The lesion can develop *de novo* or as a secondary reaction to preexisting lesions, such as chondroblastoma, osteoblastoma, giant cell tumor, and fibrous dysplasia.[27] Although plain radiographs are usually sufficient to evaluate the lesion, other modalities such as conventional tomography, CT, and radionuclide bone scan can be of further assistance.

Histologically, the lesion consists of multiple

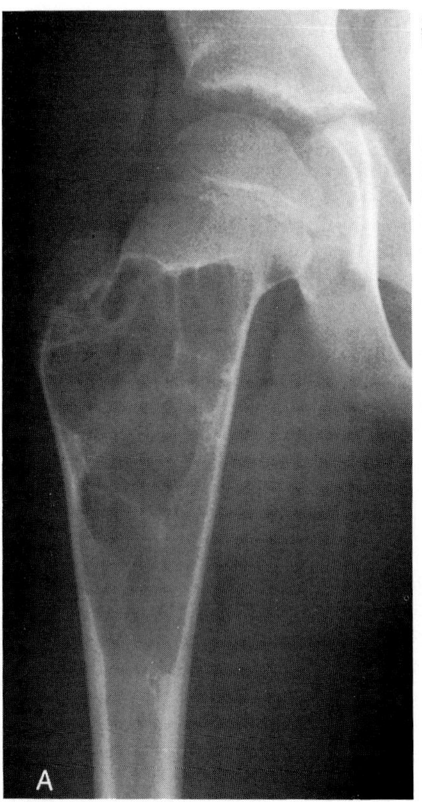

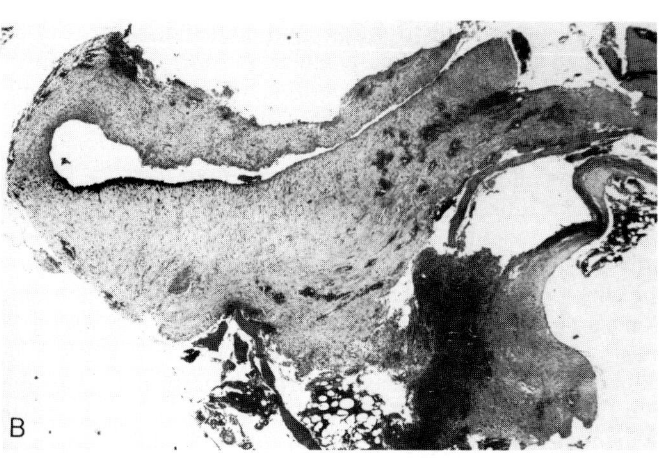

FIGURE 2–32. Simple bone cyst. *A,* Radiolucent lesion with sclerotic borders is centrally located in the proximal diaphysis of the right femur. Note the slight thinning of the cortex and the lack of periosteal reaction. *B,* Flattened fibrous lining containing a few sparse osseous fragments (×20).

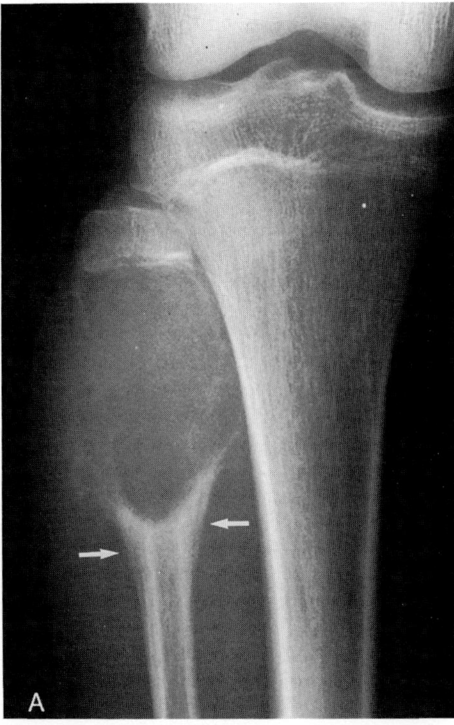

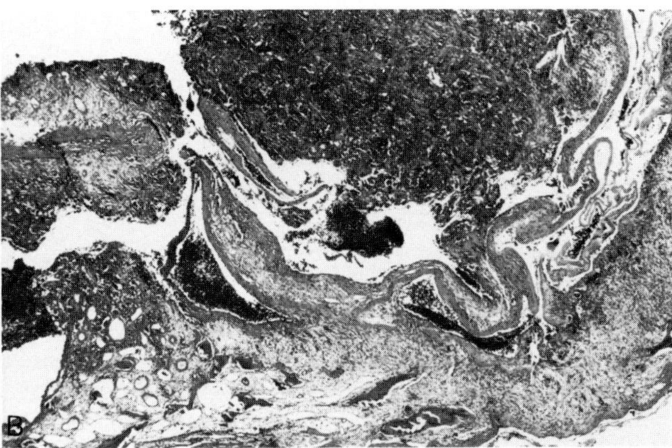

FIGURE 2–33. Aneurysmal bone cyst. *A,* Expansile, radiolucent lesion is seen in the metaphysis of the proximal fibula. Note the blown-out appearance and the buttress of periosteal response (arrows). *B,* Multiple sinusoid spaces containing blood, some of which have bony walls. Solid area (top center) contains spindle cells, irregular multinucleated giant cells, and organizing hemorrhage (×20).

blood-filled sinusoid spaces alternating with more solid areas.[129] The solid tissue, which is composed of fibrous elements containing numerous multinucleated giant cells, is richly vascular, showing a progression from tiny to large vessels.[27] The sinusoids have fibrous walls, often containing osteoid tissue or even mature bone; multinucleated giant cells are also seen, some of which are present in the fibrous lining (Fig. 2–33*B*). Some of the sinusoids are lined by flattened cells resembling endothelium, but continuous endothelial spaces, as seen in normal vascular structures, are not completely formed in aneurysmal bone cyst.

Adamantinoma

A rare malignant tumor occurring with equal frequency in males and females between the second and fifth decades, adamantinoma has a predilection to involve the tibia in 90% of cases. Well-delineated, elongated osteolytic defects of different sizes are separated by areas of sclerotic bone, occasionally imparting a soap bubble appearance (Fig. 2–34*A*). A sawtoothed area of cortical destruction, when present, is quite distinctive of this tumor. At times, the entire bone may be affected with multiple satellite lesions.

Histologically, the tumor is biphasic and

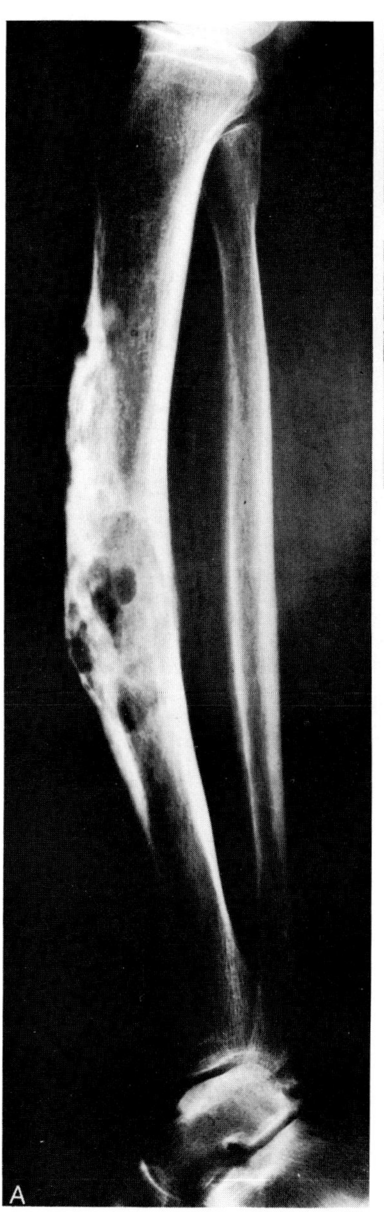

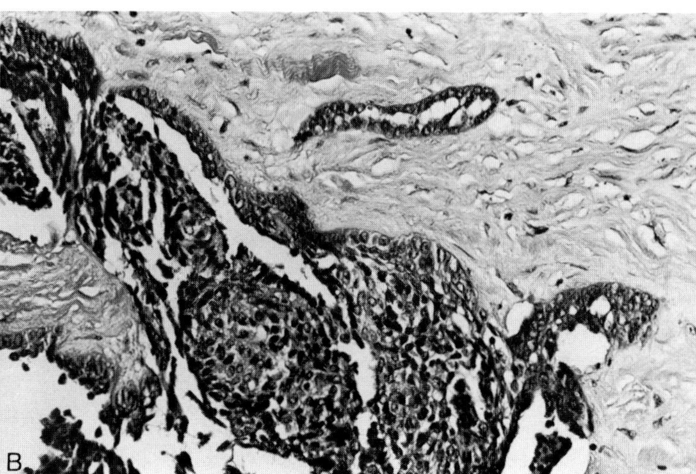

FIGURE 2–34. Adamantinoma. *A*, Destructive multicystic lesion affects predominantly the anterior aspect of the tibia and demonstrates osteolytic and sclerotic foci, creating a soap bubble appearance. (From Greenspan A: Orthopedic Radiology. Philadelphia, JB Lippincott, 1988.) *B*, A biphasic pattern of sparsely cellular, fibrous tissue containing glandular and squamoid epithelial tumorous elements characterizes this tumor (×200).

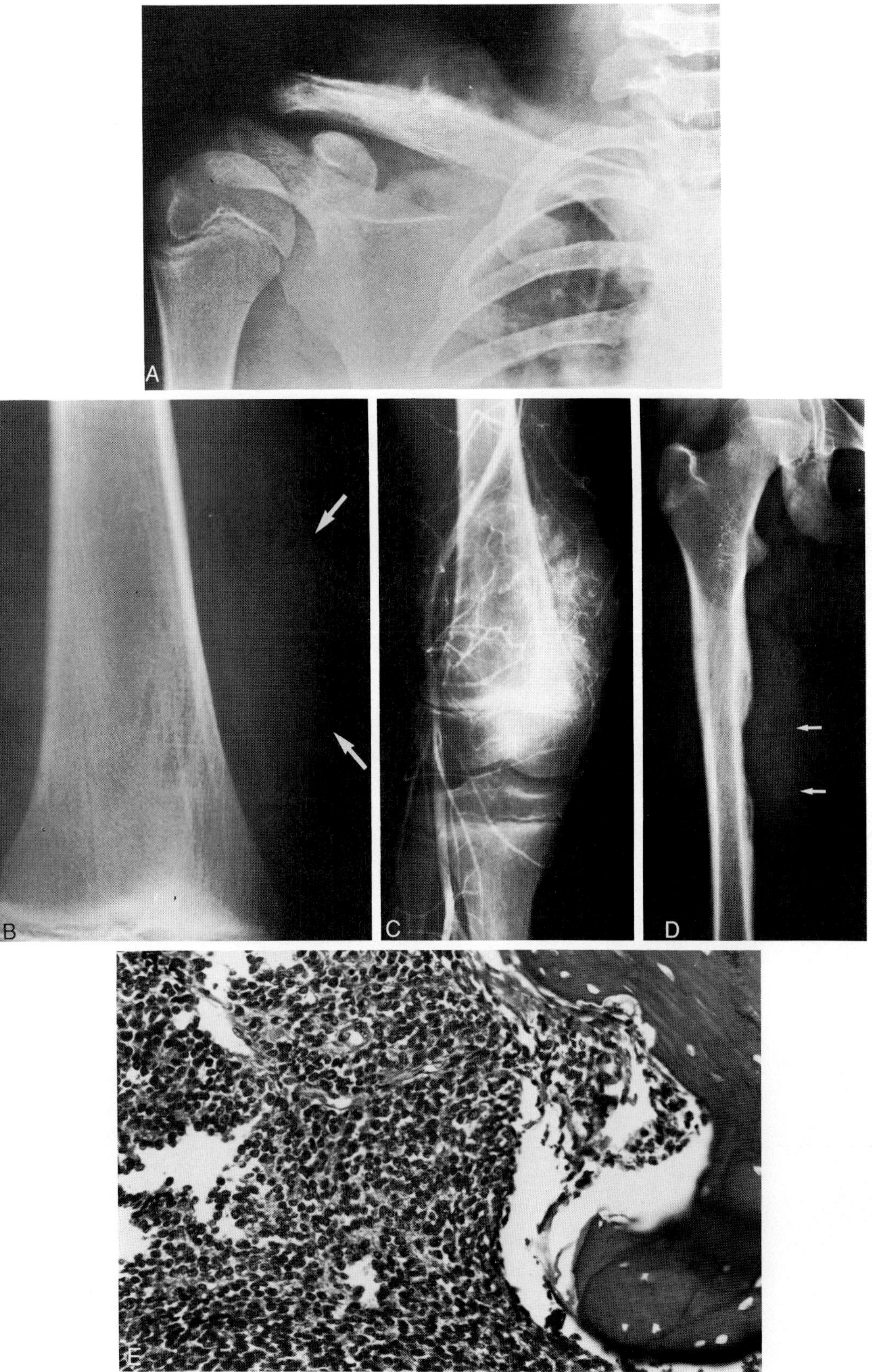

FIGURE 2–35. *See legend on opposite page.*

consists of an epithelial component intimately admixed in varying proportions with a fibrous component. The epithelial component usually consists of islands of polyhedral cells in glandlike spaces or in pavemented nests showing peripheral nuclear palisading and a looser, myxoid inner zone resembling the stellate reticulum of odontogenic tissue (Fig. 2–34*B*). Squamous metaplasia is sometimes seen, and if it is extensive, the lesion may be erroneously interpreted as squamous cell carcinoma. The fibrous component consists of spindle cells, which usually show only slight atypia. Occasionally, the epithelial spaces and stroma become highly vascularized, and the lesion may resemble a vascular tumor. Although it has been speculated that adamantinoma represents a form of vascular neoplasm, ultrastructural and immunohistochemical evidence points toward an epithelial derivation.[46, 114, 115] Despite this interpretation, it is still hard to conceive how an epithelial neoplasm could still be primary in bone.

A relationship of adamantinoma with osteofibrous dysplasia (Kempson-Campanacci lesion) and fibrous dysplasia has been suggested by some investigators. This remains a controversial matter; however, adamantinoma may contain a fibro-osseous component that, on pathologic examination, resembles both fibrous and osteofibrous dysplasias.

Ewing's Sarcoma

This is a highly malignant primitive round cell tumor, predominantly affecting children and adolescents. About 90% of cases occur before the patient is 20 years of age. The tumor is more common in males and is only exceptionally seen in black individuals. Diaphyses of the long bones, the ribs, and the flat bones, such as the scapula and the pelvis, are the sites of predilection.[36, 88]

The radiographic presentation in most cases is quite characteristic and consists of an ill-defined lesion with permeative or moth-eaten type of bone destruction associated with an aggressive type of periosteal response and a large soft tissue mass (Fig. 2–35*A*). Occasionally, the lesion in the bone is almost imperceptible, and the only prominent finding is a soft tissue mass (Fig. 2–35*B, C*). Ewing's tumor may mimic metastatic neuroblastoma, eosinophilic granuloma, and osteomyelitis. At times, it creates a typical "saucerization" of the cortex, a feature once thought to be virtually pathognomonic of this tumor (Fig. 2–35*D*). The phenomenon of saucerization may be related to the combination of destruction of the periosteal surface of bone by the tumor and an associated extrinsic pressure effect by the large soft tissue mass. Recently, this sign was reported in other tumors and even in osteomyelitis; however, the presence of saucerization in association with a permeative lesion and a soft tissue mass favors the diagnosis of Ewing's sarcoma.

Histologically, Ewing's sarcoma consists of a uniform array of small cells with round, hyperchromatic nuclei; scant cytoplasm; and ill-defined cell borders (Fig. 2–35*E*). At times, the cytoplasm contains a moderate amount of glycogen demonstrable with the periodic acid–Schiff stain. The mitotic rate is high, and necrosis is frequently extensive. The differential diagnosis includes malignant lymphoma, metastatic neuroblastoma, and other small round cell tumors such as rhabdomyosarcoma. Although neuroblastomas are generally tumors of early childhood accompanied by elevated levels of urinary catecholamines, and lymphomas usually affect an older age group and have larger cells, the histologic distinctions blur in practice. The demonstration of glycogen, which at one time was considered an absolutely distinctive marker for Ewing's sarcoma,[119] has fallen into disfavor, because in not all Ewing's sarcomas can glycogen be demonstrated. Moreover, malignant lymphoma as well as primitive neural tumors may at times contain glycogen. Since the advent of immunohistochemistry, lymphomas are usually separable

FIGURE 2–35. Ewing's sarcoma. *A,* Poorly defined, destructive lesion in the right clavicle is associated with lamellated and sunburst types of periosteal reaction and a large soft tissue mass. (From Greenspan A: Orthopedic Radiology. Philadelphia, JB Lippincott, 1988.) *B,* Bone destruction is almost imperceptible on this magnification study of the distal femoral diaphysis of a 10-year-old girl. The soft tissue mass is adjacent to the medial cortex (arrows). (From Greenspan A: Orthopedic Radiology. Philadelphia, JB Lippincott, 1988.) *C,* Femoral arteriogram (same patient as in *B*) demonstrates a large soft tissue mass and tumor vessels. *D,* "Saucerization" of the medial cortex of the femoral diaphysis is frequently seen in this tumor. Note also a large soft tissue mass (arrows). (From Greenspan A: Orthopedic Radiology. Philadelphia, JB Lippincott, 1988.) *E,* Sheets of uniform, round nuclei practically devoid of cytoplasm compose this tumor. At right there is a devitalized bone trabecula with several resorption bays (×200).

from Ewing's sarcomas by demonstrating leukocyte common antigen.

Neural tumors are marked by a positive reaction for neuron-specific enolase and positive test result for neural filament proteins, and electron microscopy may demonstrate the presence of neurosecretory granules in tumors of neural origin. Recent immunocytochemical analyses suggested, however, that Ewing's sarcoma cells are derived from primitive pluripotential cells capable of differentiating into cells with mesenchymal, epithelial, and even neural features;[101] and tissue culture studies of five Ewing's sarcoma cell lines treated with cyclic adenosine monophosphate or phorbol 12-myristate 13-acetate induced marked neural differentiation.[23] These investigations led to speculation that Ewing's sarcoma may in fact be regarded as a primitive neural tumor affecting bone.

Chordoma

Chordoma is a malignant bone tumor arising from developmental remnants of the notochord. It is seen only in those sites where notochordal remnants are not normally present; hence, although it is a midline lesion of the axial skeleton, it never occurs in the nuclei pulposi. It is most frequently discovered between the fourth and seventh decades and is slightly more common in males. The three commonest sites for this tumor are the sacrococcygeal area, the spheno-occipital area, and the second cervical vertebra. It is a locally aggressive neoplasm, and, in most reported series, metastases were rare and occurred late in the course of the disease.

The radiographic appearance is that of a highly destructive, lytic lesion with irregular, scalloped borders, occasionally with matrix calcifications, which are probably due to extensive tumor necrosis (Fig. 2–36*A*). Soft tissue masses are commonly associated with the lesion. Although conventional radiography, including tomography, delineates the tumor well, CT scan is important to demonstrate the soft tissue extension and myelography frequently demonstrates invasion of the spinal canal.

Histologically, the tumor consists of loose aggregates of mucoid material separating cordlike arrays and lobules of large polyhedral cells with vacuolated cytoplasm and vesicular nuclei (Fig. 2–36*B*), referred to as physaliphorous (from Greek for bubble bearing).

Skeletal Metastases

Skeletal metastases are the most frequent variety of bone tumors and should always be considered in differential diagnosis, particularly in older patients. The incidence varies with the type of primary neoplasm and the duration of disease. Some malignant tumors demonstrate a far greater predilection for osseous involvement than others. In males, carcinoma of the prostate has been reported to account for nearly 60% of all bone metastases,

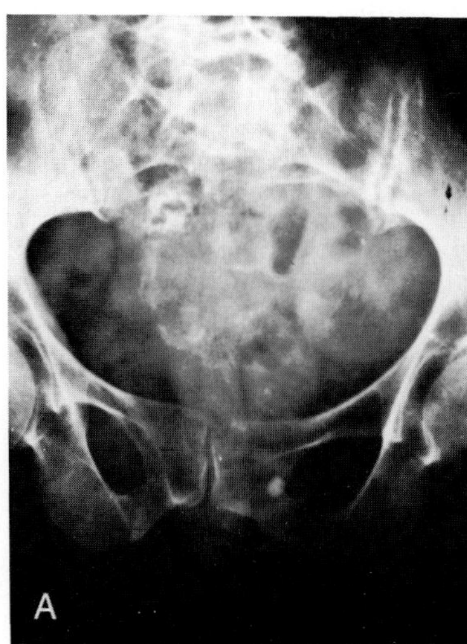

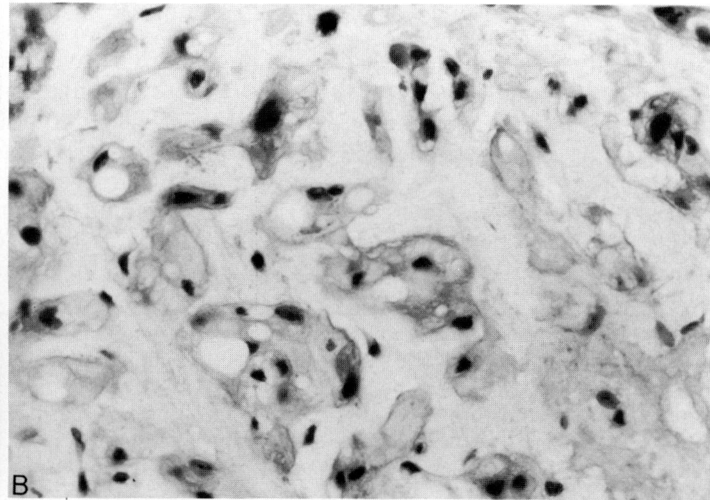

FIGURE 2–36. Chordoma. *A*, Destructive lesion is seen in the sacrum, demonstrating scalloped, partially sclerotic borders and amorphous calcifications in the tumor matrix. *B*, Clusters of physaliphorous (bubble-bearing) cells are characteristic of this tumor (×360).

whereas in women, carcinoma of the breast is responsible for nearly 70% of all metastatic lesions.[1] Other primary tumors commonly responsible for bone metastases include carcinomas of the lung, the kidney, the thyroid, and the stomach. Because of their frequency, cancers of the breast, the lung, and the prostate result in the majority of bone metastases. Most skeletal metastases are "silent." If metastases are symptomatic, pain is the main clinical feature and only occasionally a pathologic fracture through the lesion may focus attention on the disease. In the spine, metastases are frequently associated with neurologic symptoms resulting from compression of the cord or nerve routes or even complete obstruction of the thecal sac. Metastases are solitary or multiple, and they may be further subdivided into purely lytic, purely blastic, and mixed lesions. Primary tumors responsible for purely osteolytic metastases are usually situated in the kidneys, the lung, the breast, the thyroid, and the gastrointestinal tract. Primary tumors responsible for osteoblastic metastases are usually situated in the prostate gland. It must be pointed out, however, that after treatment (radiation therapy, chemotherapy, or hormonal therapy), purely lytic lesions may become sclerotic. Metastases usually involve the axial skeleton (skull, spine, and pelvis) and the most proximal segments of limb bones. Only in extremely rare cases are metastatic tumors seen distal to the elbows and the knees. Although metastases in the skeleton may appear similar, irrespective of their primary source, instances may occur in which their location, distribution, and morphologic appearance may suggest a site of origin.[134] For example, 50% of skeletal metastases distal to the elbows and the knees, although unusual, are due to either bronchogenic or breast carcinoma. An expansile, blown-out appearance of a lesion is typical of metastatic renal carcinoma (Fig. 2–37*A*). Multiple round, dense foci or diffuse increases in bone density are seen frequently in metastatic carcinoma of the prostate (Fig. 2–37*B*). In women, sclerotic metastases are usually from breast carcinoma.

Recently, characteristic cortical metastases were reported in bronchogenic carcinoma.[39, 54, 55] They produce a type of cortical destruction termed "cookie bites" or "cookie cutter" lesions. The usual way of spread of malignant cells to involve the skeleton is via hematogenous route. In such instances, the bulk of the tumor lodges in the marrow and spongy bone. Thus the initial radiographic appearance of metastatic lesions in the skeleton consists of destruction of cancellous bone, and only after further tumor growth is the cortex affected. An anastomosing vascular system in the cortex originating in the overlying periosteum probably serves as a pathway by which malignant cells from bronchogenic carcinoma reach the compact bone and produce initial cortical destruction.

Single metastatic bone lesions have to be distinguished from primary malignant and even benign bone tumors. One typical feature may be helpful in making the distinction: a metastatic lesion usually presents without or with only a small soft tissue mass, and periosteal reaction is absent unless the mass breaks through the cortex. In some reported series, however, more than 30% of metastatic lesions demonstrated periosteal response, particularly metastases from carcinoma of the prostate. In the spine, metastatic lesions usually destroy the pedicle, a useful feature to distinguish this lesion from myeloma or neurofibroma eroding the vertebra.

Detection of skeletal metastases is not always possible on routine radiographs, because destruction of the bone may not be visible. Radionuclide bone scan is the best screening method in early detection of metastatic tumors, and it detects lytic as well as blastic lesions. CT and MRI may also be helpful in this respect.

Histologically, metastatic tumors are easier to diagnose than many primary tumors because of their essentially epithelial pattern. Biopsies of suspected metastases are useful for diagnosis in patients with known primary tumors, but only unusually are they helpful in specifying an exact site for an unknown primary tumor. A pathologist may be fortunate enough to specify adenocarcinoma if gland formation is present and make a list of differential diagnoses by comparing the morphologic features with the statistical likelihood of similarity in a primary tumor (Fig. 2–37*C*). Occasionally, the only identifying feature in the marrow spaces is a desmoplastic fibrotic reaction to tumor, and if a bone biopsy reveals predominantly mature bone trabeculae with intertrabecular fibrosis, the differential diagnosis of metastatic carcinoma should be considered. Exceptionally, a metastatic lesion may demonstrate a morphologic pattern that strongly suggests a primary tumor, such as the clear cells of renal carcinoma, or the pigment production of melanoma. A few neoplasms are associated with the production of enzymes or antigens that can

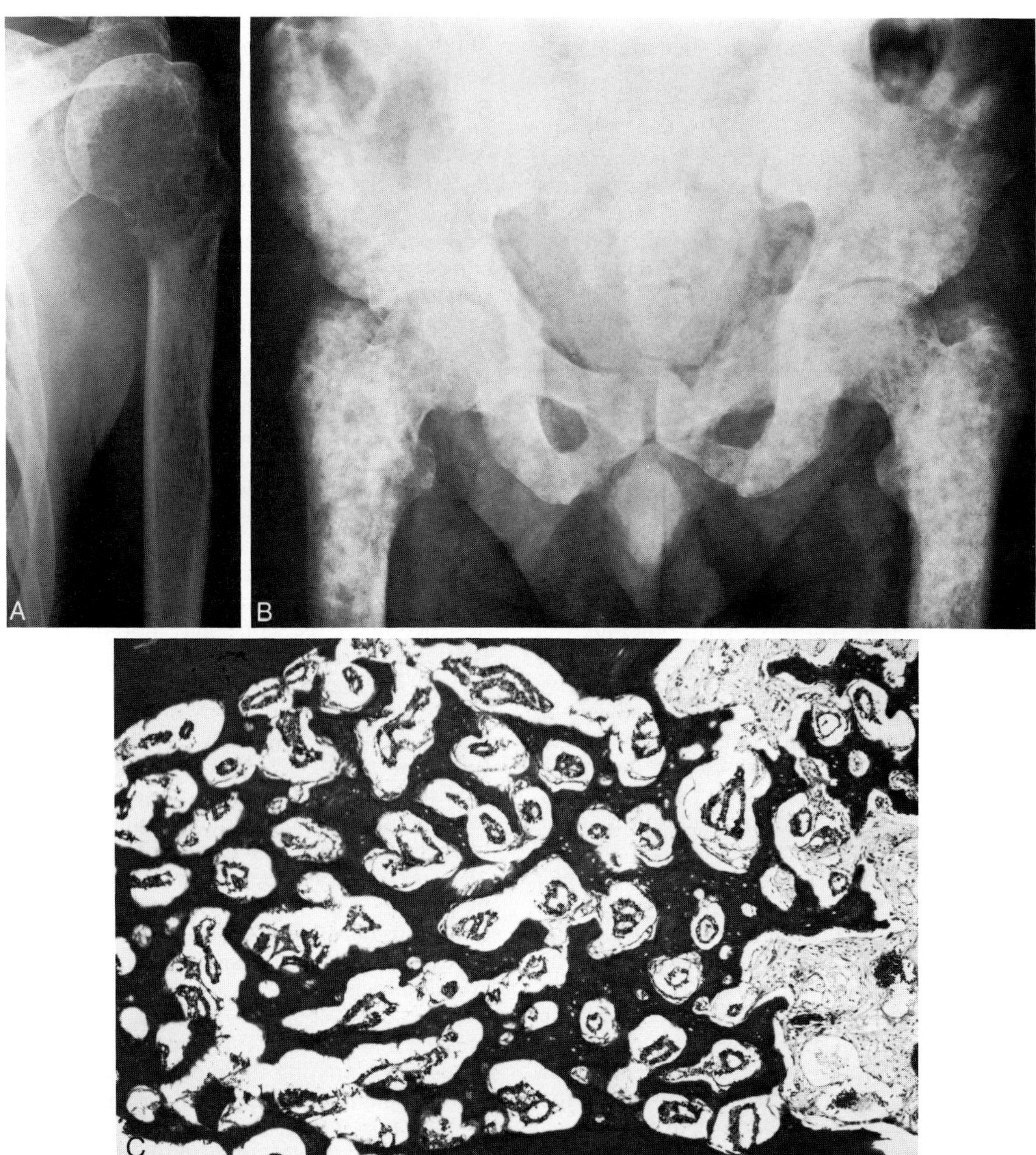

FIGURE 2–37. Metastasis. *A,* Purely osteolytic, destructive lesion with ill-defined borders is seen in the left humeral head and neck in a 50-year-old woman with renal cell carcinoma. *B,* Multiple sclerotic foci are scattered throughout the pelvis and the proximal femora of a 55-year-old man with blastic metastases from carcinoma of the prostate. *C,* Uniform cribriform glandular structures of metastatic prostate adenocarcinoma causing secondary osteoblastic activity (×50).

be detected after the decalcification procedure, so it is possible, for example, to perform a prostate-specific antigen study to delineate a primary site in the prostate. Currently, however, this method is used only rarely, and until specific antigens to other organ types become widely available, it has a limited practical value.

References

1. Abrams HL: Skeletal metastases in carcinoma. Radiology 55:534, 1950.
2. Ahuja SC, Villacin AB, Smith J, et al: Juxtacortical (parosteal) osteogenic sarcoma: Histological grading and prognosis. J Bone Joint Surg 59A:632, 1977.
3. Aisen AM, Martel W, Braunstein EM, et al: MRI and CT evaluation of primary bone and soft-tissue tumors. AJR 146:749, 1986.
4. Albright F, Butler AM, Hampton AO, et al: Syndrome characterized by osteitis fibrosa disseminata, areas of pigmentation and endocrine dysfunction with precocious puberty in females. N Engl J Med 216:727, 1937.
5. Amstutz HC: Multiple osteogenic sarcomata—metastatic or multicentric? Cancer 24:923, 1969.
6. Angervall L, Kindblom LG: Clear cell chondrosarcoma. A light and electron microscopic and histochemical study of two cases. Virchows Archiv (Pathol Anat) 389:27, 1980.
7. Barnes GR, Gwinn JL: Distal irregularities of the femur simulating malignancy. AJR 122:180, 1974.
8. Barnes R, Catto M: Chondrosarcoma of bone. J Bone Joint Surg 45B:729, 1966.
9. Bergsagel DE: Plasma cell myeloma. Cancer 30:1588, 1972.
10. Bertoni F, Boriani S, Laus M, et al: Periosteal chondrosarcoma and periosteal osteosarcoma. J Bone Joint Surg 64B:370, 1982.
11. Bertoni F, Picci P, Bacchini P, et al: Mesenchymal chondrosarcoma of bone and soft tissue. Cancer 52:533, 1983.
12. Bjornsson J, Unni KK, Dahlin DC, et al: Clear cell chondrosarcoma of bone: Observations in 47 cases. Am J Surg Pathol 8:223, 1984.
13. Bloem JL, Bluemm RG, Taminiau AHM, et al: Magnetic resonance imaging of primary malignant bone tumors. Radiographics 7:425, 1987.
14. Bloem JL, Mulder JD: Chondroblastoma: A clinical and radiological study of 104 cases. Skeletal Radiol 14:1, 1985.
15. Bohndorf K, Reiser M, Lochner B, et al: Magnetic resonance imaging of primary tumors and tumor-like lesions of bone. Skeletal Radiol 15:511, 1986.
16. Boston HC Jr, Dahlin DC, Ivins JC, et al: Malignant lymphoma (so-called reticulum cell sarcoma) of bone. Cancer 34:1131, 1974.
17. Brower AC, Culver JC, Keats TE: Histological nature of medial posterior distal femoral metaphysis in children. Radiology 99:389, 1971.
18. Brown TS, Paterson CR: Osteosclerosis in myeloma. J Bone Joint Surg 55B:621, 1973.
19. Burmester GR, Winchester RJ, Dimitriu-Bona A, et al: Delineation of four cell types comprising the giant cell tumor of bone. J Clin Invest 71:1633, 1983.
20. Campanacci M: Osteofibrous dysplasia of the long bones. A new clinical entity. Ital J Orthop Traumatol 2:221, 1976.
21. Campanacci M, Guernelli N, Leonessa C, et al: Chondrosarcoma: A study of 133 cases. Ital J Orthop Traumatol 1:387, 1975.
22. Campanacci M, Laus M: Osteofibrous dysplasia of the tibia and fibula. J Bone Joint Surg 63A:367, 1981.
23. Cavazzana AO, Miser JS, Jefferson J, et al: Experimental evidence for a neural origin of Ewing's sarcoma of bone. Am J Pathol 127:507, 1987.
24. Clarke BE, Xipell JM, Thomas DP: Benign fibrous histiocytoma of bone. Am J Surg Pathol 9:806, 1985.
25. Codman EA: Epiphyseal chondromatous giant cell tumors of the upper end of the humerus. Surg Gynecol Obstet 52:543, 1931.
26. Cohen EK, Kressel HY, Frank TS, et al: Hyaline cartilage-origin bone and soft-tissue neoplasms: MR appearance and histologic correlation. Radiology 167:477, 1988.
27. Dahlin DC: Bone tumors: General aspects and data on 6221 Cases, 3rd ed. Springfield, IL, Charles C Thomas, 1981.
28. Dahlin DC: Malignant osteoblastic tumors. *In* Taveras JM, Ferrucci JT (eds): Radiology: Diagnosis—Imaging—Intervention, Vol 5. Philadelphia, JB Lippincott, 1986.
29. Dahlin DC, Beabout JW: Dedifferentiation of low grade chondrosarcomas. Cancer 28:461, 1971.
30. Dahlin DC, Coventry MB: Osteogenic sarcoma: A study of six hundred cases. J Bone Joint Surg 49A:101, 1967.
31. Dahlin DC, Henderson ED: Mesenchymal chondrosarcoma: Further observations on a new entity. Cancer 15:410, 1962.
32. Dahlin DC, Ivins JC: Benign chondroblastoma. Cancer 30:401, 1972.
33. Dahlin DC, Ivins JC: Fibrosarcoma of bone: A study of 114 cases. Cancer 23:35, 1969.
34. Dahlin DC, Johnson EW Jr: Giant osteoid osteoma. J Bone Joint Surg 36A:559, 1956.
35. Dahlin DC, Unni KK: Osteosarcoma of bone and its important recognizable varieties. Am J Surg Pathol 1:61, 1977.
36. Dahlin DC, Unni KK: Bone Tumors, 4th ed. Springfield, IL, Charles C Thomas, 1986.
37. Dahlin DC, Unni KK, Matsuno T: Malignant (fibrous) histiocytoma of bone—fact or fancy? Cancer 39:1508, 1977.
38. DeLange EE, Pope TL Jr, Fechner RE: Dedifferentiated chondrosarcoma: Radiographic features. Radiology 160:489, 1986.
39. Deutsch A, Resnick D: Eccentric cortical metastases to the skeleton from bronchogenic carcinoma. Radiology 137:49, 1980.
40. Dorfman HD, Norman A, Wolff H: Fibrosarcoma complicating bone infarction in a caisson worker. A case report. J Bone Joint Surg 48A:528, 1966.
41. Dorfman HD, Weiss SW: Borderline osteoblastic tumors: Problems in the differential diagnosis of aggressive osteoblastoma and low-grade osteosarcoma. Semin Diagn Pathol 1:215, 1984.
42. Dosoretz DE, Raymond AK, Murphy GF, et al: Primary lymphoma of bone: The relationship of morphologic diversity to clinical behavior. Cancer 50:1009, 1983.
43. Edeiken J, Hodes PJ, Caplan LH: New bone production and periosteal reaction. AJR 97:708, 1966.
44. Edeiken J, Raymond AK, Ayala AG, et al: Small cell osteosarcoma. Skeletal Radiol 16:621, 1987.

45. Ehman RL, Berquist TH, McLeod RA: MR imaging of the musculoskeletal system: A 5-year appraisal. Radiology 166:313, 1988.
46. Eisenstein W, Pitcock JA: Adamantinoma of the tibia: An eccrine carcinoma. Arch Pathol Lab Med 108:246, 1984.
47. Evans HL, Ayala AG, Romsdahl MM: Prognostic factors in chondrosarcoma of bone. Cancer 40:818, 1977.
48. Feldman F, Hecht HI, Johnston AD: Chondromyxoid fibroma of bone. Radiology 94:249, 1970.
49. Feldman F, Lattes R: Primary malignant fibrous histiocytoma (fibrous xanthoma) of bone. Skeletal Radiol 1:145, 1977.
50. Frassica FJ, Unni KK: Dedifferentiated chondrosarcoma. J Bone Joint Surg 68A:1197, 1986.
51. Freiberger RH, Loitman BS, Halpern M, et al: Osteoid osteoma: Report of 80 cases. AJR 82:194, 1959.
52. Gardner EJ, Richards RE: Multiple cutaneous and subcutaneous lesions occurring simultaneously with hereditary polyposis and osteomatosis. Am J Hum Genet 5:139, 1953.
53. Greenspan A, Elguezabel A, Bryk D: Multifocal osteoid osteoma. A case report and review of the literature. AJR 121:103, 1974.
54. Greenspan A, Klein MJ, Lewis MM: Skeletal cortical metastases in the left femur arising from bronchogenic carcinoma. Skeletal Radiol 11:297, 1984.
55. Greenspan A, Norman A: Osteolytic cortical destruction: An unusual pattern of skeletal metastases. Skeletal Radiol 17:402, 1988.
56. Hall RB, Robinson LH, Malawer MM, et al: Periosteal osteosarcoma. Cancer 55:165, 1985.
57. Helms CA: Osteoid osteoma. The double density sign. Clin Orthop 222:167, 1987.
58. Henderson ED, Dahlin DC: Chondrosarcoma of bone: A study of 280 cases. J Bone Joint Surg 45A:1450, 1963.
59. Dahlin DC, Henderson ED: Mesenchymal chondrosarcoma: further observations on a new entity. Cancer 15:410, 1963.
60. Hudson TM, Chew FS, Manaster BJ: Scintigraphy of benign exostoses and exostotic chondrosarcomas. AJR 140:581, 1983.
61. Hudson TM, Hamlin DJ, Enneking WF, et al: Magnetic resonance imaging of bone and soft-tissue tumors: Early experience in 31 patients compared with computed tomography. Skeletal Radiol 13:134, 1985.
62. Hudson TM, Hawkins IF Jr: Radiological evaluation of chondroblastoma. Radiology 139:1, 1981.
63. Hudson TM, Spriengfield DS, Spanier SS, et al: Benign exostoses and exostotic chondrosarcomas: Evaluation of cartilage thickness by CT. Radiology 152:595, 1984.
64. Huvos AG: Bone Tumors, Diagnosis, Treatment and Prognosis. Philadelphia, WB Saunders Co, 1979.
65. Huvos AG, Higinbotham NL: Primary fibrosarcoma of bone. A clinicopathologic study of 130 patients. Cancer 35:837, 1975.
66. Jaffe HL: Osteoid osteoma. Arch Surg 31:709, 1935.
67. Jaffe HL, Lichtenstein L: Non-osteogenic fibroma of bone. Am J Pathol 18:205, 1942.
68. Jaffe HL: Hereditary multiple exostosis. Arch Pathol 36:335, 1943.
69. Jaffe HL: Aneurysmal bone cyst. Bull Hosp J Dis Orthop Inst 11:3, 1950.
70. Jaffe HL: Benign osteoblastoma. Bull Hosp J Dis Orthop Inst 17:141, 1956.
71. Jaffe HL: Tumors and Tumorous Conditions of the Bones and Joints. Philadelphia, Lea & Febiger, 1968.
72. Jaffe HL, Lichtenstein L: Solitary unicameral bone cyst with emphasis on the roentgen picture, pathologic appearance and pathogenesis. Arch Surg 44:1004, 1942.
73. Jaffe HL, Lichtenstein L: Benign chondroblastoma of bone: Reinterpretation of so-called calcifying or chondromatous giant cell tumor. Am J Pathol 18:969, 1942.
74. Jaffe HL, Lichtenstein L: Chondromyxoid fibroma of bone: A distinctive benign tumor likely to be mistaken especially for chondrosarcoma. Arch Pathol 45:541, 1948.
75. Kempson RL: Ossifying fibroma of the long bones. A light and electron microscopic study. Arch Pathol 82:218, 1966.
76. Kenney PJ, Gilula LA, Murphy WA: The use of computed tomography to distinguish osteochondroma and chondrosarcoma. Radiology 139:129, 1981.
77. Kricun ME: Radiographic evaluation of solitary bone lesions. Orthop Clin North Am 14:39, 1983.
78. Kumar R, David R, Cierney G III: Clear cell chondrosarcoma. Radiology 154:45, 1985.
79. Kyriakos M, Land VJ, Penning HL, et al: Metastatic chondroblastoma: Report of a fatal case with review of the literature on atypical, aggressive and malignant chondroblastoma. Cancer 55:1770, 1985.
80. Laredo JD, Reizine D, Bard M, Merland JJ: Vertebral hemangioma: Radiologic evaluation. Radiology 161:183, 1986.
81. Levine E, De Smet AA, Huntrakoon M: Juxtacortical osteosarcoma: A radiologic and histologic spectrum. Skeletal Radiol 14:38, 1985.
82. Lewis MM: The use of an expandable and adjustable prosthesis in the treatment of childhood malignant bone tumors of the extremity. Cancer 57:499, 1986.
83. Lewis MM, Schneider R: Percutaneous needle biopsy of bone. *In* Taveras JM, Ferrucci JT (eds): Radiology: Diagnosis—Imaging—Intervention, Vol 5. Philadelphia, JB Lippincott, 1986.
84. Lewis MM, Sissons HA, Norman A, Greenspan A: Benign and malignant cartilage tumors. *In* Instructional Course Lectures, Chicago, American Academy of Orthopaedic Surgeons, 1987, p 87.
85. Lichtenstein L, Hall JE: Periosteal chondroma: A distinctive benign cartilage tumor. J Bone Joint Surg 34A:691, 1952.
86. Lichtenstein L, Jaffe HL: Fibrous dysplasia of bone. Arch Pathol 33:777, 1942.
87. Lichtenstein L, Jaffe HL: Chondrosarcoma of bone. Am J Pathol 19:553, 1943.
88. Lichtenstein L, Jaffe HL: Ewing's sarcoma of bone. Am J Pathol 23:43, 1947.
89. Lindell MM Jr, Shirkhoda A, Raymond AK, et al: Parosteal osteosarcoma: Radiologic-pathologic correlation with emphasis on CT. AJR 148:323, 1987.
90. Ling L, Klein MJ, Sissons HA, et al: Expression of Ia and monocyte-macrophage lineage antigens in giant cell tumor of bone and related lesions. Arch Pathol Lab Med 112:65, 1988.
91. Lodwick GS: A systematic approach to the roentgen diagnosis of bone tumors. *In* Anderson Hospital and Tumor Institute: Tumors of the Bone and Soft Tissue. Chicago, Year Book Medical Publishers, 1965.
92. Lodwick GS, Wilson AJ, Farell C, et al: Determining growth rates of focal lesions of bone from radiographs. Radiology 134:577, 1980.
93. Marsh BW, Bonfiglio M, Brady LP, Enneking WF: Benign osteoblastoma: Range of manifestations. J Bone Joint Dis 57A:1, 1957.

94. Matsuno T, Unni KK, McLeod RA, et al: Telangiectatic osteogenic sarcoma. Cancer 38:2538, 1976.
95. McCarty EF, Dorfman HD: Chondrosarcoma of bone with dedifferentiation: A study of 18 cases. Hum Pathol 13:34, 1982.
96. McKenna RJ, Schwinn CP, Soong KY, et al: Osteogenic sarcoma arising in Paget's disease. Cancer 17:42, 1964.
97. McLeod RA, Beabout JW: The roentgenographic features of chondroblastoma. AJR 118:464, 1973.
98. Mirra JM, Gold R, Downs J, et al: A new histologic approach to the dedifferentiation of enchondroma and chondrosarcoma of the bones. Clin Orthop 201:214, 1985.
99. Mirra JM, Gold RH, Marcove RC: Bone Tumors, Diagnosis and Treatment. Philadelphia, JB Lippincott, 1980, p 186.
100. Mirra JM, Kendrick RA, Kendrick RE: Pseudomalignant osteoblastoma vs. arrested osteosarcoma. Cancer 37:2005, 1976.
101. Moll RH, Lee I, Gould VE, et al: Immunocytochemical analysis of Ewing's tumors. Am J Pathol 127:288, 1987.
102. Moser RP, Madewell JE: An approach to primary bone tumors. Radiol Clin North Am 25:1049, 1987.
103. Murray RO, Jacobson HG: The Radiology of Bone Diseases, 2nd ed. New York, Churchill Livingstone, 1977.
104. Norman A: Tumor and tumor-like lesions of the bones of the foot. Semin Roentgenol 5:407, 1970
105. Norman A: Persistence or recurrence of pain: A sign of surgical failure in osteoid osteoma. Clin Orthop 130:263, 1978.
106. Norman A, Abdelwahab IF, Buyon J, et al: Osteoid osteoma of the hip stimulating an early onset osteoarthritis. Radiology 158:417, 1986.
107. Norman A, Dorfman HD: Osteoid osteoma inducing pronounced overgrowth and deformity of bone. Clin Orthop 110:233, 1975.
108. Norman A, Sissons HA: Radiographic hallmarks of peripheral chondrosarcoma. Radiology 151:589, 1984.
109. Petterson H, Gillepsy T, Hamlin DJ, et al: Primary musculoskeletal tumors: Examination with MR imaging compared with conventional modalities. Radiology 164:237, 1987.
110. Petterson H, Slone RM, Spanier S, et al: Musculoskeletal tumors: T1 and T2 relaxation times. Radiology 167:783, 1988.
111. Reiter FB, Ackerman LV, Staple TW: Central chondrosarcoma of the appendicular skeleton. Radiology 105:525, 1972.
112. Richardson ML, Kilcoyne RF, Gilespy T III, et al: Magnetic resonance imaging of musculoskeletal neoplasms. Radiol Clin North Am 24:259, 1986.
113. Rock MG, Pritchard DJ, Unni KK: Metastases from histologically benign giant cell tumor of bone. J Bone Joint Surg 66A:269, 1984.
114. Rosai J: Adamantinoma of the tibia: Electron microscopic evidence of its epithelial origin. Am J Clin Pathol 51:786, 1969.
115. Rosai J, Pinkus GS: Immunohistochemical demonstration of epithelial differentiation in adamantinoma of the tibia. Am J Surg Pathol 6:427, 1982.
116. Sanerkin NG, Gallagher P: A review of the behavior of chondrosarcoma of bone. J Bone Joint Surg 61B:395, 1979.
117. Sanerkin NG, Woods CG: Fibrosarcomata and malignant fibrous histiocytomata arising in relation to enchondromata. J Bone Joint Surg 61B:366, 1979.
118. Schajowicz F: Tumors and Tumor-like Lesions of Bone and Joints. Berlin, Springer-Verlag, 1981.
119. Schajowicz F: Ewing's sarcoma and reticulum cell sarcoma of bone: With special reference to the histochemical demonstration of glycogen as an aid to differential diagnosis. J Bone Joint Surg 41A:394, 1959.
120. Schajowicz F: Juxtacortical chondrosarcoma. J Bone Joint Surg 59B:473, 1978.
121. Schajowicz F: Chondromyxoid fibroma: Report of three cases with predominant cortical involvement. Radiology 164:783, 1987.
122. Schajowicz F, Gallardo H: Epiphyseal chondroblastoma of bone: A clinicopathological study of 69 cases. J Bone Joint Surg 42B:205, 1970.
123. Schajowicz F, Gallardo H: Chondromyxoid fibroma. J Bone Joint Surg 53B:198, 1971.
124. Schajowicz F, Lemos C: Osteoid osteoma and osteoblastoma. Acta Orthop Scand 41:272, 1970.
125. Schajowicz F, McGuire MH, Santini E, et al: Osteosarcomas arising on the surfaces of long bones. J Bone Joint Surg 70A:555, 1988.
126. Schreiman JS, Crass JR, Wick MR, et al: Osteosarcoma: Role of CT in limb-sparing treatment. Radiology 161:485, 1986.
127. Sim FH, Unni KK, Beabout JW, et al: Osteosarcoma with small cells simulating Ewing's tumor. J Bone Joint Surg 61A:207, 1979.
128. Sissons HA, Kancherla PL, Lehman WB: Ossifying fibroma of bone. Report of two cases. Bull Hosp Jt Dis Orthop Inst 43:1, 1983.
129. Spjut HJ, Dorfman HD, Fechner RE, et al: Tumors of bone and cartilage. *In* Atlas of Tumor Pathology, Series 2 Fascicle 5. Washington, DC, Armed Forces Institute of Pathology, 1971.
130. Steiner GC: Benign cartilage tumors. *In* Taveras JM, Ferrucci JT (eds): Radiology: Diagnosis—Imaging—Intervention, Vol 5. Philadelphia, JB Lippincott, 1986.
131. Strauchen JA, Dimitriu-Bona A: Malignant fibrous histiocytoma: Expression of monocyte-macrophage differentiation antigens detected with monoclonal antibodies. Am J Pathol 124:303, 1986.
132. Sundaram M, McGuire MH, Herbold DR, et al: Magnetic resonance imaging in planning limb-salvage surgery for primary malignant tumors of bone. J Bone Joint Surg 68A:809, 1986.
133. Tetu B, Ordonez NG, Ayala AG, et al: Chondrosarcoma with additional mesenchymal component (dedifferentiated chondrosarcoma). An immunohistochemical and electron microscopic study. Cancer 58:287, 1986.
134. Thrall JH, Ellis BI: Skeletal metastases. Radiol Clin North Am 25:1155, 1987.
135. Unger EC, Kessler HB, Kowalyshyn MJ, et al: MR imaging of Maffucci syndrome. AJR 150:351, 1988.
136. Unni KK: Osteosarcoma of bone. *In* Unni K (ed): Bone Tumors. New York, Churchill Livingstone, 1988, p 107.
137. Unni KK, Dahlin DC, Beabout JW: Periosteal osteogenic sarcoma. Cancer 37:2476, 1976.
138. Unni KK, Dahlin DC: Premalignant tumors and conditions of bone. Am J Surg Pathol 3:47, 1979.
139. Unni KK, Dahlin DC, Beabout JW, et al: Chondrosarcoma: Clear cell variant: A report of 16 cases. J Bone Joint Surg 58A:676, 1976.
140. Unni KK, Dahlin DC, Beabout JW, et al: Parosteal osteogenic sarcoma. Cancer 37:2466, 1976.

141. Unni KK, Dahlin DC, McLeod RA: Intraosseous well-differentiated osteosarcoma. Cancer 40:1337, 1977.
142. Van Der Heul RO, Von Ronnen JR: Juxtacortical osteosarcoma: Diagnosis, differential diagnosis, treatment, and an analysis of eighty cases. J Bone Joint Surg 49A:415, 1967.
143. Watt I: Isotope scanning of the musculoskeletal system. Curr Orthop 1:324, 1987.
144. Wester SM, Beabout JW, Unni KK, et al: Langerhans cell granulomatosis (histiocytosis X) of bone in adults. Am J Surg Pathol 6:413, 1982.
145. Wilner D: Radiology of Bone Tumors and Allied Disorders. Philadelphia, Lea & Febiger, 1982.
146. Wold LE: Fibrohistiocytic tumors of bone. *In* Unni KK (ed): Bone Tumors. New York, Churchill Livingstone, 1988, p 183.
147. Wold LE, Unni KK, Beabout JW, et al: High grade surface osteosarcomas. Am J Surg Pathol 8:181, 1984.
148. Wold LE, Unni KK, Beabout JW, et al: Dedifferentiated parosteal osteosarcoma. J Bone Joint Surg 66A:53, 1984.
149. Wood GS, Beckstead JH, Turner RR, et al: Malignant fibrous histiocytoma cells do not express the antigenic or enzyme histochemical features of cells of monocyte/macrophage lineage. Lab Invest 52:78A, 1985.
150. Yabut MS, Kenan S, Sissons HA: Malignant transformation of fibrous dysplasia. Clin Orthop 228:281, 1988.
151. Zimmer WD, Berquist TH, McLeod RA, et al: Bone tumors: Magnetic resonance imaging versus computed tomography. Radiology 155:709, 1985.

CHAPTER 3

Principles of Pediatric Oncology

BEVERLY R. RYAN

The topography of pediatric oncology has undergone dramatic changes in the past 25 years. Many advances made through cooperative group clinical research and basic research have given the clinician in this specialty the means to decrease mortality significantly.

Cancer in the child represents slightly less than 1% of the malignancies diagnosed per year in the United States.[46] This is approximately 6000 to 7000 new cases, or 12 per 100,000 population younger than the age of 15 years.[23] The predominant type of cancer is leukemia, which constitutes 30 to 40% of diagnoses. Acute lymphoblastic leukemia (ALL) accounts for 80% of all leukemias seen in children: chronic leukemias represent 1% or less of all leukemias in children. Tumors of the central nervous system (CNS) are the second most common malignancy, with an overall incidence of 20%. The incidence of CNS tumors is somewhat lower in those younger than 5 years of age, and higher in those 5 to 10 years old. Lymphomas have an incidence of 12% of malignant tumors, and Hodgkin's disease accounts for 45% of malignant lymphomas. The incidence of other tumor types is as follows: bone sarcoma, 7%; Wilms' tumor, 5%; neuroblastoma, 5%; soft tissue sarcoma, 5%; retinoblastoma, 3%; and other types, 10%.[16, 18, 23, 33]

Except for accidents, cancer is the leading cause of childhood mortality, accounting for 11.3% of childhood deaths in 1981.[16] Childhood deaths from cancer have, in turn, decreased by 50% since 1965.[34] Death rates have decreased by 80% in Hodgkin's disease, 68% in Wilms' tumor, and 50% from leukemia and bone sarcomas.[34]

Today, childhood cancer is approached with the attitude that it is curable. Survival statistics support this optimism. For leukemia in the mid-1960s, the median survival was less than 1 year, with fewer than 1% of patients alive 5 years from the time of diagnosis.[31] For ALL, up to 60% of children with currently diagnosed disease can expect to remain disease free for more than 5 years, with an excellent chance of being cured.[39] For solid tumors, the overall 2-year survival rate is 60%, as compared with below 20% in 1940. This figure is as high as 90% for Wilms' tumor and 80% for Hodgkin's disease.[18]

The reasons that pediatric malignancies have become curable are the basis for understanding the field as a whole. Although there have been many contributions and accomplishments, some are recognized by pediatric oncologists as being singularly significant. Because incidence numbers are small, it has taken the collaboration of many to collect, process, analyze, and build on the results obtained through clinical protocols. These protocols are developed, are monitored, reach statistical significance, and are used for the development of newer protocols for increased efficacy and decreased toxicity under the auspices of a cooperative group. There are two such national groups in the United States today: Children's Cancer Study Group and Pediatric Oncology Group.[45] It has been shown that children treated according to nationally recognized protocols have significantly improved survival.[27, 29, 46]

The realization that combination chemotherapy increases efficacy and impedes the emergence of drug resistance improved the basic therapeutic approach to the child with cancer. Another major contribution was the use of prophylactic CNS therapy in ALL as a protection against CNS relapse. The use of intrathecal drugs and, in selected subsets of patients, cranial irradiation as prophylaxis has decreased the incidence of CNS leukemia from 40% to between 2 and 8%. This should result in fewer bone marrow relapses and an improved cure rate.[32]

The concepts of tailoring therapy to certain subgroups within the same tumor type and treating children with unfavorable tumor characteristics more aggressively have become well recognized. This not only increases the chances of survival in poor-risk patients, but also avoids unneeded toxicity in patients who would respond well with lesser therapy. Prognostic variables for many pediatric tumor types, enable the selection of patients (by risk) for the purpose of adjusting the intensity of therapy (Table 3–1). The variables change as more is understood about the tumor's biologic features and lose significance as therapy becomes more effective.[39] However, their use has allowed some sets of patients to be treated more intensively, thereby increasing survival as well as knowledge of supportive care. Advances in the treatment modalities of surgery, radiation therapy, and chemotherapy have significantly added to the curability of childhood cancer.

DIFFERENCES BETWEEN ADULT AND PEDIATRIC MALIGNANCIES

Children are not microcopies of adults. The differences between children and adults are nowhere more notable than in the practice of pediatric oncology. Appreciating these differences expands the understanding of malignant tumors in children.

Tumor Types

Carcinomas account for 85% of the tumors seen in adults, yet they are rare neoplasms in children. Childhood malignancies arise predominantly in lymphoreticular, CNS, and connective tissue and viscera.[29] Many are embryonal tumors such as Wilms' tumor, neuroblastoma, medulloblastoma, retinoblastoma, and hepatoblastoma, with peak incidence in patients younger than 5 years of age. In general, tumors are heritable in a small percentage of cases; however, up to 40% of retinoblastomas may be inherited. This becomes important for surveillance and detection purposes, because children with heritable forms of tumors are at greater risk for second malignant neoplasms. As the capacity of molecular genetic study increases, DNA probes will identify high-risk groups, thereby improving surveillance and early detection.

Detection and Screening

In children, tumors are often deep seated and thus are sometimes discovered accidentally at an advanced stage. In addition, childhood tumors are not as amenable to screening programs as are some adult malignancies.

Surveillance should be more stringent for those who may have a predisposition to the development of a malignancy. This includes children with the following conditions:

1. Chromosome instability syndromes (e.g., telangiectasia, xeroderma pigmentosum, Fanconi's syndrome, Bloom's syndrome)
2. Immunodeficiency states
3. Chromosomal abnormalities, such as Down's syndrome
4. Congenital abnormalities (e.g., hemihypertropy is associated with an increased risk for Wilms' tumor)
5. Neurocutaneous syndromes, such as neurofibromatosis
6. Cancer family syndromes[17]

Because the incidence of childhood cancer is low, an increased index of suspicion is necessary for earlier detection. Malignancy should be included in the differential diagnosis of any prolonged or unexplained fever, pain, or mass, especially if it is progressive.[24] Also arousing

TABLE 3–1

Prognostic Variables in Common Pediatric Malignancies

Tumor Type	Prognostic Variable	Expected Effect on Outcome
Acute lymphoblastic leukemia[31]	Age	
	<12 mo	Poor
	2–10 y	Good
	White blood cell count	
	Low (<10,000)	Good
	High (>50,000)	Poor
	Bulky disease at presentation	Poor
	Thoracic mass	
	Adenopathy >3 cm	
	Liver/spleen at or below umbilicus	
	Cytogenetics	
	Hyperdiploid	Good
	Hypodiploid	Poor
	Translocations	Poor
	Immunophenotype	
	B cell precursors	Good
	Undifferentiated	Poor
	Biphenotypic	Poor
	Mature T/B cell	Poor
	Rapid response to therapy: <5% blasts in marrow at d 14	Good
	Presence of immunodeficiency syndrome at diagnosis	Poor
Medulloblastoma[14]	Age: <4 y	Poor
	Dissemination	Poor
	Large tumor at presentation (T3, T4 Chang classification)	Poor
	Residual tumor after initial surgery	Poor
Wilms' tumor[15]	Unfavorable histologic findings	
	Anaplasia stage II–IV	Poor
	Clear cell, II–IV	Poor
Neuroblastoma[13]	Age: <1 y	Good
	Extent of disease	
	Stage I, II, IV	Good
	Stage III, IV	Poor
	*N-*myc* oncogene amplification	Poor
	*Neuron-specific enolase level elevation	Poor

*Actual impact on survival still under investigation.

suspicion should be pallor; purpura; changes in balance, gait, or personality; and squinting or changes in the eye.[12]

Neuroblastoma is an example of a tumor that presents with extensive disease in 60% of cases. Neuroblastoma arises from neuroectodermal tissue and has an incidence of 8 per 1 million population per year and a peak incidence in those younger than 4 years of age. There is a 10% long-term survival rate if advanced disease is diagnosed when the child is older than 1 year of age. Because, in more than 90% of cases, neuroblastoma secretes degradation products of tyrosine metabolism in the urine, it has become a prototype pediatric tumor in which mass screening may offer early detection and change the survival rates. Such mass screening was undertaken in Sapporo City, Japan, using urine obtained by filter paper for quantitative analysis of vanillylmandelic acid/homovanillic acid ratios.[37] From 1981 to 1986, 73,226 infants were screened. Eleven cases of neuroblastoma were detected by screening. More importantly, the 48-month survival rate improved from 21.3 to 87.5%, with early-stage disease at presentation (stages I, II, and IV) increasing from 22.9 to 61.1%. The survival in another area of the country not screened only improved from 21.1 to 28.1%.[37] Although the numbers are small, the expenditures are justified in that the cost of a large-scale screening to detect one case of neuroblastoma amounts to between 10 and 33% of the treatment costs of just one case.[17]

Tumor Response

Even children with advanced disease generally respond well to therapy, with cure rates greater than 50%. This may relate to the doubling time of pediatric tumors. It is known that, to be clinically appreciated by imaging studies or physical examination, a tumor mass must be at least 0.5 cm in diameter. In cell numbers, this represents 1.5×10^8 cells. Assuming that one cell gives rise to two equally prolific cells, this represents 27 doublings. Approximately 40 doublings result in 1.1×10^{12} cells, or a 1-kg mass. Success of chemotherapy, which is most effective for rapidly dividing cells, is related to the tumor growth rate (volume doubling time):

Group I: doubling times <30 days
Group II: doubling times ≥30 days to ≤80 days
Group III: doubling times ≥80 days

Virtually all the tumor types seen in pediatrics are group I, which may explain the chemosensitivity of most childhood cancers.[1]

Multidisciplinary Team

Childhood malignant tumors are considered a chronic disease. Therapy is intensive, is prolonged, and requires the concerted efforts of pediatric oncologists, radiotherapists, surgeons, pathologists, and radiologists. However, personnel from ancillary disciplines are also highly visible in the care of the child with cancer to ensure a functional cure. These include oncology nurses, psychologists, social workers, play therapists, nutritionists, and a school liaison/advocate (preferably a teacher on the team).

These resource personnel can best be gathered and supported at a regional medical center, often defined as a member or an affiliate of a national pediatric oncology cooperative group.[46] Often, care is shared between the patient's local pediatrician and personnel at a medical referral center to lessen the nonmedical expenses of care, which have been shown to amount to potentially more than 25% of weekly family income.[33] However, it has been shown that children's outcomes are better when they are treated by established protocols and risk is increased when patients are treated without support from a multidisciplinary team.[29]

Etiology

The etiology of most childhood cancers remains an enigma. Genetic predispositions have been theorized. Environmental carcinogens may induce tumor genesis through gene mutation. Because the number of pediatric tumors is small, epidemiologic studies have been hampered. Case reports have established that there is an increased risk of cancer associated with 200 different types of single-gene disorders. Environmental agents with strong links to the risk of cancer development include prenatal exposure to diethylstilbestrol and postnatal irradiation.

ONCOGENES

As scientists have become more proficient at deciphering the 6 billion pairs of DNA that make up a cell's genome, there has been an explosion of knowledge regarding the role of individual genes in initiating, maintaining, and directing growth and differentiation of cells. It seems implausible that a gene composed of 5000 nucleotide base pairs can alter the growth of a cell with a millionfold-larger genome, but that, in fact, has been observed in experimental models. Genetic material introduced by injection (viral genome insertion) or transfection (the transfer of DNA from tumor to normal cell) can transform a normally functioning cell into a malignant one unleashed from its regular constraints of growth and differentiation.[4, 48]

Strong evidence is accumulating that cancer is a genetically engineered alteration of normal growth and differentiation.[10, 41] The evolution from an initial event to a macroscopic tumor is probably a multistep process. In the early 1970s, work with tumor viruses seemed to clarify one element in that process. It was shown that DNA from the papovavirus simian virus 40 (SV40) and polyomavirus could insert into the genome of individual cultured cells, giving them the potential for malignant growth, and that after the DNA took up permanent residence, its continued presence was required to maintain the transformed state.[48] This viral gene or oncogene (so called because of oncogenic potential) closely resembled genes already found in vertebrate organisms. These genes, normally found also in humans if triggered by viral or nonviral mechanisms, could cause tumorigenesis. The mechanisms for triggering these human cancer-inducing genes (proto-oncogenes, cellular oncogenes) include mutation, translocation, amplification, and chromosome deletion. To date, about 50 oncogenes are known; however, oncogenes have been detected in only 15 to 20% of human tumors.[48]

It is speculated that cellular oncogenes function in growth and differentiation through the production of proteins. A variety of proteins have been found to be encoded by viral oncogenes as well. These protein products have included growth factors and cell surface receptors, proteins that function in controlling cellular proliferation and differentiation.[31] It is attractive to theorize about a cancer therapeutic agent targeted to oncogenes and their cellular products, because, unlike surface protein antigens that may modulate, oncogenes and their products must remain associated with the transformed cell and active to ensure its malignant growth.[27]

An often-used example of oncogene expression is Burkitt's lymphoma, in which a translocation changes the position of the c-*myc* oncogene from chromosome 8 to a locus adjacent to one of the immunoglobulin genes. In Burkitt's lymphoma, the promotor, which controls immunoglobulin production, assumes control of the transcription of c-*myc,* whose gene product functions normally but whose expression is altered by its new location.[41]

A malignant transformation may not only be actively expressed but may also occur secondarily to failure of normal suppression. Recently, genes whose deletions unleashed tumorigenesis were discovered. Although these genes have been functionally described as growth suppressor genes, they have also been called antioncogenes. Just such a gene has been isolated in the chromosome's 13q14 region and represents the first human recessive cancer gene ever cloned.[5] Deletion of both alleles at this location was found in some cases of retinoblastoma and osteosarcoma. A single locus deletion may be found in germ cells and passed from one generation to the next, being the initial event required for the subsequent development of retinoblastoma. The 40% of retinoblastomas that are hereditary may be activated by an acquired insult: deletion of the remaining gene may result in alteration to a malignant clone. The loss of suppressor genes may be common in the development of cancer. Deletion of these genes in the germ cell might confer a lifelong increased risk of cancer development.[47]

CHROMOSOMAL ABNORMALITIES

As noted, chromosomal changes may trigger or reflect an insult that ultimately is a link in the chain of events leading to a malignancy. However, these changes have also served as markers and prognostic variables, allowing the individualization of therapy to fit the risk.[40]

In ALL, 40% of children have demonstrated hypoploidy or hyperploidy. Pseudodiploidy (translocations) are found in 10 to 20%. Thirty-five per cent have normal diploid cells. Children demonstrating translocation or hypoploidy have had shorter disease-free survival. Translocations reported in ALL have included t(4;11), occurring predominately in children younger than 1 year at diagnosis; t(9;22), a Philadelphia chromosome associated with a poorer prognosis, which is seen in 3 to 4% of cases of ALL; and t(11;14), with an appearance in about 25% of T cell ALL.[31]

The field of molecular genetics continues to enlighten scientists about the biologic characteristics of the cancerous cell. Clinical application of these discoveries may help prevent, detect earlier, diagnose, and destroy a cancerous clone of cells.

IMMUNE SURVEILLANCE

Although the search for the cause and control of cancer has included genetic theories, the immune surveillance theory remains an attractive hypothesis and a force in creating new therapeutic options.[38] The main tenets are that cancer cells are antigenic, they can be destroyed by an immune response, and immunosuppression is associated with the development of cancer.

There is the suggestion that immune surveillance may operate only in those tumors induced by oncogenic viruses and ultraviolet radiation. Evidence in support of this comes from studies showing that tumors induced by carcinogens and those arising spontaneously vary in their ability to induce protective immunity. However, in a large number of tumor models, tumor-associated cellular neoantigens are identified.[21] Research is ongoing in using these antigens as targets for monoclonal antibodies alone or for conjugating antibodies with radioisotopes or toxins.

A problem with immune therapies may arise because of variable antigen expression and also ineffectual host immune response. Although poor immune response was previously thought to be due solely to circulating blocking factors, there is evidence for an immune suppressor cell network in cancer, which would enhance tumor growth. In general, these reactions, possibly mediated by macrophage-like cells or T cells, seem related to total body tumor burdens. In mice, there is evidence that suppressor cell activity rapidly declined after tumor was excised.[8] The extrapolation and application of these theories to human cancer remains an ongoing challenge.

Therapy

Surgery, radiation, and chemotherapy are the primary and conventional therapeutic modalities in pediatric oncology. Often, they are used in combination. Chemotherapy, used as adjuvant therapy, is known to be more effective in small-bulk disease and micrometastatic foci than in large-bulk disease. In a review of its surviving population, a major pediatric cancer center found that 80% of the children had received some combination of surgery, radiation, and chemotherapy; 30% had received all thrcc.[25]

Advances in and wider application of all three modalities have helped increase the survival statistics in pediatric cancers. For instance, even though first reported in 1939, resection of pulmonary metastasis in osteogenic sarcoma only became accepted as effective therapy in the 1980s, with 5-year survival rates of 40%.[20]

The practice of placing right atrial catheters (Hickman, Broviac, or implantation reservoirs) has alleviated much discomfort and distress for the child by allowing easy access for drawing blood and administering chemotherapy and supportive care. Infection and clotting associated with catheters are problems that need close surveillance but have been manageable.[20, 42]

RADIATION THERAPY

Radiation therapy is tolerated fairly well in the child. However, the late effects may be more pronounced than those in adults. In planning therapy, special emphasis is placed on possible growth, endocrine, neuropsychologic, and neoplastic sequelae. Attention is also paid to the concurrent use of drugs that may enhance radiation effect and/or toxicity, such as the radiosensitizers actinomycin D and the anthracyclines. Radiotherapy equipment with greater capabilities and treatment planning using a simulator have brought greater sophistication to the use of radiotherapy for the pediatric patient.[44]

CHEMOTHERAPY

Principles

The effectiveness of chemotherapy in pediatric oncology has accounted for a substantial number of successes in overcoming previously low survival rates. Significant increases in survival rates with the use of adjuvant therapy have been noted for Wilms' tumor, lymphomas, leukemia, and rhabdomyosarcomas. The introduction of new drugs and drug combination protocols has been greatly facilitated by rigorously monitored investigational studies. Before its conventional use, a drug is assessed in phase I, II, and III studies to determine its efficacy and toxicity (Table 3–2).

In using a chemotherapeutic drug or combinations, certain well-known principles are utilized; one is that drugs are used in maximally tolerated doses. The hypothesis of Shipper, Schabel, and Wilcox is that these drugs obey first-order kinetics; i.e., increasing the drug dosage leads to an exponential decrease in the percentage of surviving cells. To increase the percentage killed, one must increase the dosage. Obviously, host toxicity limits dosage. However, using drugs in combination can add efficacy and may even delay the emergence of drug resistance.[1]

Therapy should be instituted as rapidly as possible. This is based on the Goldie Goldman hypothesis that the number of resistant cells increases with time. Tumors with large volumes are probably more resistant.[1]

TABLE 3–2
Clinical Trials

Phase I	New drug is evaluated for maximally tolerated dose and toxicity. Trials test clinical pharmacology. Drug dosages are increased in sequential groups of patients.
Phase II	Drugs are screened for their effectiveness in variety of tumor types. Disease must be measurable and evaluable to assess response.
Phase III	Drugs are used alone or in combination to establish firmly efficacy and their role in therapy.

In using combinations, one should select drugs with different mechanisms of action, toxicities, and durations or peaks of toxic effect. In selecting drug combinations with different mechanisms of action, drug classification is considered. A drug cannot always be strictly classified; however, three general categories are recognized:

Class I: drugs that kill proliferating and nonproliferating (resting) cells, i.e., independent of cell cycles

Class II: drugs particularly effective in one phase, usually the S phase of protein synthesis in the cell cycle

Class III: drugs that are cycle specific, killing proliferating cells but not as effective for resting cells.[1]

Class II drugs may have greater affinity for tumor cells because tumors may have more cells in S phase than normal tissue does. However, with drugs in both classes II and III, normal tissue sparing is lost because exposure time is increased.

Norton and Simon's proposal indicates that the growth-inhibiting effect of a therapy is proportional to the growth rate of untreated tumor.[1] This helps support the inclination to effect a rapid initial decrease in tumor bulk, treat known sanctuary sites, apply vigorous combination therapy for maintenance, and consider a late intensification phase. These principles have been used with success in patients with poor-risk leukemia and osteogenic sarcoma.[1]

Side Effects

Commonly used chemotherapeutic agents, their actions, side effects, and indications are outlined in Table 3–3.

Because all chemotherapeutic agents lack absolute specificity for tumor cells, normal cells (especially those in organ systems with rapid turnover) are affected. Side effects are acute, delayed, and late. Late effects involve growth disturbances, hormonal dysfunction, increased risk of second malignant neoplasms, and neuropsychologic alterations.

Acute effects are predominantly nausea and vomiting. Antiemetics, singly or in combination, are used to manage this distressing symptom, which is triggered by both local and central mechanisms. A few drugs, including cytarabine (Ara-C) and bleomycin, can induce fever. There is always the possibility of an acute allergic reaction with L-asparaginase.

Delayed effects include bone marrow suppression and immunosuppression, stomatitis, disruption of small bowel villi, hair loss, and specific organ effects of certain drugs. This latter effect may be influenced by cumulative dosages. The anthracylines may cause ventricular failure and arrhythmias. Methotrexate and 6-mercaptopurine are hepatotoxic, and their administration may lead to varying degrees of hepatic fibrosis. Cyclophosphamide (Cytoxan) can cause hemorrhagic cystitis, with development of hematuria months to years after its use. The nitrosoureas, busulfan, bleomycin, cyclophosphamide, and methotrexate may cause interstitial pneumonitis and late pulmonary fibrosis.

SUPPORTIVE CARE

The principles of chemotherapy and impressive advances in survival have supported the use of aggressive therapy in selected situations. The problems of this approach require diligent surveillance, immediate response, and institutional resources.

Susceptibility to infection is a major concern. This susceptibility is increased by the myelosuppressive effects of chemotherapy and the breakdown of protective barriers, which occurs in gastrointestinal muscosal ulceration and with the use of central venous catheters. The use of prophylactic oral trimethoprim-sulfa, using a 3 day per week regimen, and prophylactic antifungal therapy has become standard in certain aggressive protocols. The surveillance of immunoglobulins and monthly administration of intravenous IgG in deficient patients have become recognized as effective adjuncts, especially in treating the infant with leukemia. Exposure to varicella in susceptible children poses the threat of disseminated disease. Some children have received prophylactic varicella vaccine; its efficacy is being demonstrated.[15a] Others receive varicella-zoster immunoglobulin as passive immunization on exposure in an attempt to modify the virulence of infection. Influenza vaccine is also tolerated and recommended in children receiving chemotherapy.

Fever and neutropenia require parenteral antibiotic therapy. Drug combinations are used for their synergistic effects, broad-spectrum coverage, and control of multiple-organism infection. The neutropenia of myelosuppression from chemotherapy often necessitates 2 to 3 weeks for recovery. A recent study of

TABLE 3–3

Commonly Used Chemotherapeutic Agents in Children

Drug	Class/Mechanism	Side Effects	Comments and Common Usage
I. Plant Alkaloids			
Vincristine (VCR; Oncovin)	Class II/S phase	Neurotoxicity (ileus; paresthesias; areflexia; jaw, leg, and abdominal pain; ptosis; changes in gait; cranial nerve palsies) Ulceration with extravasation Alopecia SIADH Seizures	All, Wilms' tumor, rhabdomyosarcoma and other soft tissue sarcomas Brain tumors
Vinblastine (VLB, Velban)	Class II/S phase	Bone marrow suppression Ulceration with extravasation, anorexia, nausea, vomiting, alopecia	Hodgkin's disease, Langhans' cell histiocytosis and testicular cancer
Etoposide (VP-16-213)	Class II	Bone marrow suppression Alopecia Nausea, vomiting *Fever *Generalized erythema *Bronchospasm Hypertension	Hodgkin's disease Neuroblastoma Rhabdomyosarcoma Testicular cancer NHL Leukemia
II. Antimetabolites			
Methotrexate (MTX)	Class II/S phase	Bone marrow suppression Mucositis/stomatitis Liver enzyme elevations/ fibrosis Alopecia Leukoencephalopathy Skin rashes Renal toxicity in high-dose schedules	ALL Burkitt's lymphoma Osteogenic sarcoma (high dose) Intrathecal administration as CNS prophylaxis in ALL
6-Mercaptopurine (6-MP)	Class II/S phase	Bone marrow suppression Stomatitis Hepatic dysfunction	ALL
Cytarabine (Ara-C, cytosine arabinoside)	Class II/S and early G_2 phase	Bone marrow suppression Nausea, vomiting, diarrhea Stomatitis Fever In high dosage, CNS dysfunction and conjunctivitis	ALL Intrathecal administration for CNS prophylaxis Very high dosages in AML and ALL relapse
III. Antibiotics			
Doxorubicin (ADM, Adriamycin)	Class III/all phases	Bone marrow/suppression Nausea, vomiting Stomatitis Alopecia Cardiac toxicity (below cumulative dose of 550 mg/ m^2 incidence of congestive heart failure $<1\%$) Pneumonitis, esophagitis, and dermatitis in previously irradiated areas Ulceration with extravasation	ALL AML NHL Osteogenic sarcoma Ewing's sarcoma Rhabdomyosarcoma Neuroblastoma Hodgkin's disease Following administration, excretion of red urine Irradiation to heart increases risk of cardiac toxicity; total cumulative dose should be reduced
Daunorubicin (daunomycin)	Class III	Toxicities similar to those with doxorubicin	ALL AML NHL

TABLE 3–3
Commonly Used Chemotherapeutic Agents in Children *Continued*

Drug	Class/Mechanism	Side Effects	Comments and Common Usage
Actinomycin D (dactinomycin)	Class III	Bone marrow suppression Nausea, vomiting, diarrhea Mucositis/stomatitis Ulceration with extravasation Skin rash Radiation recall	Wilms' tumor Rhabdomyosarcoma Ewing's sarcoma Testicular tumors
Bleomycin (Blenoxane)	Class III	Pulmonary toxicity (dyspnea, cough, rales) Fibrosis (incidence increases sharply with cumulative doses >400 mg) Cutaneous lesions (induration/erythema of fingers, hands, and areas of previous irradiation) Alopecia Nausea Fever	Hodgkin's disease Testicular tumors Carcinomas of head or neck
IV. Alkylating agents			
Cyclophosphamide (CTX, Cytoxan)	Class III	Bone marrow suppression Nausea, vomiting Hemorrhagic cystitis SIADH Alopecia	ALL Burkitt's lymphoma Rhabdomyosarcoma Ewing's sarcoma Hodgkin's disease NHL Neuroblastoma Brain tumors
Mechlorethamine (nitrogen mustard, mustargen)	Class III	Bone marrow suppression Alopecia Nausea, vomiting Ulceration with extravasation	Hodgkin's disease
Carmustine (bischloroethylnitrosourea, BCNU)	Class I	Delayed bone marrow suppression (4–6 wk) Nausea, vomiting	Brain tumors Lymphomas
Cisplatin (*cis*-diamminedichloroplatinum, CDDP)	Class III	Bone marrow suppression Nausea and vomiting Neurotoxicity Renal toxicity Ototoxicity	Neuroblastoma Osteogenic sarcoma Brain tumors Ovarian/testicular tumors
Dacarbazine (dimethyltriazenoimidazolecarboxamide, DTIC)	Class III	Bone marrow suppression Nausea, vomiting Alopecia Influenza syndrome (fever, myalgia, malaise)	Soft tissue sarcomas Neuroblastoma
V. Enzymes			
L-Asparaginase (L-asp)	G_1 phase	Hypersensitivity reaction Pancreatitis Hyperglycemia Liver dysfunction Coagulation abnormalities (decreased fibrinogen, factor IX, and antithrombin III levels) CNS problems (lethargy, somnolence, confusion)	ALL

*Responsive to antihistamine and discontinuation of infusion.

ALL, acute lymphocytic leukemia; AML, acute myelogenous leukemia; CNS, central nervous system; NHL, non-Hodgkin's lymphoma; SIADH, syndrome of inappropriate antidiuretic hormone.

Data from Adelson HT: Cancer chemotherapy. *In* Nathan DG, Oski FH (eds): Hematology of Infancy and Childhood, 3rd ed. Philadelphia, WB Saunders Co, 1987; and Niski M, Miyake H, Taneda T, et al: Effect of mass screening of neuroblastoma in Sapporo City. Cancer 60:433–436, 1987.

recombinant human granulocyte-macrophage colony-stimulating factor (RhGM-CSF) showed a significant increase in white blood cell counts and granulocyte counts in patients with leukemia using a central venous infusion.[2] There is future promise using RhGM-CSF for safer and perhaps more efficient administration of chemotherapy.

Bleeding may be a problem because of decreased platelet counts and coagulation factor abnormalities as a result of therapy or as a manifestation of disseminated intravascular coagulation. The aggressive use of irradiated blood products has facilitated correction of these complications.

Other supportive measures include total parenteral nutrition, magnesium replacement during and after cisplatin therapy, administration of mesna as a uroprotective agent for the hemorrhagic cystitis that may accompany cyclophosphamide (Cytoxan) or ifosfamide therapy, hydration with the use of cyclophosphamide and cisplatin, and parenteral and/or epidural narcotic infusions for severe pain.

BONE MARROW TRANSPLANT

There are groups of patients still being defined in whom the risk/benefit ratio of bone marrow transplant outweighs that of salvage chemotherapy. In patients with acute myelogenous leukemia with an HLA-matched sibling in first bone marrow remission, the advantage is apparent. Those patients with ALL who sustain a bone marrow relapse while receiving initial therapy have a grim prognosis with chemotherapy alone. Recently, a 30% salvage rate was obtained with aggressive chemotherapy in patients who experienced relapse 18 months or longer after diagnosis. However, prolonged disease-free survival was 20% or less in those who had relapsed early in treatment. Patients receiving allogeneic bone marrow transplant while in second remission have a prolonged disease-free survival of 60%. The recommendation is for either an allogeneic or an autologous (with marrow purging) bone marrow transplant in those ALL patients with bone marrow relapse occurring during therapy or within 12 months of completing therapy.[32]

Another area of investigation is the use of marrow transplantation in the child older than 1 year of age with advanced-stage neuroblastoma. Results of one study showed that, for patients treated after initial therapy but before disease progression, 8 of 13 were alive at 3 years.[3] Results are preliminary with this modality and await further clinical trials.

Therapy of poor-risk patients remains a challenge for the pediatric oncologist. In addition, there is the responsibility for the development and application of new and innovative therapies, which would improve the efficacy and decrease the toxicity of currently used regimens.

Future directions in therapy include the investigation of monoclonal antibodies for imaging and therapy, new chemotherapeutic agents, intraoperative radiation and autologous purging in bone marrow transplantation.

LATE EFFECTS

In 1980, the projection was made that by 1990 1 in 1000 children reaching the age of 20 years would be a survivor of childhood cancer.[28] This added emphasis to assessing the late effects of therapy. Not only pediatric oncologists but also all health care providers should be familiar with the sequelae of therapy in a growing population of survivors.

The effects often relate to the modality of therapy used. For instance, linear growth in children receiving only chemotherapy is usually normal. However, in children who received cranial irradiation for brain tumors or CNS leukemia prophylaxis and/or therapy, growth problems are common.[9, 26] In assessing late effects, the areas of concern are

1. Growth
2. Thyroid function
3. Gonadal function
4. Neuropsychologic effects
5. Second malignant neoplasm
6. Specific late organ damage, such as liver fibrosis

Growth impairment may be attributed to the direct effect of radiation therapy, deficient growth hormone levels, decreased somatomedin production (either primary or secondary to decreased growth hormone production), and the general effects of chronic disease. The direct effects of radiation therapy on growing bone, especially the spine, are most evident in the younger child (younger than 6 years old) and during puberty. If only a portion of the vertebral body is irradiated, scoliosis may occur, whereas damage to the growth center ultimately results in a decrease in sitting height, especially when doses in excess of 20 Gy are given.[9] It is estimated that 15% of children having prolonged survival after cranial irradiation will show growth abnormalities.[9] Children's heights should be followed closely. Any child showing less than 4 cm in height gain per year should be assessed by provocative testing for growth hormone deficiency.

Thyroid abnormalities in the irradiated child have long been recognized. Decreases of thyroxine and/or increases of thyroid-stimulating hormone levels are not uncommon. Abnormalities have been reported in 17% of children receiving 26 Gy or less and in 78% of those receiving more than 26 Gy to the thyroid area.[9] Benign and malignant neoplasms may be late sequelae as well. In follow-up studies, the thyroid gland should be carefully palpated with each examination, and thyroid function studies should be obtained periodically.

Ovaries and testes are at risk for damage from cancer therapy. Infertility and hormonal dysfunction are known sequelae related to the type and intensity of therapy administered. The prepubertal female patient may experience the delay of secondary sex characteristics with elevations of gonadotropins and decreased serum estradiol levels. The postpubertal female patient may experience amenorrhea and menstrual irregularities. In pregnancies after previous cancer therapy, no significant changes in the occurrence of spontaneous abortion or abnormal offspring were found.[26] In male patients, azoospermia, oligospermia, decreased libido, impotence, gynecomastia, and elevated gonadotropin and decreased testosterone concentrations have been cited.[26]

Perhaps the most studied sequelae of therapy have been the neuropsychologic effects. Special emphasis has been placed on sequelae in children after cranial irradiation for brain tumors and after irradiation as treatment and/or prophylaxis for CNS leukemia. Recently, a study of 15 patients with brain tumor (6 to 19 years old) examined at a median of 20 months after diagnosis showed that 50% experienced major academic, motor, sensory, cognitive, and emotional problems. An interesting finding was that the deficits were irrespective of whether irradiation was part of therapy. In addition, the testing results had little correlation with functional ratings made by their physicians, who judged 80% as having excellent or good functional status.[22]

Increased disabilities have been related to age of younger than 3 years at diagnosis and tumor extension to the hypothalamus. In a study of 38 patients (1 to 16 years old) with brain tumor, performance status was rated good to excellent in 89%. Six patients (17%) had IQs of 69 or less. This related to younger age, but not to brain volume irradiated, because all had had local field irradiation.[11]

Children receiving cranial irradiation as prophylaxis and/or treatment for CNS leukemia have been and continue to be studied to assess differences in functioning after varying prophylactic doses, as well as after additional therapy for relapse. It seems apparent that children who were treated aggressively for CNS relapse (i.e., having received two courses of radiation therapy), and who were younger at the time of treatment had an increased risk of neuropsychologic sequelae. In a recent study, 40 children with ALL and an isolated CNS relapse were studied at a median of 6.1 years after the relapse. Mean scores for IQ as well as their academic performance in reading, spelling, and mathematics were below those expected for children of comparable age; 20% had IQs within the mentally retarded range.[35]

Since the 1970s, there have been reports that prophylactic cranial radiation did not of itself result in neuropsychologic deficiency.[43] Two recent studies support this view.[36, 49] However, an interesting finding in one study assessing 40 children 5 years after CNS prophylaxis either with or without 18 Gy of cranial radiation was that, within the entire group, scores were lower than age-corrected norms. Perhaps the neuropsychologic deficits are related more to the effects of systemic disease, chronic illness, or systemic therapy than to radiation therapy.[36] Another study of 18 children with ALL treated with (24 Gy) or without prophylactic irradiation showed that there were no substantial differences in functioning related to radiation, but also showed that these children had decreased performance scores when compared with population norms.[49]

These studies illustrate that ALL survivors have neuropsychologic sequelae. Therapy is continually being reassessed to find the regimen that is the least toxic without jeopardizing efficacy. Prophylactic use of cranial irradiation is being evaluated, and not just for certain high-risk groups for CNS disease (e.g., those with high white blood cell counts at diagnosis or T cell leukemia).

The risk of a second malignant neoplasm in cancer survivors appears to be 10 to 20 times greater than in age-matched individuals.[25] The Late Effect Study Group with members from North American and European pediatric cancer centers evaluated 292 cases of primary childhood malignancy with 308 secondary malignancies. Genetic factors and specific therapies appear to play a role.[6, 7, 19, 30] Twenty-five per cent of individuals developing a second tumor (73 of 292) had an underlying factor contributing to the development of cancer. Retinoblastoma was the most frequent of these underlying factors, followed by neurofibromatosis. Of the second malignant neoplasms, bone sarcomas were the most common, with 52 of 67 occurring in previously irradiated sites. Soft tissue sarcomas were second in frequency, with approximately 36 of 59 being radiation associated. Acute leukemia was the most common secondary malignancy in those patients who did not undergo radiation therapy.[30] Overall, it appears that the risk of developing subsequent cancer in childhood survivors of cancer falls between 3 and 20% at 20 years from diagnosis.[25]

NORMALIZATION

Health care providers for the child with cancer have been involved in a rapidly changing, progressive field. In many instances, the goal of therapy has changed from one of increasing a poor survival percentage to that of maintaining an improved cure rate using the least toxic therapy. The therapy often is intensive and prolonged: what years ago may have been an acute illness necessitating short-term care for a terminally ill child has changed to a chronic disease with a significant cure rate. The implementation of a multidisciplinary team approach for health care has paralleled medical advances. It is recognized that the truly cured child must be returned to his or her peers after progressing along the continuum of growth and development unique to childhood. The health care team and the family must be advocates for the child, ensuring that as normal as possible socialization and education occur during treatment.

Cure of childhood cancer has become an expected outcome. The sequelae from therapy and the effects of chronic disease have become important considerations in treatment planning. Society's acceptance of the cancer survivor must be encouraged, allowing the least restrictive schooling situations and equal insurance and employment opportunities. With functional as well as medical cure being attainable, there are brighter and better tomorrows for children with cancer.

References

1. Abelson HT: Cancer chemotherapy. *In* Nathan DG, Oski FA (eds): Hematology of Infancy and Childhood, 3rd ed. Philadelphia, WB Saunders Co, 1987.
2. Antman KS, Griffin JD, Elias A, et al: Effect of recombinant human granulocyte-macrophage colony-stimulating factor on chemotherapy-induced myelosuppression. N Engl J Med 319:593–598, 1988.
3. Appelbaum FR: Intensive chemotherapy or chemo radiotherapy with autologous marrow support as treatment for patients with solid tumors. Hematol Oncol Clin North Am 2:345–352, 1988.
4. Baltimore D: Immunoglobulin gene expression. Adv Oncol 3:3–7, 1987.
5. Benedict WF, Fung YK, Murphree AL: The gene responsible for the development of retinoblastoma and osteosarcoma. Cancer 62:1691–1694, 1988.
6. Boivin JF, O'Brien K: Solid cancer risk after treatment of Hodgkin's disease. Cancer 61:2541–2546, 1988.
7. Breslow NE: Second malignant neoplasms in survivors of Wilms' tumors: A report from the National Wilms' Tumor Study. J Natl Cancer Inst 80:592–595, 1988.
8. Broder S, Waldmann TA: The suppression-cell network in cancer. Part 1. N Engl J Med 299:1281–1284, 1978.
9. Byrd R: Late effects of treatment of cancer in children. Pediatr Clin North Am 32:835–857, 1985.
10. Dana BW: Treating malignancies with curative intent: Understanding growth and differentiation. Hematol Oncol Clin North Am 2:337–343, 1988.
11. Danoff BF, Cowchock FS, Marquette C, et al: Assessment of the long term effects of primary radiation therapy for brain tumors in children. Cancer 49:1580–1586, 1982.
12. Fernback DJ: The role of the family physician in the care of the child with cancer. CA 35:258–270, 1985.
13. Finklestein JZ: Neuroblastoma: The challenge and frustration. Hematol Oncol Clin North Am 1:675–694, 1987.
14. Finlay JL, Goins SC, Uteg R, Giese WL: Progress in the management of childhood brain tumors. Hematol Oncol Clin North Am 1:753–776, 1987.
15. Ganick DJ: Wilms' tumor. Hematol Oncol Clin North Am 1:695–719, 1987.

15a. Gershon A: Live attenuated varicella vaccine. J. Pediatr. 110:154–157, 1987.

16. Greenberg RS, Shuster JL: Epidemiology of cancer in children. Epidemiol Rev 7:22–48, 1985.
17. Hammond D: Opportunities for cancer preventions and early detection among children. Cancer 62:1829–1932, 1988.
18. Hammond D, Chard RL, D'Angio GJ, et al: Pediatric malignancies. *In* Hoogstraten B (ed): Cancer Research: Impact of Co-operative Groups. New York, Masson, 1980, p 1–23.
19. Hutter JJ Jr: Late effects in children with cancer. Role of the pediatrician. Am J Dis Child 140:17–19, 1986.
20. Kaufman BH: Progress in pediatric solid tumors. Mayo Clin Proc 61:269–277, 1986.
21. Kripke ML: Immunoregulation of carcinogenesis: Past, present and future. J Natl Cancer Inst 80:722–727, 1988.
22. LeBaron S, Zelter PM, Zelter LK, et al: Assessment of quality of survival in children with medulloblastoma

and cerebellar astrocytoma. Cancer 62:1251–1222, 1988.

23. Li FP, Bader JL: Epidemiology of cancer in childhood. *In* Nathan DG, Oski FA (eds): Hematology of Infancy and Childhood, 3rd ed. Philadelphia, WB Saunders Co, pp 918–941.
24. Mauer AM, Simone JV, Pratt CB: Current progress in the treatment of the child with cancer. J Pediatr 91:523–539, 1977.
25. Meadows AT, Hobbie WL: The medical consequences of cure. Cancer 58:524–528, 1986.
26. Meadows AT, Silber J: Delayed consequences of therapy for childhood cancer. 35:271–286, 1985.
27. Meadows AT, Kramer S, Hopson R, et al: Survival in childhood acute lymphocytic leukemia: Effect of protocol and place of treatment. Cancer Invest 1:49–55, 1983.
28. Meadows AT, Krymas NL, Belasco JB: The medical cost of cure: Sequelae in survivors of childhood cancer. *In* Van Eys J, Sullivan MP (eds): Status of the Curability of Childhood Cancers. New York, Raven Press, 1980, pp 263–276.
29. Meadows AT, Hopson R, Lustbader E, et al: Survival in childhood acute lymphocytic leukemia (ALL): The influence of protocol and place of treatment. Proc Am Soc Clin Oncol 20:425, 1979.
30. Meadows AT, Baum E, Fossati-Bellani F, et al: Second malignant neoplasms in children: An update from the Late Effects Study Group. J Clin Oncol 3:532–538, 1985.
31. Mellic DR: Childhood acute lymphoblastic leukemia: 1. Biological features and their use in predicting outcome of treatment. Am J Pediatr Hematol Oncol 10:163–173, 1989.
32. Miller DR: Childhood acute lymphoblastic leukemia: 2. Strategies and innovations for producing more cures. Am J Pediatr Hematol Oncol 10:174–179, 1988.
33. Miller LP, Miller DR: The pediatrician's role in caring for the child with cancer. Pediatr Clin North Am 31:119–131, 1984.
34. Miller RW, McKay FW: Decline in US childhood cancer mortality 1950 through 1980. JAMA 251:1567–1570, 1984.
35. Mulhern RK, Ochs J, Fairclough D, et al: Intellectual and academic achievement status after CNS relapse; a retrospective analysis of 40 children treated for acute lymphoblastic leukemia. J Clin Oncol 5:933–940, 1987.
36. Mulhern RK, Wasserman AL, Fairclough D, Ochs J: Memory function in disease free survivors of childhood acute lymphocytic leukemia given CNS prophylaxis with or without 1800cGy cranial irradiation. J Clin Oncol 6:315–320, 1988.
37. Niski M, Miyake H, Taheda T, et al: Effect of mass screening of neuroblastoma in Sapporo City. Cancer 60:433–436, 1987.
38. Old LJ: Cancer immunology. Sci Am 236:62–70, 72–73, 76, 79, 1977.
39. Pinkel D: Curing children of leukemia. Cancer 59:1683–1691, 1987.
40. Sandberg AA: The usefulness of chromosome analysis in clinical oncology. Oncology 1:21–38, 1987.
41. Shapiro JR: Biology of gliomas: Heterogeneity, oncogenes, growth factors. Semin Oncol 13:4–15, 1986.
42. Shulman RJ: A totally implanted venous access system in pediatric patients with cancer. J Clin Oncol 5:137–140, 1987.
43. Soni SS, Marten GW, Pitner SE, et al: Effects of central-nervous-system irradiation on neuropsychologic functioning of children with acute lymphocytic leukemia. N Engl J Med 293:113–118, 1975.
44. Tarbell NJ, Cassady JR: Radiation therapy. *In* Nathan DG, Oski FA (eds): Hematology of Infancy and Childhood, 3rd ed. Philadelphia, WB Saunders Co, 1987, pp 918–941.
45. Van Eys J, Viettie TJ: Pediatric co-operative trial groups in the eighties—challenges and opportunities. Cancer Bull 34:117–120, 1982.
46. Van Eys J, Bowman WP, Britton HA, et al: Pediatric cancers. Texas Med 83:24–45, 1987.
47. Weinberg RA: Finding the anti-oncogene. Sci Am 88:44–51, 1988.
48. Weinberg RA: The genetic origins of human cancer. Cancer 61:1963–1968, 1988.
49. Whitt JK: Cranial radiation in childhood acute lymphocytic leukemia—neuro psychologic sequelae. Am J Dis Child 138:730–736, 1989.

CHAPTER 4

Childhood Tumors That May Result in Metastatic Bone Disease

MICHAEL A. WEINER

In pediatric and adolescent patients, malignant bone lesions are most frequently primary bone tumors such as osteogenic sarcoma and Ewing's sarcoma.[161] In contrast to the situation in adults, skeletal metastases in children and adolescents are rare, and when they occur, they frequently represent either an initial symptom at the time of diagnosis or a manifestation of widely metastatic end-stage disease.[97] Characteristically, metastatic bone lesions present as areas of bone loss with indistinct margins; however, osteolytic defects or fusiform areas are usually found in the metaphyseal region of the bone. Additional evidence of periosteal reaction and cortical destruction occurs when long bones are involved. The former may give a radiographic appearance of an onionskin lamination or, less commonly, a sunburst phenomenon. When cortical destruction is present, the tumor mass may extend into the adjacent soft tissues. If metastases are generalized, the destructive lesions may resemble osteoporosis with diffuse loss of bone mass, such as is seen in acute leukemia. In addition, pathologic fractures are commonplace.

The most frequent presenting complaint for patients with malignant bone tumors is pain. In a series of 39 patients with metastatic skeletal disease reported by Leeson and colleagues, 95% had pain at the time of diagnosis;[90] other symptoms were local tenderness and reduced function. Eleven patients of the group had pathologic fractures; 6 of these had vertebral body compression, and another 3 had acute spinal cord compression. The bones most frequently involved, in order of decreasing frequency, were the spine, the ribs, the skull, the femur, the pelvis, the humerus, and the tibia; 80% of the patients had multiple bone involvement.[90]

The diagnosis of metastatic bone lesions is not difficult to make. A radionuclide bone scan is the most reliable diagnostic procedure, although plain radiography, computed tomography (CT), and nuclear magnetic resonance imaging (MRI) techniques are often utilized. The treatment and the prognosis of the various lesions depend on the specific primary tumor.

This chapter presents an overview of the most common malignant solid tumors of childhood that produce skeletal metastases or have a predilection to arise in the extremities or the trunk. Rhabdomyosarcoma (RMS), Wilms' tumor, non-Hodgkin's lymphoma (NHL), and Hodgkin's disease are discussed. The emphasis is on the differential diagnosis, biologic features, treatment, and prognosis.

Rhabdomyosarcoma

Rhabdomyosarcoma, the most common soft tissue tumor in the pediatric and adolescent age groups, accounts for 5 to 8% of all cases of cancer in people younger than 21 years of age. RMSs arise from primitive mesenchymal cells scattered throughout the body.

The etiology of primary RMS remains uncertain. Interaction among genetic and environmental factors needs to be defined. A number of studies found cytologic abnormalities in the tissues of patients with RMS. Chromosomal perturbations that have been identified include alterations of modal number and marker chromosomes 5q+, 9q+, 16p+, and 17p+ as well as a nonrandom alteration, 3p14–21.[129, 149] Of possible significance is that the locus of the oncogene c-*ras* was found to coincide with the common fragile site locus of the 3p chromosome.[76] The precise structure and biologic function of this common fragile site with respect to causation of malignancy remain speculative; nevertheless, a surprisingly frequent association of fragile sites and the loci of human cell oncogenes exists.[89, 163]

HISTOPATHOLOGY

Although RMS is the most common soft tissue sarcoma, it may be difficult to establish the precise diagnosis. Entities that must be differentiated from RMS include extraosseous Ewing's sarcoma, primitive neuroectodermal tumors, synovial sarcoma, fibrosarcoma, malignant fibrous histiocytoma, and hemangiopericytoma. The presence of cross striations that simulate skeletal muscle is the light microscopic feature that is most helpful in making the distinction.[71, 145] Immunocytochemical methods have been developed to aid in diagnosis; monoclonal antibodies directed against skeletal muscle actin and desmin, as well as Z band protein and creatine kinase, are frequently utilized.[2, 31, 151] Finally, the identification of sarcomeric differentiation into actin-myosin bundles by electron microscopy may be extremely useful.[33]

After the diagnosis is established, most cases of RMS may be categorized into histologic subtypes. The Intergroup Rhabdomyosarcoma Study (IRS) pathology committee recently reviewed histopathologic material from 1626 eligible patients entered in the IRS-I and IRS-II studies.[117] They considered the four types of RMS according to the criteria of Horn and Enterline:[71] embryonal, alveolar, botryoid, and pleomorphic. In addition, they included extraosseous Ewing's sarcoma and a group of undifferentiated small round cell sarcomas and tumors that were unclassifiable but clearly sarcomas. Table 4–1 demonstrates the frequency of each histopathologic subtype. The classification of RMS and the soft tissue sarcomas of childhood will continue to evolve as new immunohistochemical, ultrastructural, and molecular biologic data become available. The pathologic description of each subtype of RMS is beyond the scope of this chapter, and the reader is referred to the literature for more comprehensive reviews.[51, 71, 117, 124]

A relationship exists between the histologic subtype and the primary site of the tumor. The most common histologic type of primary tumors occurring in the extremities and the trunk is alveolar RMS. Table 4–2 presents the correlation between the pathologic subtype and the primary site as reported by IRS-I and IRS-II.[117] Recently, a case of an embryonal RMS primary tumor in bone was reported; however, this is exceedingly rare.[72] The IRS investigators similarly demonstrated that, regardless of stage or clinical group, a relationship exists between histologic subtype and survival. The estimated proportions of patients surviving for 3 years are 88% for botryoid, 75% for extraosseous Ewing's sarcoma and pleomorphic subtypes, 68% for embryonal, and 53% for alveolar tumors.[117] Clearly, other factors influence survival, such as primary site and stage, and not every investigator agrees that histologic subtypes independently predict survival.[53, 99] There does appear to be agree-

TABLE 4–1

Frequency of Histopathologic Subtypes of Rhabdomyosarcoma

	Number	Percentage
Embryonal	877	54
Botryoid	88	5
Alveolar	343	21
Pleomorphic	11	1
Extraosseous Ewing's sarcoma	84	5
Small round cell sarcoma	135	8
Unclassified sarcoma	88	6
TOTAL	1626	100

Modified from Newton WA Jr, Soule EH, Hamoudi AB, et al: Histopathology of childhood sarcomas, Intergroup Rhabdomyosarcoma Studies I and II: Clinicopathologic correlation. J Clin Oncol 6:67–75, 1988.

TABLE 4–2

Correlation of Primary Anatomic Site and Pathologic Subtype in Rhabdomyosarcoma

	Percentage by Primary Anatomic Site			
Histopathologic Subtype	*Genitourinary*	*Head and Neck*	*Extremity*	*Trunk*
Embryonal	71	71	24	19
Alveolar	2	13	50	30
Pleomorphic	1	0	2	2
Botryoid	20	2	0	0
Extraosseous Ewing's sarcoma	1	3	7	19
Small round cell sarcoma	2	6	11	20
Unclassified sarcoma	4	5	6	10

Modified from Newton WA Jr, Soule EH, Hamoudi AB, et al: Histopathology of childhood sarcomas, Intergroup Rhabdomyosarcoma Studies I and II: Clinicopathologic correlation. J Clin Oncol 5:67–75, 1988.

ment that alveolar and pleomorphic disease is associated with the poorest prognosis.[66, 139] The discrepancy between histopathologic findings and prognosis prompted others to develop alternative classification schemes. Palmer and Foulkes suggested that RMS tissue with nuclear anaplasia and a monomorphic cell type is associated with a decreased survival; all other types, including alveolar RMS, are clinically less aggressive and may have a better outcome.[121]

CLINICAL MANIFESTATIONS

The clinical presentation of RMS depends on its anatomic site of origin. Extremity or truncal primary tumors usually appear as mass lesions, which may grow to considerable size before detection. They spread along fascial planes and may involve contiguous structures. Extremity lesions represent approximately 20% of all cases of primary RMS, whereas tumors of the trunk occur in 10% of newly diagnosed cases. Extremity tumors have a greater frequency of regional lymph node involvement than truncal neoplasms have. As stated above, nearly one half of the extremity lesions exhibit alveolar histologic patterns.

The assessment of tumor extent is paramount because treatment and prognosis depend on the degree of spread of the primary lesion. After the diagnosis is established, the evaluation for metastases should include plain radiographs, CT scans, ultrasonograms, radionuclide bone scans, and a bone marrow aspirate and biopsy. MRI has considerable promise in delineating tumor extent, but sufficient data regarding its utility are presently not available.[79]

Essentially two staging systems are used. The first is based on a surgical pathologic system, which is weighted by the impact of operative removal of the primary tumor (if possible).[54] The IRS committee adopted such a clinical grouping system:[102] Group I patients have local, completely resected disease. Group II patients have microscopic residual and/or regional lymph node involvement. Group III patients have gross residual disease. Group IV patients have distant metastases at diagnosis.[102]

The second system, proposed by the International Union Against Cancer, is based on a TNM (tumor, node, metastasis) classification, whereby pretreatment assessment of tumor extent without regard to surgical removal is employed.[65] This system emphasizes tumor size, invasiveness, nodal status, and the presence or absence of metastatic spread.[35] A study using the TNM staging system found that, in a multivariate analysis, both T and M were strong predictors of relapse, whereas histologic subtype and primary site had little impact.[127]

THERAPEUTIC CONSIDERATIONS

Improved survival in patients with RMS resulted when multicenter trials were able to register large numbers of patients to conduct randomized studies, enabling refinements of treatment and heightened knowledge of tumor biologic features and prognostic factors. The IRS committee was formed in 1972 when members of the Children Cancer Study Group and the pediatric divisions of the Southwest Oncology Group and Cancer Acute Leukemia Group B banded together. From single-agent and phase II studies, the IRS committee recognized the need for a multimodality approach of surgery, radiation therapy, and chemotherapy.

For primary tumors of the extremity and the trunk, gross surgical removal should be accomplished, provided the limb can be preserved. Lymph node sampling is an essential part of the operative procedure. For patients whose tumors are not amenable to gross resection, debulking surgery to reduce the tumor volume should be performed, chemotherapy and/or radiation therapy should be initiated, and a delayed resection of the residual primary tumor should be attempted after the first 20 weeks of treatment.

Radiation therapy helps eradicate microscopic and/or gross residual tumor if surgical management alone is unable to ablate the lesion. High rates of local control with radiation therapy after surgery, ranging from biopsy only to gross resection, have been reported, with and without chemotherapy.[75, 116] As local control rates improved with the advent of chemotherapy, however, the need for radiation therapy in group I patients with tumor-negative margins was questioned. The IRS-I study confirmed that radiation therapy (50 Gy) did not confer either an improved disease-free survival or increased length of survival in group I patients who also received VAC (vincristine, actinomycin D, and cyclophosphamide) chemotherapy.[102] On the other hand, nonirradiated group I patients with alveolar histologic lesions of the extremity had a higher local recurrence rate than did patients with favorable histologic findings.[147] It has also been demonstrated that, for patients with group II disease, local control rates exceed 92% when a minimum of 40 Gy is administered.[146] At present, patients with group I lesions with nonalveolar histologic pattern do not receive radiation therapy. Patients with group II disease receive 40 to 55 Gy, depending on their age and the size of the primary tumor.

The rationale for the use of combination chemotherapy in conjunction with surgery and radiation therapy was crystallized when it became known that patients who died had distant metastases. However, despite this approach, 10 to 70% of the patients with group I to IV disease, respectively, had a locoregional recurrence or metastasis, and 95% of this cohort died.[130] Initially, the chemotherapeutic agents that were beneficial in patients with RMS included actinomycin D, cyclophosphamide, vincristine, doxorubicin (Adriamycin), and dacarbazine. Newer drugs that have recently been tested include cisplatin, ifosfamide, and etoposide.[131] Theoretical data exist to support the concept of incorporating as many active agents as possible into a protocol scheme to prevent multiple drug resistance.[56] The duration of chemotherapy is between 1 year for patients with early-stage disease and 2 years for patients with more advanced disease. Table 4–3 is a modification of the therapeutic recommendations of the IRS-III committee.

The outcome for patients with RMS has improved significantly with each new IRS study. The overall survival rate at 3 years for all registered patients, irrespective of any prognostic variable, was 60% for IRS-I, 67% for IRS-II, and 73% for IRS-III.[105] In addition, the committee performed a preliminary analysis of the 2-year disease-free survival for patients with nonmetastatic extremity primary tumors and found that in IRS-I it was 72%; in IRS-II, 78%; and in IRS-III, 87%.[104]

Directions for the future must include new therapeutic approaches for tumors with unfavorable histologic pattern and advanced clinical stage to increase patient survival. In patients in whom the results of treatment are acceptable, the goal must be to increase the benefit/risk ratio and to reduce the acute and long-term complications of treatment.

Wilms' Tumor

Wilms' tumor is the most common intraabdominal tumor of childhood, representing between 5 and 6% of all newly diagnosed malignancies in the pediatric age group.[92] Its incidence is 7 cases per million children younger than 16 years of age per year.[162] The age distribution at diagnosis peaks at approximately 3 years of age, and new cases occur equally in both sexes.[15] A relationship exists between certain congenital anomalies, such as malformations of the genitourinary tract, aniridia, and hemihypertrophy, and the development of Wilms' tumor.[107] In addition, children with neurofibromatosis and the Beckwith-Wiedemann syndrome have an increased risk of Wilms' tumors.[6, 142]

Progress in molecular biology has demonstrated that, although patients with Wilms' tumor have normal karyotypes, they may possess a recessive mutant allele at the 11p13 locus, which might, in turn, play a role in the evolution of the tumor.[83, 84] Knudson and Strong proposed a two-stage model, based on epidemiologic data, for the origin of several pediatric cancers, including Wilms' tumor.[82] With the advent of newer molecular biologic techniques, this hypothesis has been expanded accordingly. Thus, tumors may originate from two events. The first is either a germinal or a

TABLE 4–3

Therapy for Rhabdomyosarcoma*

Clinical Group	Histologic	Surgical Management	Radiation Therapy	Chemotherapy (duration)
I	Nonalveolar	Complete resection	None	AMD, VCR (1 y)
	Alveolar	Complete resection	41.4 Gy	VCR, CPPD, ADR, CTX, AMD (1 y)
II	Nonalveolar	Complete gross resection with microscopic residual or regional node extension	41.4 Gy	VCR, AMD ± ADR (1 y)
	Alveolar		41.4 Gy	VCR, CPPD, ADR, CTX, AMD (1 y)
III	Any	Biopsy only or incomplete resection Second-look attempt at complete resection	45–50.4 Gy	VCR, CPPD, ADR, CTX, AMD ± VP-16-213
IV	Any		45–50.4 Gy	

*Recommendations of Intergroup Rhabdomyosarcoma Study III.

AMD, actinomycin D; VCR, vincristine; CPPD, cisplatin; CTX, cyclophosphamide; ADR, Adriamycin; VP-16-213, etoposide.

Modified from Raney RB Jr, Hays DM, Tefft M, et al: Rhabdomyosarcoma and the undifferentiated sarcomas. *In* Pizzo PA, Poplack DG (eds): Principles and Practice of Pediatric Oncology. Philadelphia, JB Lippincott, 1989, pp 635–658.

somatic cell mutation, perhaps a deletion at the 11p13 locus. The second event is a somatic cell chromosomal nondisjunction or recombination. In hereditary cases, the first event occurs in a germ cell. For sporadically occurring cases, it resides in a somatic cell. The hereditary cases tend to be bilateral and to occur at an earlier age than do the nonhereditary cases. Approximately 15 to 20% of Wilms' tumor cases are believed to be hereditary.[80]

CLINICAL PRESENTATION

Wilms' tumor most commonly occurs as an asymptomatic mass that grows insidiously. Approximately 25% of the patients experience lethargy, abdominal pain, hematuria, or hypertension, which may be caused by heightened renin release.[52] Occasionally, a child has a rapidly enlarging abdomen, fever, and anemia, symptoms that relate to a subcapsular hemorrhage, and the child may be acutely ill. The primary consideration in the differential diagnosis should be neuroblastoma. Characteristically, Wilms' tumors are intrarenal and distort the collecting system of the kidney, whereas neuroblastoma arises in the adrenal gland and displaces the kidney. Less common renal malignancies include mesoblastic nephroma, renal cell carcinoma, and rarely, NHL or RMS and other soft tissue sarcomas. Multicystic kidney disease and renal hamartomas are benign processes that must be ruled out.

The diagnostic evaluation includes a careful physical examination to ascertain the presence or absence of any congenital anomalies that are associated with Wilms' tumor. The radiographic assessment should focus on gathering data that are important to the surgeon, such as the function of the contralateral kidney and the presence of intravascular tumor growth in the renal veins or the inferior vena cava. An abdominal real-time ultrasonogram is the best test to perform to gain information.[25, 106] Although not essential, abdominal CT scans are frequently obtained; occasionally, inferior venacavography is performed specifically to delineate tumor thrombus extension above the level of the diaphragm. At present, MRI has unknown benefits. The complete metastatic work-up should include an assessment of the lungs with a plain radiograph; lung tomography and chest CT should be performed if clinically indicated. The abdominal CT scan is sufficient for the identification of liver involvement. In patients with the histologic variant of clear cell sarcoma, a radionuclide bone scan is required, and in those patients with the rhabdoid subtype, brain CT scanning or MRI is obligatory.[98, 122] The staging system employed to determine the extent of disease at diagnosis is based on surgical pathologic principles. Table 4–4 is a simplified modification of the staging system recommended by the National Wilms' Tumor Study (NWTS) committee.[45]

HISTOPATHOLOGY

Wilms' tumors display histologic diversity, with a wide range of cell types. The tumor is derived from the primitive metanephric blastema, but it may contain tissue such as skeletal muscle and cartilage as well as epithelial cells. Grossly, Wilms' tumors may arise anywhere within the kidney and are pale gray to tan. Cysts are common, and hemorrhage and necrosis are frequently found and, if of long duration, may induce calcification. Microscopically, Wilms' tumors rarely present diagnostic problems. The classic pathologic changes are triphasic, including stromal, epithelial, and blastemic elements.[8] The reader is referred to the literature for a more definitive histopathologic explanation.[59]

There is a strong relationship between the histopathologic features of Wilms' tumors and prognosis. The triphasic pattern with tubular differentiation, the most common variant, is associated with an increased survival,[24, 87] and tumors with this pattern have been termed "favorable histology Wilms' tumors" by the NWTS pathology committee.[6] The NWTS group also identified an unfavorable histologic subset, which includes anaplastic and sarcomatous variants.[7]

TABLE 4–4

Clinicopathologic Staging System for Wilms' Tumors

Stage	Description
Stage I	Tumor limited to kidney and completely excised; renal capsule is intact and no residual tumor is apparent.
Stage II	Tumor extends beyond kidney, capsule is violated, but it is completely excised. No residual tumor is apparent.
Stage III	Residual nonhematogenous tumor confined to abdomen defined by positive lymph nodes, peritoneal implants or tumor spillage, or incomplete resection with tumor at margins of excision.
Stage IV	Hematogenous metastases: lung, liver, bone, brain.
Stage V	Bilateral renal involvement at diagnosis.

Modified from Farewell VT, D'Angio GJ, Breslow N, et al: Retrospective validation of a new staging system for Wilms' tumor. Cancer Clin Trials 4:167–171, 1981.

The anaplastic histologic variant represents approximately 5% of the newly diagnosed cases of Wilms' tumor. It is more common in children younger than 5 years of age and is more frequently observed in black than in Caucasian patients.[10] It is characterized by hyperdiploid mitotic figures, enlarged nuclear content, and hyperchromatic nuclei. Douglas and colleagues demonstrated by flow cytometric analysis that the DNA content of anaplastic cells was 1.7 to 3.2 times that found in normal diploid cells; in addition, they found extreme hyperdiploidy, with more than 70 chromosomes and numerous complex translocations in the tumor tissue.[39]

Another subtype is the clear cell sarcoma. Histologically, there are a variety of features, including capillaries, sclerosis, liquefaction, cysts, epithelial cells, stroma, hyalinization, and angiectasis.[7, 136] It is associated with a poor outcome, is classified as an unfavorable histologic pattern, and has a distinct predilection to metastasize to bone and brain.[63, 98]

The rhabdoid tumor of the kidney is a monomorphous tumor and, like the clear cell sarcoma, was identified by the NWTS pathologists.[7] Its cell of origin remains speculative; it is usually seen in infants and is associated with early relapse and death. Thus, it too is classified as unfavorable histologic type of Wilms' tumor.

In addition to the favorable versus unfavorable histologic variable as a predictor of outcome in patients with stage I, II, or III Wilms' tumor, the second most important prognostic factor is the presence or absence of abdominal lymph node involvement, the former portending a shorter survival. Other factors associated with poor outcome, although not statistically significant, include operative tumor spillage, tumor thrombi in the renal vein or the inferior vena cava, and intrarenal vascular invasion.[8] NWTS investigators studied patients with stage IV disease at diagnosis to determine if prognostic variables existed in this cohort. They found that only 12% of all registered patients had evidence of hematogenous spread and that patients with renal vein and lymph node involvement were more likely to have advanced disease at diagnosis and to have a higher rate of recurrence and death. Survival was also poor for patients with stage IV tumors with unfavorable histologic findings.[18]

THERAPEUTIC CONSIDERATIONS

Total surgical resection of a Wilms' tumor is the initial goal of treatment. The procedure must include examination of the contralateral kidney, total nephrectomy, subtotal ureterectomy, lymph node sampling, and placement of radiopaque titanium clips to delineate unresectable tumors.[88] In patients who undergo biopsy initially or in those whose tumor is deemed unresectable, cytoreductive therapy should be administered and a second-look operation should be performed to attempt to excise the lesion completely.[62]

Although the use of radiotherapy may be successful in eradicating residual disease in the tumor bed and in achieving local control, the advent of effective chemotherapeutic agents has diminished its role. NWTS-1 and NWTS-2 concluded that patients with stage I or II favorable-histology lesions did not require postoperative radiotherapy provided they received both vincristine and actinomycin D. For patients with stage III disease, 10 Gy appears to be sufficient to ensure local control when doxorubicin (Adriamycin) is added to vincristine and actinomycin D.[148]

The formation of the NWTS was based on the same motivating principles as that of the IRS committee. The goals of the NWTS have been to maximize the cure rate while simultaneously modifying the intensity and duration of treatment. As with all cooperative group efforts, such studies build on the data obtained from the outcomes of the previous study. Table 4–5 is a modification of the therapy appropriate for patients registered in NWTS-3.

The 2-year disease-free survival for patients with stage I or II favorable-histology disease exceeds 90%. For those with stage III favorable-histology lesions, it is approximately 82%, and for those with stage IV lesions or any tumors with unfavorable histologic pattern, it is about 65%.[28]

Neuroblastoma

Metastatic neuroblastoma diagnosed in children older than 1 year of age has one of the highest mortality rates of all the childhood cancers, and although neuroblastoma has been studied intensively, effective treatment remains an enigma. Neuroblastoma is the third most common malignancy of childhood, representing 7 to 10% of all newly diagnosed cases of cancer; only acute leukemia and brain tumors are diagnosed more frequently. It is essentially a tumor of early life. The median age at diagnosis is 2 years, and nearly 80% of the cases are diagnosed before the patient is 5 years of age.[161]

Rudolf Virchow, in 1864, was the first to describe neuroblastoma.[154] In 1881, Marchand noted the resemblance of this tumor to the embryonic central nervous system and recognized the histologic similarities between the adrenal gland and the tissues of the sympathetic nervous system.[96] This theory was confirmed in 1910 by Wright, who demonstrated that the microscopic pattern of neuroblastoma coincides with that of the embryonic adrenal medulla.[159] In 1965, Greenfield and Shelly established that the pathologic features of neuroblastoma, ganglioneuroblastoma, and ganglioneuroma recapitulate the normal differentiation of neural crest stem cells.[61] The primitive neural crest cells give rise to ganglion cells, glial and arachnoid cells, and the sympathogonia, which differentiate and mature to become the sympathetic ganglion cells and the chromaffin cells of the adrenal medulla.

The pathogenesis of neuroblastoma is consistent with the Knudson and Strong two-stage hypothesis.[81] As with Wilms' tumors, in neu-

TABLE 4–5

Therapy for Wilms' Tumor*

Stage/Histologic Type	Chemotherapy (duration)	Radiotherapy
I/FH	AMD + VCR (10 wk–6 mo)	None
II/FH	AMD + VCR (15 mo)	None
III/FH	AMD + VCR + ADR (15 mo)	10 Gy
IV/FH	AMD + VCR + ADR ± CTX (15 mo)	20 Gy
I–IV/UH	AMD + VCR + ADR ± CTX (15 mo)	20 Gy

*Recommendations of National Wilms' Tumor Study 3.

FH, favorable histology; UH, unfavorable histology; AMD, actinomycin D; VCR, vincristine; ADR, Adriamycin; CTX, cyclophosphamide.

roblastoma cases believed to be hereditary, the initial occurrence causes a deletion or mutation in a germ cell allele; a subsequent event results in the loss or inactivation of the homologous gene on the sister chromosome. In the absence of both alleles, discordant growth transpires, and a clone of aberrant neuroblasts forms. Affected patients have an earlier onset of disease and may have multiple primary foci. In the nonhereditary, sporadic cases, both mutations occur in somatic cells as postzygotic events; the disease is usually diagnosed at an older age and the propensity for multiple primary foci is absent.[80–82]

Neuroblastomas may arise from any site where elements of the sympathetic nervous system are found. Therefore, the adrenal medulla or any segment of the sympathetic chain of the neck, the thorax, the abdomen, and the pelvis, as well as the aortic and carotid ganglia and the organs of Zuckerkandel, may be sites of origin. The commonest site of origin is the abdomen, with 40% of neuroblastomas arising from the adrenal medulla and 25% from the paraspinal sympathetic ganglia. Thoracic, pelvic, and cervical ganglia are sites of origin in 15, 5, and 3% of the patients, respectively.[40] Most children with neuroblastoma appear ill at the time of diagnosis and have evidence of systemic disease, such as weight loss, fever, failure to thrive, pain, and anemia. More specific symptoms and signs depend on the site of origin of the primary tumor and the presence or absence of metastatic dissemination.

Neuroblastomas originating in the cervical sympathetic chain of the head and neck may produce signs and symptoms such as a cranial nerve palsy, proptosis, nasal obstruction, or Horner's syndrome. Intrathoracic neuroblastomas emanating from the sympathetic ganglion primarily occur in the posterior superior mediastinum. Symptoms associated with neuroblastomas in this location include cough, respiratory dysfunction, chest pain, paresthesia, weakness, and paralysis of a limb. Primary tumors arising from either the abdomen or the pelvis have symptoms referable to a retroperitoneal mass, which may include bowel and/or bladder dysfunction, pain, and neurologic findings resulting from spinal cord compression. When a patient has findings compatible with a neuroblastoma, the diagnostic evaluation should proceed in a logical fashion to establish the diagnosis, quantify tumor markers, and detect the extent of disease.

CT is presently the radiographic technique of choice. It is superior to conventional radiography and sonography in detecting the sites of disease involvement.[57] The use of MRI may further improve disease delineation in patients with neuroblastoma.[34] For detection of skeletal disease, radionuclide bone scans are more sensitive than radiographic skeletal surveys.[82] Metaiodobenzylguanidine (MIBG) and iodine-131 radioisotopes, which are chemically similar to catecholamines,[47] and the radiolabeled murine monoclonal antibodies UJ13A and 3F8 are potentially useful diagnostic tools to detect not only primary neuroblastoma at diagnosis but also residual disease after treatment has been initiated.[58, 108]

To confirm the diagnosis, histopathologic analysis of tumor tissue is mandatory. However, the triad of a characteristic clinical picture, a bone marrow infiltrated with neuroblasts arranged in syncytial clumps, and biochemical markers is considered sufficient evidence to establish a diagnosis. Recently, Brodeur and colleagues reported the findings from the International Criteria for Neuroblastoma Committee and established the recommended minimal work-up required for diagnosis.[19] Excessive urinary excretion of catecholamines, in particular vanillylmandelic acid (VMA) and homovanillic acid (HVA), is found in up to 95% of all patients with newly diagnosed neuroblastoma. Heightened levels of these biochemical markers, found in ganglionic sympathetic nerve fibers, are metabolic products of norepinephrine synthesis from phenylalanine.[86] Other markers, although not specific for neuroblastoma, include increased levels of neuron-specific enolase a cytoplasmic enzyme;[164] disialoganglioside, a surface-like lipid antigen; and serum ferritin.[43]

HISTOPATHOLOGY

Pathologically, the hallmark of neuroblastoma is rosette formation and neurofibrils. When these features are absent, the light microscope alone may be inadequate to distinguish neuroblastomas from other small round cell tumors of childhood, such as RMS, lymphoma, Ewing's sarcoma, and primitive neuroectodermal tumors. Cytochemical methods, identification of biochemical markers, electron microscopy demonstrating neurosecretory granules, and the clinical picture must be employed to establish the proper diagnosis.

Three major variants of tumors of the sympathetic nervous system, which represent a biologic spectrum, are recognized. The neuroblastoma, which is composed of sympathoblasts and is the least differentiated, consists of sheets of primitive cells with scant cytoplasm and dark-stained nuclei. The tumor cells and their fibrillar processes form so-called Homer-Wright rosettes. The ganglioneuroblastoma shows signs of differentiation and maturation; it is composed of both primitive neuroblasts and mature ganglion cells.[1] The ganglioneuroma is a mature tumor composed of fully differentiated ganglion cells embedded in Schwann cell sheaths. It is benign and lacks metastatic potential.[46]

Shimada and coworkers described a classification system for neuroblastoma and ganglioneuroblastoma based on the morphologic features of the primary tumor.[139] The three variables that they assessed were the degree of differentiation, the nuclear morphologic features of the neuroblastic cells, and the organizational pattern of the stromal tissue. With respect to nuclear morphologic pattern, the tumors are graded by the number of cells that were mitotic and/or karyorrhectic; a mitosis/karyorrhexis index (MKI) is determined. Correlation between the Shimada classification and prognosis is postulated. A stroma-rich differentiated tumor with a low MKI is similar to a ganglioneuroblastoma or an immature ganglioneuroma, whereas the traditional neuroblastoma is stroma poor, is undifferentiated, and has an increased MKI.[139]

CLINICAL MANIFESTATIONS

After the diagnosis is established and the metastatic evaluation is complete, a clinical stage is assigned to the patient. Evans and coworkers developed a staging scheme in 1971.[41] However, the International Criteria for Neuroblastoma committee established staging criteria that were based on clinical, radiographic, and surgical data that permitted consistency and comparison of therapeutic results.[19] Table 4–6 is a simplified version of this staging system. At the time of diagnosis, approximately 65 to 70% of the patients have stage III or IV disease.[16]

An assessment of the pretreatment prognostic factors for a patient with newly diagnosed disease is crucial in formulating an effective therapeutic approach. The following prognostic factors are statistically significant predictors of outcome: age of the patient, stage of the lesion, level of neuron-specific enolase, ferritin levels, pathologic findings, and the VMA/HVA ratio.[43] Research has determined that the presence of homogeneously staining regions and double minute chromosomes present in karyotypic analysis of the neuroblastoma tissue may be a hallmark of a patient with a poor prognosis.[73] Similarly, the identification of n-*myc* oncogene amplification contained in the homogeneously staining regions and double minutes may predict a reduced curative potential.[20, 137] Table 4–7 defines the relevant prognostic variables in patients with neuroblastoma.

TABLE 4–6

International Staging System for Neuroblastoma

Stage	Description
Stage I	Tumor is localized to site of origin and is grossly resected.
Stage II	Tumor is completely resected. Ipsilateral lymph nodes positive or negative; contralateral lymph nodes negative.
Stage III	Tumor crosses midline, regional lymph nodes involved.
Stage IV	Tumor dissemination to distant lymph nodes, bone, bone marrow, liver, etc.
Stage IVS	Primary tumor as defined for stage I or II with dissemination limited to liver, skin, bone marrow. (Patients usually <1 y of age.)

Modified from Brodeur GM, Seeger RC, Barrett A, et al: International criteria for diagnosis, staging and response to treatment in patients with neuroblastoma. J Clin Oncol 6:1874–1881, 1988.

Knowledge of prognostic markers permitted pediatric oncologists to stratify patients with neuroblastoma into two therapeutic categories: those who do well with minimal treatment and those who require intensive and novel therapeutic strategies. Children with early-stage, localized disease without lymph node involvement fall into the first group, whereas those with advanced disease are in the latter category. When the tumor is totally excised and only microscopic residual disease exists, survival rates are between 80 and 100% with surgery alone; the addition of chemotherapy with or without radiation therapy has not significantly improved outcome.[30, 41] Infants younger than 1 year of age with stage IVS disease and without evidence of prognostic variables that portend an unfavorable outcome also have a relatively high cure rate, between 60 and 90% with minimal or, in some situations, no treatment.[42, 118]

For patients with advanced-stage neuroblas-

TABLE 4–7

Predictors of a Favorable Outcome in Children with Neuroblastoma

Variable	Comment
Age	<1–2 y of age
Stage	I, II, IVS
Primary site	Mediastinum
Histopathologic findings	Favorable
Catecholamine levels	VMA/HVA ratio >1
Neuron-specific enolase level	Normal (1–100 ng/ml)
Ferritin level	Normal (1–150 ng/ml)
Gene amplification	Single copy of n-*myc* oncogene
DNA index	Aneuploidy >1

VMA, vanillylmandelic acid; HVA, homovanillic acid.

toma, aggressive, multimodal therapy is employed. Cell kinetic research has shown that a steep linear dose-response relationship exists between neuroblastoma and chemotherapeutic agents; thus, at least in animal models, drug resistance may be reversed by high-dose schedules.[67] Historically, the 2-year disease-free survival of these patients is 40 and 15% for stage III and stage IV, respectively.[16] Several groups of investigators reported promising preliminary results for these patients, utilizing maximal tolerated dosages of cyclophosphamide, cisplatin, doxorubicin (Adriamycin), vincristine, and teniposide (epipodophyllotoxin, VM-26). Complete response and good partial response rates achieved with these regimens are between 65 and 100%. However, it is too early to determine whether the 2-year disease-free survival and ultimate cure rate were improved when compared with results of previous studies.[60, 85, 138]

Another treatment modality presently under investigation is bone marrow transplantation. Both allogeneic and autologous methods have been employed. Patients at high risk with poor prognosis receive ablative therapy with alkalating agents such as cyclophosphamide, busulfan (Myleran), or thiotepa with or without the addition of total body irradiation. Patients undergoing allogeneic transplants then receive infusions of marrow from a donor with matched tissue, usually a sibling. In the case of an autologous procedure, the patient's own marrow is harvested and then purged *ex vivo* with either pharmacologic agents, monoclonal antibodies, or plant lectins to deplete it of contaminated neuroblasts.[133, 134, 150] At present, a survival advantage with the use of an allogeneic marrow transplant instead of an autologous procedure has not been demonstrated.[27] Similarly, it is too early to determine whether a bone marrow transplant procedure will improve the cure rate of patients when compared with intensive chemotherapy alone. This issue is presently being studied in a randomized protocol by the Pediatric Oncology Group.

Non-Hodgkin's Lymphoma

Collectively, the lymphomas are the third most common malignant tumor of childhood, representing 13 to 15% of all newly diagnosed disease. In the United States NHL constitutes 60% of the lymphomas, and Hodgkin's disease constitutes 40%.[161] Epidemiologically, both NHL and Hodgkin's disease have a male preponderance, with a ratio of 2:1 to 3:1; the median age at diagnosis for the former is 9 years, whereas for the latter, it is in early adolescence.[48, 113]

The clinical presentation of a child with NHL is quite variable and depends on the anatomic site of origin and the extent of disease. Although any lymphoid tissue of the body may be involved, the majority of children have extranodal involvement. Murphy tabulated data from several series and concluded that 14% had peripheral node disease, whereas 35% had primary foci in the abdomen, 26% in the mediastinum, and 13% in the head and neck. Approximately 2 to 5% had primary bone involvement.[113]

Painless lymphadenopathy is the most common presentation for the patient with peripheral node disease. The adenopathy may be solitary or multiple or may reflect regional or systemic disease. NHL of the head and neck may involve the sinuses, the orbit, the jaw, or structures of the nasopharynx. The systemic signs and symptoms of disease in this region may appear trivial and are frequently misdiagnosed as a common childhood illness. Patients with mediastinal involvement exhibit

TABLE 4–8

Staging of Childhood Non-Hodgkin's Lymphoma

Stage I	Single anatomic site.
Stage II	Single anatomic site with regional node involvement or two or more sites above or below diaphragm.
Stage III	Two or more sites above and below diaphragm. Extensive intrathoracic. Extensive intraabdominal.
Stage IV	One of above with bone marrow and/or central nervous system involvement

cough, stridor, and dyspnea; they may require emergency intervention for superior vena caval syndrome. Abdominal NHL is associated with a mass lesion, pain, weight loss, nausea, vomiting, and signs of intestinal obstruction at the ileocecal junction. The presence of pain and swelling is the hallmark of primary bone tumors.

After the diagnosis is established by a lymph node biopsy, a thorough investigation should proceed to determine the anatomic extent of disease. The work-up should include a complete blood count, a chemical profile, assessment of hepatic and renal function, a bone scan, a bone marrow aspirate, and a lumbar puncture. CT scans and MRI are necessary but should be obtained only if clinically indicated. A formal staging laparotomy and a splenectomy are not necessary.

The traditional Ann Arbor staging system utilized for patients with Hodgkin's disease is clinically inadequate for use in patients with NHL because it does not take into account the frequency of advanced disease, intraabdominal disease, and the increased likelihood of a leukemic evolution.[110] Several investigators attempted to provide alternative staging approaches. They are all applicable to NHL, are relatively simple, and make no distinction between nodal and extranodal primary sites.[113, 158, 165] Table 4–8 presents a simplified compilation of the clinical staging systems in use. A distribution according to stage at the time of diagnosis reveals that fewer than 30% of the lesions are stage I or II; the remaining 70% are stage III or IV.[95]

The multitude of histopathologic classification schemes utilized in adult patients with NHL are not applicable for categorizing the pediatric population, in which NHL is virtually limited to three subtypes: lymphoblastic, undifferentiated, and histiocytic or large cell.[112, 114, 115] Nodular or follicular lymphomas originating from germinal centers are rare.[49] Interestingly, as is the case with RMS, there is a relationship of histologic type, immunophenotype, and the anatomic site of the primary tumor (Table 4–9).

Primary Non-Hodgkin's Lymphoma of Bone

Primary non-Hodgkin's lymphoma of bone (PNHLB) is a rare but well-recognized clinicopathologic entity. Oberling first described the disorder in 1928,[119] and Parker and Jackson detailed the first series of cases, gleaned from the National Tumor Registry, in 1939.[123] Originally, PNHLB was referred to as reticulum cell sarcoma; however, it is now recognized as a malignant lymphoid tumor histologically identical to NHL arising from either nodal or extranodal sites.

Ostrowsky and coworkers reported a natural history study of 422 patients at the Mayo Clinic.[120] They identified that their patients had either solitary PNHLB or multifocal disease. There was a male preponderance of 1.6:1, and the median age of their patients was 46 years. In their review, a wide variety of bony sites was appreciated; the most frequently involved bones were the femur, the pelvis, the spine, the maxilla, and the mandible. Marugg and colleagues and Spagnolia and coworkers reported that PNHLB is more prevalent in appendicular bones and that axillary sites are more often affected when the disease has metastasized.[100, 141] Clearly, PNHLB is more prevalent in the adult population than in the pedi-

TABLE 4–9

Relationship of Histology, Immunophenotype, and Primary Site in Childhood Non-Hodgkin's Lymphoma

Histologic Subtype	Immunophenotype	Primary Site	Frequency
Lymphoblastic	T cell	Mediastinum	35%
Undifferentiated (Burkitt's and non-Burkitt's)	B cell	Abdomen	45%
Histiocytic or large cell	B cell	Variable	20%

atric and adolescent age groups, where it probably represents between 3 and 5% of all newly diagnosed cases of malignant lymphoma in children.[112]

Radiographically, PNHLB has been described as having a moth-eaten or permeative appearance; other findings include periosteal new bone formation, pathologic fractures, cortical defects, and soft tissue masses.[115, 128, 157] It is histologically and immunophenotypically similar in its appearance and frequency to lymphomas of nodal or extranodal sites. A solitary lesion would be stage I; multifocal presentations would be stage II or III, depending on whether the lesions were on one or both sides of the diaphragm, respectively.

Although the addition of radiation therapy to nonablative surgery permitted acceptable local tumor control and preserved adequate function, it did not improve overall survival because failure of distant tumor eradication occurred in up to 50% of the patients.[38, 74, 115]

In 1939, Parker and Jackson reported a 42% survival for patients with PNHLB treated with amputations.[123] More recently, in an attempt to improve survival, chemotherapy in addition to involved-field radiation therapy has been employed. Investigators at the Instituto Ortopedica Rizzoli reported that 80 to 85% of their patients treated with vincristine, doxorubicin (Adriamycin), and cyclophosphamide plus 40 to 50 Gy to the whole bone were continuously disease free more than 5 years after diagnosis.[4, 5] Loeffler and associates reported similar results with vincristine, prednisone, doxorubicin, and comparable radiation therapy. However, 2 of 11 patients developed second malignancies in the irradiated bone; one, a pleomorphic sarcoma and the second, a malignant fibrous histocytoma.[94]

The issue of second malignancies is not trivial, especially in children, who, if cured of their primary cancer, may have a life expectancy of an additional 50 to 60 years. Although aggressive multimodal treatment results in increased survival rates for patients with malignant disease, questions have been raised about the late sequelae of treatment. Therefore, the present goals of therapy for PNHLB are to continue the high cure rate but to diminish toxicity. These intentions have been realized, as recent reports cite excellent results with reduced chemotherapy[3, 50] plus radiation therapy, or more aggressive chemotherapy but without radiation therapy. In a study of the latter protocol in patients with localized PNHLB, there have been no relapses, no local recurrences, and no second malignant tumors with a mean follow-up of 5 years.[64]

Hodgkin's Disease

Hodgkin's disease is slightly less common than NHL; its annual incidence (based on data from the National Cancer Institute) is approximately 5.7 cases per million children younger than the age of 15 years.[161] However, unlike the situation with NHL, Hodgkin's disease in the pediatric age group is similar to the disease in adults with respect to clinical presentation, histopathologic pattern, and treatment.

Hodgkin's disease was first described by Thomas Hodgkin in 1832 in his historic paper "On Some Morbid Appearances of the Absorbent Glands and Spleen."[69] Since its first description, the entity has been the subject of intense scientific and clinical investigation. The accumulated knowledge about the disease exemplifies the way in which research is applied to patient care and translated into lengthened survival.

In the vast majority of patients, a painless enlargement of the cervical lymph nodes is the initial complaint. Other symptoms include fever, night sweats, and weight loss. When any or all of these symptoms are present, the patient is considered to have systemic signs of disease and is classified as possessing B symptoms; approximately 20% of all children have B symptoms at diagnosis. The absence of systemic signs and symptoms confers an A classification.

An excisional biopsy of the enlarged lymph node is the management of choice when a suspicion of Hodgkin's disease exists. The normal architecture of the lymph node is usually lost and is replaced by the malignant process. The Reed-Sternberg cell, first described in 1900, is the hallmark of Hodgkin's disease.[132, 144] Most experts agree that the Reed-Sternberg cell is the neoplastic cell of Hodgkin's disease and must be present to confirm the diagnosis. The origin of the Reed-Sternberg cell remains speculative. It has been proposed that it may be derived from either interdigitating reticulum cells or macrophage-histiocytes, both of which are found in the microenvironment in the thymus-dependent areas of lymph node tissue.[23, 77, 125] Other investigators suggested that it is of lymphoid origin[13, 37] or is perhaps a fusion of B lymphocytes, reticulum cells, and Hodgkin's cells.[126] The initiation of this fusion may occur in a genetically predisposed individual in whom induction by a virus occurs.[21] There is evidence of the presence of Epstein-Barr viral genomes in Reed-Sternberg cells from patients with Hodgkin's disease.[156] Intensive research is being performed to elucidate the answer to this problem.

Four histopathologic subtypes of Hodgkin's disease are recognized in accordance with the Rye classification scheme developed in 1965. In order of decreasing frequency, they are nodular sclerosis, mixed cellularity, lymphocyte predominance, and lymphocyte depletion.[78] In general, the histologic type corresponds to the extent of disease, in that lymphocyte depletion and mixed cellularity tend to be found in patients with advanced disease and lymphocyte predominance is more frequently associated with early-stage involvement; nodular sclerosis is intermediate.[55]

After the diagnosis is established by lymph node biopsy, it is imperative that all patients undergo a diagnostic assessment to delineate the extent of disease. Mandatory tests include a careful history and physical examination to determine the presence of B symptoms, a complete blood count, erythrocyte sedimentation rate, serum copper determination, chemical profile, and hepatic and renal function tests. Radiologic studies, such as a chest x-ray film and CT scans of the thorax, the abdomen, and the pelvis, are necessary, and a lymphangiogram to assess lower abdominal and pelvic lymph node areas is recommended. A bone scan to detect the presence of skeletal involvement and a gallium citrate ^{67}Ga scan (as an adjunct to the CT scan for mediastinal disease) should both be performed.

In the absence of clinically advanced disease, an exploratory laparotomy to precisely define the pathologic stage is presently employed by most oncologists.[35, 109] Surgically, a staging laparotomy consists of a splenectomy, wedge and needle biopsies of the liver, a trephine-needle bone marrow biopsy, and a sampling of lymph nodes in the upper abdominal, porta hepatis, splenic hilum, paraaortic, mesenteric, iliac, and inguinal groups. In addition, in females, an oophoropexy (ovariopexy) to move the ovaries behind the uterus is performed to maintain reproductive function. Before performing the splenectomy, the polyvalent pneumococcal vaccine is administered, and postoperatively, all patients should be given prophylactic penicillin to prevent bacterial sepsis.

At the completion of the entire work-up, the patient is assigned a pathologic stage in accordance with the guidelines established at the Ann Arbor Symposium in 1971.[22] Patients with bone involvement are considered to have advanced disease and thus are classified as stage IV.

With respect to bone involvement, the appendicular skeleton is more frequently the site of disease than is the axial skeleton. Radiographically, the lesions are destructive in nature and quite similar in appearance to those of PNHLB. Similarly, no correlation exists between the histologic subtype and bone manifestations of disease. However, because bone involvement connotes advanced disease, patients with bone involvement are more likely to have systemic signs and symptoms (B symptoms).

Several prognostic variables are helpful in predicting outcome. In general, children and adolescents and females have a better prognosis than adults and males, respectively.[26, 135] Other variables considered to indicate a poor prognosis include excessive tumor volume, advanced stage, bulky mediastinal disease with a mediastinal mass/thoracic diameter ratio in excess of 0.33,[93, 101] B symptoms, and a lymphocyte depletion histologic pattern.[11]

The goal of treatment for patients with Hodgkin's disease is cure, but one must adopt a philosophy that "more is not better." Thus, one should administer the minimal therapy required to ensure a high survival rate but to minimize complications and untoward sequelae. In patients with stage IA or II disease, subtotal nodal radiotherapy is curative in more than 90% of the cases.[70] Patients with stage IB or IIB disease and those with bulky disease or a mediastinal mass/thoracic diameter ratio greater than 0.33 should receive four to six courses of chemotherapy plus subtotal nodal radiation therapy (30 to 35 Gy). The relapse-free survival is 80 to 85%.

The optimal management of patients with stage III disease remains unresolved. Most investigators stratify IIIA disease into two subsets the basis of intraabdominal location: $IIIA_1$ signifies upper abdominal involvement, and $IIIA_2$ indicates lower abdominal and/or pelvic involvement.[32] Patients with $IIIA_1$ disease, when treated with subtotal or total nodal irradiation, have survival rates comparable with those of patients with stage IIA disease.[110] Another approach is to use low-dose total nodal irradiation (20 Gy) plus four to six cycles of chemotherapy with MOPP (mechlorethamine [Mustargen], vincristine [Oncovin], pro-

TABLE 4–10

Therapy for Pediatric Patients with Hodgkin's Disease

Stage	Patient Characteristics	Recommended Therapy
IA, IB, IIA	Pubertal, without unfavorable signs	RT (IF or EF): 35–40 Gy
	Prepubertal, mediastinal mass >⅓ of thoracic diameter	Chemotherapy: 4–6 courses + RT (IF or EF): ≤25 Gy
IIB, $IIIA_1$	Pubertal, without unfavorable signs	RT (TNLI ± liver, spleen): 35–44 Gy
	Prepubertal, mediastinal mass >⅓ of thoracic diameter	Chemotherapy: 4–6 courses + RT (IF or EF): ≤25 Gy
$IIIA_2$, IIIB, IVA, IVB		Chemotherapy: 8–12 courses *or* Chemotherapy: 6 courses + RT (IF or EF): 35–44 Gy *or* Chemotherapy: 6 courses + RT (TNLI): ≤25 Gy

RT, radiotherapy; IF, involved field; EF, extended field; TNLI, total nodal lymphoid irradiation.

carbazine, and prednisone) and/or ABVD (doxorubicin [Adriamycin], bleomycin, vinblastine [Velban], and dacarbazine). On the other hand, patients with stage $IIIA_2$ or IIIB disease require combination chemotherapy with or without irradiation.[143] Italian investigators at the Milan Cancer Institute have reported a 94% 7-year survival using ABVD plus total nodal irradiation as opposed to only 67% survival when MOPP alone was combined with radiation therapy.[135]

The treatment of patients with stage IV disease must include full-dose chemotherapy, and most investigators include total nodal irradiation as well. Eight to 12 cycles of alternating MOPP and ABVD, two non–cross-resistant regimens, are superior to either regimen alone, with a long-term survival of 70 to 80%.[11] Patients with bone involvement do not, as a rule, require radiation therapy for the bone lesions, except to alleviate symptoms. A recent, as yet unpublished study conducted by the Pediatric Oncology Group of patients with advanced-stage disease utilizes alternating MOPP and ABVD plus low-dose (20 Gy) total nodal irradiation and has a projected 2-year disease-free survival of 86%.[155] Table 4–10 presents a summary of the therapeutic strategies employed in the management of patients with Hodgkin's disease.

The treatment strategy must also include a consideration of the iatrogenic morbidity. Clearly, the most significant toxicity is the development of a second malignancy, particularly acute nonlymphocytic leukemia and solid tumors. In a long-term follow-up study of more than 1300 patients with Hodgkin's disease, the actuarial risk of leukemia was 3 to 4%, whereas the risk of solid tumors was between 10 and 17%.[9, 153] It appears that the alkylating agents used in MOPP, mechlorethamine (Mustargen) and procarbazine, are the most likely offenders for the induction of secondary leukemia, because when these agents are not used, the risk is insignificant.[153] Interestingly, with respect to solid tumors, there is no relationship between the malignancy and the radiation therapy field or dosage, and in patients who receive chemotherapy, solid cancers are generally not found.[9]

Other late effects of treatment include growth disturbances, cardiopulmonary dysfunctions, hypothyroidism, and sterility.[91]

References

1. Adam A, Hochholzer L: Ganglioneuroblastoma of the posterior mediastinum, a clinicopathologic review of 80 cases. Cancer 47:373–381, 1981.
2. Altmannsberger M, Weber K, Droste R, et al: Desmin is a specific marker for rhabdomyosarcoma of human and rat origin. Am J Pathol 118:85–95, 1985.
3. Anderson JR, Wilson JF, Jenkin DT, et al: Childhood non-Hodgkin's lymphoma. The results of a randomized therapeutic trial comparing a 4 drug regimen (COMP) with a 10 drug regimen (LSA_2–L_2). N Engl J Med 308:559–565, 1983.
4. Bacci G, Jaffe N, Emiliani E, et al: Staging, therapy and prognosis of primary non-Hodgkin's lymphoma of bone and a comparison of results with localized Ewing's sarcoma: Ten years experience at the Instituto Ortopedico Rizzoli. Tumori 71:345–354, 1985.
5. Bacci G, Picci P, Bertoni F, et al: Primary non-Hodgkin's lymphoma of bone. Results of 15 patients treated by radiotherapy combined with systemic chemotherapy. Cancer Treat Rep 66:1859–1862, 1982.
6. Beckwith JB: Macroglossia, omphalocele, adrenal

cytomegaly, gigantism and hyperplastic visceromegaly. Birth Defects 5:188–916, 1969.

7. Beckwith JB, Palmer NF: Histopathology and prognosis of Wilms' tumor. Results from the National Wilms' Tumor Study. Cancer 41:1937–1948, 1978.
8. Bennington JL, Beckwith JB: Tumors of the kidney, renal pelvis and ureter. Atlas of Tumor Pathology, 2nd series, Fascicle 12. Washington, DC, Armed Forces Institute of Pathology, 1975.
9. Boivin JF, O'Brien K: Solid cancer risk after treatment of Hodgkin's disease. Cancer 61:2541–2546, 1988.
10. Bonadio JR, Storer B, Norkool P, et al: Anaplastic Wilms tumor: Clinical and pathological studies. J Clin Oncol 3:513–520, 1985.
11. Bonadonna G, Santoro A, Viviani S, Valagussa P: Treatment strategies for Hodgkin's disease. Semin Hematol 25:51–57, 1988.
12. Bonadonna G, Valagussa P, Santoro A: Prognosis of bulky Hodgkin's disease treated with chemotherapy alone or combined with radiotherapy. Cancer Surv 4:439–458, 1985.
13. Borowitz M, Croker B, Metzgar R: Immunohistochemical analysis of the distribution of lymphocyte subpopulation in Hodgkin's disease. Cancer Treat Rep 66:667–674, 1982.
14. Boston HC, Dahlin DC, Ivin JC, et al: Malignant lymphoma (so-called reticulum cell sarcoma) of bone. Cancer 34:1131–1137, 1974.
15. Breslow NE, Beckwith JB: Epidemiologic features of Wilms' tumor: Results of the National Wilms' Tumor Study. J Natl Cancer Inst 68:429–436, 1982.
16. Breslow N, McCann B: Statistical estimation of prognosis for children with NB. Cancer Res 31:2098–2103, 1976.
17. Breslow N, Churchill G, Beckwith JB: Prognosis of Wilms' tumor patients with non-metastatic disease at diagnosis—results of the Second National Wilms' Tumor Study. J Clin Oncol 3:521–531, 1985.
18. Breslow NE, Churchill G, Newmith B: Clinicopathologic features and prognosis for Wilms' tumor patients with metastases at diagnosis. Cancer 58:2501–2511, 1986.
19. Brodeur GM, Hayes FA, Green AA, et al: Consistent n-*myc* copy number in simultaneous or consecutive neuroblastoma samples from sixty individual patients. Cancer Res 47:4248–4253, 1987.
20. Brodeur GM, Seeger RC, Barrett A, et al: International criteria for diagnosis staging and response to treatment in patients with neuroblastoma. J Clin Oncol 6:1874–1881, 1988.
21. Bucsky P: Origin of Hodgkin's and Reed-Sternberg cells. N Engl J Med 303:284–285, 1980.
22. Carbone PP, Kaplan HS, Masshof KM, et al: Report of the Committee on Hodgkin's Disease Staging Classification. Cancer Res 31:1860–1861, 1971.
23. Carbone A, Manconi R, Poletti A, Sulfaro S, et al: Reed-Sternberg cells and their micro environment in Hodgkin's disease with reference to macrophage-histiocytes and interdigitating reticulum cells. Cancer 60:2662–2665, 1987.
24. Chatten J: Epithelial differentiation in Wilms' tumor—a clinicopathologic appraisal. Perspect Pediatr Pathol 3:225–254, 1976.
25. Cohen MD, Siddiqui A, Weetman R, et al: A rational approach to the radiologic evaluation of children with Wilms' tumor. Cancer 50:887–892, 1982.
26. Crynkovich MJ, Hoppe RT, Rosenberg SA: Stage IIB Hodgkin's disease: The Stanford experience. J Clin Oncol 4:472–479, 1986.
27. D'Angio GJ, August C, Elkins W, et al: Metastatic neuroblastoma managed by supralethal therapy and bone marrow reconstitution (BMRc): Results of a four-institution children's cancer study group pilot study. *In* Evans A, D'Angio GJ, Seeger RC (eds): Advances in Neuroblastoma Research. New York, Alan R Liss, 1985.
28. D'Angio GJ, Evans AE, Breslow N, et al: Results of the Third National Wilms' Tumor Study (NWTS-3): A preliminary report. Proc Am Assoc Cancer Res 25:183, 1984.
29. D'Angio GJ, Tefft M, Breslow N, et al: Radiation therapy of Wilms' tumor: Results according to dose, field, post-operative timing and histology. Int J Radiat Oncol Biol Phys 4:769–780, 1978.
30. de Bernardi B, Rogers D, Carli M: Localized NB: Surgical and pathologic staging. Cancer 60:1066–1072, 1987.
31. DeJong ASH, Van Kessel–Van Vark M, Albus-Lutter CE, et al: Skeletal muscle actin as a tumor marker in the diagnosis of rhabdomyosarcoma in childhood. Am J Surg Pathol 9:467–474, 1986.
32. Desser RK, Colomb HM, Ultman JE, et al: Prognostic classification of Hodgkin's disease in pathologic stage III, based on anatomic considerations. Blood 49:883–893, 1977.
33. Dickman PS: Electron microscopy for diagnosis of tumors in children. Perspect Pediatr Pathol 9:171–213, 1987.
34. Dietrich RB, Kangarloo H, Lemarsky C, et al: Neuroblastoma: The role of MR imaging. Am J Radiol 148:937–942, 1987.
35. Donaldson SS, Belli JA: A rational clinical staging system for childhood rhabdomyosarcoma. J Clin Oncol 2:135–139, 1984.
36. Donaldson SS, Kaplan HS: A survey of pediatric Hodgkin's disease at Stanford University. Results of therapy and quality of survival. *In* Rosenberg S, Kaplan H (eds): Malignant Lymphomas. New York, Academic Press, 1982, p 575.
37. Dorreen MS, Habeshaw HA, Stansfeld AG, et al: Characterization of Sternberg-Reed and related cells in Hodgkin's disease. An immunohistologic study. Br J Cancer 49:465–476, 1984.
38. Doseretz DE, Murphy GF, Raymond K, et al: Radiation therapy for primary lymphoma of bone. Cancer 51:44–46, 1983.
39. Douglas EC, Look AT, Webber B, et al: Hyperdiploidy and chromosomal rearrangements define the anaplastic variants of Wilms tumor. J Clin Oncol 4:975–981, 1986.
40. Evans AE: Natural History of Neuroblastoma Research. New York, Raven Press, 1980.
41. Evans AE, Brand W, de Lorimier A, et al: Results in children with local and regional NB managed with and without vincristine, cyclophosphamide and imidazole carboxamide. Am J Clin Oncol 6:3–7, 1984.
42. Evans AE, Chatten J, D'Angio GJ, et al: A review of 17 IV-S neuroblastoma patients at the Children's Hospital of Philadelphia. Cancer 45:833–839, 1980.
43. Evans AE, D'Angio GJ, Propert K, Anderson J, Hann HWL: Prognostic factors in neuroblastoma. Cancer 59:1853–1859, 1987.
44. Evans AE, D'Angio GJ, Randolph J: A proposed staging for children with neuroblastoma: Children's Cancer Study Group A. Cancer 27:374–378, 1971.
45. Farewell VT, D'Angio GJ, Breslow N, et al: Retrospective validation of a new staging system for Wilms' tumor. Cancer Clin Trials 4:167–171, 1981.
46. Feigin I, Cohen M: Maturation and anaplasia in

neuronal tumors of the peripheral nervous system with observation on the glial-like tissues in the ganglioneuroblastoma. J Neuropathol Exp Neurol 36:748–763, 1977.

47. Feine U, Muller Schauenburg W, Treuner J, et al: Metaiodobenzylguanidine (MIBG) labeled with ^{123}I/^{131}I in neuroblastoma diagnosis and follow-up treatment with a review of the diagnostic results of the International Workshop of Pediatric Oncology. Rome, 1986.
48. Fraumeni JF, Li FP: Hodgkin's disease in childhood: An epidemiologic study. J Natl Cancer Inst 42:681–691, 1969.
49. Frizzera G, Murphy SB: Follicular (nodular) lymphoma in childhood: A rare clinical-pathologic entity. Cancer 44:2218–2235, 1979.
50. Furman WL, Fitch S, Huster HO, et al: Primary lymphoma of bone in children. J Clin Oncol 7:1275–1280, 1989.
51. Gaiger AM, Soule EH, Newton WA Jr: Pathology of rhabdomyosarcoma: Experience of the Intergroup Rhabdomyosarcoma Study 1972–78. Natl Cancer Inst Monogr 56:19–27, 1981.
52. Ganguly A, Gribble J, Tune B, et al: Renin-secreting Wilms' tumor with severe hypertension; report of a case and brief review of renin-secreting tumors. Ann Intern Med 79:835–837, 1973.
53. Gehan EA, Glover FN, Maurer HM, et al: Prognostic factors in children with rhabdomyosarcoma. Natl Cancer Inst Monogr 56:83–92, 1981.
54. Ghavimi F, Exelby PR, Lieberman PH, et al: Multidisciplinary treatment of embryonal rhabdomyosarcoma in children: A progress report. Natl Cancer Inst Monogr 56:111–120, 1981.
55. Gilchrist GS, Evans RG: Contemporary issues in pediatric Hodgkin's disease. Pediatr Clin North Am 32:721–734, 1985.
56. Goldie JH, Coldman AJ: The genetic origin of drug resistance in neoplasms: Implications for systemic therapy. Cancer Res 44:3643–3653, 1984.
57. Golding SJ, McElwain TJ, Husband JE: The role of computed tomography in the management of children with advanced neuroblastoma. Br J Radiol 57:661–666, 1984.
58. Goldman A, Gordon I, Kemshead J: Immunolocalization of neuroblastoma using radiolabeled monoclonal antibody UJ13A. J Pediatr 105:252–256, 1984.
59. Gonzalez-Crussi F: Wilms' Tumor (Nephroblastoma) and Related Renal Neoplasms of Childhood. Boca Raton, FL, CRC Press, 1984.
60. Green AA, Hayes FA, Rao B: Disease control and toxicity of aggressive 4 drug therapy for children with disseminated neuroblastoma. Proc ASCO 5:210, 1986.
61. Greenfield LJ, Shelley WM: The spectrum of neurogenic tumors of the sympathetic nervous system: Maturation and adrenergic function. J Natl Cancer Inst 35:215–226, 1965.
62. Grosfeld JL, Ballantine TVN, Baehnev RL: Experience with "second-look" operations in pediatric solid tumors. J Pediatr Surg 13:275–280, 1978.
63. Haas JE, Bonadio JF, Beckwith JB: Clear cell sarcoma of kidney with emphasis on ultrastructural studies. Cancer 54:2978–2987, 1984.
64. Haddy TB, Keenan AM, Jaffe ES, Magrath IT: Bone involvement in young patients with non-Hodgkin's lymphoma: Efficacy of chemotherapy without local radiotherapy. Blood 72:1141–1147, 1988.
65. Harmer MH (ed): TNM Classification of Pediatric Tumors. Geneva, International Union Against Cancer, 1982, pp 23–28.
66. Harms D, Schmidt D, Treuner J: Soft-tissue sarcomas in childhood: A study of 262 cases including 169 cases of rhabdomyosarcoma. Z Kinderchir 40:140–145, 1985.
67. Hayes FA, Green AA, Casper J, Cornet J, Evans WE: Clinical evaluation of sequentially scheduled cisplatin and VM26 in neuroblastoma: Response and toxicity. Cancer 48:1715–1718, 1981.
68. Heisel MA, Miller JH, Reid BS, et al: Radionuclide bone scan in neuroblastoma. Pediatrics 71:206–209, 1983.
69. Hodgkin T: On Some Morbid Appearances of the Absorbent Glands and Spleen. Med Chirurg Trans 17:68–114, 1832.
70. Hoppe RT, Coleman CN, Cox RS, et al: The management of stage I-II Hodgkin's disease with irradiation alone or combined modality therapy: The Stanford experience. Blood 59:455–465, 1982.
71. Horn RC Jr, Enterline HT: Rhabdomyosarcoma: A clinicopathologic study and classification of 39 cases. Cancer 11:181–199, 1958.
72. Hsueh S, Hsih SN, Kuo TT: Primary rhabdomyosarcoma of long bone. Orthopedics 9:705–707, 1986.
73. Israel MA: The evolution of clinical molecular genetics: Neuroblastoma as a model tumor. Am J Pediatr Hematol Oncol 8:163, 1986.
74. Ivins JC, Dahlin DC: Malignant lymphoma (reticulum cell sarcoma of bone). Mayo Clin Proc 38:375–385, 1963.
75. Jereb B, Cham W, Lattin P, et al: Local control of embryonal rhabdomyosarcoma in children by radiation therapy when combined with concomitant chemotherapy. Int J Radiat Oncol Phys 1:217–225, 1976.
76. Jhanan SC, Neel BG, Hayward WS, et al: Localization of c-*ras* oncogene family on human germ-line chromosomes. Proc Natl Acad Sci USA 80:4794–4797, 1983.
77. Kadin ME: Possible origin of the Reed-Sternberg cell from an interdigitating reticulum cell. Cancer Treat Rep 66:601–608, 1982.
78. Kaplan HS: Hodgkin's Disease, 2nd ed. Cambridge, MA, Harvard University Press, 1980.
79. Kneeland JB, Lee BCP, Whalen JP, et al: NMR: The new frontier in diagnostic radiology. Adv Surg 18:37–65, 1984.
80. Knudson AG: Genetics and the child cured of cancer. *In* Van Eys J, Sullivan MP (eds): Status of the Curability of Childhood Cancers. New York, Raven Press, 1980, pp 295–305.
81. Knudson AG: Hereditary cancer, oncogenes, and antioncogenes. Cancer Res 45:1437–1443, 1985.
82. Knudson AG, Strong LC: Mutation and cancer. A model for Wilms' tumor of the kidney. J Natl Cancer Inst 48:313–324, 1978.
83. Koufas A, Hansen MF, Copeland IV, et al: Loss of heterozygosity in three common embryonal tumors suggests common pathogenetic mechanism. Nature 316:330–334, 1985.
84. Koufas A, Hansen MF, Lamplin BC, et al: Loss of alleles at loci on human chromosome 11 during genesis of Wilms' tumor. Nature 309:170–172, 1984.
85. Kushner BH, Helson L: Coordinated use of sequentially escalated cyclophosphamide and cell-cycle-specific chemotherapy (the N4SE protocol) for advanced neuroblastoma. Experience with 100 patients. J Clin Oncol 5:1746–1751, 1987.
86. Laug WE, Siegel SE, Shaw KNF, et al: Initial urinary catecholamine metabolite concentrations and prognosis in neuroblastoma. Pediatrics 62:77, 1978.
87. Lawler W, Marsden HB, Palmer MK: Wilms' tu-

mor—histologic variation and prognosis. Cancer 36:1122–1126, 1975.
88. Leape LL, Breslow NE, Biship HC: The surgical treatment of Wilms' tumor: Results of the National Wilms' Tumor Study. Ann Surg 187:351–356, 1978.
89. LeBeau MM, Rowley JD: Heritable fragile sites in cancer. Nature:607–608, 1984.
90. Leeson MC, Makley JT, Carter JR: Metastatic skeletal disease in the pediatric population. J Pediatr Orthop 5:261–267, 1985.
91. Leventhal BG, Donaldson SS: Hodgkin's disease. *In* Pizzo PA, Poplack DG (eds): Principles and Practice of Pediatric Oncology. Philadelphia, JB Lippincott, 1988, p 457.
92. Li FP: Cancers in children. *In* Schottenfeld D, Fraumeni JF: Cancer Epidemiology and Prevention. Philadelphia, WB Saunders, 1982, pp 1012–1024.
93. Liew KH, Easton D, Horwich A, et al: Bulky mediastinal Hodgkin's disease. Management and prognosis. Hematol Oncol 2:45–59, 1984.
94. Loeffler JS, Tarbell NJ, Kozakewich H, et al: Primary lymphoma of bone in children: Analysis of treatment results with Adriamycin, prednisone, Oncovin (APO) and local radiation therapy. J Clin Oncol 4:496–501, 1986.
95. Malpas JS: Lymphomas in children. Semin Hematol 19:301–314, 1982.
96. Marchand F: Beitrage zur Kenntnis der Normalen und Patholgoischen Anatomie der Glandula Carotica und der Nebenneiren. Virchows Arch 5:578, 1981.
97. Maroteaux P: Metastatic malignant tumors of the skeleton. *In* Maroteaux P: Bone Diseases of Children. Philadelphia, JB Lippincott, 1979, pp 411–420.
98. Marsden HB, Lawler W, Kuman PM: Bone metastasizing renal tumor of childhood. Morphological and clinical features and differences from Wilms' tumor. Cancer 42:1922–1928, 1978.
99. Marsden HB, Steward JK (eds): Connective tissue tumors. *In* Recent Results in Cancer Research: Tumors in Children. Heidelberg, Springer-Verlag, 1976, pp 282–326.
100. Marugg S, Berchtold C, Elke M: Evaluation of bone lesions in malignant lymphoma. Radiologe 25:587–593, 1985.
101. Mauch P, Gorshein D, Cunningham J, et al: Influence of mediastinal adenopathy on site and frequency of relapse in patients with Hodgkin's disease. Cancer Treat Rep 66:809–817, 1982.
102. Maurer HM: The Intergroup Rhabdomyosarcoma Study (N.I.H.): Objectives and clinical staging classification. J Pediatr Surg 10:977–978, 1975.
103. Maurer HM: The Intergroup Rhabdomyosarcoma Study II: Objectives and study design. J Pediatr Surg 15:371–372, 1980.
104. Maurer HM: Personal communication, 1990.
105. Maurer HM, Gehan E, Crist W, et al: Intergroup rhabdomyosarcoma Study (IRS)–III: A preliminary report of overall outcome. Proc Am Soc Clin Oncol, 8:296, 1989.
106. Miller JH: Imaging in Pediatric Oncology. Baltimore, Williams & Wilkins, 1985.
107. Miller RW, Fraumeni JF Jr, Manning MD: Association of Wilms' tumor with aniridia, hemihypertrophy and other congenital malformations. N Engl J Med 270:922–927, 1964.
108. Miraldi FD, Nelson AD, Kraly C, et al: Diagnostic imaging of human neuroblastoma with radiolabeled antibody. Radiology 161:413–418, 1986.
109. Muraji T, Hays DM, Siegel SE, et al: Evaluation of the surgical aspects of staging laparotomy for Hodgkin's disease in children. J Pediatr Surg 17:843–848, 1982.
110. Murphy SB: Prognostic features and obstacles to cure of childhood non-Hodgkin's lymphoma. Semin Oncol 4:265–271, 1977.
111. Murphy SB: Classification, staging and end results of treatment of childhood non-Hodgkin's lymphoma: Dissimilarities from lymphomas in adults. Semin Oncol 7:332–339, 1980.
112. Murphy SB, Frizzera G, et al: A study of childhood non-Hodgkin's lymphoma. Cancer 36:2121–2131, 1975.
113. Murphy SB, Husta HO: A randomized trial of combined modality therapy of childhood non-Hodgkin's lymphoma. Cancer 45:630–637, 1980.
114. Nathwani BN: A critical analysis of the classifications of non-Hodgkin's lymphomas. Cancer 44:347–384, 1979.
115. Nathwani BN, Kim H, Rappaport H, et al: Non-Hodgkin's lymphomas. A clinicopathologic study comparing two classifications. Cancer 41:303–325, 1978.
116. Nelson AJ III: Embryonal rhabdomyosarcoma: Report of twenty-four cases and study of the effectiveness of radiation therapy upon the primary tumor. Cancer 22:64–68, 1968.
117. Newton WA Jr, Soule EH, Hamoudi AB, et al: Histopathology of childhood sarcomas, Intergroup Rhabdomyosarcoma Studies I and II: Clinicopathologic correlation. J Clin Oncol 6:67–75, 1988.
118. Nickerson HJ, Nesbit ME, Grosfeld JL, et al: Comparison of stage IV and IV-S neuroblastoma in the first year of life. Med Pediatr Oncol 13:261, 1985.
119. Oberling C: Les reticulosarcomes et les reticuloendotheliosarcomes de la moelle aasseuse. Bull Assoc Fr Etude Cancer 17:259–296, 1928.
120. Ostrowski ML, Unni KK, Banks PM, Shives TC, Evans RG, O'Connell MJ, Taylor WF: Malignant lymphoma of bone. Cancer 58:2646–2655, 1986.
121. Palmer N, Foulkes M: Histopathology and prognosis in the Second Intergroup Rhabdomyosarcoma Study (IRS-II). Proc Am Soc Clin Oncol 2:229, 1983.
122. Palmer NF, Sutow W: Clinical aspects of the rhabdoid tumor of the kidney: A report of the National Wilms' Tumor Study Group. Med Pediatr Oncol 11:242–245, 1983.
123. Parker FW, Jackson J: Primary reticulum cell sarcoma of bone. Surg Gynecol Obstet 68:45–53, 1939.
124. Patton RB, Horn RC Jr: Rhabdomyosarcoma: Clinical and pathologic features and comparison with human fetal and embryonal skeletal muscle. Surgery 52:572–584, 1962.
125. Payne SV, Wright DH, Jones KJM, Judd MA: Macrophage origin of Reed-Sternberg cells: An immunohistochemical study. J Clin Pathol 35:159–166, 1982.
126. Peckham MJ, Cooper EH: Cell proliferation in Hodgkin's disease. Natl Cancer Inst Monogr 36:179–189, 1973.
127. Pedrick TJ, Donaldson SS, Cox RS: Rhabdomyosarcoma: The Stanford experience using a TNM staging system. J Clin Oncol 4:370–378, 1986.
128. Phillips WC, Kattapuram SV, Doseretz DE, Raymond AK, Schiller AL, Murphy G, Wyshak G: Primary lymphoma of bone: Relationship of radiographic appearance and prognosis. Radiology 144:285–290, 1982.
129. Potluri VR, Gilbert F: A cytogenetic study of embryonal rhabdomyosarcoma. Cancer Genet Cytogenet 14:169–173, 1985.

130. Raney RB Jr, Crist WM, Maurer HM, et al: Prognosis of children with soft tissue sarcoma who relapse after achieving a complete response: A report from the Intergroup Rhabdomyosarcoma Study I. Cancer 52:44–50, 1983.
131. Raney RB Jr, Hays DM, Tefft M, et al: Rhabdomyosarcoma and the undifferentiated sarcomas. *In* Pizzo PA, Poplack DG (eds): Principles and Practice of Pediatric Oncology. Philadelphia, JB Lippincott, 1989, pp 635–658.
132. Reed DM: On the pathologic changes in Hodgkin's disease with special reference to its relation to tuberculosis. Johns Hopkins Hosp Rep 10:133–196, 1902.
133. Reynolds CP, Reynolds DA, Frankel EP, et al: Selective toxicity of 6-hydroxydopamine and ascorbate for human neuroblastoma *in vitro:* A model for clearing marrow prior to autologous transplant. Cancer Res 42:1331–1336, 1982.
134. Saarinen U, Coccia PF, Gersen SL, et al: Eradication of neuroblastoma cells *in vitro* by monoclonal antibody and human complement: Method for purging autologous bone marrow. Cancer Res 45:5969–5975, 1985.
135. Santoro A, Bonadonna G, Valagussa P, et al: Long-term results of combined chemotherapy-radiotherapy approach in Hodgkin's disease: Superiority of ABVD plus radiotherapy v MOPP plus radiotherapy. J Clin Oncol 5:27–37, 1987.
136. Schmidt D, Harms D, Evers KG, et al: Bone metastasizing renal tumor (clear cell sarcoma) of childhood with epithelioid elements. Cancer 56:609–613, 1985.
137. Seeger RC, Brodeur GM, Sather H, Dalton A, Siegel SE, Wong KY, Hammond D: Association of multiple copies of the n-*myc* oncogene with rapid progression of neuroblastomas. N Engl J Med 313:1111–1116, 1985.
138. Shafford EA, Rogers DW, Pritchard J: Advanced neuroblastoma: Improved response rate using a multiagent regimen (OPEC) including sequential cisplatin and VM-26. J Clin Oncol 2:742–747, 1984.
139. Shimada H, Chatten J, Newton WA Jr, et al: Histopathologic prognostic factors in neuroblastic tumors: Definition of subtypes of ganglioneuroblastoma and an age-linked classification of neuroblastomas. J Natl Cancer Inst 73:405–416, 1984.
140. Shimada H, Newton WA Jr, Soule EH, et al: Pathology of fatal rhabdomyosarcoma: Report from the Intergroup Rhabdomyosarcoma Study (IRS-I and II). Cancer 59:459–465, 1987.
141. Spagnoli I, Gattoni F, Viganotti G: Roentgenographic aspect of non-Hodgkin's lymphoma presenting with osseous lesions. Skeletal Radiol 8:39–41, 1982.
142. Stay EJ, Vawter G: The relationship between nephroblastoma and neurofibromatosis (von Recklinghausen's disease). Cancer 39:2550–2555, 1977.
143. Stein RS, Golomb HM, Wiernik PH, et al: Anatomic substages of stage IIIA Hodgkin's disease. Follow-up of a collaborative study. Cancer Treat Rep 66:733–741, 1982.
144. Sternberg C: Uber eine Eigenartige unter dem Bilde der Pseudoleukamie verlaufende Tuberculose des Lymphatischen Apparates. Z Heilk 19:21–90, 1898.
145. Stout AP: Rhabdomyosarcoma of the skeletal muscles. Ann Surg 123:447–472, 1946.
146. Tefft M, Lattin PB, Jereb B, et al: Acute and late effects on normal tissue following combined chemo and radiotherapy for childhood rhabdomyosarcoma and Ewing's sarcoma. Cancer 37:1201–1217, 1976.
147. Tefft M, Wharam M, Ruymann F, et al: Radiotherapy for rhabdomyosarcoma in children: A report from the Intergroup Rhabdomyosarcoma Study #2 (IRS-2). Proc Am Soc Clin Oncol 4:234, 1985.
148. Thomas PRM, Tefft M, Farewell VT, et al: Abdominal relapses in irradiated Second National Wilms' Tumor Study Patients. J Clin Oncol 2:1098–1101, 1984.
149. Trent J, Casper J, Meltzer P, et al: Nonrandom chromosome alterations in rhabdomyosarcoma. Cancer Genet Cytogenet 16:189–197, 1985.
150. Treleaven JG, Gibson FM, Ugelstad J, et al: Removal of neuroblastoma transplant cells from bone marrow with monoclonal antibodies conjugated to magnetic microspheres. Lancet 1:70, 1984.
151. Tsokos M, Howard R, Costa J: Immunohistochemical study of alveolar and embryonal rhabdomyosarcoma. Lab Invest 48:148–155, 1983.
152. Bucsky P: Origin of Hodgkin's and Reed-Sternberg cells. N Engl J Med 303:284–285, 1980.
153. Valagussa P, Santoro A, Fossati-Bellani F, et al: Second acute leukemia and other malignancies following treatment for Hodgkin's disease. Clin Oncol 4:830–837, 1986.
154. Virchow R: Hyperlasie der Zirbel und der Nebennieren. *In* Die Krankhaffen Geschwulste, Vol 2. Berlin, A Hirschwald, 1864–1865.
155. Weiner MA, Leventhal BG, Marcus R, et al: Intensive chemotherapy (MOPP plus ABVD) and low dose total nodal irradiation for the treatment of advanced stage Hodgkin's disease in pediatric patients: A Pediatric Oncology Group study. J Clin Oncol (in press).
156. Weiss LM, Movahed LA, Warnke RA, et al: Detection of Epstein-Barr viral genomes in Reed-Sternberg cells of Hodgkin's disease. N Engl J Med 320:502–506, 1989.
157. Wilson TW, Pugh DG: Primary reticulum cell sarcoma of bone, with emphasis on roentgen aspects. Radiology 65:343–351, 1955.
158. Wollner N, Burchenal JH, Lieberman PH, et al: Non-Hodgkin's lymphoma in children. A comparative study of two modalities of therapy. Cancer 37:123–134, 1976.
159. Wright JH: Neurocytoma or neuroblastoma, a kind of tumor not generally recognized. J Exp Med 12:556–561, 1910.
160. Wu ZL, Schwartz E, Seeger R, et al: Expression on GD_2 ganglioside by untreated primary human neuroblastomas. Cancer Res 46:440–443, 1986.
161. Young J, Miller R: Incidence of malignant tumors in U.S. children. J Pediatr 1:254–258, 1975.
162. Young JL, Miller RW: Incidence of malignant tumors in children. J Pediatr 86:254–258, 1979.
163. Yunis JJ: Fragile sites and predisposition to leukemia and lymphoma. Cancer Genet Cytogenet 12:85–88, 1984.
164. Zeltzer PM, Marangos PJ, Evans AE, et al: Serum neuron-specific enolase in children with neuroblastoma. Relationship to stage and disease course. Cancer 57:1230–1234, 1986.
165. Ziegler J, Magrath I: Burkitt's lymphoma. Pathobiol Annu 4:129–142, 1974.

CHAPTER 5

Pediatric Ewing's Sarcomas, Osteosarcomas, and Primitive Neuroectodermal Tumors

MICHAEL B. HARRIS

Ewing's sarcomas, osteosarcomas, and primitive neuroectodermal tumors (PNETs) (neuroepitheliomas) are the predominant primary malignant bone tumors of childhood. During the past 25 years, substantial progress has been made in the treatment of these disorders. Treatment regimens that relied on surgery, with or without radiation therapy, usually yielded only 10 to 20% long-term disease-free survival.[27, 32, 48, 94, 122, 143] With the advent of intensive multiagent chemotherapy, at least 60% of children with either osteosarcoma or Ewing's sarcoma are expected to be long-term survivors.[65, 132]

The progress in the treatment of bone tumors has been made with the cooperation of orthopedists interested in oncology, radiotherapists, pathologists, and pediatric oncologists. Together, these physicians have defined the natural history of these tumors, prognostic factors, and the principles of combined modality treatment necessary to improve the survival rates of children with these rare neoplasms.

Clinical Evaluation

Pain at the primary site, with or without swelling or warmth, is usually the initial manifestation of bone tumors. An x-ray film of the area usually reveals the nature of the problem better than computed tomography (CT) and magnetic resonance imaging (MRI) and is the most important tool for diagnosis before the biopsy. The clinical evaluation (Table 5–1) that should take place before biopsy includes the following:[120, 163]

Detailed history to identify symptoms such as fever, weight loss, location of pain, loss of neurologic function, and paresthesias

Careful physical examination, including neurologic assessment in suspected pelvic and/or vertebral or paravertebral lesions

Peripheral blood studies including complete blood count, erythrocyte sedimentation rate, coagulation profile, chemistry screen (with special attention to lactate dehydrogenase (LDH) and alkaline phosphatase levels), and hepatitis screen and varicella titers (to judge susceptibility to these diseases before the onset of chemotherapy)

Bone marrow aspiration

Radiologic examinations, including CT and MRI of the primary lesion to judge the extent of intraosseous and soft tissue involvement by tumor. Bone scan, chest x-ray film, and CT of the chest are necessary

TABLE 5–1

Diagnostic Work-up of Bone Tumors

History
- Pain, swelling, erythema, fever, weight loss, neurologic function

Physical Examination
- Careful neurologic examination in patients with pelvic and central lesions

Blood Studies
- Complete blood count, erythrocyte sedimentation rate, chemical screen (lactic dehydrogenase, alkaline phosphatase), blood cultures

Bone Marrow Aspiration and Biopsy
- (for Ewing's sarcoma and PNET)

Radiologic Studies
- Plain x-ray films—primary site and chest
- CT and or MRI—primary site; CT of chest
- Bone scan

Pathologic Studies
- Hematoxylin and eosin evaluation
- Cytochemistry
- Electron microscopy
- Immunocytochemistry
- Determination of cytogenetics and oncogenes

to evaluate for metastases. Finally, if a pelvic, vertebral, or paravertebral mass is present, intravenous pyelogram, barium enema study, and/or myelogram may be necessary.

This evaluation, before biopsy, aids the clinician in ascertaining the clinical stage of the disease. The gathering of data such as LDH and alkaline phosphatase levels and tumor volume from CT scans may be useful in determining prognosis. Staging enables appropriate therapy for a particular patient or prospective controlled studies to improve on the current treatment results.

Pathology and Staging

The biopsy yields the definitive diagnosis and histologic subtype. The subtype (see later) may be of prognostic significance regarding the outcome of treatment in Ewing's sarcoma and osteosarcoma. The tissue obtained at biopsy should be prepared for routine hematoxylin and eosin evaluation, histochemical stains, and electron microscopy, and for cytogenetic evaluation, which may help in determining the diagnosis and prognosis.[10, 117, 182, 183] In addition, monoclonal antibodies raised against specific tumor antigens may prove helpful in differentiating a number of small round cell tumors from each other and thus help in the initial pathologic diagnosis of difficult cases.[38]

When the clinical and pathologic evaluation is completed, treatment of the tumor should be planned with the orthopedic surgeon, the oncologist, and when appropriate, the radiotherapist. Before the advent of neoadjuvant chemotherapy (i.e., chemotherapy given before the definitive surgical procedure), surgery was usually performed at this point and stage of tumor would be assigned according to the criteria of Enneking and associates.[42] This staging schema was in many ways the most important indicator of how a patient would fare clinically before the advent of aggressive chemotherapeutic regimens. In pediatric patients, this system has been used less often to determine prognosis, and at present, other criteria are used to aid in this determination.

Pediatric Ewing's Sarcoma

Ewing's sarcoma is the second most common primary malignant bone tumor in children (after osteosarcoma) and the fourth most common malignant tumor of bone, constituting approximately 7% of cases of malignant bone tumors (i.e., in adults and children). Ewing's sarcoma, neuroblastoma, lymphoma, and neuroepithelioma are the primary round cell tumors of bone that occur during childhood through the young adult years. Ewing's sarcoma must also be differentiated from chronic osteomyelitis.

The peak incidence of Ewing's sarcoma is during the second decade of life, with a male preponderance of approximately 1.6:1.[9, 17, 28, 37, 46, 50, 51, 59, 70, 72, 74, 137, 146, 153, 184] This particular tumor occurs rarely in blacks.[22, 65, 77, 153]

The most common presenting symptoms are pain (in approximately 90% of patients) and swelling (in about 70% of patients).[17, 146, 184] These symptoms are usually present for 2 to 3 months before the patient seeks medical advice, but some patients do not come to a physician for as long as 2 years from the onset of symptoms. Patients with Ewing's sarcoma may also have fever (20 to 30%) and pathologic fractures (15 to 25%). Finally, 15 to 35% of patients have metastases at the time of diagnosis, with an increased incidence seen in patients with larger tumors, fever, and delays in diagnosis.

Ewing's sarcoma most frequently occurs in

TABLE 5–2

Distribution of Primary Sites of Ewing's Sarcoma and Osteosarcoma

	Ewing's Sarcoma		Osteosarcoma*	
	Number	*(%)*	*Number*	*(%)*
Foot	20	(5.0)	11	(0.9)
Tibia				
Distal	9	(2.2)	21	(1.6)
Mid	1	(0.2)	18	(1.4)
Proximal	20	(5.0)	197	(15.5)
Fibula				
Distal	6	(1.5)	4	(0.3)
Mid	8	(2.0)	2	(0.2)
Proximal	17	(4.2)	30	(2.4)
Femur				
Distal	19	(4.7)	405	(31.8)
Mid	30	(7.5)	70	(5.5)
Proximal	41	(10.2)	66	(5.2)
Hand	1	(0.2)	3	(0.2)
Radius	5	(1.2)	11	(0.9)
Ulna	7	(1.8)	6	(0.5)
Humerus				
Distal	7	(1.8)	9	(0.7)
Mid	10	(2.5)	12	(0.9)
Proximal	29	(7.2)	106	(8.3)
Pelvis	71	(17.7)	109	(8.5)
Scapula	21	(5.2)	19	(1.5)
Sacrum	19	(4.7)	12	(0.9)
Vertebrae	13	(3.2)	32	(2.5)
Ribs	31	(7.7)	16	(1.3)
Clavicle	10	(2.5)	5	(0.4)
Face and head	7	(1.8)	110	(8.6)
TOTAL	402	(100)	1274	(100)

*Excluding parosteal osteosarcoma.

Adapted from Dahlin DC, Unni KK: Bone Tumors. General Aspects and Data on 8,542 Cases, 4th ed. Springfield, IL, Charles C Thomas, 1986, pp 269–305.

the long bones and the pelvis (Table 5–2). When it occurs in the long bones, it usually involves the diaphysis. The sites of Ewing's sarcoma can be divided into three distinct areas, and the incidence of occurrence in these areas is as follows:

1. Central (pelvis, vertebrae, sternum, ribs, scapula, clavicle, face, head)—45%
2. Proximal (femur, humerus)—30%
3. Distal (tibia, fibula, radius, ulna, hands, feet)—25%

The majority of patients with Ewing's sarcoma have tumors of the larger bones (i.e., pelvis, femur, tibia, humerus), accounting for 65% of all the primary sites at presentation.

PROGNOSIS

The major prognostic factors in Ewing's sarcoma are site, volume of tumor, histologic characteristics, metastases at diagnosis, and, perhaps, chemotherapy effect (Table 5–3). These act as independent variables in prognosis, but site and tumor volume may be difficult to separate from each other.

TABLE 5–3

Prognostic Factors in Ewing's Sarcoma

	Prognosis Good	Prognosis Poor
Location	Distal Head/face	Pelvic Distal vertebrae
Size	<10 cm	≥10 cm
Volume	<100 ml	≥100 ml
Tissue extension	Absent	Present
Histologic features at diagnosis		Filigree Necrosis
Chemotherapy response	Present	Absent
Metastases at diagnosis	Absent	Present

For prognostic purposes, the site of origin of Ewing's sarcoma can be divided into central, proximal, and distal areas[153](see above). Patients with distal primary lesions fare significantly better than those with central lesions, and those with proximal lesions have a better prognosis than those with pelvic lesions.[51, 56, 153] In the many series that have been published, patients with Ewing's sarcoma of the rib and the head have a much better prognosis than patients with pelvic tumors, even though both are central in location.[22, 160, 170]

In many ways, site reflects the initial size of the tumor. This is especially true for primary tumors in pelvic and proximal sites where tumors may become larger before clinical detection. Size plays a significant role in the eventual outcome of treatment. In some series, patients with neoplasms of 10 cm or larger do significantly worse than those with tumors of less than 10 cm[20, 43] whereas in other studies, tumors greater than 8 cm carry a poorer prognosis.[72, 123] This finding can be further refined by measuring tumor volume with CT scans. Individuals having a tumor with a volume of 100 ml or greater have significantly poorer prognosis than do those with tumor volumes less than 100 ml.[58, 158] In measuring tumor size or volume, the clinician also determines the extent of local tissue invasion, which in turn is correlated by some investigators with a poor prognosis[9, 42, 131] but not by other researchers.[184] Tumors with greater tissue extension tend to be in more unfavorable sites (e.g., pelvis and distal spine) and have a higher proportion of metastases at the time of diagnosis. This is further substantiated by analyzing prognosis by size and site of tumors and noting that tumors of 100 ml or greater yield a poorer prognosis regardless of the site of origin.[158] A chemical correlate of size is serum LDH concentration, which is often elevated in patients with Ewing's sarcoma. Some investigators have noted a poorer outcome with an LDH level of 200 U/L or greater.[57] Increased levels of LDH were associated with centrally located tumors, perhaps reflecting the size of the primary tumors at these locations and the increased amount of necrosis seen with larger tumors. LDH level also was an independent variable and portended a poorer disease-free survival if 200 U/L or greater in patients with distal tumors was found. Elevated LDH level is not universally accepted as indicating a poor prognosis[22, 153] but may be a marker for recurrence.[45]

Ewing's sarcoma has a number of histologic patterns including diffuse, filigree, lobular, and trabecular.[177] In addition, a subgroup of patients may have a predominance of large cells or endothelial appearing cells.[115] Histologically, the two features associated with a poor prognosis are a filigree pattern and necrosis, with the latter indicative of a rapidly growing neoplasm.[35, 115]

Patients who demonstrate a good clinical and/or pathologic response to chemotherapy have a better prognosis than those who do not.[65, 138] Adequate responses to chemotherapy can be judged by a decrease in the size of the tumor mass on physical examination, by the results of radiologic assessment, and by the amount of residual viable tumor seen on pathology examination of surgically excised tumors. Tumors that respond to chemotherapy may be easier to remove with good surgical margins. They may be easier to irradiate because they are smaller and less likely to have areas missed during radiotherapy and a good response in areas where micrometastases have occurred is more likely. Thus, good chemotherapy response may yield better local and distant control of Ewing's sarcoma.

Metastatic disease at the time of diagnosis is a poor prognostic sign. These patients, however, may survive with aggressive management that includes chemotherapy together with surgery and/or radiation treatment of residual metastatic deposits.[72] In a small series from the National Cancer Institute (NCI), patients with less than four metastatic nodules removed do better than those with four or more tumor nodules removed or in those not rendered disease free at thoracotomy.[107]

TREATMENT

The goal of treatment in Ewing's sarcoma is to achieve control of distant metastases and local disease with the least amount of short- and long-term morbidity. The problems in management are compounded because Ewing's sarcoma is sensitive to both ionizing radiation and multiple chemotherapeutic agents. The role of each, in relation to one another and to surgery, is still undergoing critical evaluation. It is indisputable, however, that chemotherapy has changed the survival of patients with Ewing's sarcoma from approximately 10% to greater than 60% in most series.

Surgery and Radiotherapy

Historically, surgery and/or radiotherapy was used to treat Ewing's sarcoma (Table 5–4).

TABLE 5–4

Modalities for Local Control of Ewing's Sarcoma

Radiation	Surgery
Total dose: 30–70 Gy	Excise expendable bone
Recommended doses	Excise tumor with or without normal tissue
Whole bone: 45–55 Gy	Biopsy only
Tumor bed boost: 10–15 Gy	

The survival of these patients was poor. A representative example is in the historical control group from the Instituto Ortopedica Rizzoli, where 83 patients were treated (1950 to 1970) with either surgery and/or radiotherapy.[9] In this series, only 4 of 83 patients survived longer than 5 years. Radiotherapy was not standardized in many of the cases and surgery was not optimal. Yet, only 11 of 83 patients had local recurrences, whereas 78 of 83 had distant metastases and 76 of 83 died of their disease (3 patients with recurrence were lost to follow-up). It is certainly possible that if the patients had survived longer more local relapses would have occurred, especially because autopsy series find a higher incidence of local recurrences than is suspected from clinical evaluation alone.[169]

The relatively poor local control achieved with radiation therapy without adjuvant chemotherapy was emphasized by Thomas and colleagues in their study of the role of radiotherapy in Ewing's sarcoma.[171] In reviewing the literature, they tabulated the results in 78 patients treated with radiation and no chemotherapy and contrasted these patients to 151 patients treated with radiation and adjuvant chemotherapy. Twenty-eight patients (35%) in the group receiving radiotherapy alone had a local recurrence as compared with only 18 patients (12%) among those who had both chemotherapy and radiation to the primary site.

Surgery without chemotherapy has almost as poor results as radiation alone. With ablative surgery (historically, this has been amputation), the incidence of local relapse is virtually nonexistent and the long-term results are slightly better than with radiotherapy alone, but never have these results exceeded 20% long-term disease-free survival. These slightly better results could well be secondary to selection bias because only patients with primary tumors that were amenable to surgery were operated on. Thus, patients with large central primary tumors tended not to have definitive surgical procedures, whereas those with smaller lesions tended to have a surgical procedure with curative intent. When surgery is combined with chemotherapy, the long-term survival approaches 60% in most series (see below).

Chemotherapy

Chemotherapy has evolved as the primary modality of therapy in Ewing's sarcoma (Table 5–5). In the earliest trials, the agents that were found to be most effective were cyclophosphamide (Cytoxan), vincristine, actinomycin D (dactinomycin), and doxorubicin (Adriamycin). After these agents were identified as effective single agents to induce responses, but for the most part not yielding long-term survival advantages when used with surgery and/or radiation therapy, several trials combined these agents into multiagent treatment regimens.[46, 74, 146] These single-institution trials gave encouraging results, with at least one series reporting a survival of 52% at 5 years (with survival rates increasing with the use of more intensive chemotherapeutic regimen).[146]

After these early trials, the Intergroup Ewing's Sarcoma Study (IESS) was mounted with the participation of 83 institutions. Because of the previous results and the determination that most patients in whom treatment failed had metastatic disease to the lungs, these workers decided to study whether four drugs (vincristine, cyclophosphamide, actinomycin D, and doxorubicin) were better than a three-drug regimen (vincristine, actinomycin D, cyclophosphamide) and whether prophylactic pulmonary irradiation produced the same or superior results to either regimen when added to the three-drug regimen.[137, 142] Originally, this study included an arm in which patients did not receive chemotherapy. This arm was closed when two of the first three patients had early relapses. During the years that this first multi-

TABLE 5–5

Chemotherapeutic Agents Used in Ewing's Sarcoma

Commonly Used	Seldom Used	New
Vincristine	BCNU (Iomustine)	Ifosfamide
Cyclophosphamide (Cytoxin)	Methotrexate	Etoposide (VP-16)
Doxorubicin (Adriamycin)	Bleomycin	
Actinomycin D	5-Fluorouracil	
	Procarbazine	

institutional trial was performed, it became apparent that the four-drug regimen was significantly better than the three-drug regimen and marginally better than the regimen that contained three drugs and prophylactic lung radiation. These investigators also observed that when the courses of drugs were shortened from 6 to 3 weeks more patients had longer disease-free survival periods.

These results have been mirrored in various other studies, thus confirming the utility of aggressive chemotherapy in the treatment of Ewing's sarcoma.[8, 9, 28, 50, 59, 70, 72, 142, 152, 153, 184, 192] In the latest Intergroup Ewing's Sarcoma Study (IESS-II) report[22] on patients with nonmetastatic, nonpelvic primary tumors, a relapse-free survival of 73% (median follow-up, 5.6 years) was obtained in patients treated with a high-dose, intermittent schedule (every 3 weeks) of vincristine; doxorubicin (75 mg/m^2), alternating with vincristine; cyclophosphamide (1400 mg/m^2); and actinomycin D (0.45 mg/m^2 for 5 days), substituted for doxorubicin after six doses of the latter. In the same study, a 56% relapse-free survival was obtained in patients treated with a less aggressive regimen that utilized weekly vincristine (1.5 mg/m^2, maximum of 2 mg) and cyclophosphamide (500 mg/m^2) for 6 weeks. After the first 6 weeks, seven additional cycles were given that included actinomycin D (0.45 mg/m^2 for 5 days) followed by a 1-week rest. Then, for 5 weeks, vincristine and cytoxan (500 mg/m^2) were given weekly, with doxorubicin (60 mg/m^2) also given on the fifth week. Patients with Ewing's sarcoma can now expect a disease-free survival of approximately 60%, with those with tumors in favorable sites exceeding 60% and those with tumors in less favorable locations experiencing less than 50% survival (Table 5–6).

TABLE 5–6

Treatment Results for Ewing's Sarcoma Using Multiagent Chemotherapy, With or Without Radiation and/or Surgery

	Number of Patients	Local Control	Disease-Free Survival	Follow-up (months)
Nonmetastatic	793	86.8%	53.3%	4–110
Special sites				
Head and neck	29	—	82.8%	7–123
Ribs	42	—	61.9%	6–82
Hands and feet	21	90.5%	57.1%	119–221
Pelvic	174	70.0%	40.1%	
Metastatic	143	—	26.2%	16–82

Special Sites

PELVIS

Ewing's sarcoma of the pelvic bones carries a poor prognosis,[43, 44, 97, 111] with most series reporting long-term survival in the range of 30 to 40%.

The problems associated with pelvic lesions are mainly due to the size of the lesion on presentation, making local control with surgery and/or radiation difficult. In addition, chemotherapeutic responses might be less than optimal because of the sheer size of the tumor. This has led investigators to attempt different treatment approaches, including aggressive chemotherapy with or without total body irradiation.[164] Whether this strategy will generate better local control and longer disease-free survival is not known.

RIBS (CHEST WALL)

Ewing's sarcoma is among the most common tumors of the chest wall and, in children, is perhaps the most frequent malignant tumor at this site.[31, 63] The disease-free survival for this group has been reported to be about 50%.[31, 170] However, in patients who are able to undergo total excision of the primary lesion, the disease-free survival may be considerably better, and this clearly is related to the size of the initial tumor.[31, 170] These patients could have an excellent prognosis with adequate local control. One approach in this group of patients is to use preoperative chemotherapy to shrink the tumor, allowing surgical excision of the tumor and avoiding radical chest wall resection. This is followed by postoperative chemotherapy with or without radiation therapy.[148]

HEAD AND NECK

The head and neck is a rare site for Ewing's sarcoma and accounts for approximately 4 to 7% of the primary lesions.[22, 161] Patients with primary tumors in this location fare well. In the IESS reports a total of 29 patients had Ewing's sarcoma of the head and neck.[161] Of these, 24 survived and 5 did not. The 5 patients who died had primary tumors of the cervical spine (3 patients) or the skull (2 patients). The patients who had either biopsies or complete excisions did much better than those who had incomplete removal of their tumors.

HANDS AND FEET

Only 12 of 377 patients with Ewing's sarcoma had tumors at these locations in the IESS experience.[160] Except for patients with primary tumors of the calcaneus, patients with these lesions do quite well with chemotherapy, surgical excision, and when needed, radiotherapy. Seven of the 12 patients are alive and 5 have died. Four of the five patients who died had primary tumors of the calcaneus.

Special attention must be given when using radiation therapy in this site, because there is little soft tissue between the primary tumor area and the skin. Careful simulation, casting to ensure reproducible treatment position, maximal sparing of normal tissue, immersion of the hand or the foot in a water bath for the administration of the first 30 to 40 Gy to improve dose homogeneity, and protection of the scar and the nail beds have been used to ensure both local control and eventual function.[101] With such careful planning, surgery can be limited to excision of the primary lesion and thus preserve the function of the patient's hand or foot.

Future Approaches to Patients with Poor Prognosis

Treatment of patients with poor prognosis (e.g., those with pelvic lesions, tumor volume greater than 100 ml, metastases at diagnosis, and recurrent disease) remains a challenge, because these patients all have less than a 40% chance to survive. In this group of patients, new chemotherapeutic agents are needed, and novel approaches to therapy must be tried.

The IESS group noted that patients with metastatic disease could be treated successfully with intensive chemotherapy and radiation to most, if not all, the metastatic sites.[178] In this group's latest report of 122 patients with metastatic disease, 70% attained either complete or partial remission. Thirty per cent of the responding patients remained disease free for more then 5 years after diagnosis. The sites of recurrence in this group of patients were equally distributed between the lungs and the bones.[24]

Although it is encouraging that a number of patients with overwhelming disease may be cured, new drugs or drug combinations are clearly needed for this group of patients. The combination of ifosfamide (an ozaphosphorine analogous to cyclophosphamide) and etoposide (VP-16) stands out as the most promising of these approaches.[133, 136] In trials on patients with recurrent sarcomas from the NCI, there were a number of long-term survivors when these agents were combined with surgery and radiation therapy.

On the basis of these encouraging results in patients with recurrent disease, ifosfamide, with or without VP-16, in newly diagnosed patients, is beginning to be used as front line therapy in patients with Ewing's sarcoma. When ifosfamide is used in combination with other drugs, but without VP-16, the results have not been any different than when compared with multiagent therapy that includes cyclophosphamide.[139] With this in mind, the current approach of two large cooperative groups (Pediatric Oncology Group [POG] and Children's Cancer Study Group [CCSG]) is to test the efficacy of ifosfamide and VP-16 compared with cyclophosphamide in a randomized trial in all patients with Ewing's sarcoma. Both arms of this study include other chemotherapeutic agents, radiotherapy, and surgery. The combined trial of POG and CCSG began in 1988, and it will take at least 5 to 7 years to determine the efficacy in patients with either good or poor-prognosis Ewing's sarcoma.

Another approach that is currently undergoing preliminary investigations is the use of autologous bone marrow transplantation (ABMT) after bone marrow ablative high-dose chemotherapy and total body irradiation. Radiotherapy in patients with recurrent disease has been used by a number of investigators with encouraging results, especially when the technique of sequential half body irradiation is used. In this technique, a single high dose of radiation is used on the half of the body where the major site of Ewing's sarcoma is, and the other half of the body is treated after a 4 to 8-week rest. With this therapy, an overall response rate of 50% was noted, with 6 of 18 patients surviving for 4 to 27 months, 3 of them without evidence of disease.[116] The use of supralethal doses of chemotherapy has also been reported in Ewing's sarcoma. Melphalan, with or without radiation therapy, followed by ABMT, was given to eight patients with recurrent disease, of whom six had a partial response that lasted for a median of 3 months.[64] A number of trials have been mounted to utilize aggressive combination chemotherapy and total body irradiation. The early results of these studies indicated that this therapy can be given, that toxicity can be manageable, and that long-term survivors can be expected with this method of treatment. Whether this will offer an advantage to patients with poor-prognosis Ewing's sarcoma, compared with the use of newer agents, needs to be addressed in future trials.[11, 16, 43, 68, 135]

Side Effects

The effects of therapy can be short term and long term (Table 5–7). The long-term effects must be addressed in an attempt to limit their impact on the patient's future functioning in life. The long-term sequelae of chemotherapy include sterility in males from cyclophosphamide and possibly decreased cardiac function from doxorubicin. In the report by Burgert and colleagues[22] of the IESS-II results, 3 of 182 children died of cardiotoxicity. An additional 14 had moderate to life-threatening cardiotoxicity. The most severe cardiac abnormalities were noted in the treatment regimen that included multiple doses of doxorubicin given at 75 mg/m^2. Another major treatment modality that has serious side effects is radiotherapy, with its effects on the musculoskeletal system, decreased fertility in females who receive pelvic irradiation, and the risk of developing secondary cancer.

A musculoskeletal grading system to assess function was developed by Jentzsch and colleagues at the NCI.[95] This system utilizes soft tissue changes, muscle function, contractures, pain, edema, leg length discrepancies, need for orthopedic appliances, history of surgical procedures, and quality of life to assess the sequelae of therapy in terms of the overall functioning of the patient. Although this system was developed for the lower extremity, it may be modified to assess the functioning of the upper extremity as well. More importantly, it points to the various complications that may arise from radiation. In the group of 29 patients treated for Ewing's sarcoma of the leg, 20 were judged to have mild to moderate (grade I–II) and 9 had severe (grade III–IV) functional defects. The worse functional results tended to occur when the tumors originated in the femur (a higher percentage of pathologic fractures) and in children younger than 16 years of age with Ewing's sarcoma (higher percentage of leg length discrepancies, fractures, contractures, and joint deformities). These results were in contrast to those reported from Memorial Sloan-Kettering Cancer Center, where more than one half of the patients had severe functional defects[110]; they were more in line with the results of the IESS-I study, where 75% of patients had adequate function.[171] The recommendation of a number of radiation therapists and surgeons is to irradiate upper extremity lesions and femoral lesions in postpubescent children, but to excise (either by amputation or limb salvage technique) tumors of the femur in younger children, expendable bones, and perhaps the small bones of the feet.[110, 171] Other researchers, however, believe that, by careful planning, radiation can be used in most patients, except those with very large destructive tumors and/or pathologic fractures at diagnosis.[100] Future studies need to be done to answer these questions.

Secondary cancers in the irradiated bone have been reported in a small percentage (1 to 2%) of survivors.[100, 171] All of these secondary tumors have been osteosarcoma, and whether this represents new malignancies in every case or an erroneous primary diagnosis is unknown.[165]

TABLE 5–7

Late Effects in Treating Ewing's Sarcoma

Limb
Soft tissue fibrosis
Contractures
Muscle function diminished
Pain, edema
Leg length discrepancies
Need for orthopedic appliances
Sterility
Cardiomyopathy
Secondary cancer

SUMMARY, CONCLUSIONS, AND FUTURE DIRECTIONS

The results from single institutions and the cooperative trials in Europe and the United States have clearly demonstrated the need for combined treatment that includes multiagent chemotherapy, surgery, and radiotherapy. With this approach, patients with Ewing's sarcoma have a survival expectancy that ranges from approximately 30% to greater than 80%, depending on the location of the primary tumor and/or the presence of metastases. In children with Ewing's sarcoma, the site of the primary tumor, the size of the initial tumor, and the presence of metastases at diagnosis are the most important features in predicting the outcome of treatment. Combining radiation therapy and multiagent chemotherapy has dramatically increased the local control rate to approximately 90%. The role of surgery in attaining both local control and disease-free survival has not been clearly delineated. There is no question that tumors originating in expendable bones, such as the clavicle and the rib, are best managed with surgical removal. However, even in these cases, radiation may be needed because it is often difficult to ascertain the adequacy of the surgical margins, especially in tumors with a large soft tissue component. Not as clear cut is the role of surgery in the primary treatment of pelvic and extremity tumors. In these children, the ability of extensive surgery to influence the eventual outcome is unknown and often left to the experience, and bias, of the treating institution. The role of surgery, especially in pelvic primary tumors, needs to be tested in a prospective trial. Treatment of poor-prognosis patients with newer therapeutic approaches, such as ABMT, must be vigorously supported.

Late effects must be decreased. The report of cardiotoxicity from the IESS-II study is particularly disheartening. The high doses of radiation needed to control Ewing's sarcoma also lead to significant morbidity. Therapeutic strategies that explore novel ways to administer useful agents, such as doxorubicin by continuous infusion, or the role of various combinations of chemotherapy to decrease the total radiation dose used should be carried out.

Finally, the origin of the Ewing's sarcoma cell is close to being discovered. If the origin is determined, perhaps the treatment might be tailored even further. The relationship of Ewing's sarcoma to other round cell tumors is discussed below. The close relationship of Ewing's sarcoma to tumors of neuroectodermal origin necessitates careful pathologic review and analysis using the latest histochemical, monoclonal antibody, electron microscopic, and cytogenetic techniques to definitely diagnose a Ewing's sarcoma.

Primitive Neuroectodermal Tumor of Bone

PNET of bone was first described by Jaffe and associates.[93] PNET of bone is similar and perhaps identical in histogenesis to Ewing's sarcoma; Askin's tumor,[4] a malignant small round cell tumor of the thoracopulmonary region; and adult peripheral neuroblastoma,[126] peripheral neuroepithelioma,[18, 182] and malignant neuroepithelioma.[69] In his discussion on the nosologic concept of peripheral PNETs, Dehner considers as peripheral PNETs not only the above tumors but also classic neuroblastoma and its variants, pigmented neuroectodermal tumor, and ectomesenchymoma.[34]

Dehner and other investigators[77] pointed out that these tumors have a number of indistinguishable ultrastructural and immunohistochemical characteristics. Cytogenetic findings have enabled a number of these tumors to be distinguished from and related to one another. Specifically, Ewing's sarcoma is closely related to PNET of bone and soft tissue. The most striking evidence for the close association and perhaps common histogenic origin of these tumors is that the same translocation, (11;22) (q24;q12), is found in both entities.[118, 182]

Further laboratory evidence for the close relationship of Ewing's sarcoma and PNET are the following:

- Indistinguishable and highly reproducible patterns of protooncogene expression of c-*myc,* n-*myc,* c-*myb,* and c-*mil*/*raf*-1 appear with equal frequency in these tumors, along with high levels of choline acetyltransferase.[128]
- Ewing's sarcoma cultured cell lines stimulated with AMP or TPA differentiate to cells that morphologically and histochemically resemble those of neural origin.[26]
- Neuron-specific enolase, neuroblastoma cell surface antigen, neuron cell surface antigen, and neurofilaments have been demonstrated by Japanese workers in Ewing's sarcoma and PNET.[174]

PATIENT CHARACTERISTICS

PNET of bone occurs primarily in the thoracopulmonary region. The distribution of PNET by the age and sex of patients and the location of the primary tumor is found in Table 5–8 as modified from Jurgens and associates.[96] The median age was 15 years, with the majority of patients older than 10 years of age. The youngest patient in this series was 9 months and the oldest was 23 years. There was a definite male preponderance. PNET rarely occurs in blacks, a situation that is similar to that in Ewing's sarcoma.[77]

Thirty-one (74%) of 42 patients had bone involvement. Among these 31 patients, only 5 had isolated involvement of bone, whereas 26 had involvement of bone with large soft tissue components. Twenty-four patients had chest wall disease. Fourteen of these patients were evaluable for pleural involvement and eight evidenced this complication. Epidural extension was seen in four of seven evaluable patients with posterior chest wall tumors.

TABLE 5–8

Characteristics of 42 Patients with PNET*

Sex	
Male	28
Female	14
Age	
<10 yr	12
10–15 yr	16
>15 yr	14
Distribution (Bone Involvement)	
Scapula	2(2)
Rib	15(15)
Sternum	2(2)
Paravertebral/vertebral	5(2)
Head and neck	4(2)
Upper arm	2(1)
Abdomen/pelvis	6(4)
Thigh	3(2)
Lower leg	3(1)
	42 (31)
Location of Metastases at Diagnosis†	
Bone	5
Lung	5
Liver	2
Bone marrow	3
Spleen	1
Lymph node	1

*Modified from data in Jurgens et al.[96]

†A total of ten patients had metastases at diagnosis. Several had more than one site involved.

Most striking was the high rate of metastases at diagnosis. Ten of 42 patients had metastases, with 6 of the 10 having multiple metastatic sites.

The series by Jurgens and associates is the most comprehensive reported to date.[96] However, as PNET becomes more easily recognized by pathologists, it is expected that tumors previously diagnosed as extraosseous Ewing's sarcoma and/or Ewing's sarcoma of bone will be recognized as PNET. As this occurs, the true incidence and mode of presentation of this tumor will be deciphered. For example, many tumors originally thought to be Ewing's sarcoma of bone have neuroectodermal origins on pathologic review.[141]

TREATMENT

The treatment of PNET is not well delineated in the literature. On retrospective analysis, Jurgens and associates culled their series of 42 patients that were treated on protocols of various European cooperative group trials from 23 different institutions. From these patients a number of important points can help plan future clinical trials:

1. Patients with tumor of volumes greater than 100 ml had the same prognosis as those with tumors of smaller volumes; however, eight of the ten patients with metastases at diagnosis had tumors with volumes greater than 100 ml. Similarly, patients with tumors with extracompartmental growth had the same outcome as those with tumors confined to one compartment.
2. Patients with metastases at diagnosis had a worse outcome, with only 1 of 10 patients in complete remission compared with 20 of 32 among those without metastases.
3. Surgical ablation is important. Ten of 12 relapses in patients with nonmetastatic disease at diagnosis occurred in those who had only marginal or intralesional resections rather than more extensive surgical procedures. The role of radiation could not be determined for this group of patients. Radiation did not improve the final results for patients who could not undergo radical surgery. However, in a study by Miser and associates,[134] radiation was used and thought to be an important adjunct to chemotherapy in this tumor (see below).
4. Active chemotherapeutic combinations for PNET are similar to those for Ewing's sarcoma and include vincristine, doxorubicin (Adriamycin), cytoxan, ifosfamide, and actinomycin D.

This was confirmed in a study from the Dana-Farber Cancer Institute of 23 children with soft tissue PNET.[66] Six of these 23 patients had metastatic disease at diagnosis. The tumor was resected completely in 8 of 23 patients at diagnosis or after chemotherapy, and 15 of 23 patients received radiation therapy. Seventeen patients (13 of whom had nonmetastatic disease) received vincristine, cyclophosphamide (Cytoxan), doxorubicin, and actinomycin D. Twelve of the 13 patients with nonmetastatic disease were failure free at the time of the report (median follow-up of 18.8 months).

Miser and colleagues[134] evaluated a treatment regimen for patients with high-risk PNET (i.e., gross residual disease or metastatic disease) and compared these results with those for an identical population of patients with Ewing's sarcoma. Patients with PNET and Ewing's sarcoma were treated with chemotherapy induction that included cyclophosphamide, doxorubicin, vincristine, and radiation to the primary tumor. The patients' bone marrow was harvested, and intensive chemotherapy with vincristine and cyclophosphamide was given, followed by total body irradiation and ABMT. Sixteen of 17 patients with PNET achieved a complete remission, with a median duration of follow-up of 18 months. Six patients experienced relapse, and there were no survival differences (disease-free survival or survival) between the patients with stage III and stage IV disease. In addition, the survival of these patients was similar to that of those with stage III and IV Ewing's sarcoma.

From these studies, it is obvious that advanced-stage PNET is curable. What is needed is more effective chemotherapeutic regimens and a better understanding of the role of surgery in this entity.

Osteosarcoma

Osteosarcoma is the most common malignant bone tumor in children and young adults and constitutes approximately 5% of all tumors in childhood. The peak age incidence is between 10 and 25 years, with disease in most patients occurring in their teenage years near the time of their pubertal growth spurt.[108] As is the case in Ewing's sarcoma, males are more commonly affected than females (1.5:1).[32] Despite the relative rarity of osteosarcoma, the treatment of this disease has undergone dramatic changes owing in large measure to the close cooperation between orthopedic surgeons and oncologists. At present, at least 60% of all patients with aggressive, but nonmetastatic, osteosarcoma will be cured of their disease (see below).

Patients with osteosarcoma present almost exclusively with pain and swelling. As opposed to patients with Ewing's sarcoma, few have fever or pathologic fractures. The location of osteosarcoma at presentation, as opposed to that of Ewing's sarcoma, is overwhelmingly in the bones of the extremities, with tumors arising in central locations (e.g., pelvis and vertebral column) seen much less frequently. The sites of presentation were excellently collated by Dahlin and Unni[33] (see Table 5–2). In their series, approximately half of the lesions involved sites that surrounded the knee. Forty-three of the 1274 patients had Paget's disease, and 52 osteosarcomas arose in previously irradiated sites.

PROGNOSIS

Attempts to correlate the patient's age, the site and size of the primary lesion, pathologic features (type and grade), duration of symptoms, spread of disease (local or regional extension, distant metastases) at diagnosis, the patient's sex, serum alkaline phosphatase and LDH levels, chromosomal number or DNA index, response to initial chemotherapy, and location of the lesion on the bone with eventual outcome have been made (Table 5–9).

Patients with metastatic disease clearly have a poor prognosis. This can include pulmonary and/or synchronous bone metastases. The reported incidence of patients with pulmonary metastases has increased with the use of CT scans and now approximates 15 to 20% of patients with newly diagnosed disease. Synchronous bone metastases at initial diagnosis are rare and involved only 3 of 1274 patients in the Mayo Clinic series.[33] Although few series include these patients in their treatment results, the cure rate for these children is very poor.[140]

The following were correlated with poor prognosis in the past: younger age at presentation, male sex, shorter duration of symptoms, osteoblastic and/or chondroblastic histologic features, larger lesions, and primary lesions of the humerus, femur, or trunk.[15, 49, 167] Utilizing these criteria, Taylor and colleagues, from the Mayo Clinic, devised a scoring system to judge the potential prognosis of a patient with osteosarcoma.[167] They assigned a 1 to poor prognosis characteristics and a 0 to good prognostic factors. The six criteria that were assigned a value of 1 were age of 9 years or younger, male sex, tumor size of 15 cm or larger, osteoblastic or chondroblastic histologic features, symptom duration of up to 2 months, and tumors originating in the femur or humerus. Patients who had a total prognosis score of 0, 1, or 2 had a longer disease-free survival than those patients with scores of 4, 5, or 6. Patients with a score of 3 were intermediate between the two.[167]

In a subsequent study, Taylor and associates analyzed the records of 444 patients with osteosarcoma who did not have metastases at diagnosis or inoperable disease.[168] The cohort of patients were treated in 13 institutions from July 1, 1977 to December 31, 1982. Few deaths and little progression of disease occurred after 3 years; therefore, data beyond 3 years from diagnosis were not analyzed. The following characteristics carried the worse prognosis: (1) osteoblastic, chondroblastic, fibroblastic, or telangiectatic histologic features (this differs from the previous study in which only osteoblastic or chondroblastic histologic features

TABLE 5–9

Prognostic Factors in Osteosarcoma

	Good Prognosis	Poor Prognosis
Parosteal location	Present	—
Metastatic disease at diagnosis	—	Present
Mayo Clinic series*		
Necrosis after chemotherapy	≥90%	<90%
Lactate dehydrogenase level	<300 U/L	≥300 U/L
E/L ratio† on CT scan	≤50%	>50%
DNA index‡	<1.1	>1.1

*See text (refs. 167, 168)

†Extent of marrow involvement/length of bone.

‡Specimens are usually heterogeneous; as long as a cell line is represented that has a DNA index of <1.1, prognosis is good.[117]

were a poor prognostic sign); (2) regional extension; (3) histologic grades 3 and 4; (4) duration of symptoms shorter than 12 months; (5) tumor size of 20 cm or larger; (6) site in the head, the spine, the sternum, the rib, or the pelvis; (7) site in the humerus, the clavicle, the scapula, or the proximal femur; and (8) weight loss of 10 lb or more. On the basis of these variables, the patients were able to be divided into four categories of outcome—low probability of disease progression or death, medium low probability, medium high probability, and high probability. Whether these indicators will withstand the test of time, especially for patients treated with current aggressive therapy, still needs to be determined.

The initial response of the tumor to chemotherapeutic agents has also been used to help decide which patients will do well and is considered by a number of workers to be one of the most important predictors of outcome. This concept, popularized first by investigators at Memorial Sloan-Kettering Cancer Center, and verified by others, assumes that patients whose tumors do not undergo significant necrosis (i.e., less than 90% destruction) with the initial chemotherapy course will have a poor outcome.[98, 149–151, 187] Controversy exists about whether the initial response can be used to tailor the patient's therapy and improve the outcome of the poor responders (see discussion of the current treatment below). Another treatment variable, the number of perioperative transfusions, has been inversely correlated with survival, with those patients who received more units of blood doing poorer than patients receiving less or no transfusions.[29]

Serum biochemical analysis, except perhaps for LDH levels, has not been especially useful in predicting outcome. Increased serum LDH levels (300 U/L or greater) (as well as black race and white blood cell count of 8000/dl or greater) were found by workers at St. Jude Children's Research Hospital to be associated with a shortened disease-free survival.[112] Increased LDH level was also noted by the POG to be predictive of a poor response.[114] Why LDH is associated with poor outcome is not clear. It might reflect a more metabolically active tumor and thus a more aggressive malignant course. Alternatively, it might be associated with larger tumor size and thus represent a tumor with more potential for spread.

Tumor size has been thought by many to be associated with a poorer prognosis. It is expected that patients with larger tumors have more aggressive and tissue-infiltrating tumors and thus have a higher incidence of occult metastatic disease at diagnosis. However, in contradistinction to the case with Ewing's sarcoma, this correlation has not been as common in osteosarcoma. The reasons for this are difficult to assess. One reason could be that, in osteosarcoma, the length of the involved bone and its relationship to the size of the tumor must be considered together. Workers have assessed intramedullary tumor encroachment and correlated this with prognosis. With the use of the attenuation coefficient of the CT scan, a ratio can be established between the extent of marrow involvement (E) and the length of the involved bone (L).[73] Among 30 patients without metastatic disease, no one with an E/L ratio of greater than 50% remained disease free for more than 14 months from diagnosis. This concept needs to be tested on a larger cohort of patients and might be able to be refined further with the use of the MRI.

Another characteristic of osteosarcoma is its ability to secrete a bone morphogenetic protein (BMP). This substance has the ability to induce new bone formation when devitalized osteosarcoma tissue is implanted subcutaneously in athymic nude mice. BMP was found in 8 of 20 patients with osteosarcoma. These patients were characterized by their relative resistance to preoperative chemotherapy (doxorubicin with high-dose methotrexate [HIMTX]) and the tendency of their tumors to metastasize to the lungs and other bones.[190]

Finally, chromosome and DNA analysis has been utilized in an attempt to predict outcome. First, with the use of microspectrophotometry, DNA content can be assessed on biopsy specimens.[105] Using this technique, workers from Sweden have been able to predict if a tissue specimen represents a benign or a malignant tumor.[10] All noncontroversial benign specimens were diploid (i.e., normal DNA content), 92 of 96 high-grade osteosarcomas were hyperdiploid (i.e., an increased, and therefore, abnormal DNA content), and the 4 low-grade parosteal specimens were diploid. Seventeen tumors were difficult to assess histologically as benign or malignant. Of these, seven were diploid and ten were hyperdiploid. None of the seven patients with diploid lesions had a local or distant recurrence, whereas eight of ten patients with hyperdiploid lesions did. Thus, ploidy determination may prove to be a powerful and useful tool in assigning biologic potential to questionable lesions.

Furthermore, DNA content as measured by flow cytometry might be valuable in stratifying patients into good and poor prognostic categories, as has been demonstrated by Look and colleagues.[117] These investigators used flow cytometric analysis to assign to tumors a DNA index. In these studies, tumor stem cell lines with a DNA index of 1.0 represented diploid content, those between 0.9 and 1.0 were considered near diploid, and those greater than 1.1 are hyperdiploid. They found that tumor cell suspensions prepared from osteosarcoma specimens were often heterogeneous and contained multiple stem cell lines. Seventeen of 26 patients remained disease free. When this survival was analyzed according to DNA content, it was noted that, with a median follow-up time of 3 years, only 2 of 16 patients who had tumors that included diploid or near-diploid cell lines had recurrences, compared with 7 recurrences among the 10 patients with only hyperdiploid cell lines. Thus, in this small series of patients, DNA content as reflected by the DNA index measured with the use of a flow cytometer was predictive of relapse-free survival. It must be cautioned that this study involved a small number of patients, and verification of these results with larger numbers of patients with longer follow-ups is needed to determine the usefulness of this method indicating prognosis.

TREATMENT

The controversy regarding the efficacy of chemotherapy for osteosarcoma occupied much of the early 1980s.[25, 39, 103, 106, 166, 167] It had always been expected that no more than 20% of patients with osteosarcoma would survive their disease if they were treated with surgery and/or radiation therapy without chemotherapy.[127, 173] This was further reflected in single-institution studies that investigated the role of chemotherapy in their patients, comparing chemotherapy results with those in the same institution using surgery and/or radiation therapy.[60, 156] The improvement noted in survival of patients with osteosarcoma was attributed by most investigators to the use of multiple chemotherapeutic agents in these patients.

This was challenged by data from the Mayo Clinic that suggested that this increased survival was due not to chemotherapy but rather to an unknown factor that had altered the natural history of this disease.[39, 167] The Mayo Clinic investigators found that survival of patients treated without chemotherapy increased from approximately 20 to 50% from 1963 to 1981 and disease-free survival from approximately 20 to 35% during the same time period.[167] In a randomized trial from this same institution, 20 patients who received chemotherapy had an identical 42% disease-free survival rate at 5 years compared with 18 patients who were treated only with ablative surgery.[39] Subsequent to this study, two randomized trials confirmed the utility of chemotherapy in osteosarcoma, with a disease-free survival that approximated 60% in those receiving chemotherapy compared with approximately 20% in patients treated with surgery alone.[41, 113] As a result, the principle that chemotherapy is needed for treating osteosarcoma is now well established, and it is up to orthopedists and oncologists to improve the treatment of this disease to attain higher cure rates.

Single agents (Table 5–10) in osteosarcoma have yielded response rates of 0 to 40%. The agents considered to yield the highest response rates have been cisplatin, doxorubicin, and HDMTX. Although single agents can cause significant regression of the primary tumor

TABLE 5–10
Chemotherapeutic Agents Used in Osteosarcoma

Methotrexate
Cisplatin
Doxorubicin (Adriamycin)
Bleomycin
Cyclophosphamide (Cytoxan)
Actinomycin D
Ifosfamide

and/or metastases and, at times, total necrosis of the tumor, which renders the patient disease free, such therapy cannot be relied on to cure the patient. As noted, the therapy of osteosarcoma has undergone an evolution during the past 20 years, so that the major roles that surgery and chemotherapy play in the treatment of this disease are well established. The timing of surgery in relation to chemotherapy, the selection and combination of chemotherapeutic agents for maximal effect, and the route of administration that is most beneficial to the patient are open to question.

Adjuvant Chemotherapy (Fig. 5–1)

Jaffe and coworkers reported the first trials using HDMTX in children with osteosarcoma.[79, 80, 81, 83, 84, 86] The impetus for their work came from the studies of Djerassi and associates, who showed that patients with lung cancer could be treated with HDMTX if folinic acid (leucovorin) rescue and vigorous hydration were used to ameliorate the toxic effects of the methotrexate.[36] From these early studies, it was shown that patients with metastatic disease could respond to HDMTX, that disease-free survival could be prolonged beyond that expected on the basis of historical controls with the administration of HDMTX after surgical ablation of the tumor, and that frequent administration of HDMTX was superior in relation to response and disease-free survival than spread-out administration. Although many of Jaffe's earlier studies utilized vincristine with HDMTX, it is now believed that vincristine offers no advantage to patients with osteosarcoma. These studies by Jaffe and coworkers were exceedingly influential in the development of most of the subsequent therapeutic trials for osteosarcoma, and HDMTX is included in nearly all treatment regimens for this disease.

As an aside, it must be pointed out that adequate trials using frequent dosing of low-dose MTX, whether intravenously or orally, have not been tried.[67] At least four studies have looked at lower doses of MTX. The first was a trial in patients with measurable metastatic disease by Waegner and associates who treated 25 evaluable patients with 80 mg/m^2 of MTX IV on days 1, 8, and 15; if response occurred, the dose was repeated on days 29 and 43; and if response was sustained by day 57, this dose was continued every 2 weeks until disease progression. Three of 25 patients achieved complete remission with duration of response of 5 to 34 weeks. Twelve patients had stable disease with a range of 6 to 20 weeks before progression ensued.[179] In the second study, the CCSG could find no difference in disease-free survival in a group of patients treated with intermediate-dose MTX (690 mg/m^2) versus a group of patients treated with HDMTX (7.5 g/m^2). In both groups of patients, they found only a 38% disease-free survival.[104] In a third study, Bacci and colleagues compared a group of patients receiving 2000 mg/m^2 with those receiving 200 mg/m^2 of MTX; both groups had an approximate 50% disease-free survival.[6] In the fourth study, Picci and colleagues reported the results of a randomized study in which patients given HDMTX (7.5 g/m^2) had a disease-free survival of 78% compared with 62% of patients treated with 750 mg/m^2 of MTX.[144] In the latter three studies, agents other than MTX were given to the patients, and MTX was used infrequently (i.e., no closer than every 3 weeks). Thus, a true trial of lower, frequent doses of MTX has not been done to establish the final effective dose of MTX. This is not a moot point, because HDMTX and leucovorin rescue treatment is expensive and necessitates an inordinate amount of nursing supervision for its effective and safe administration.

Regardless of the final role of MTX in the treatment of osteosarcoma, combination adjuvant chemotherapy has been established as the single most important reason for the improved survival in this disease. In their excellent literature review of methotrexate-containing chemotherapeutic regimens, Grem and coworkers pointed out that a prolonged disease-free survival of 55% to 78% can be expected with the use of multiagent chemotherapy[65] (Fig. 5–1). The agents most often used in combination with HDMTX are cisplatin; doxorubicin; bleomycin, cyclophosphamide, and actinomycin D in combination (BCD); and, most recently, ifosfamide. The contribution of each of these agents to the final

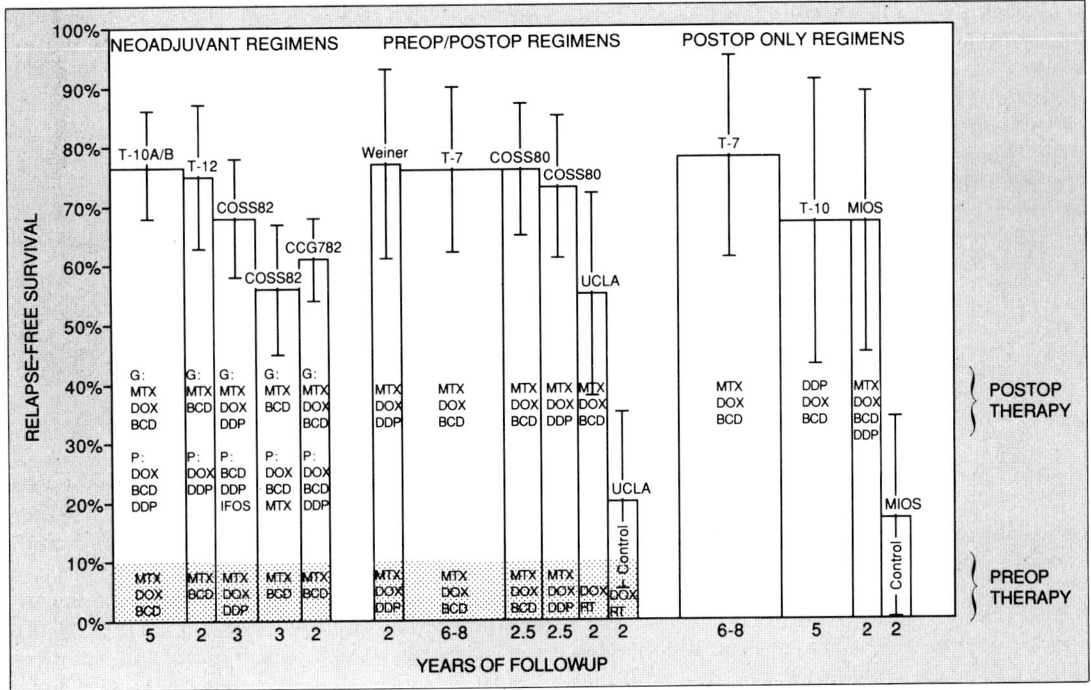

FIGURE 5–1. Relapse-free survival on recently conducted trials in osteogenic sarcoma. Bars denote 95% confidence interval. Shaded area shows drugs used preoperatively. Drugs listed outside shaded area refer to postoperative therapy. For neoadjuvant studies, G refers to good histologic response (extensive tumor necrosis) and P refers to poor histologic response (minimal or no effect). (From Grem JL, King SA, Wittes RE, Leyland-Jones B: The role of methotrexate in osteosarcoma. J Natl Cancer Inst 80:626–656, 1988.) BCD, bleomycin, cytoxan, and actinomycin D; DDP, cisplatin; Dox, doxorubicin; IFOS, ifosfamide; MTX, methotrexate; RT, radiotherapy.

results in these studies is still largely unknown and has been the subject of a number of prospectively randomized studies.

Patients with osteosarcoma who receive the major portion of the calculated dose of chemotherapy (as per protocol) do better than those who do not. This was first noted by Cortes and colleagues in patients treated with doxorubicin as the sole chemotherapeutic agent.[30] They reported that approximately 30% of patients survived disease free at 5 years if there was an inappropriate reduction in the dose of doxorubicin or surgical procedure, compared with a 61% disease-free survival in patients who did not have any deviations from their protocol. This was confirmed in multiagent chemotherapy for osteosarcoma by Bacci and associates.[7] They noted that patients who received at least 80% of their prescribed chemotherapeutic doses had a disease-free survival of 87% compared with only 65% disease-free survival among patients who received less than 80% of the calculated dose (median follow-up, 2 years).

Bacci and associates highlighted that the calculated dose intensity included not only the total dose given but also the time interval between courses.[7] Thus, it must be stressed in treating osteosarcoma, as is true of all cancers, that reduction in the doses of chemotherapy and delays in the cycles of chemotherapy be avoided to achieve the maximal disease-free survival.

When the diagnosis of osteosarcoma has been established, a decision must be made when to initiate chemotherapy. Many surgeons urge that surgery be delayed for 2 to 3 months from diagnosis and that chemotherapy be administered. This request is made because of the desire to shrink the size of the tumor to make large lesions amenable to resection, to facilitate limb sparing, and in selected cases, to give time for customized prostheses to be made.

Preoperative chemotherapy gained impetus from the reports of Rosen and colleagues[155] and Jaffe and coworkers.[87] Both groups of investigators found that it was possible to successfully administer chemotherapy before surgery, shrink the tumor, and carry out *en bloc* resections of primary tumors without loss of the limb. These workers also believed that a number of primary tumors that were considered nonresectable were rendered resectable by the use of presurgical chemotherapy. Finally, and most importantly, they did not believe that delaying the eventual surgical ablation of the tumor compromised the patient's outcome. Indeed, an advantage was thought to exist with this approach in that patients with micrometastases at diagnosis were beginning treatment as soon as the diagnosis of osteosarcoma was made without the extra delay in chemotherapy caused by an amputation or limb salvage procedure.

Neoadjuvant Chemotherapy

From this work arose a new concept in the treatment of tumors, neoadjuvant chemotherapy. The principle of this mode of treatment is that chemotherapy given before ablative surgery can be used to determine the efficacy of the treatment regimen, in addition to aiding the surgeon in limb-sparing therapy. Neoadjuvant chemotherapy, by utilizing chemotherapeutic agents before surgery, enables the clinician to gain insight into the tumor's sensitivity to the agents used by the clinical decrease in pain and tumor size. More importantly, the pathologist can determine the amount of tumor destruction caused by the drugs. Thus, by dispensing the medications before surgery, the oncologist performs an *in vivo* drug sensitivity test. Patients with a poor histologic response to preoperative chemotherapy tend to do worse than those with a good response. This led a number of investigators to attempt to tailor therapy by replacing drugs that appear ineffective with drugs that had not been used initially to treat the osteosarcoma. Whether this strategy improves the disease-free and overall survival of patients with osteosarcoma is still in need of control trials.

A number of groups have published their results using the neoadjuvant approach to treating osteosarcoma. Rosen and colleagues reported on the use of preoperative chemotherapy with HDMTX with citrovorum rescue, doxorubicin, and a combination of bleomycin, cyclophosphamide, and actinomycin D (BCD) given for 4 to 16 weeks before the surgery for the primary tumor (T-10) or without the use of doxorubicin in the preoperative regimen (T-12).[150, 155] Other differences between these two protocols were that in T-10 the patients undergoing amputation did so at the end of 4 weeks after having received only HDMTX, whereas those who had a limb salvage with an endoprosthesis received doxorubicin and BCD until the sixteenth week. In T-12, all patients received HDMTX and BCD (without the use of doxorubicin) and were operated on during the tenth week. In addition, in T-12, patients with a good histologic response were treated for only a total of two more cycles and had their therapy stopped at the end of 15 weeks. Patients with a poor response to therapy were treated with doxorubicin and cisplatin without HDMTX and BCD for an additional 17 weeks (i.e., 27 total weeks of chemotherapy). In the earlier T-10 protocol, patients were randomized to receive or not receive vincristine (no difference noted), and patients who had a poor response to preoperative chemotherapy were treated with doxorubicin, cisplatin, and BCD, but without HDMTX. Both the good and poor histologic responders were treated for approximately another 30 weeks after the definitive surgery. Patient's histologic responses were graded according to the classification of Huvos and coworkers.[76] This classification is as follows: grade I, little or no necrosis; grade II, a partial response to chemotherapy with greater than 50% tumor necrosis noted attributable to preoperative chemotherapy; grade III, greater than 90% tumor necrosis; and grade IV, total tumor necrosis with no viable tumor cells seen. Either grade III or IV was considered a satisfactory histologic response, indicating a tumor sensitive to the chemotherapeutic regimen. Approximately 45% of patients achieved greater than 90% necrosis with their initial chemotherapy and were continued on their original regimen. The overall disease-free survival with this regimen was approximately 80%, with the initial good responders and poor responders achieving approximately the same results. Among the poor responders from a previous study (T-7), only 2 of 13 patients survived. The investigators reasoned from their experience that neoadjuvant chemotherapy can be utilized in the treatment of osteosarcoma to tailor therapy for maximal survival.[150, 155]

As encouraging as these results are, a word of caution must be given. Both the CCSG[147] and the Cooperative German/Austrian Osteosarcoma Studies (COSS)[185–187] failed to substantiate the outstanding results that Rosen and colleagues[150, 155] obtained by substituting different agents in poor responders. CCSG utilized a nearly identical regimen to T-10 and found that those patients with greater than

95% necrosis constituted 30% of the entire group and had a disease-free survival of 91%. Twenty-nine per cent of patients were intermediate responders (50 to 95% necrosis) and were switched from their initial regimen, as were T-10 patients. Their disease-free survival was 83%. Finally, 41% of patients had tumor necrosis of less than 50%. These patients had a disease-free survival of only 40%, despite the use of tailored therapy. Because these results were reported within 1 year of closure of the study, more relapses than those already reported are expected.

In the COSS series, patients with tumor necrosis of less than 90% did poorly (48% disease-free survival) when compared with the 81% disease-free survival of patients with tumor necrosis of greater than 90%. The poor responders in the COSS-82 study were treated with a regimen that included no drugs that were used in the initial regimen, and it failed to improve the disease-free survival of these patients.[187] Therapy in the COSS-82 lasted for a total of 18 to 22 weeks. One important result from this study was the major influence of aggressive preoperative therapy on the eventual outcome. In COSS-82, patients were randomized to receive before surgery either doxorubicin, cisplatin, and HDTMX or BCD and HDTMX. The good response rate with the former was 60% and that with the latter was only 26%. The poor responders were then treated with either cisplatin and doxorubicin (for those who initially received BCD and HDTMX) or cisplatin, ifosfamide, and BCD (for those who initially received cisplatin, doxorubicin, and HDTMX). Despite this therapy, the poor responders did poorly. The importance of obtaining an excellent initial response with aggressive chemotherapy and eradicating resistant tumor cells early in the treatment is underscored by this study. Attempts to decrease toxicity initially by starting with less toxic agents may not be warranted at present. After obtaining a good histologic response, the question of whether less aggressive chemotherapy and/or a shorter course of treatment should be tried is still unanswered.

Preoperative chemotherapy was shown, in a preliminary report from the Istituto Ortopedica Rizzoli,[145] to make limb salvage feasible in patients who might not have been candidates for this procedure and (by grading the histopathologic response) to predict which patients are at a greater risk for local recurrence. In this study of 205 patients, 52 underwent amputation and 153 were managed by a limb-sparing procedure. Of the 153 patients, 123 survived for a minimum of 18 months and were evaluated for local recurrence. Only 1% of patients whose histopathologic tumor necrosis was graded as greater than 90% had a local recurrence, whereas 23% of patients with 60 to 90% tumor necrosis and 50% of those with less than 60% necrosis had local recurrences. In patients with 60 to 90% tumor necrosis, the surgical margins were important in determining the local recurrence rate. Thus, 4% of patients with a wide surgical margin had local recurrences, whereas 83% of those with "marginal" surgical margins and 50% of those with contamination of the surgical field had local recurrences. In patients with less than 60% tumor necrosis, the local recurrence rate was 43 (wide surgical margin), 50 (marginal surgical margins), and 100% (contaminated surgical margins). Picci and coworkers concluded that patients whose tumor necrosis is less than 60% should have an amputation, and in those with 60 to 90% necrosis, wide surgical margins must be obtained.

In summary, neoadjuvant therapy has not adversely affected patients and has allowed the surgeons time to await construction of custom-made prostheses. Preoperative chemotherapy also helps to determine which patients do well with the chemotherapeutic regimen chosen. It has not yet been decisively confirmed that changing chemotherapeutic agents in patients who have an initial poor response will be of benefit. Further studies to address this question must be carried out. Patients who do not respond favorably with the initial drugs may be ideal candidates to try newer agents or approaches in the future.

Intraarterial Therapy

Intraarterial therapy has been tried by a few investigators in an attempt to achieve high tissue concentrations of chemotherapeutic agents within the tumor. In their review of intraarterial therapy, Jaffe and associates[82] noted that Akahoshi and coworkers[1] were the first to try intraarterial therapy in osteosarcoma. Akahoshi and coworkers used mitomycin C, 5-fluorouracil, and methotrexate and observed significant tumor necrosis in a number of patients. In addition, Akahoshi and coworkers reported that survival was 44% in patients who had infusions that lasted for more than 3 weeks as compared with 26% in those whose infusion was administered for less than 3 weeks. Eilber and coworkers administered doxorubicin as intraarterial therapy for 72 hours (90 mg/m^2 total dose) followed by 35 Gy of radiation.[41] They observed 90 to 100% necrosis in approximately 50% of the primary tumors. After surgery, the patients received vincristine, HDMTX, and doxorubicin. Of the patients treated, only one had a local recurrence, and the 5-year survival was 55%. In their own experience from MD Anderson Hospital and Tumor Institute, Jaffe and associates used either doxorubicin, HDMTX, or cisplatin as intraarterial therapy in successive trials and found that the best results are obtained when cisplatin was used intraarterially for more than three courses.[90] In a comparison of intraarterial MTX versus intraarterial cisplatin, cisplatin was superior. In fact, HDMTX administered by the conventional route yielded the same results as when it was administered intraarterially.[88] Intraarterial cisplatin was also associated with fewer complications than intraarterial doxorubicin. The complications of this intraarterial therapy include necrosis at the surgical site, lymphedema, vascular damage, local induration, and erythema.

Jaffe and associates embarked on a therapeutic approach using intraarterial therapy as the initial treatment for all patients with osteosarcoma.[82, 88, 89] They hoped that this approach would not only yield a superior histologic response but also allow a number of patients to forego amputation or limb-sparing procedures. In an update of this treatment method, they noted that the best results were obtained among those patients who had a minimum of four intraarterial courses of cisplatin at a dosage of 150 mg/m^2 given every 2 to 3 weeks.[90] Thirty-three patients received at least four courses and 17 had greater than 90% necrosis. After surgery, the poor responders were treated with continuation therapy that consisted of HDMTX and doxorubicin, whereas the good responders were treated with those agents and IV cisplatin. Thirty patients not included in the study had an excellent clinical response, did not undergo ablative surgery, were treated with continuation therapy, and are being followed for the incidence of local recurrences and metastases.[90] In an earlier report on similarly treated patients, these authors mentioned that those who had a complete or partial response (i.e., 60 to 100% necrosis) had a 64% disease-free survival, whereas those with less necrosis experienced a 34% disease-free survival.[89]

In a group of older patients from the same institution, Benjamin and colleagues reported that, with preoperative cisplatin intraarterial therapy followed by postoperative, tailored chemotherapy, approximately 70% 3-year disease-free survival was expected.[14] In addition, they believe that such therapy will allow more than 80% of patients to be candidates for limb salvage surgery when only 8% were considered eligible for such surgery at presentation.[14]

Caution once again must be stated. First, as impressive as these studies are, an adequate control study has not been mounted to compare intraarterial therapy with IV therapy. Second, many studies have shown that impressive necrosis can be obtained with the use of IV chemotherapy, and these results seem to be equal to those obtained by the MD Anderson group. Third, for a period of up to 12 weeks, these patients may be getting only one drug, cisplatin, and thus the opportunity for tumor cells to become resistant to this agent might be enhanced. Fourth, the rate of only 8% limb salvage candidates before any chemotherapy seems low and may be a function of institutional bias. Finally, intraarterial therapy necessitates an invasive procedure for each administration and a sophisticated team of physicians and nurses in attendance with each course. Such a team is not available at many institutions that are more than adequately able to treat patients with osteosarcoma with the most advanced chemotherapeutic regimens. Whether such a team is necessary must await further, critical evaluation.

Radiotherapy

Osteosarcoma is not exquisitely sensitive to radiotherapy, hence the role of radiotherapy is not as clearly defined as in Ewing's sarcoma. The early attempts at using radiation therapy for primary osteosarcoma did not yield any better results than were achieved with amputation. The question arose whether radiation to the lungs could delay or permanently suppress metastases. In an initial randomized study, Rab and colleagues[147a] failed to show an advantage of 15 Gy given to the lungs as adjuvant therapy. In a study from the European Organization for Research on Treatment of Cancer (EORTC) Radiotherapy Cooperative Group, a suggestion of an advantage to pulmonary radiation was noted.[19] These authors used 20 Gy to the lungs and up to 80 Gy to the primary tumor in an attempt at limb salvage in some centers. In other centers, the regimen was used to delay amputation for 4 to 6 months until it could be determined that metastases had not occurred. Zaharia and coworkers had no survivors in a group of seven patients treated with 20 Gy to the lungs alone, but an approximate 35% disease-free survival in patients treated with radiation and doxorubicin.[191]

Radiotherapy for osteosarcoma was finally tested in a multiinstitutional trial run by the EORTC and the Societe Internationale d'Oncologie Pediatrique (SIOP).[21] This study noted a particularly poor disease-free survival of only 24%. The survival of 43% at 4 years was most likely due to the chemotherapy regimen also given to these patients. The important points of this study were that 20 Gy administered electively to the lungs yielded the same survival as did chemotherapy alone. In patients who eventually experienced lung metastases, those who were given radiation to the lungs had lesions that were more amenable to resection. In this study, 37 patients received radiation to the primary tumor rather than surgical ablation, and 23 did not have a local recurrence. Data on 21 of these 23 patients are known. Three patients kept normal limb function, ten patients had moderate disability, and eight had severe dysfunction. Among these eight patients, three underwent amputation. This is a rather high local recurrence rate (i.e., 14 of 37), and it might have been higher if patients survived for a longer period of time. Therefore, radiation to the primary tumor cannot be recommended as treatment of the primary lesion. The results of this study were surprising in that the patients receiving radiation did as well as those given chemotherapy, although the chemotherapy was not a successful regimen and the results are not better than those for many historical controls. On the other hand, the study raises the possibility for radiation therapy to the lungs in patients who have a poor initial response to chemotherapy and in whom occult metastases will likely not be controlled with the available chemotherapy. This, of course, needs to be evaluated in a controlled study before it can be suggested for use in patients with osteosarcoma.

Radiation therapy with intraarterial infusion of the radiosensitizer 5-bromodeoxyuridine and systemic chemotherapy has also been used to treat patients with unresectable primary tumors or those who refused amputation. Local control was achieved in seven of nine patients, and four patients survived free of disease from 6 to 10½ years after initial treatment (one of these patients had lung metastases and continues to survive after treatment with high-dose lung irradiation and chemotherapy). Obviously, further trials are needed to test this modality of therapy.[124]

The toxicity of radiation can be considerable. To reach doses that are effective for the primary tumor, more than 80 Gy has been used. This dose can lead to significant morbidity to the extremity, including lymphedema, contractures, fibrosis, and radiation necrosis to the bone with an increased risk of pathologic fractures. In addition, breast cancer has been described in two long-term survivors who received elective whole lung irradiation for treatment of osteosarcoma approximately 15 years earlier while they were adolescents.[78]

Limb Salvage

There is no doubt that limb salvage has a definite place in the treatment of osteosarcoma of the extremities. "Will I lose my leg?" is the question most frequently asked of the pediatric oncologist by the child. Children, especially teenagers, assume that their lives will be saved; they fear most the disfigurement of an amputation and the limitation on their life style that such an operation will have. The parents are usually more concerned with the issues surrounding life and death, but after these are resolved, they often participate in therapeutic decisions, which are based heavily on the ability to save the limb. The role of the oncology team is to try to put the desires of the patient and the family into proper perspective and to put "life before limb."

In a review on limb salvage, Simon pointed out that, to judge limb salvage procedures, survival, morbidity, function, and psychologic outcome all must be compared with those with amputation.[162] Most of what is found in the literature are retrospective evaluations of these points, and an adequate prospective trial has not been done.

As mentioned above, neoadjuvant treatment allows time for surgeons to perform limb salvage procedures. The COSS group sounded a warning that limb salvage procedures might be detrimental to the patient in that in their initial evaluation of patients undergoing such techniques indicated that these patients had a worse disease-free survival when compared with those who underwent standard amputations.[185] The same group later refuted their own findings and, at present, can find no difference in disease-free survival between those who undergo limb salvage and those who have had a standard amputation.[187] This has been substantiated in practically every study that included patients who have had limb salvage procedures. The current belief is that, if the limb salvage is done by an experienced orthopedic tumor surgeon, the overall results of limb salvage and amputation are the same, albeit patients undergoing limb-sparing procedures might have a slightly increased chance for a local recurrence.

Patients who have limb salvage procedures do have more morbidity. They often require extensive hospitalizations during the initial surgical phase. They need aggressive physical therapy to ensure proper function; and they need occasional to frequent treatment of local complications such as infections, contractures, and revisions or lengthenings. This demands a major time commitment by patients, families, and medical personnel as well as a significant expenditure of financial resources. On the other hand, if this leads to a better quality of life for the patient, such an effort is desirable and justified.

Function, as pointed out by Simon, has not been routinely assessed by investigators in the field of limb salvage surgery.[162] Most workers agree that an upper limb should be salvaged if possible. Debate among workers exists regarding which type of procedure is best for lower extremity lesions and these issues have been addressed in other chapters of this textbook. For good function to result from any limb salvage procedure, a highly motivated patient who carries through on all aspects of the postsurgical rehabilitation period is needed. This can be difficult, for during this time the patient is usually receiving aggressive chemotherapy that carries its own morbidity of nausea, vomiting, stomatitis, pancytopenia, and so on. Oncologists and rehabilitation therapists must coordinate their efforts and be prepared to give as much psychologic support as the situation demands.

Finally, an assessment of psychologic adjustment to limb salvage versus amputation must be considered. The only appraisals of psychologic outcome have been retrospective and have not shown an advantage to limb salvage.[162, 181] This type of evaluation may not be able to yield the definitive answer for patients in either group (i.e., amputation or limb salvage) who were assigned to that type of surgery largely through patient and/or physician preference and thus may have been more prepared for the specific type of surgery and its outcome.

Whether a controlled trial can be mounted to scientifically assess the benefits of limb salvage versus amputation is questionable, given the prejudices that exist among oncologists, surgeons, and patients regarding these issues. If such a study is not designed and carried out, perhaps better tools of assessment can be developed that will help answer the questions posed by the use of limb salvage. The only word of caution that pediatric oncologists always add is that excessive delays in initiating postoperative chemotherapy must be avoided, even if the outcome of the limb salvage will be compromised.

METASTATIC DISEASE

Metastatic disease may be present at the time of diagnosis, during treatment, or after therapy. It has been estimated that approximately 15% of patients have metastases at the time of diagnosis and almost all die of their disease. As stated above, approximately 65% of patients with osteosarcoma of the extremities who do not have metastases survive without recurrences. Thus, only about 55% of patients with osteosarcoma can be expected to survive free of any disease and/or recurrence.

Metastases usually occur in the lungs or bones; there are occasional reports of patients with liver, skin, soft tissue, heart, mediastinal, or central nervous system metastases. Before the advent of chemotherapy for the treatment of osteosarcoma, practically all patients developed pulmonary metastases as their initial site of relapse. Most centers now are seeing more patients with extrapulmonary metastases both as the initial site of recurrence or in simultaneous association with pulmonary metastases.[54] In addition, it is apparent that patients who receive chemotherapy and experience lung metastases do so at a later time interval from diagnosis and with fewer nodules than those who did not have chemotherapy.[91]

It has become evident that aggressive and repeated pulmonary resections could be used to prolong the survival of patients with pulmonary metastases.[47, 53, 125, 154] With this approach, a prolonged survival of approximately 20 to 40% is noted by many investigators.[13, 61, 75, 99, 157, 159] In reviewing the data generated from these reports, it is apparent that patients with isolated pulmonary metastases and complete resection (including free microscopic margins and no pleural involvement) have the best chance for a prolonged survival. In the past, it was reported that patients with less than five pulmonary lesions on conventional linear tomography (1-cm cuts) also had a better survival than those with more lesions.[157] The significance of this finding with the newer techniques of scanning is not known. Certainly, earlier detection of pulmonary metastases is occurring because of the use of CT and this may lead to increased survival of patients with this complication.

The role of chemotherapy in recurrent disease is unknown and needs to be assessed in a prospective fashion. Many workers have noted that unresectable pulmonary lesions almost always lead to the death of the patient, regardless of chemotherapy.[61] In addition, patients with metastases to areas other than the lungs usually succumb to their disease.

An approach to the patient who develops metastases has recently been proposed by Chawla and colleagues.[28] They treated 16 patients with recurrent disease after HDMTX, doxorubicin, and cisplatin administration with high-dose ifosfamide (starting dose of 2g/m^2, followed by 2 g/m^2 per day for 6 days by continuous infusion with equal doses of mesna for uroprotection). Complete clinical remission was seen in two patients, and eight patients had a partial remission. These results are particularly impressive in view of a POG study that failed to show a response to ifosfamide (2.4 g/^{2} for 5 days given by a 1-hour infusion) in patients with recurrent osteosarcoma.[67a]

Patients with metastases traditionally do poorly and usually die. However, Winkler and colleagues reported on patients who had metastases and were treated using the chemotherapy regimens in the COSS-80 and COSS-82 studies.[188] Fifty-nine (14%) of 421 patients had metastatic disease; 42 of these cases were confined to the lungs. After chemotherapy and surgery to the primary tumor, 15 (48%) of 31 patients whose lung lesions could be totally removed are surviving for 4 to 8 years compared with only 1 of 22 patients whose metastases could not be ablated. Thus, it seems that these patients may follow the same pattern as those who experience relapse, in that survival depends on total removal of all metastatic deposits.

PAROSTEAL OSTEOSARCOMA

Osteosarcoma that occupies a parosteal (juxtacortical) location is a rare and distinct entity.[23, 52, 109, 119, 168, 172, 176, 189] Parosteal osteosarcoma accounted for about 4.5% of the approximately 1200 cases of osteosarcoma seen at the Mayo Clinic.[189] These tumors are not included in trials of chemotherapy because ablative surgery, with generous surgical margins, is curative in the majority of cases. The reasons for this successful outcome are apparently associated with the occurrence of this tumor on the surface of the bone, their relatively low histologic grade of malignancy, and in the majority, a lack of medullary involvement.[23, 119, 172] It is important to stress these factors, because if they are not present, the outcome is not as favorable, and treatment must include chemotherapy.

These facts were stressed by Campanacci and coworkers in a retrospective analysis of 35 evaluable patients treated at the Istituto Ortopedica Rizzoli.[23] These researchers stressed that adequate surgery must be performed, regardless of the histologic grade of the tumor, to ensure adequate local control. They noted that patients (13 patients) with histologic grade I tumors fared quite well, with no distant metastases noted (even if there was intramedullary involvement) and with a high salvage rate after local recurrence. Patients with tumors of histologic grade II (14 patients) had an intermediate prognosis, and those with tumors with grade III pathologic characteristics (8 patients) had the worst outcome. Distant metastases in these last two grades occurred only when there was intramedullary involvement and this was found with increasing frequency the higher the grade. Finally, others reported that parosteal osteosarcoma from patients with multiple local recurrences can undergo dedifferentiation to a higher, more malignant tumor with a predilection for distant metastases.[176, 189]

Thus, the majority of patients with parosteal osteosarcoma can be cured without chemotherapy if careful pathologic analysis, surgical staging, and adequate surgery are performed. Adjuvant chemotherapy should be reserved for those patients with grade III histologic tumors.

SIDE EFFECTS OF THERAPY

The major side effects of therapy are confined to those from chemotherapy and surgery (Table 5–11). With the use of aggressive chemotherapy, the immediate side effects of nausea and vomiting (especially with cisplatin and doxorubicin) must be addressed adequately, for these side effects cause the most immediate

TABLE 5–11

Late Effects in Osteosarcoma

Cardiomyopathy
Nephropathy
Decreased pulmonary function
Auditory damage
Leukoencephalopathy
Limb sequelae
- Amputation—need for prosthesis
- Limb sparing
  - Infection
  - Decreased range of motion from fibrosis and nerve and muscle damage
  - Instability of internal prosthesis
  - Pain

consternation and lack of compliance by the adolescents who are being treated. Obviously, the other known side effects of the agents most commonly used in the treatment of osteosarcoma must be watched for, including pancytopenia with accompanying fever, stomatitis, bleeding, and weakness; kidney damage (associated with cisplatin and/or HDMTX)[62, 85]; decreased pulmonary function (especially decreased diffusion capacity with bleomycin); auditory damage (with cisplatin); and cardiac damage (associated with doxorubicin). HDMTX has been associated with leukoencephalopathy[2, 55] and transient neurologic disturbances.[1a, 92, 180] The issue of sterility was addressed and noted not to be a problem in males, despite the use of cyclophosphamide in regimens that include BCD.[130]

The morbidity and problems associated with limb salvage were addressed above.

SUMMARY, CONCLUSIONS, AND FUTURE DIRECTIONS

A majority of patients with osteosarcoma survive their disease, but approximately 30 to 40% eventually die. Although the roles of surgery and chemotherapy have been delineated during the past 20 years in treating patients with osteosarcoma, how best to treat these patients must be determined and newer approaches to the therapy of this disease must be developed. The following conclusions and questions arise when treating children with osteosarcoma:

Biopsy should be done with the subsequent surgery in mind, and an adequate sample must be obtained and evaluated by an experienced pathologist. This becomes crucial when cooperative, multiinstitutional studies are done.[12, 121] The role of needle biopsy in the diagnosis of this disease needs to be further assessed but might be one way of reducing morbidity.[5]

The place of chemotherapy in the treatment of osteosarcoma is well established and no longer controversial. With the use of HDMTX, cisplatin, doxorubicin, bleomycin, cyclophosphamide, and actinomycin D, the disease-free survival rate has increased from 20% to at least 60%. Ifosfamide, a newer agent, has not increased the disease-free survival. Which of these agents will eventually prove to be the most important and how much MTX per dose is necessary (e.g., is HDMTX really needed, or can lower, but more continuous doses be used?) are issues that still need to be addressed.

Neoadjuvant chemotherapy has been used to assess the response of the tumor to the agents employed, and to give the surgeon time to have a prosthesis made for limb salvage. Whether the necrosis of the tumor secondary to chemotherapy can be used as a deciding factor in tailoring chemotherapy is still debatable and in need of further study. Also still to be agreed on is the need for preoperative chemotherapy in making previous unsalvageable limbs salvageable.

How long a patient must be treated is still unknown, although studies indicate that shorter periods of therapy may be adequate, and therapy for no more than 6 to 8 months may become standard.

Advantages of limb salvage techniques, especially for lower extremity primary tumors, need to be further assessed. This includes not only the type of limb-sparing procedure performed, but whether such a procedure offers any real functional and psychologic advantage to the patient.

Intraarterial cisplatin has been used extensively at the MD Anderson Hospital and Tumor Institute.[14, 82, 89, 90] The results of these studies indicated that such therapy is feasible to administer and that significant tumor necrosis is obtained in the primary site with this particular modality of treatment. Whether this yields better results than does conventional IV administration of chemotherapeutic agents is not known, as a controlled study has not been carried out to investigate the potential superiority of this approach.

The role of radiotherapy, long consigned to oblivion in the treatment of osteosarcoma, should have another look. Studies from Europe opened up the questions of the utility of prophylactic pulmonary radiation given with chemotherapy.[147a] In a novel strategy for limb salvage surgery, there may be a role for extracorporeal irradiation of the bone involved with the primary lesion followed by reimplantation.[175]

Finally, in an attempt to improve on the current cure rate, there has been renewed interest in interferon[40] and the use of other classes of biologic modifiers such as liposomal muramyl-tripeptide, an agent that might enhance the ability of pulmonary macrophages to attack metastatic tumor cells.[102] Monoclonal antibodies have also been developed that are specific for osteosarcoma cells.[129] These antibodies may be used to help in the detection of occult metastases if tagged with radioactive tracers[3] or in the treatment of disease by either direct action or delivery to the tumor cells of chemotherapeutic agents or cellular poisons.

References

1. Akahoshi Y, Takehchi S, Chen SH, Nishimoto T, Kikiki A, Yonezawa H, Yamamuro T: The results of surgical treatment combined with intra-arterial infusion of anti-cancer agents in osteosarcoma. Clin Orthop 120:103–109, 1976.

1a. Allen JC, Rosen G: Transient cerebral dysfunction following chemotherapy for osteogenic sarcoma. Ann Neurol 3:441–444, 1978.

2. Allen JC, Rosen G, Mehta BM, Horten B: Leukoencephalopathy following high-dose IV methotrexate chemotherapy with leucovorin rescue. Cancer Treat Rep 64:1261–1273, 1980.

3. Armitage NC, Perkins AC, Pimm MV, Wastie M, Hopkins JS, Dowling F, Baldwin RW, Hardcastle JD: Imaging of bone tumors using a monoclonal antibody raised against human osteosarcoma. Cancer 58:37–42, 1986.

4. Askin FB, Roasi J, Dehner LP, McAlister WH: Malignant small cell tumor of thoracopulmonary region in childhood. A distinctive clinicopathologic entity of uncertain histogenesis. Cancer 43:2348–2351, 1979.

5. Ayala AG, Zornosa J: Primary bone tumors: Percutaneous needle biopsy. Radiology 149:675–679, 1983.

6. Bacci G, Gherlinzoni F, Picci P, Van Horn JR, Jaffe N, Guerra A, Ruggieri P, Biagini R, Capanna R, Toni A, Mercuri M, Dallari D, Campanacci M: Adriamycin-methotrexate high dose versus Adriamycin-methotrexate moderate dose and adjuvant chemotherapy for osteosarcoma of the extremities: A randomized study. Eur J Cancer Oncol 22:1337–1345, 1986.

7. Bacci G, Picci P, Avella M, Dallari D, Ferrari S, Prasad R, Di Scioscio M, Malaguti C, Caldora P: The importance of dose-intensity in neoadjuvant chemotherapy of osteosarcoma: A retrospective analysis of high-dose methotrexate, cisplatinum and Adrimaycin used preoperatively. J Chemother 2:127–135, 1990.

8. Bacci G, Picci P, Gherlinzoni F, Capanna F, Calderoni P, Putti C, Mancini A, Campanacci M: Localized Ewing's sarcoma of bone: Ten years' experience at the Instituto Ortopedico Rizzoli in 124 cases treated with multimodal therapy. Eur J Cancer Clin Oncol 21:163–173, 1985.

9. Bacci G, Picci P, Gitelis S, Borghi A, Campanacci M: The treatment of localized Ewing's sarcoma: The experience at the Instituto Ortopedico Rizzoli in 163 cases treated with and without adjuvant chemotherapy. Cancer 49:1561–1570, 1982.

10. Bauer HCF, Kriecbergs A, Silfversward C, Tribukait B: DNA analysis in the differential diagnosis of osteosarcoma. Cancer 61:2532–2540, 1989.

11. Baumgartner C, Bleher EZ, Brun del Re G, Bucher U, Deubelbeiss KA, Greiner R, Hirt A, Imbach P, Luthy A, Odavic R, Wagner HP: Autologous bone marrow transplantation in the treatment of children and adolescents with advanced malignant tumors. Med Pediatr Oncol 12:104–111, 1984.

12. Becker W, Ramach W, Delling G: Problems of biopsy and diagnosis in a cooperative study of osteosarcoma. J Cancer Res Clin Oncol (Suppl) 106:11–13, 1983.

13. Belli L, Scholl S, Livartowski A, Ashby M, Palangie T, Levasseur P, Pouillart P: Resection of pulmonary metastases in osteosarcoma. A retrospective analysis of 44 patients. Cancer 63:2546–2550, 1989.

14. Benjamin RS, Chawla SP, Carrasco C: Arterial infusion in the treatment of osteosarcoma. Dev Oncol 55:269–274, 1988.

15. Bentzen SM, Poulsen HS, Kaae S, Myhre Jenson O, Johansen H, Mouridsen HT, Daugaard S, Arnoldi C: Prognostic factors in osteosarcomas. Cancer 62:194–202, 1988.

16. Berry MP, Jenkin DT, Harwood AT, Cummings BJ, Quirt IC, Sonley MJ, Rider WD: Ewing's sarcoma: A trial of adjuvant chemotherapy and sequential half-body irradiation. Int J Radiat Oncol Biol Phys 12:19–24, 1986.

17. Bhansali SK, Desai PB: Ewing's sarcoma. Observations on 107 cases. J Bone Joint Surgery 45A:541–553, 1963.

18. Bohen JW, Thorning D: Peripheral neuroepithelioma: A light and electron microscopic study. Cancer 46:2456–2462, 1980.

19. Breur K, Cohen P, Schweisguth O, Hart AAM: Irradiation of the lungs as a adjuvant therapy in the treatment of osteosarcoma of the limbs. Eur J Cancer 14:461–471, 1978.

20. Brown AP, Fixsen JA, Plowman PN: Local control of Ewing's sarcoma; An analysis of 67 patients. Br J Radiol 60:261–268, 1987.

21. Burgers JMV, van Glabberk M, Busson A, Cohen P, Mazzbraud AR, Abbatucci JS, Kalifa C, Tubaina M, Lemerle JS, Voute PA, van Oosterom A, Waegner TH, van der Werf-Messing B, Somers R, Pons A, Duez N: Osteosarcoma of the limbs. Report of the EORTC–SIOP 03 Trial 20781 investigating the value of adjuvant treatment with chemotherapy and/ or prophylactic lung irradiation. Cancer 61:1024–1031, 1988.

22. Burgert EO Jr, Nesbit EM, Garnsey LA, Gehan EA, Herrmann J, Vietti TJ, Cangir A, Tefft M, Evans R, Thomas P, Askin FB, Kissane JM, Pritchard DJ, Neff J, Makley JT, Gilula L: Multimodal therapy for the management of nonpelvic localized Ewing's sarcoma of bone: Intergroup study IESS–II. J Clin Oncol 8:1517–1524, 1990.

23. Campanacci M, Picci P, Gherlinzoni F, Guera A,

Bertoni F, Neff JR: Parosteal osteosarcoma. J Bone Joint Surgery 66B:313–321, 1984.
24. Cangir A, Vietti TJ, Gehan EA, Burgert O, Thomas P, Teftt M, Nesbit M, Kissane J, Pritchard D: Ewing's sarcoma metastatic at diagnosis. Results and comparisons of two intergroup Ewing's sarcoma studies. Cancer 66:887–893, 1990.
25. Carter SK: Adjuvant chemotherapy in osteogenic sarcoma: The triumph that isn't? J Clin Oncol 2:147–148, 1984.
26. Cavazzana AO, Miser JS, Jefferson J, Triche TJ: Experimental evidence for a neural origin of Ewing's sarcoma of bone. Am J Pathol 127:507–518, 1987.
27. Chan PYM, Gilbert HA, Stein JJ, et al: The role of early diagnosis and radiation therapy in the management of Ewing's sarcoma. Front Radiat Ther Oncol 141–151, 1975.
28. Chawla SP, Rosen G, Lowenbraun S, Morton D, Eilber F: Role of high dose ifosfamide (HDI) in recurrent osteosarcoma. Proc ASCO 9:310, 1990.
29. Chesi R, Cazzola A, Baci G, Borghi B, Balladelli A, Urso G: Effect of perioperative transfusions on survival in osteosarcoma treated by multimodal therapy. Cancer 64:1727–1737, 1989.
30. Cortes EP, Holland JF, Glidewell O: Osteogenic sarcoma studies by the cancer and leukemia group B. Natl Cancer Inst Monogr 56:207–209, 1981.
31. Cummings WA, Sabbah R: Large unilateral chest tumors in children. J Can Assoc Radiol 36:116–118, 1985.
32. Dahlin DC, Coventry MB: Osteogenic sarcoma. A study of 600 cases. J Bone Joint Surg 49A:101–110, 1967.
33. Dahlin DC, Unni KK: Bone Tumors. General Aspects and Data on 8,542 Cases, 4th ed. Springfield, IL, Charles C Thomas, 1986, pp 269–305.
34. Dehner LP: Peripheral and central primitive neuroectodermal tumors. A nosologic concept seeking a consensus. Arch Pathol Lab Med 110:997–1005, 1986.
35. de Stefani E, Carzoglio J, Deneo-Pellegrini H, Olivera L, Cendan M, Kasdorf H: Ewing's sarcoma: Value of tumor necrosis as a predictive factor. Bull Cancer 71:16–21, 1984.
36. Djerassi I, Rominger CJ, Kim JS, Suvansri U, Hughers D: Phase I study of methotrexate with citrovorum factor in patients with lung cancer. Cancer 30:22–30, 1972.
37. Donaldson S, Krischer J: POG protocol #8346. Unpublished data.
38. Donner L, Triche TJ, Israel MA, et al: A panel of monoclonal antibodies which discriminate neuroblastoma from Ewing's sarcoma, rhabdomyosarcoma, neuroepithelioma, and hematopoietic malignancies. Prog Clin Biol Res 75:347–366, 1985.
39. Edmonson JH, Green SI, Ivins JC, Gilchrist GS, Creagan ET, Pritchard DJ, Smithson WA, Dahlin DC, Taylor WF: A controlled study of high-dose methotrexate as postsurgical adjuvant treatment for primary osteosarcoma. J Clin Oncol 2:152–156, 1984.
40. Edmonson JH, Long HJ, Frytak S, et al: Phase II study of recombinant Alph-2a interferon in patients with advanced bone sarcomas. Cancer Treat Rep 71:747–748, 1987.
41. Eilber F, Giuliano A, Eckardt GJ, Moseley PS, Goodnight J: Adjuvant chemotherapy of osteosarcoma: A randomized prospective trial. J Clin Oncol 5:21–26, 1987.
42. Enneking WF, Spanier SS, Goodman MA: A system for the surgical staging of musculoskeletal sarcoma. Clin Orthop 153:106–120, 1980.
43. Evans R, Burgert EO, Gilchrist GS, Smithson WA, Pritchard DJ, Bruckman JE: Sequential half-body irradiation (SHBI) and combination chemotherapy as salvage treatment for failed Ewing's sarcoma—a pilot study. Int J Radiat Oncol Biol Phys 10:2363–2368, 1984.
44. Evans E, Nesbit M, Askin F, Burgert O, Cangir A, Foulkes M, Gehan E, Gilula L, Kisane J, Makely J, Neff J, Perez C, Pritchard D, Tefft M, Thomas P, Vietti T: Local recurrence rate and sites of metastases and time to relapse as a function of treatment regimen, size of primary and surgical history in 62 patients presenting with nonmetastatic Ewing's sarcoma of the pelvic bones. Int J Radiat Oncol Biol Phys 11:129–136, 1985.
45. Farley FA, Healey JH, Caparros-Sison B, Godbold J, Lane JM, Glasser DB: Lactase dehydrogenase as tumor marker for recurrent disease in Ewing's sarcoma. Cancer 59:1245–1248, 1987.
46. Fernandez CH, Lindberg RD, Sutow WW, Samuels ML: Localized Ewing's sarcoma—treatment and results. Cancer 34:143–148, 1974.
47. Flye MW, Woltering G, Rosenber SA: Aggressive pulmonary resection for metastatic osteogenic and soft tissue sarcomas. Ann Thorac Surg 37:123–127, 1984.
48. Frei E, Jaffe N, Gero M, Skipper H, Watts H: Guest editorial: Adjuvant chemotherapy of osteogenic sarcoma. Progress and perspective. JNCI 60:3–10,1978.
49. French Bone Tumor Study Group: Age and dose of chemotherapy as major prognostic factors in adjuvant therapy of osteosarcoma combining two alternating drug combinations and early prophylactic lung irradiation. Cancer 61:1304–1311, 1988.
50. Gasparini M, Lombardi F, Gianni C, Fossati-Bellani F: Localized Ewing's sarcoma: Results of integrated therapy and analysis of failures. Eur J Cancer Clin Oncol 17:1205–1209, 1981.
51. Gehan EZ, Nesbit ME, Burgert EO, Vietti TJ, Tefft M, Perez CA, Kissane J, Hempel C: Prognostic factors in children with Ewing's sarcoma. Natl Cancer Inst Monogr 56:273–278, 1981.
52. Geschickter CF, Copeland MM: Parosteal osteoma of bone: A new entity. Ann Surg 133:790–807, 1951.
53. Giritsky AS, Eteubanas E, Mark JBD: Pulmonary resection in children with metastatic osteogenic sarcoma: Improved survival with surgery, chemotherapy and irradiation. J Thorac Cardiovasc Surg 75:354, 1978.
54. Giuliano AE, Feig S, Eilber FR: Changing metastatic patterns of osteosarcoma. Cancer 54:2160–2164, 1984.
55. Glass JP, Lee Y-Y, Bruner J, Fields WS: Treatment-related leukoencephalopathy. A study of three cases and literature review. Medicine 65:154–162, 1986.
56. Glaubinger DL, Makuch R, Schwarz J, Levine AS, Johnson RE: Determination of prognostic factors and their influence on therapeutic results in patients with Ewing's sarcoma. Cancer 45:2213–2219, 1980.
57. Glaubinger DL, Makuch RW, Schwarz J: Influence of prognostic factors on survival in Ewing's sarcoma. Natl Cancer Inst Monogr 56:285–288, 1981.
58. Gobel V, Jurgens H, Etspuler G, Kemperdick H, Jungblut RM, Stienen U, Gobel U: Prognostic significance of tumor volume in localized Ewing's sarcoma of bone in children and adolescents. J Cancer Res Clin Oncol 113:187–191, 1987.
59. Goldman A: Ewing's sarcoma: Treatment with high-dose radiation and adjuvant chemotherapy. Recent Results Cancer Res 80:115–119, 1980.

60. Goorin AM, Delorey M, Gelber RD, Price K, Vawter G, Jaffe N, Watts H, Link M, Frei E, Abelson HT: Dana-Farber Cancer Institute/The Children's Hospital adjuvant chemotherapy trials for osteosarcoma; Three sequential studies. Cancer Treat Symposia 35:155–159, 1985.
61. Goorin AM, Delorey MJ, Lack EE, Gelber RD, Price K, Cassady JR, Levey R, Tapper D, Jaffe N, Link M: Prognostic significance of complete surgical resection of pulmonary metastases in patients with osteogenic sarcoma: Analysis of 32 patients. J Clin Oncol 2:425–431, 1984.
62. Goren MP, Wright RK, Horowitz ME, Meyer WH: Enhancement of methotrexate nephrotoxicity after cisplatin therapy. Cancer 58:2617–2621, 1986.
63. Graeber GM, Snyder RJ, Fleming AW, Head HD, Lough FC, Parker JS, Zajtchuk R, Brott WH: Initial and long term results in the management of primary chest wall neoplasms. Ann Thorac Surg 34:664–673, 1982.
64. Graham-Pole G, Lazarus HM, Herzig RH, Gross S, Coccia P, Weiner R, Strandjord S: High-dose melphalan therapy for the treatment of children with refractory neuroblastoma and Ewing's sarcoma. Am J Pediatr Hematol Oncol 6:17–26, 1984.
65. Grem JL, King SA, Wittes RE, Leyland-Jones R: The role of methotrexate in osteosarcoma. J Natl Cancer Inst 80:626–656, 1988.
66. Grier HE, Tarbell NJ, Perez-Atayde AR, Shamberger RC, Blattner SR: Treatment of soft tissue primitive neuroectodermal tumors (PNET): Favorable early results. Proc Annu Meet Am Soc Clin Oncol 9:294, 1990.
67. Harris MB: Osteosarcoma—is there a role for oral low-dose methotrexate. Cancer Invest 7:357–360, 1989.
67a. Harris MB: POG study 8759. Unpublished data.
68. Hartman O, Oberlin O, Kalifa C, Patte C, Brugieres L, Lemerle J: Repeated high-dose chemotherapy (HDC) followed by autologous bone marrow transplantation as consolidation therapy in metastatic Ewing's sarcoma. Proc Annu Meet Am Soc Clin Oncol 7:260 (A-1008), 1988.
69. Hashimoto H, Enjoji M, Nakajima T, Kryer H, Daimaru Y: Malignant neuroepithelioma (peripheral neuroblastoma): A clinicopathologic study of 15 cases. Am J Surg Pathol 7:309–318, 1983.
70. Hayes FA, Thompson EI, Hustu HO, Kumar M, Coburn T, Webber B: The response of Ewing's sarcoma to sequential cyclophosphamide and Adriamycin induction therapy. J Clin Oncol 1:45–51, 1983.
71. Hayes FA, Thompson EI, Meyer WH, Kun L, Parham D, Rao B, Hancock M, Parvey L, Magill L, Hustu HO: Therapy for localized Ewing's sarcoma of bone. J Clin Oncol 7:208–213, 1989.
72. Hayes FA, Thompson EI, Parvey L, Rao B, Kun L, Parham D, Hustu HO: Metastatic Ewing's sarcoma: Remission induction and survival. J Clin Oncol 5:1199–1204, 1987.
73. Herman G, Leviton M, Mendelson D, Norton K, Harris M, Weiner M, Lewis M: Osteosarcoma: Relation between extent of marrow infiltration on CT and frequency of lung metastases. AJR 149:1203–1206, 1987.
74. Hustu OH, Pinkel D, Pratt CB: Treatment of clinically localized Ewing's sarcoma with radiotherapy and combination chemotherapy. Cancer 30:1522–1527, 1972.
75. Huth JF, Eckardt JJ, Eilber FR: Patterns of recurrence following primary resection of osteosarcoma of the extremity: Strategies for treatment of metastases (meeting abstract). Forty-first Annual Cancer Symposium of the Society of Surgical of Head and Neck Surgeons 1988, p 204. May 22–25, 1988, New Orleans, LA, p 204, 1988.
76. Huvos AG, Rosen G, Marcove RC: Primary osteogenic sarcoma. Pathologic aspects in 20 patients after treatment with chemotherapy, *en bloc* resection and prosthetic bone replacement. Arch Pathol Lab Med 101:14–18, 1977.
77. Israel MA, Miser JS, Triche TJ, Kinsella T: Neuroepithelial tumors. *In* Pizzo PA, Poplack DG (eds): Philadelphia, JB Lippincott, 1989, pp 623–634.
78. Ivins JC, Taylor WF, Wold LE: Elective whole-lung irradiation in osteosarcoma treatment: Appearance of bilateral breast cancer in two long-term survivors. Skeletal Radiol 16:133–135, 1987.
79. Jaffe N: Progress report on high-dose methotrexate (NSC–740) with citrovorum rescue in the treatment of metastatic bone tumors. Cancer Chemother Rep 58:275–280, 1974.
80. Jaffe N, Frei E: Osteogenic sarcoma: Advances in treatment. CA 26:351–359, 1976.
81. Jaffe N, Paed D: Recent advances in the chemotherapy of metastatic osteogenic sarcoma. Cancer 30:1627–1631, 1972.
82. Jaffe N, Bowman R, Wang Y-M, Cangir A, Ayala A, Chaung VP, Wallace S, Murray J: Chemotherapy for primary osteosarcoma by intra-arterial infusion. Cancer Bull 36:37–41, 1984.
83. Jaffe N, Frei E, Traggis D Bishop Y: Adjuvant methotrexate and citrovorum-factor treatment of osteogenic sarcoma. N Engl J Med 291:994–997, 1974.
84. Jaffe N, Goorin A, Link M, Watts H, Frei E, Vawter G, Fellows KE, Beardsley PG, Abelson HT: High-dose methotrexate in osteogenic sarcoma adjuvant chemotherapy and limb salvage results. Can Treat Rep (Suppl 1) 65:99–106, 1981.
85. Jaffe N, Keifer R, Robertson R, Cangir A, Wang A: Renal toxicity with cumulative doses of *cis*-diamminedichloroplatinum-II in pediatric patients with osteosarcoma. Effect on creatinine clearance and methotrexate excretion. Cancer 59:1577–1581, 1987.
86. Jaffe N, Paed D, Farber S, Traggis D, Geiser C, Kim BS, Das L, Frauenberger G, Djerassi I, Cassady JR: Favorable response of metastatic osteogenic sarcoma to pulse high-dose methotrexate with citrovorum rescue and radiation therapy. Cancer 31:1367–1373, 1973. Cancer 39:45–50, 1977.
87. Jaffe N, Paed D, Frei E, Traggis D, Watts H: Weekly high-dose methotrexate–citrovorum factor in osteogenic sarcoma. Cancer 39:45–50, 1977.
88. Jaffe N, Prudich J, Knapp J, Wang Y-M, Bowman R, Cangir A, Ayala A, Chaung V, Wallace S: Treatment of primary osteosarcoma with intra-arterial and intravenous high-dose methotrexate. J Clin Oncol 1:428–431, 1983.
89. Jaffe N, Raymond AK, Ayala A, Carrasco H, Sesaki K, Wallace S, Murray J, Robertson R, Wang A: Intra-arterial *cis* diamminedichloroplatinum-II in pediatric osteosarcoma: Relationship of effect on primary tumor to survival. Dev Oncol 55:275–282, 1988.
90. Jaffe N, Raymond K, Ayala A, Carrasco CH, Wallace S, Robertson R, Griffiths M, Wang Y-M: Effect of cumulative courses of intra-arterial *cis*-diamminedichloroplatin-II on the primary tumor in osteosarcoma. Cancer 63:63–67, 1989.
91. Jaffe N, Smith E, Abelson HT: Osteogenic sarcoma: Alteration in the pattern of pulmonary metastases

with adjuvant chemotherapy. J Clin Oncol 1:251–254, 1983.

92. Jaffe N, Takaue Y, Anzai T: Transient neurologic disturbances induced by high-dose methotrexate treatment. Cancer 56:1356–1360, 1985.
93. Jaffe R, Santamaria M, Yunis EJ, Tannery NH, Agostini RM Jr, Medina J, Goodman M: The neuroectodermal tumor of bone. A M J Surg Pathol 8:885–898, 1984.
94. Jenkin RDT: Ewing's sarcoma; A study of treatment methods. Clin Radiol 92:97–106, 1966.
95. Jentzsch K, Binder H, Cramer H, Glaubiger DK, Kessler RM, Bull C, Pomeroy TC, Gerber NL: Leg function after radiotherapy for Ewing's sarcoma. Cancer 47:1267–1278, 1981.
96. Jurgens H, Bier V, Harms D, Beck J, Brandeis W, Etspuler G, Gadner H, Schmidt D, Treuner J, Winkler K, Gobel U: Malignant peripheral neuroectodermal tumors. A retrospective analysis of 42 patients. Cancer 61:349–357, 1988.
97. Jurgens H, Exner U, Gadner H, Harms D, Michaelis J, Sauer R, Treuner J, Voute T, Winkelmann W, Winkler K, Gobel U: Multidisciplinary treatment of primary Ewing's sarcoma of bone: a six year experience of a European cooperative trial. Cancer 61:23–32, 1988.
98. Jurgens H, Kosloff C, Nirenberg A, Mehta BM, Huvos AG, Rosen G: Prognostic factors in the response of primary osteogenic sarcoma to preoperative chemotherapy (high-dose methotrexate with citrovorum factor). Natl Cancer Inst Monogr 56:221–226, 1981.
99. Kadota RP, Gilchrist GS, Pairolero PC, Taylor WF, Telander RL: Pulmonary metastases in osteosarcoma: A review of treatment and outcome in 88 pediatric patients. Proc Annu Meet Am Soc Clin Oncol 4:239, 1985.
100. Kinsella TJ, Lichter AS, Miser J, Gerber L, Glatstein E: Local treatment of Ewing's sarcoma: Radiation therapy versus surgery. Cancer Treat Rep 68:695–701, 1984.
101. Kinsella TJ, Loeffler JS, Fraass BA, Tepper J: Extremity preservation by combined modality therapy in sarcomas of the hand and foot: An analysis of local control, disease free survival and functional result. Int J Radiat Oncol Biol Phys 9:1115–1119, 1983.
102. Kleinerman E: Personal communication.
103. Kolata GB: Dilemma in cancer treatment. Science 209:792–794, 1980.
104. Krailo M, Ertel I, Makley J, et al: A randomized study comparing high-dose methotrexate with moderate-dose methotrexate as components of adjuvant chemotherapy in childhood non-metastatic osteosarcoma: A report from the Children's Cancer Study Group. Med Pediatr Oncol 15:69–77, 1987.
105. Kreicbergs A, Brostrom LA, Cewrien G, Einhorn S: Cellular DNA content in human osteosarcoma. Aspect on diagnosis and prognosis. Cancer 50:2476–2481, 1982.
106. Lange B, Levine AS: Is it ethical to conduct a prospectively controlled trial of adjuvant chemotherapy in osteosarcoma? Cancer Treat Rep 2:1699–1704, 1982.
107. Lanza LA, Miser JS, Pass HI, Roth JA: The role of resection in the treatment of pulmonary metastases from Ewing's sarcoma. J Thorac Cardiovasc Surg 94:181–187, 1987.
108. Larsson S-E, Lorentzon R: The incidence of malignant primary bone tumours in relation to age, sex, and site: A study of osteogenic sarcoma, chondrosarcoma, and Ewing's sarcoma diagnosed in Sweden from 1958 to 1968. J Bone Joint Surg 56B:534–540, 1974.
109. Levine E, DeSmet AA, Huntrakoon M: Juxtacortical osteosarcoma: A radiologic and histologic spectrum. Skeletal Radiol 14:38–46, 1985.
110. Lewis RJ, Marcove RC, Rosen G: Ewing's sarcoma—functional effects of radiation therapy. J Bone Joint Surg 59A:325–331, 1977.
111. Li WK, Lane JM, Rosen G, Marcove RC, Caparraos B, Huvos A, Groshen S: Pelvic Ewing's sarcoma: Advances in treatment. J Bone Joint Surg 65A:738–747, 1983.
112. Liddell RH, Meyer WH, Dodge RK, Green AA, Pratt CB: Prognostic indicators for patients with osteosarcoma (OS) treated with adjuvant chemotherapy. Proc Annu Meet Am Assoc Cancer Res 29:A900, 1988.
113. Link MP, Goorin AM, Miser AW: The effect of adjuvant chemotherapy on relapse-free survival in patients with osteosarcoma of the extremity. N Engl J Med 314:1600–1606, 1986.
114. Link MP, Schustrer JJ, Goorin AM, Miser A, Meyer WH, Kingston JE, Belasco J, Baker AR, Ayala AG, Vietti T: Adjuvant chemotherapy in the treatment of osteosarcoma: Results of multi-institutional osteosarcoma study: recent concepts in sarcoma treatment. *In* Rya J, Baker LH (eds): International Symposium on Sarcomas, Tarpon Springs, FL, October 8–10, 1987. Drodrecht, Netherlands, Kluwer Academic Publishers, 1988, p 283–290.
115. Llombart-Borsch A, Contesso G, Henry-Amar M, Lacombe MJ, Oberlin O, Dubousset J, Rouesse J, Sarrazin K: Histopathological predictive factors in Ewing's sarcoma of bone and clinicopathological correlations. A retrospective study of 261 cases. Virchows Arch (A) 409:627–640, 1986.
116. Lombardi F, Lattuada A, Gasparini M, Gianni C, Marchesini R: Sequential half-body irradiation as systemic treatment of progressive Ewing's sarcoma. Int J Radiat Oncol Biol Phys 8:1679–1682, 1982.
117. Look AT, Douglass EC, Meyer WH: Clinical importance of near-diploid tumor stem lines in patients with osteosarcoma of an extremity. N Engl J Med 318:1567–1572, 1988.
118. Lopez-Gines C, Pellin A, Llombart-Bosch A: Two new cases of primary peripheral neuroepithelioma of soft tissue with translocation (11,22) (q24;q12). Cancer Genet Cytogenet 33:291–297, 1988.
119. Lorentzon R, Larsson SE, Boquist L: Parosteal (juxtacortical) osteosarcoma. J Bone Joint Surg 62B:86–92, 1980.
120. Mankin HJ, Gebhardt MC: Advances in the management of bone tumors. Clin Orthop Res 200:73–84, 1985.
121. Mankin HJ, Lange TA, Spanier SS: The hazards of biopsy in patients with malignant primary bone and soft tissue tumors. J Bone Joint Surg 64A:1121–1127, 1982.
122. Marcove RC, Mike V, Hajek JV, Levin AG, Hutter R: Osteogenic sarcoma under the age of twenty-one: A review of 145 operative cases. J Bone Joint Surg 52A:411–423, 1970.
123. Marcus RB Jr, Million RR: The effect of primary tumor size on the prognosis of Ewing's sarcoma. Int J Rad Oncol Biol Phys 10(Suppl 2):88, 1984.
124. Martinez A, Goffinet DR, Donaldson SS, Bagshaw MA, Kaplan HS: Intra-arterial infusion of radiosensitizer (BUDR) combined with hypofractionated ir-

radiation of chemotherapy for primary treatment of osteogenic sarcoma. Int J Radiat Oncol Biol Phys 11:123–214, 1985.

125. Martini N, Huvos AG, Mike V, et al: Multiple pulmonary resections in the treatment of osteogenic sarcoma. Ann Thorac Surg 12:271, 1971.
126. McKay B, Luna MA, Butler JJ: Adult neuroblastoma. Electron microscopic observations in nine cases. Cancer 37:1334–1351, 1976.
127. McKenna RJ, Schwinn CP, Soong KY, Higinbotham NL: Sarcomata of the osteogenic series (osteosarcoma, fibrosarcoma, chondrosarcoma, parosteal osteogenic sarcoma, and sarcomata arising in abnormal bone). J Bone Joint Surg 48A:1–26, 1966.
128. McKeon C, Thiel CJ, Ross RA, Kwan M, Triche TJ, Iser JS, Israel MA: Indistinguishable patterns of protooncogene expression in two distinct but closely related tumors. Ewing's sarcoma and neuroepithelioma. Cancer Res 48:4307–4311, 1988.
129. McKlay EF, Slovin SF: Immunotherapeutic approaches to the treatment of bone and soft tissue sarcomas. Semin Oncol 16:328–332, 1989.
130. Meistrich ML, Chawla SP, Da Cunha MF, Johnson SL, Plager C, Papadopoulous NE, Lipshultz LI, Benjamin RS: Recovery of sperm production after chemotherapy for osteosarcoma. Cancer 63:2115–2123, 1989.
131. Mendenhall CM, Marcus RB Jr, Enneking WF, Springfield DS, Thar TL, Million RR: The prognostic significance of soft tissue extension in Ewing's sarcoma. Cancer 51:913–917, 1983.
132. Meyers PA: Malignant bone tumors in children: Ewing's sarcoma. Hematol Oncol Clin North Am 1:667–673, 1987.
133. Miser J, Kinsella T, Triche T, Jaronski P, Magrath I: Treatment of recurrent sarcomas in children and young adults: The use of a multimodality approach including ifosfamide (IFF) and etopside (VP-16). Proc Annu Meet Am Soc Clin Oncol 7:258 (A-999), 1988.
134. Miser JS, Kinsella TJ, Triches TJ, Steis R, Tsokos M, Wesley R, Horvath K, Belasco J, Longo DL, Glatstein E, Israel MA: Treatment of peripheral neuroepithelioma in children and young adults. J Clin Oncol 5:1752–1758, 1987.
135. Miser JS, Kinsella TJ, Triche TJ, Tsokos M, Forquer R, Wesley R, Horvath K, Belasco J, Longo DL, Steis R, Glatstein E, Pizzo PA: Preliminary results of treatment of Ewing's sarcoma of bone in children and young adults: Six months of intensive combined modality therapy without maintenance. J Clin Oncol 6:484–490, 1988.
136. Miser JS, Kinsella TJ, Triche TJ, Tskos M, Jaronski P, Forquer R, Wesley R, Magrath I: Ifosfamide with mesna uroprotection and etopside: An effective regimen in the treatment of recurrent sarcomas and other tumors of children and young adults. J Clin Oncol 5:1191–1198, 1987.
137. Nesbit ME, Perez CA, Tefft M, Burgert EO, Vietti TJ, Kissane J, Pritchard DJ, Gehan EA: Multimodal therapy for the management of primary, non-metastatic Ewing's sarcoma of bone: An intergroup study. Natl Cancer Inst Monogr 56:255–262, 1981.
138. Oberlin O, Patte C, Demeocq F, Lacombe MJ, Brunat-Mentigny M, Demaille MC, Tron P, Bui BN, Lemerle J: The Response to initial chemotherapy as a prognostic factor in localized Ewing's sarcoma. Eur J Cancer Clin Oncol 21:463–467, 1985.
139. Oberlin O, Zucker JM, Demeocq F, Demaille MC, Brunatmentigny M, Boutard P, Vannier JP: Ifosfamide (IFO) in Ewing's sarcoma (ES) no clear benefit of IFO vs cyclophosphamide but significant toxicity. A report from the French Society of Pediatric Oncology (SFOP). Proc Annu Meet Am Soc Clin Oncol 7:256 (A-993), 1988.
140. Parham DM, Pratt CB, Parvey LS, Webbrer BL, Champion J: Childhood multifocal osteosarcoma. Cancer 55:2653–2658, 1985.
141. Perez-Atayde AR, Grier H, Weinstein H, Belarey M, Neslie N, Vawter G: Neuroectodermal differentiation in bone tumors presenting as Ewing's sarcoma. Proceedings of SIOP Meeting XIX, 1985, p 61.
142. Perez CA, Razek A, Tefft M, Nesbit M, Burgert EO, Kissane J, Vietti T, Gehan EA: Analysis of local tumor control in Ewing's sarcoma: Preliminary results of a cooperative intergroup study. Cancer 40:2864–2873, 1977.
143. Phillips TL, Sheline GE: Radiation of malignant bone tumors. Radiology 92:1537–1545, 1969.
144. Picci P, Bacci G, Capanna R, et al: Neoadjuvant chemotherapy for localized osteosarcoma of the extremities. Experience related to 103 cases treated between March 83–March 86. *In* Fifth International Conference on the Adjuvant Therapy of Cancer, Tuscon, Arizona, 1987, p 35.
145. Picci P, Bacci G, Neff JR, Capanna R, Baldini N, Banassi NS, Prasad R, Mercuri R, Ruggieri P, Biagini R, Ferruzzi A, Ferraro A, De Cristofaro R, Casadei R, Campanacci M: The influence of preoperative chemotherapy (POC) in the surgical planning in patients (PTS) with osteosarcoma (OS). A histopathologic study of 205 PTS. Proc Annu Meet Am Soc Clin Oncol 9:310, 1990.
146. Pomeroy TC, Johnson RE: Combined modality therapy of Ewing's sarcoma. Cancer 35:36–47, 1975.
147. Provisor A, Nachman J, Krailo M, Etinger L, Hammond D: Treatment of non-metastatic osteogenetic sarcoma (OS) of the extremities with pre- and postoperative chemotherapy. Proc Annu Meet Am Soc Clin Oncol 6:A855, 1987.

147a. Rab GT, Ivins JC, Childs DS, Cupps RE, Pritchard DJ: Elective whole lung irradiation in the treatment of osteogenic sarcoma. Cancer 38:939–942, 1976.

148. Rao BN, Hayes FA, Thompson EI, Kumar AP, Fleming ID, Green AA, Austin BA, Pate JW, Hustu HO: Chest wall resection for Ewing's sarcoma of the rib: An unnecessary procedure. Ann Thorac Surg 46:40–44, 1988.
149. Raymond AK, Chawla SP, Carrasco CH, Ayala AG, Fanning CV, Brice B, Armen T, Plager C, Papadopoulos NEJ, Edeiken J, Wallace S, Jaffe N, Murray JA, Benjamin RS: Osteosarcoma chemotherapy effect: A prognostic factor. Semin Diagn Pathol 4:212–236, 1987.
150. Rosen G, Nirenberg A: Neoadjuvant chemotherapy for osteogenic sarcoma: A five year follow-up (T-10) and preliminary report of new studies (T-12). *In* Wagner T, et al. (eds.): Primary Chemotherapy in Cancer Medicine. Alan R Liss, New York, 1985, pp 39–51.
151. Rosen G, Caparros B, Huvos AG, Kosloff C, Nirenberg A, Cacavio A, Marcove RC, Lane JM, Mehta B, Urban C: Preoperative chemotherapy of osteogenic sarcoma. Cancer 49:1221–1230, 1982.
152. Rosen G, Caparros B, Mosende C, McCormick B, Huvos AG, Marcove RC: Curability of Ewing's sarcoma and considerations for future therapeutic trials. Cancer 41:888–899, 1978.
153. Rosen G, Caparros B, Nirenberg A, Marcove RC,

Huvos AG, Kosloff C, Lane J, Murphy ML: Ewing's sarcoma; Ten-year experience with adjuvant chemotherapy. Cancer 47:2204–2213, 1981.
154. Rosen G, Huvos AG, Mosende E, Beattie EJ Jr, Exelby PR, Capparos B, Marcove RC: Chemotherapy and thoracotomy for metastatic osteogenic sarcoma. A model for adjuvant chemotherapy and rationale for the timing of thoracic surgery. Cancer 41:841, 1978.
155. Rosen G, Murphy ML, Huvos AG, Gutierrez M, Marcove RC: Chemotherapy *en bloc* resection, and prosthetic bone replacement in the treatment of osteogenic sarcoma. Cancer 37:1–11, 1976.
156. Rosenberg SA, Chabner BA, Young RC, Seipp CA, Levine AS, Costa J, Hanson TA, Head GC, Simon RM: Treatment of osteogenic sarcoma: I. Effect of adjuvant high-dose methotrexate after amputation. Cancer Treat Rep 63:739–751, 1979.
157. Roth JA, Putnam JB, Wesley MN, Rosenberg SA: Differing determinants of prognosis following resection of pulmonary metastases from osteogenic and soft tissue sarcoma patients. Cancer 55:1361–1366, 1985.
158. Sauer R, Jurgens H, Burgers JM, Dunst J, Hawlicek R, Michaelis J: Prognostic factors in the treatment of Ewing's sarcoma. The Ewing's Sarcoma Study Group of the German Society of Paediatric Oncology CESS 81. Radiother Oncol 10:101–110, 1987.
159. Schaller RT, Haas J, Schaller J, Morgan A, Bleyer A: Improved survival in children with osteosarcoma following resection of pulmonary metastases. J Pediatr Surg 17:546–550, 1982.
160. Shirley SK, Askin FB, Gilula LA, Vietti TJ, Thomas PR, Siegal GP, Reinus WR, Kissane JM, Nesbit ME: Ewing's sarcoma in bones of the hands and feet: A clinicopathologic study and review of the literature. J Clin Oncol 3:686–697, 1985.
161. Siegal GP, Oliver WR, Reinus WR, Gilula LA, Foulkes MA, Kissane JM, Askin FB: Primary Ewing's sarcoma involving the bones of the head and neck. Cancer 60:2829–2940, 1987.
162. Simon MA: Current concepts review; Limb salvage for osteosarcoma. J Bone Joint Surg 70A:307–310, 1988.
163. Sims FH; Musculoskeletal oncology: State of the art. Orthopedics 10:1673–1684, 1987.
164. Stea B, Kinsella T, Triche TJ, Horvath K, Glatstein E, Miser J: Treatment of pelvic sarcomas in adolescents and young adults with intensive combined modality therapy. Int J Radiat Oncol Biol Phys 13:1797–1805, 1987.
165. Strong LC, Herson J, Osborne B, Sutow WW: Risk of radiation-related subsequent malignant tumors in survivors of Ewing's sarcoma. J Natl Cancer Inst 62:1401–1406, 1979.
166. Taylor WF, Ivins JC, Dahlin DC, et al: Trends and variability in survival from osteosarcoma. Mayo Clin Proc 53:695–700, 1978.
167. Taylor WF, Ivins JC, Pritchard DJ, Dahlin DC, Gilcrist GS, Edmonson JH: Trends and variability in survival among patients with osteosarcoma: A 7-year update. Osteosarcoma and related survival. Mayo Clin Proc 60:91–104, 1985.
168. Taylor WF, Ivins JC, Unni K, Beabout JW, Golenzer JH, Black LE: Prognostic variables in osteosarcoma: A multi-institutional study. J Natl Cancer Inst 81:21–30, 1989.
169. Telles NC, Rabson AS, Pomeroy TC: Ewing's sarcoma: An autopsy series. Cancer 41:2321–2329, 1978.
170. Thomas PRM, Foulkes M, Gilula LA, Burgert EO, Evans RG, Kissane J, Nesbit ME, Pritchard DJ, Tefft M, Vietti TJ: Primary Ewing's sarcoma of the ribs: A report from the Intergroup Ewing's Sarcoma Study. Cancer 51:1021–1027, 1983.
171. Thomas PRM, Perez CA, Neff JR, Nesbit ME, Evans RG: The management of Ewing's sarcoma: Role of radiotherapy in local tumor control. Cancer Treat Rep 68:703–710, 1984.
172. Unni KK, Dahlin DC, Beabout JW, Ivins JC: Parosteal osteogenic sarcoma. Cancer 37:2466–2475, 1976.
173. Uribe-Botero G, Russell WO, Sutow WW, Martin RG: Primary osteosarcoma of bone. A clinicopathologic investigation of 243 cases, with necropsy studies in 54. Am J Clin Pathol 67:427–435, 1977.
174. Ushigome S, Shimoda T, Takaki K, Nikaido T, Takakuwa AT, Ishikawa E, Spjut HJ: Immunocytochemical and ultrastructure studies of the histogeneses of Ewing's sarcoma and putatively related tumors. Cancer 64:52–62, 1989.
175. Uyttendaele D, De Schryver A, Claessens H, Roels H, Berkvens P, Mondelaers W: Limb conservation in primary bone tumours by resection, extracoporeal irradiation and reimplantation. J Bone Joint Surg 70B:348–353, 1988.
176. van Oven MW, Molenaar WM, Freling NJM, Koops H, Muis N, Dam-Meiring A, Oostehuis JW: Dedifferentiated parosteal osteosarcoma of the femur with aneuploidy and lung metastases. Cancer 63:807–811, 1989.
177. Variend S: Small cell tumors in childhood: A review. J Pathol 145:1–25, 1985.
178. Vietti TJ, Gehan EA, Nesbitt ME, Burgert EO, Pilepich M, Tefft M, Kissane J, Pritchard DJ: Multimodal therapy in metastatic Ewing's sarcoma: An intergroup study. Natl Cancer Inst Monogr 56:279–284, 1981.
179. Waegner DJT, van Oosterom AT, Mulder JH, Somer SR, Mouridsen HT, Cortes Foanes H, Thomas D, Sylvester R: Phase II study of low-dose methotrexate in advanced osteosarcoma followed by escalation after disease progression: A study of the soft tissue sarcoma group of the European Organization of Research of Cancer. Cancer Treat Rep 70:615–618, 1986.
180. Walker RW, Allen JC, Rosen G, Caparros B: Transient cerebral dysfunction secondary to high-dose methotrexate. J Clin Oncol 4:1845–1850, 1986.
181. Weddington WW, Segraves KB, Simon MA: Psychological outcome of extremity sarcoma survivors undergoing amputation or limb salvage. J Clin Oncol 3:1393–1400, 1985.
182. Whang-Peng J, Triche TJ, Knutsen T, Miser J, Kao-Shan S, Tsai S, Israel MA: Chromosome translocation in peripheral neuroepithelioma. N Engl J Med 311:584–585, 1984.
183. Whang-Peng J, Triche TJ, Knutsen T, Miser J, Kao-Shan S, Tsai S, Israel MA: Chromosome characterization of selected, small round cell tumors of childhood. Cancer Genet Cytogenet 21:185–208, 1986.
184. Wilkins RM, Pritchard DG, Burgert EO, Unni KK: Ewing's sarcoma of bone. Experience with 140 patients. Cancer 58:2551–2555, 1986.
185. Winkler K, Beron G, Kotz R, Salzer-Kuntschik M, Beck J, Beck W, Brandeis W, Ebell W, Erttman R, Gobel U, Havers W, Henze G, Hinderfeld L, Hocker P, Jobke A, Jurgens H, Kabisch H, Preusser P, Prindull G, Ramach W, Ritter J, Sekera J, Treuner J, Wust G, Landbeck G: Neoadjuvant chemotherapy

for osteogenic sarcoma: Results of a cooperative German/Austrian study. J Clin Oncol 2:617–624, 1984.

186. Winkler K, Beron G, Kotz R, Salzer-Kuntschik M: Adjuvant and neoadjuvant chemotherapy of osteosarcoma: Experience of the German-Austrian Cooperative Osteosarcoma studies (COSS). *In* van Osstrom AT, van Unnik JA (eds): Management of Soft Tissue and Bone Sarcoma. New York, Raven Press, 1986, pp 275–288.

187. Winkler K, Beron G, Delling G, Heise U, Kabisch H, Purfurst C, Berger J, Ritter J, Jurgens H, Gerein V, Graf N, Russe W, Gruemayer ER, Ertelt W, Kotz R, Preusser P, Prindull G, Brandeis W, Landbeck G: Neoadjuvant chemotherapy of osteosarcoma. J Clin Oncol 6:329–337, 1988.

188. Winkler K, Torggler S, Beron G, Bode U, Gerein V, Jurgens H, Kusnierz-Glaz C, Kotz R, Salzer-Kuntschik M, Schmoll HJ, et al: Results of treatment in primary disseminated osteosarcoma. Analysis of the follow-up of patients in the cooperative osteosarcoma studies COSS-80 and COSS-82 (abstract). Onckologie 12(2):92–96, 1989.

189. Wold LE, Unni KK, Beabout JW, Sim FH, Dahlin DC: Dediffentiated parosteal osteosarcoma. J Bone Joint Surg 66A:53–59, 1984.

190. Yoshikawa H, Takaoka K, Hamada H, Ono K: Clinical significance of bone morphogenetic activity in osteosarcoma. A study of 20 cases. Cancer 56:1682–1687, 1985.

191. Zaharia M, Caceres E, Valdivia S, Moran M, Tejda F: Postoperative whole lung irradiation with or without Adriamycin in osteogenic sarcoma. Int J Radiat Oncol Biol Phys 12:907–910, 1986.

192. Zucker JM, Henry-Amar M, Sarrazin D, Blache R, Patte C, Schweisguth O: Intensive systemic chemotherapy in localized Ewing's sarcoma in childhood: A historical trial. Cancer 52:415–423, 1983.

CHAPTER 6

Adult Oncology

CHARLES FORSCHER
DIANA WILLIAMSON
RONALD H. BLUM
JAMES F. HOLLAND

Primary malignant tumors involving the bones and the soft tissues, despite their relative rarity, have served as models in the development of interdisciplinary approaches to the management of human cancer. Cooperative efforts among medical, orthopedic, and radiation oncologists have altered the previously grim prognoses for many patients, and techniques such as limb preservation and the use of preoperative chemotherapy for these rare cancers have also proved useful in many other oncologic settings. This chapter discusses the medical management of both primary bone and soft tissue sarcomas and metastatic disease to bone.

Bone Sarcomas

OSTEOSARCOMA

Osteosarcoma is a malignant connective tissue tumor characterized by the production of bone or osteoid (see Chapter 5). Approximately 30% of osteosarcomas occur in patients outside the pediatric age group. Although it is sometimes stated that osteosarcoma has a bimodal age distribution (one large peak in the second decade and a second smaller one in the sixth decade), in a Mayo Clinic series, there was a small but consistent percentage of cases after the age of 35 years[1]; this ranges from 2 to 6% of the total number of cases per decade. In younger patients, these sarcomas most frequently occur *de novo*. Although *de novo* occurrence also predominates in the adult age group, osteosarcoma arising secondary to Paget's disease[2, 3] or to prior radiation therapy may compose between 20 and 56% of cases in some series.[4] Osteosarcoma in adults also tends to involve locations more frequently associated with a poorer prognosis such as the pelvis, the axial skeleton, and extraosseous sites.[4, 5] Osteosarcoma of the jaw is also more common in the adult population.[6]

Sarcoma arising in association with Paget's disease often occurs in patients with extensive polyostotic disease of long standing. The exact incidence of sarcomatous degeneration is probably in the range of 1% of all cases, but the risk may be as high as 27% in advanced cases. Most series have reported poor survival. Mirra reported seven cases, all terminating fatally within six months of diagnosis.[7] Huvos reported three long-term survivors among 65 patients with Paget's sarcoma at Memorial Sloan-Kettering Cancer Center.[2] Several possible reasons for the poor outcome include multicentricity at diagnosis, metastases at diagnosis, and the presence of disease at unresectable sites.

Radiation-induced osteosarcoma usually occurs in the irradiation field in patients successfully treated for other cancers. In some patients, the sarcomas may actually arise adjacent to the portal, suggesting that, although a high dose of radiation may be curative, the lower dose of radiation present as scatter at the edge of a portal may have a higher sarcomagenic potential. The average interval before the development of a sarcoma was 15 years in the Mayo Clinic series, with a range of 2.75 to 55 years.[8] The dose of radiation was variable, but few cases have been described with radiation exposures less than 20 Gy. Osteosarcoma arising after successful combined modality treatment for other bone sarcomas, particularly Ewing's sarcoma, has also been noted.[9] Treatment of radiation-induced sarcoma has usually been surgical, with locally recurrent disease being a major problem, as these tumors often involve the sternum, the chest wall, or the thoracic vertebrae (the sites of prior radiation). Little information on the chemosensitivity of these tumors is available, but the Memorial Sloan-Kettering Cancer Center series did not show a survival benefit with the use of high-dose methotrexate in comparison with historical controls treated with surgery alone.[9] The authors have seen responses in osteosarcoma arising in regions irradiated for retinoblastoma and agree with Rosen that attempts to employ aggressive primary chemotherapy for these patients should continue.[56]

Osteosarcoma of the jaw is a distinct clinicopathologic entity seen almost exclusively in the adult population. It is distinct from osteosarcoma at other sites because radical surgery alone can be associated with an 80% disease-free survival. Less than radical surgery is associated with poorer survival. In addition, patients who experience treatment failure tend to die from uncontrolled local disease rather than from metastatic disease (as is true for classic osteosarcoma). Chemotherapy has generally been applied for recurrent or locally unresectable disease and is therefore difficult to evaluate.

Little formal information is available on the treatment of adults with osteosarcoma. It is not uncommon for trials to exclude those with radiation-induced sarcoma, patients with Paget's sarcoma, or those beyond the pediatric age group. Some series are purely descriptive[10] and provide neither the type of treatment employed nor the results obtained. Other series that include adult patients do not provide response criteria by age and have median ages in the adolescent age range. However, from the relatively small pool of data, it is possible to draw several conclusions. In those adult patients with *de novo* osteosarcoma who can tolerate treatment with aggressive chemotherapeutic regimens involving agents such as high-dose methotrexate (8 to 12 g/m^2), doxorubicin (Adriamycin), cisplatin, and a combination of bleomycin, cyclophosphamide, and actinomycin D (dactinomycin) (BCD), results closely paralleling those achieved in children can be obtained. In one study, a 44% disease-free survival with a median of 1 year has been observed using preoperative chemotherapy for patients treated between ages 19 and 60 years (Holland JF, Forscher C, personal communication). The Mount Sinai Medical Center regimen includes the first three agents initially and utilizes the BCD combination only at recurrence. Complete responses to preoperative chemotherapy can be observed in adult patients with the same favorable implications for long-term survival as in the pediatric age group. Other investigators reported similar results. Siegel and colleagues reported a superior continuous disease-free survival for a small number of adult patients with osteosarcomas treated with adjuvant chemotherapy of varying composition compared with that achieved with surgery only.[11]

Treatment of radiation-induced sarcoma, Paget's sarcoma, and sarcoma arising in elderly patients unable to receive aggressive regimens because of poor performance status or impaired renal or cardiac function remains unsatisfactory, and new approaches are needed. Although some authors have questioned whether the prognosis for osteosarcoma has improved for those older than 25 years,[12] one must determine how many of these patients received effective modern chemotherapy. As has been learned through painful experience in children, the natural history of osteosarcoma has not changed over time and the impact of chemotherapy in this disease for both children and adults is undeniable.

The same principles of aggressive surgery for pulmonary metastatic disease commonly used in children also apply to adult patients.[13] Indeed, some older patients may tolerate thoracotomy with less difficulty than certain forms of chemotherapy, and long-term disease-free survival is possible in a small but definite cohort of these patients. Chemotherapy-treated patients have fewer pulmonary nodules at recurrence than their untreated counterparts.[14] In addition, patients treated with chemotherapy appear to be at higher risk for unusual, extrapulmonary sites of recurrence, suggesting that chemotherapy has an impact on the natural history of osteosarcoma. Persons with recurrent or unresectable disease should be considered candidates for newer agents such as ifosfamide or investigational regimens.

CHONDROSARCOMA

Chondrosarcomas are malignant tumors that produce cartilage. In most series, chondrosarcoma ranks second to osteosarcoma as the most common bone tumor.[15] The incidence increases with age, with a peak in the sixth decade. Primary chondrosarcomas, which occur in normal bone, outnumber secondary chondrosarcomas, which occur in preexisting lesions such as osteochondromas, by 4:1. The pelvis, the femur, and the humerus are the most common sites. Treatment is usually surgical, as these tumors are generally considered to be resistant to both radiation and chemotherapy. Repeated local recurrence is frequently a problem in managing chondrosarcomas, and an increasingly anaplastic histologic pattern is often noted in the recurrences.[16, 17] The metastatic rate of moderate-grade lesions is 15 to 40%, and in high-grade chondrosarcomas, it is 75%.[18]

One uncommon variant, mesenchymal chondrosarcoma, characterized by the presence of small spindle cells intermixed in chondroid tissue, may be sensitive to combination chemotherapy regimens similar to those designed for childhood Ewing's disease.[19]

Clear cell chondrosarcomas are the rarest form. They are slow-growing, locally recurrent tumors occurring in adults. They tend to metastasize after several local recurrences. The treatment is surgery with a wide excision. Systemic chemotherapy plays no role.

MALIGNANT FIBROUS HISTIOCYTOMA OF BONE

It has been recognized that malignant fibrous histiocytoma, a tumor more usually associated with a presentation in the soft tissues, may occur as a primary bone lesion. Unlike osteosarcoma, it is more common in adults than in children. Although it bears some similarities to osteosarcoma, it differs in several key ways. Virtually all cases exhibit lytic bone lesions. Serum alkaline phosphatase level is invariably normal, and malignant osteoid, by definition, is absent. Despite these differences, several reports have documented the chemosensitivity of this tumor using both adjuvant and preoperative regimens similar to those used for osteosarcoma.[20–24]

Other Tumors

MYELOMA

Multiple myeloma, a plasma cell neoplasm of hematopoietic origin, is the most common primary malignant tumor of bone.[25] Approximately 11,800 new cases are seen each year, with 8900 deaths attributable to the disease annually. A full discussion of all aspects of myeloma is beyond the scope of this chapter; however, certain critical points are discussed.

Myeloma usually occurs in multiple bone sites. The most common appearance in bone is either as a lytic lesion or as an area of osteoporosis. Skeletal survey is more accurate in assessing the extent of bone involvement than is bone scintigraphy. Skeletal examination also helps differentiate myeloma from a related entity, monoclonal gammopathy of uncertain significance, as the latter is not associated with lytic bone disease.

In addition to radiography, complete blood count determination, serum electrophoresis, quantitative immunoglobulin determination to identify the M component, bone marrow examination, and evaluation of renal function and urinary excretion of Bence Jones protein are used in determining the stage of disease. Newer measures such as labeling index and serum β_2-microglobulin levels may have prognostic utility as well.[26, 27] The presence of lytic bone disease automatically places lesions in the most advanced stage in the Salmon-Durie system (stage III).[28]

Treatment with chemotherapy is usually indicated for patients with advanced disease. Combinations of alklyating agents and steroids, such as melphalan and prednisone[29] or the Memorial Sloan-Kettering Cancer Center M-2 regimen of multiple alkylators with vincristine and prednisone,[30] are most commonly used. Responses usually occur in approximately 50% of patients, and treatment is continued until the maximal response occurs. A plateau phase uninfluenced by further chemotherapy ensues, which is then followed by the reappearance of disease that is increasingly resistant to therapy. Reports of the use of a doxorubicin-based salvage regimen (infusional vincristine, doxorubicin, and dexamethasone [VAD]) provide a basis for some limited optimism.[31] In addition, several groups described significant prolongation of the plateau phase of the disease with the use of recombinant interferon-α either alone or in combination with chemotherapy.[32, 33] There have also been reports of the ability of calcium channel blockers such as verapamil to reverse drug resistance in myeloma.[34] In younger patients who have shown significant responses to chemotherapy, highly aggressive approaches, including bone marrow transplantation, may be considered.[35, 36]

Although these new developments hold promise, for most patients the median survival time with standard treatments is approximately 40 months, and myeloma remains an incurable disease. Judicious use of radiation therapy both for symptomatic pain relief and for stabilization of weight-bearing bones can play a useful palliative role in this disease.

Rarely, myeloma occurs as a solitary focus in bone without other associated findings. With time, progression to frank myeloma invariably ensues, usually within the first few years after diagnosis. This is a more common presentation in younger patients. Treatment is often initially radiotherapy, with chemotherapy employed for recurrence or dissemination. In comparison with that in disseminated disease, overall survival is prolonged, often approaching 10 years. In addition, some younger patients do not manifest progressive disease.[37, 38]

PRIMARY LYMPHOMA OF BONE

Approximately 5% of extranodal non-Hodgkin's lymphomas occur initially at bone sites. This appears to be a distinct clinical entity, which was previously called reticulum cell sarcoma of bone. They are defined as lymphomatous infiltrates within bone with or without cortical invasion or extension into contiguous soft tissue, but without concurrent involvement of regional lymph nodes or distant viscera within 6 months of diagnosis.[39] During work-up, patients thought to have primary lymphoma are often found to have extensive extraosseous disease. A retrospective review from the National Cancer Institute (NCI) emphasized this point; of 14 cases initially believed to be limited disease (stage IE or IIE), 12 (86%) demonstrated extensive disease after full evaluation.[40]

Diffuse large cell lymphoma is the pathologic subtype reported most frequently in most series,[41] but virtually any category of lymphoma may be seen. In addition, any bone may be involved by this process.

Work-up should include plain radiography and computed tomography (CT) or magnetic resonance imaging (MRI) of the involved sites. In addition, a complete blood count, Coombs test, serum protein electrophoresis, bone marrow examination, and bone and gallium scans are recommended. Additional noninvasive staging by chest and abdominal CT is also helpful in determining the true extent of disease, and lymphangiography may occasionally be necessary. Laparotomy for full staging should be considered if chemotherapy is not included in the initial management. Lastly, lumbar puncture has been advocated for lymphomas that involve bone sites in the head and neck region because of a high risk of central nervous system involvement.

Results of treatment depend on the extent of disease at presentation. Truly isolated bone lymphoma may be treated with radiation therapy alone, particularly if it occurs in a distal location. However, earlier series that utilized radiation alone often reported early dissemination and death. Dolan's series noted an 87% mortality rate.[42] This extremely poor result was most likely caused by incomplete staging. More recent series utilizing combined modality approaches have fared far better. In the Instituto Ortopedico Rizzoli experience, an 88% disease-free survival was observed with a median follow-up of 86 months.[43] This was superior to results with radiation alone in a smaller group of patients at the same institution. Mayo Clinic researchers reported a large series spanning 7 decades with 5-year disease-free survival rates of 58% for bone-only disease, 22% for bone and soft tissue and/or nodal disease, and 42% for multifocal osseous disease.

Chemotherapy is usually based on doxorubicin-containing regimens such as cyclophosphamide, doxorubicin, vincristine, and prednisone (CHOP) or bleomycin, doxorubicin, cyclophosphamide, vincristine, and prednisone (BACOP), although the regimen used in the NCI series, cyclophosphamide, vincristine, procarbazine, and prednisone (C-MOPP), does not incorporate doxorubicin. At Mount Sinai Medical Center, the authors currently employ the CHOP regimen, usually in combination with radiation therapy.

Although most lymphomas are not generally thought of as surgically treatable diseases, judicious use of surgery can be necessary for bone lymphoma (for example, when lymphoma causes a pathologic fracture in a weight-bearing limb).

Bone involvement may also frequently be

seen in the recently described leukemia-lymphoma syndrome attributed to human T cell lymphoma virus 1 (HTLV-1).[44] In these cases, lytic bone involvement is often present at multiple sites, along with a distinctive pattern of fever, hypercalcemia, leukocytosis, and malignant cells exhibiting a cloverleaf nucleus. This entity is to be distinguished from the aforementioned lymphomas, as treatment responses are often brief, despite aggressive therapy.

Bone involvement can also occur in the natural history of lymphomas that do not initially occur in bone. Management by either radiation or chemotherapy depends on the overall extent of disease.

CHORDOMA

Chordoma is a rare neoplasm that is seldom suspected. It arises from notochordal remnants in the midline of the neural axis and involves the adjacent bone. The most common site is at the ends of the spine; its onset here is completely free from symptoms. Early detection is practically impossible, and when the lesion is discovered, it is already large. Of all chordomas, 50% occur at the sacrococcygeal junction, and 35%, at the skull base. Chordomas are very often fatal because of their high rate of local recurrence and complications. Local disease is the most common cause of death.[45] Gray and associates reviewed 222 cases from the literature and found only two patients who were disease free at 10 years. The average survival for the group was 5.7 years.[46]

Patients with sacrococcygeal chordomas represent a special subset. Dull pain is the most common compliant. Constipation, loss of bladder control, and sensory losses are late complications. CT scan is necessary for accurate diagnosis. Localio and coworkers reported a series of patients whose chordomas were resected via the abdominosacral approach.[47]

The best chance of cure is with the first surgical procedure, because if there is local recurrence, there is little chance of control with additional surgical procedures. Radiation therapy is an integral treatment modality because local recurrence is so common.[48] Chemotherapy has no proven role for this local-regional disease.

Metastases

METASTATIC BONE CARCINOMA

Metastatic bone tumors far outnumber the primary malignant bone tumors. In approximately 90% of cases, metastases are present at multiple bone sites, with or without evidence of other organ involvement.[49, 50] A solitary bone metastasis should raise the possibility of a focus in the thyroid gland or the kidney. Presentation in the axial skeleton and long bones predominates, with disease being seen only rarely at distal bone sites. The spine is the most frequent site. The most common carcinomas to involve bone arise from primary lesions in the breast, the prostate, the lung, the thyroid, the kidney, and the stomach. Malignant melanoma may also spread to bone; indeed, virtually any cancer may involve bone. Often, there is a clear history of an antecedent tumor, but in some cases, metastatic presentation in bone may actually precede identification of the primary neoplasm, and rarely, no definite primary neoplasm can be found. Most skeletal metastases are either osteolytic or display a mixed osteolytic-osteoblastic pattern. Purely osteoblastic lesions are characteristic of prostate cancer, Hodgkin's disease, and carcinoid tumor.

Assessing response to therapy in skeletal metastases is more difficult than at other sites with current tools.[51–54] Indeed, some protocols specifically exclude patients whose only site of metastatic disease is osseous. Neoplastic tissue may be completely killed by chemotherapy without significant alteration in the appearance of bone films. Bone healing or recalcification, when evident, can be a slow process, lagging far behind the antitumor response. MRI may give a more accurate picture of the degree of viability at a particular metastatic site, but it is not yet routinely applied for this purpose and is inefficient for evaluating multiple sites of disease. Healing bone may actually intensify the appearance of carcinoma on bone scan, making scanning of limited use in assessing treatment response, especially in the absence of progressive symptoms.[55] Even the appearance of new areas of uptake may represent inapparent osteolytic lesions that have begun to heal, rather than the evidence of new metastatic disease.

Thus, the usual criteria of response to chemotherapy, such as complete response, partial response, improvement, stable disease, and progression, are more difficult to employ for metastatic disease to bone. The approach to osteosarcoma, which was described by Rosen and colleagues,[56] of actual histologic evaluation of response in resected specimens could potentially be used for metastatic sites when resection is feasible.

SPECIFIC METASTATIC TUMORS

Breast Carcinoma

The incidence of skeletal metastases in breast carcinoma varies from 50 to 85%.[57, 58] A subset of patients have disease limited to bone. Several series documented a more favorable outcome in this group, with a median survival time of 48 months and a 5-year survival rate of 37%.[59] In contrast, breast carcinoma metastatic to nonosseous sites is usually associated with 5-year survival in the 10% range and a median survival time of less than 2 years. The majority of these patients with bone-only disease are postmenopausal and have tumors positive for estrogen/progesterone receptors. Thus, these patients are often candidates for initial treatment by hormonal manipulation.[60, 63]

Available agents include the antiestrogen tamoxifen[62] and progestins such as megestrol acetate (Megace).[63] Promising work with the gonadotropin-releasing hormone agonists such as goserelin and leuprolide is in progress.[64, 65] Aminoglutethimide, which induces a chemical adrenalectomy, has also been used for palliation.[66] Response rates for initial hormonal intervention in the 45 to 60% range may be observed, and initial response to hormonal therapy tends to predict for subsequent benefit from later endocrine manipulations. Premenopausal patients were previously offered oophorectomy as initial hormonal treatment, but emerging data suggest that tamoxifen may be equally effective. Response to hormonal treatment may be slow, necessitating a minimum of 6 to 12 weeks to assess response. One may also observe treatment responses at the discontinuation of a given hormonal regimen, making it advisable to wait a period of weeks before instituting an alternative therapy.

Breast carcinoma also responds to a variety of chemotherapeutic agents given either individually or in combination.[67] Cyclophosphamide, methotrexate, 5-fluorouracil, vincristine, doxorubicin, and mitomycin C are all active as single agents. Combinations of these agents—such as cyclophosphamide, methotrexate, and 5-fluorouracil (CMF)[68]; cyclophosphamide, methotrexate, 5-fluorouracil, vincristine, and prednisone (CMFVP)[69]; and cyclophosphamide, doxorubicin, and 5-fluorouracil (CAF)[70]—have been associated with response rates in the 50% range. Intensive use of doxorubicin in escalating doses as a single agent has been reported to have an overall response rate of 85%, with 38% of the responses complete, although tumors in soft tissue sites responded more frequently than those in bone.[71] Response to salvage chemotherapy after disease progression is usually poor and of brief duration. Combinations of chemotherapeutic and hormonal agents have also been reported to be active.[72]

Prostate Carcinoma

Bone metastases occur in more than 90% of patients with advanced prostate cancer.[73] The pelvis is the most frequently involved bone site. Laboratory studies that suggest distant spread include increased serum prostatic acid phosphatase and prostatic specific antigen levels. As for metastatic carcinoma at other sites, pain is the most common presenting symptom.

Therapy is usually initiated with hormonal manipulation.[74] Available approaches include orchiectomy, administration of synthetic hormones such as diethylstilbestrol (usual dosage 1 to 3 mg/day), and the use of gonadotropin-releasing hormone analogues such as leuprolide. The combination of leuprolide and the antiandrogen flutamide has been reported to yield results superior to those with previous forms of hormonal therapy, with higher response rates and modest prolongation in the time to tumor progression and in survival time.[75]

Unlike the situation with breast cancer, progression after initial response to hormone treatment in prostate cancer is usually refractory to subsequent attempts at further hormonal manipulation. This has led to the use of chemotherapy in this setting. Initial studies by the National Prostatic Cancer Group established the superiority of single agents such as 5-fluorouracil and cyclophosphamide over standard therapy (which included alternative hormonal treatments and palliative radiation) in achieving symptomatic relief and in delaying tumor progression.[76] Later trials showed activity for additional agents such as dacarbazine, doxorubicin, hydroxyurea, cisplatin, and CCNU (lomustine). Combinations of these agents have also been employed with modest results. Both single-agent and combination chemotherapy studies have generally reported objective responses in the range of 20%.[77]

The survival benefit with any of these interventions in the setting of advanced disease is marginal at best, yet patients may derive significant palliation from the judicious use of chemotherapy, often in combination with radiation therapy. Those whose serum markers, such as the acid phosphatase level, fall to normal appear to enjoy the greatest benefit. However, with 5-year survival only in the range of 10%, better approaches to the management of advanced prostate cancer are clearly needed. Recent reports that suramin, an antiparasitic drug that blocks the action of several growth factors, is effective in refractory prostate cancer suggest one possible future direction.[78]

Lung Carcinoma

Bone metastases occur in approximately 20 to 40% of patients with lung cancer.[79] In the setting of small cell lung carcinoma, chemotherapy with combinations such as etoposide (VP-16) and cisplatin[80] or cyclophosphamide, doxorubicin, and vincristine have been used.[81] Although overall response rates can be in the 60 to 85% range, relapses may be seen, median survival is less than 1 year, and 5-year survival for extensive small cell lung carcinoma is in the 1% range. The situation is no better for non–small cell lung carcinoma. Unlike with breast carcinoma, there appears to be no favorable prognostic implication for bone involvement in lung carcinoma.

Renal Carcinoma

Metastatic renal cell cancer can involve bone in approximately 25 to 35% of cases.[73] These tumors can often be solitary and, if so, may be amenable to surgical excision.[82] No effective chemotherapy currently exists for diffuse bone disease. Although response rates between 15 and 35% have been reported for interleukin 2 (with or without lymphokine-activated killer cells) in advanced renal cancer, responses in bone sites were either rare or not observed.[83]

Thyroid Carcinoma

Skeletal metastases can occur in 12 to 50% of patients with metastatic thyroid cancer.[73, 84] Treatment depends on the histologic subtype. For follicular thyroid cancer and for certain well-differentiated papillary thyroid cancers, treatment with radioactive iodine is employed.[85] This should be done after it is determined that the metastases take up radioactive iodine. In addition, normal thyroid function must first be ablated. The 5-year survival may range as high as 50%.

Refractory disease and disease with unfavorable histologic findings such as anaplastic thyroid cancer may be treated with chemotherapy. Doxorubicin is the most active single agent, with a response rate of 35%.[86] Other agents with activity include bleomycin, vincristine, melphalan, and cisplatin.[87, 88] Combinations of doxorubicin and cisplatin also appear to be active.[89] Most responses are partial, but some complete responses with long-term survival have been reported.

Melanoma

Although the incidence of bone involvement is low, the detection of a bone lesion, particularly at presentation, is associated with a poor prognosis.[90]

Colorectal Carcinoma

Skeletal metastases occur in only 4% of patients. These are usually seen late in the course of disease.[91] The most common palliation is radiation therapy.

Soft Tissue Sarcomas

Approximately 5700 soft tissue sarcomas are diagnosed annually in the United States, with an estimated overall mortality rate approaching 55%.[92] Almost half of these sarcomas arise in the extremities, more commonly in the lower extremities than in the upper limbs. The usual presentation is as a palpable often painless mass. Pain, if present, is the result of impingement on adjacent structures, such as nerve or bone. Any mass that causes pain, rapidly increases in size, or reaches a diameter of 5 cm or greater should be brought to the attention of trained orthopedic and medical personnel.

Most soft tissue sarcomas arise without clear antecedent risk factors, but several predisposing factors have been identified. As with the bone sarcomas, prior exposure to radiation has been linked to soft tissue sarcomas.[93] A variety of chemical exposures have been implicated as risk factors, particularly chlorophenol and phenoxyacetic acid preparations.[94, 95] The former are constitutents of wood preservatives; the latter are components of herbicides such as Agent Orange. These agents have been implicated on the basis of somewhat conflicting epidemiologic reports.[96, 97] For example, a case-control study conducted by Kang and associates found no increased risk of soft tissue sarcomas among Vietnam War veterans compared with veterans of the same era who had not served in Vietnam. However, in veterans who did serve in Vietnam and were estimated to have greater opportunities for Agent Orange exposure, a statistically nonsignificant increased risk could be identified.[98]

Often, a previous history of trauma can be elicited, but the exact significance of this finding is not clear. Rarely, sarcomas have been reported to arise in association with foreign body material.[99] The role of infectious agents, particularly viruses, and the interaction between infection and host immunity may play an etiologic role, as exemplified by the occurrence of Kaposi's sarcoma in the acquired immunodeficiency syndrome (AIDS).[100] Immune suppression or altered immune surveillance may also be a factor in the development of lymphangiosarcomas seen in the setting of chronic lymphedema after mastectomy (the Stewart-Treves syndrome).[101]

Genetic abnormalities are being increasingly identified in association with the soft tissue sarcomas. Neurofibromatosis, a disorder with autosomal dominant inheritance, is a well-recognized risk factor for the development of malignant neurosarcomas.[102–104] The risk increases with patient age and with the extent and severity of the disease. Sarcomas have also been reported in association with Gardner's syndrome.[105] For other sarcomas, specific chromosomal abnormalities have been identified. These include the x:18 translocation in synovial sarcoma,[106] the 2:13 translocation in alveolar rhabdomyosarcoma,[107] and the 12:16 translocation in myxoid liposarcoma.[108] Genetic distinctions may have therapeutic implications in the future.

Preoperative evaluation should include plain radiographs, CT or MRI scans of the affected area, and a CT scan of the chest to rule out metastatic disease. Bone scanning may be performed if there is a question of local bone involvement, but abnormal bone scans may reflect a reactive process rather than true bone invasion. Angiography may be necessary to assess the relationship of the tumor to vascular structures. The incisional biopsy should be performed by the surgeon who will undertake the definitive resection, so as not to compromise the potential for limb-sparing surgery.

A variety of prognostic factors have been identified for the soft tissue sarcomas. By far the most important is the pathologic grade of the tumor. The histologic grading system of the American Joint Committee on Cancer (AJCC) is subjective but is based on the quantitative criteria of the mitotic rate, the nuclear morphologic appearance, the degree of cellularity, nuclear pleomorphism, and the presence of necrosis.[111, 113] Costa and colleagues proposed a different classification system, with overall prognosis based on features of histologic type, number of mitoses, degree of necrosis, pleomorphism, and cellularity.[112] In a multivariate analysis, tumor necrosis was the single histopathologic variable that best predicted both time to recurrence and overall survival. Therefore, a grading system was proposed using the degree of necrosis to distinguish between aggressive tumors and less aggressive tumors. High-grade tumors were differentiated by the extent of necrosis. Tumors with no or minimal necrosis were grade 2, whereas those with moderate to marked necrosis were grade 3.[112] Coindre and associates used a similar approach and were able to confirm that necrosis was the most important prognostic variable,[109] but unfortunately, there was only a 64% concordance rate with that previously reported by Costa. Lindberg et al compared the NCI and AJCC histopathologic grading systems and found that there were differences that could account for variations in outcome.[171]

Low-grade tumors have both a decreased risk of local recurrence and a diminished risk of metastatic spread when compared with their intermediate-grade and high-grade counterparts. A 5-year survival in the 75% range is common with the low-grade sarcomas, dropping to 56% for the intermediate-grade sarcomas, and falling to 26% for the high-grade tumors.[113] Sarcomas with metastases at presentation fare poorly, with less than 5% 5-year survival.

The other factor considered important for prognosis is staging. There are many staging systems for soft tissue sarcomas. Perhaps the most widely accepted is the AJCC system outlined in the manual of 1987.[111] In this revision, histologic grade was the main determinant of stage. Grade 1, or low grade of malignancy, is stage I: grade 2, or moderate histologic grade of malignancy, is stage II; and grade 3, or high histologic grade of malignancy, is stage III. Within the staging system, A designates tumors less than 5 cm, and B, tumors more than 5 cm in diameter. Patients with stage IVA disease have involvement of regional nodes, and patients with stage IVB disease have clinically diagnosed distant metastases. For extremity sarcomas, grade and stage correlated with 5-year local disease control, disease-free survival, and overall survival.

Enneking and associates proposed an alternative system for staging sarcomas of bone or soft tissue, particularly of the extremity.[114] Stage I was defined as low-grade histologic appearance and no metastases, and stage II, as high-grade histologic appearance without metastases. Stage III refers to regional and/or distant metastases. Within stages I and II, differentiation between A and B was based on whether the disease was intracompartmental or extracompartmental, respectively. Staging systems for other anatomic locations, such as the trunk, the retroperitoneum, and the head and neck, were less well defined. There was also significant correlation between size and actuarial control rates of distant disease and 5-year survival. Although acceptance of specific staging systems is not generally standardized, there is agreement that histopathologic grade of the tumor is as important as the more conventional criteria of tumor size, anatomic extent of disease, the presence or absence of regional or distant metastatic disease, and to a lesser extent, the presence of disease in regional lymph nodes.

The type of surgery performed can also have prognostic importance, with marginal or intralesional excisions associated with a greater risk of recurrence.[115]

Despite the large number of different histologic subtypes of soft tissue sarcoma, they tend to behave in generally similar fashions, and treatment approaches are generally determined by stage. Exceptions to this rule include tumors such as rhabdomyosarcoma and synovial sarcoma, which are high-grade tumors by definition. In general, liposarcomas may behave in a somewhat less aggressive fashion; however, certain liposarcomas, particularly the round cell variant of liposarcoma, are highly aggressive tumors with 5-year survival rates of 20%.[116] Alveolar soft tissue sarcomas tend to behave less aggressively than other sarcomas. A 5-year survival of 60% has been reported, even in the presence of metastatic disease. Certain vascular tumors such as hemangiopericytoma may also have protracted courses, with 10-year and even 20-year survival in the face of metastatic disease.[117]

Local recurrence and hematogenous dissemination, usually to lung or bone, are the major concerns in the management of most patients with sarcoma. Involvement of regional lymph nodes is less common but can be seen with more than 20% of rhabdomyosarcomas and synovial sarcomas. Local growth is usually defined by a pseudocapsule composed of the compressed normal surrounding tissues, but extensive growth along fascial planes can be seen with synovial sarcomas or epithelioid sarcomas.

CHEMOTHERAPY FOR SOFT TISSUE SARCOMAS

Although adjuvant chemotherapy is now accepted practice for osteosarcoma, its use for soft tissue sarcomas is controversial. Single-agent and combination chemotherapy for the soft tissue sarcomas both for metastatic disease and in the adjuvant setting are discussed below.

The most active single drug for treating the soft tissue sarcomas has been doxorubicin. Overall response rates from 13 to 34% have been reported, with a complete response rate of 6%.[118–120] A dose-response relationship exists, with higher responses at dosages of 75 mg/m^2 than at 50 mg/m^2 given every 3 weeks.[121] The major dose-limiting toxicity of doxorubicin is cardiomyopathy, with a 30% incidence at cumulative doses in excess of 550 mg/m^2.[122–124] This toxicity may be lessened by continuous infusion administration without a demonstrable loss of efficacy while delivering cumulative doses of doxorubicin of up to 1 g/m^2.[125, 126] Previously, cardiomyopathy after doxorubicin exposure was thought to be irreversible and poorly responsive to medical treatment; however, there have been several reports of improvement in cardiac function.[127, 128] The use of cardioprotective agents such as ICRF-187, a free radical scavenger, is also under active investigation in an effort to determine methods of limiting cardiotoxicity while maintaining drug efficacy.[129] Analogues of doxorubicin with less potential for cardiotoxicity are also being studied; one analogue, epirubicin, appears to be as active as the parent compound in European trials.[130, 131]

Ifosfamide, a cyclophosphamide analogue, is also clearly active in the sarcomas.[132] In European studies, it was more active than cyclophosphamide with less myelosuppression.[133] Given at dosages of 5 to 12.5 g/m^2 usually in divided doses during 1 to 5 days, it has yielded responses in the range of 15 to 38% in patients who had progressed while on previous therapy.[134–136] It can be given either as a short bolus or as a continuous infusion for 24 hours. It is one of the few agents capable of producing complete responses in patients previously exposed to doxorubicin. The major toxicity of ifosfamide is hemorrhagic cystitis caused by the production of acrolein. Mesna (sodium 2-mercaptoethanesulfonate) must be administered with ifosfamide to prevent this complication. When given as a continuous infusion, ifosfamide and mesna may be combined in the same infusion at a 1:1 ratio. Other toxicities encountered with ifosfamide include lethargy, confusion, azotemia, and renal tubular dysfunction.[137] These toxicities usually resolve on discontinuation of treatment. Given the current complexities of ifosfamide administration, it has generally been limited to impatient use.

Dacarbazine (DTIC) has a response rate of 17% as a single agent.[138] It is usually given at a dose of 1 g/m^2 divided over 4 to 5 days. Emesis, often severe, is the dose-limiting toxicity. Emesis may be diminished when DTIC is given as a continuous infusion.

Cyclophosphamide,[139, 140] cisplatin,[141–143] mitomycin, vincristine,[145] actinomycin D,[146] bleomycin,[147] etoposide,[148] and methotrexate[149–151] have been employed as single agents for the soft tissue sarcomas, with response rates generally in the 10 to 15% range.

Biologic agents such as interferon[152] and interleukin 2[153] have so far shown little activity as single agents in the soft tissue sarcomas.

Combination chemotherapy, which has been clearly superior to single-agent treatment of most malignancies, has been more difficult to evaluate in the sarcomas. Trials comparing doxorubicin and DTIC with doxorubicin alone have usually shown a higher response rate with the combination but no effect on overall survival and have shown greater toxicity with the combination.[154, 155] The combination of cyclophosphamide, vincristine, doxorubicin, and DTIC (CyVADIC) was initially reported to produce a 50% response rate.[156]

However, studies evaluating the addition of either vincristine or cyclophosphamide alone to the doxorubicin-DTIC combination have shown no advantage with the three-drug regimens.[157, 158] In addition, a study comparing doxorubicin alone; doxorubicin, cyclophosphamide, and vincristine; and cyclophosphamide, vincristine, and actinomycin D concluded that doxorubicin alone was the most active and the least toxic.[159]

Ifosfamide is now being incorporated into regimens with doxorubicin (and sometimes DTIC) for the treatment of the advanced sarcomas.[160–162] As with the earlier experience with CyVADIC, initial reports produced high response rates, often in the 50% range. No firm data are yet available on comparisons between ifosfamide and doxorubicin–based combinations and doxorubicin alone. However, preliminary data from the European Organization for Research and Treatment of Cancer (EORTC), which has undertaken a randomized trial comparing doxorubicin, ifosfamide and doxorubicin, and cyclophosphamide, vincristine, doxorubicin, and DTIC, has so far produced similar response rates of 24%, 27%, and 28%, respectively.[163] Furthermore, a lower incidence of leukopenia and vomiting was observed with doxorubicin alone. A trial comparing doxorubicin and DTIC with or without the addition of ifosfamide has been undertaken as an intergroup study by the major United States cooperative groups (Cancer and Leukemia Group B, Southwest Oncology Group, and Eastern Cooperative Oncology Group), but results are not yet available. One of the reasons for this seeming paradox may be the problem of dose attenuation for doxorubicin when it is combined with other agents. In this light, the trial of doxorubicin, ifosfamide, and DTIC given in combination with the growth factor granulocyte-macrophage colony-stimulating factor[164] may provide the direction for further investigations in these diseases, as this approach allows for full doses of drugs to be administered in combination, with the granulocyte-macrophage colony-stimulating factor protecting against undue hematologic toxicity.

One explanation for the relatively low response rates with any regimen used in the soft tissue sarcomas may be related to problems of drug resistance in these tumors. The P-glycoprotein is a 170-kDa cell surface constituent that is overexpressed in tumors displaying resistance to multiple chemotherapeutic agents. A study found increased expression of the P-glycoprotein in 6 of 25 sarcomas.[165] Three of these sarcomas had not been exposed to chemotherapy at the time of testing, suggesting inherent drug resistance. Other, as yet unrecognized mechanisms of resistance may also be operative.

Currently, doxorubicin-based therapy should be employed as standard treatment of the advanced sarcomas. The addition of DTIC and/or ifosfamide can be considered. Clearly, new agents are needed to affect significantly the survival of this group of patients, as the overwhelming majority of patients with metastatic sarcoma still die from their disease.

Although local failure rates for extremity sarcomas have decreased to the range of 10% with continuing improvements in limb-sparing surgery and radiation therapy techniques, in most series, 40 to 60% of patients with intermediate- and high-grade sarcomas still die from metastatic disease, usually within 5 years of diagnosis. Given this situation, it is understandable that adjuvant treatment designed to eliminate micrometastatic disease present at diagnosis would be considered for the sarcomas. Indeed, nonrandomized single-institution trials provided data suggesting a role for adjuvant therapy. However, larger randomized trials with arms using concurrent observation only rather than historical controls have yielded conflicting data.

There are 10 major randomized trials of the role of adjuvant chemotherapy in the sarcomas. Although the exact chemotherapy regimens differed slightly in some series, all regimens contained doxorubicin.

Gherlinzoni reported a benefit with the use of doxorubicin given at 75 mg/m^2 for six cycles compared with no treatment in patients with high-grade extremity lesions from the Instituto Ortopedico Rizzoli.[166] Patients were divided into two groups. The first group, candidates for limb-sparing surgery, received two cycles of preoperative chemotherapy with doxorubicin and radiotherapy (45 Gy) and were then randomized to receive no further chemotherapy or an additional four cycles of doxorubicin. The second group included patients who were not deemed suitable for conservative surgery; they underwent immediate surgery and were then randomized to receive or not receive chemotherapy at the same doses as the previous group. Disease-free survival was 73% with chemotherapy and 45% with observation (P <0.02). Overall survival rates were 91% and 70% (P <0.05), respectively. No significant cardiac toxicity was reported in this trial.

The NCI conducted several sequential trials of adjuvant chemotherapy versus observation in high-grade sarcomas, which have included substantial numbers of patients with extremity lesions.[167–170] The initial trial employed a regimen of doxorubicin at 50 mg/m^2 and cyclophosphamide at 500 mg/m^2 given in escalating doses. When the maximal cumulative dose of doxorubicin was reached (500 to 550 mg/m^2), high-dose methotrexate was substituted for an additional six cycles. The subsequent trial eliminated the methotrexate and capped the cumulative dose of doxorubicin at 350 mg/m^2. The first reports of the initial trial showed a disease-free survival and overall survival benefit for the patients with extremity sarcomas who received chemotherapy (P <0.01). However, with additional follow-up, disease-free survival remains improved, but overall survival was no longer better to a statistically significant degree. Part of the reason may be related to a 14% incidence of doxorubicin-induced cardiomyopathy. The subsequent trial with a lower cumulative dose of doxorubicin yielded disease-free survival and overall survival rates similar to those with the higher-dose regimen, suggesting no loss of potency with decreased toxicity. Of note in these trials, patients with retroperitoneal sarcomas who received chemotherapy did not fare as well as control patients.

Studies from MD Anderson Hospital randomized patients between observation and chemotherapy with a combination of cyclophosphamide, doxorubicin, vincristine, and actinomycin D with local irradiation at 6500 cGy (VACAR). Initial reports suggested poorer disease-free and overall survival rates for the chemotherapy-treated group.[171] However, more mature data with a median follow-up of 10 years revealed improved disease-free survival and a trend toward improved overall survival for the group that received chemotherapy.[172]

Two additional randomized studies utilizing the CyVADIC regimen have been reported. A large study from the EORTC with more than 400 patients found no significant differences in disease-free or overall survival between chemotherapy-treated patients and untreated controls.[173] However, a smaller study with 59 patients from a single institution in France, Foundation Bergonie, using the same regimen found both disease-free and overall survival benefit for chemotherapy-treated patients (disease-free survival 65% versus 37%, P <0.003; overall survival 83% versus 43%, P <0.002).[174] What accounts for the differing results of these studies is not immediately clear.

Studies conducted by the International Sarcoma Study Group, the Eastern Cooperative Oncology Group, and the Dana-Farber Cancer Institute and the Massachusetts General Hospital all using doxorubicin alone at doses ranging from 70 to 90 mg/m^2 found no significant differences between the treated and untreated patient groups.[175–178]

A study from Scandinavia, which also randomized treatment between doxorubicin alone at a slightly lower dose (60 mg/m^2 for nine cycles) and observation, found no advantage for the chemotherapy-treated group.[179] Compliance in this trial was problematic, as more than 50% of patients did not complete treatment. An additional doxorubicin trial from University of California at Los Angeles, which incorporated preoperative local radiotherapy and intraarterial doxorubicin for all patients with a subsequent randomization to further chemotherapy versus observation, found no benefit with the postoperative chemotherapy.[180] The authors of this trial did not believe that the fact that all patients received some chemotherapy was a confounding variable.

Lastly, a trial of sarcoma treatment from the Mayo Clinic, which included patients primarily with extremity lesions, found no difference in overall survival with treatment with doxorubicin, vincristine, actinomycin D, and cyclophosphamide.[181] However, these investigators did note a decreased risk of pulmonary recurrence in the chemotherapy-treated groups. Survival was equal in both groups because of effective salvage thoracotomy.

Thus, all these studies taken together tend to shed more heat than light. If possible, patients with intermediate- to high-grade sarcomas should be considered for entry into investigational protocols, which may help resolve the issue of the role of chemotherapy in these diseases. It is difficult to make a firm recommendation regarding the use of chemotherapy outside of a protocol setting.

Whether or not patients receive chemotherapy, they should be monitored closely for recurrence, particularly pulmonary recurrence. The Mayo Clinic study and other reports from the NCI[182] document the significant role of resection of pulmonary nodules by thoracotomy in effectively treating patients with soft tissue sarcomas. Further, long-term disease-free survival may be possible for 20 to 40% of patients.

Conclusion

The interaction between medical oncologists and their colleagues in orthopedic surgery and radiation oncology involves virtually the entire spectrum of the malignant diseases. Refinements of current techniques, development of new agents, and an increased understanding of the molecular biology of the malignant process will accelerate the progress already made against these diseases.

References

1. Dahlin DC, Unni KK: Bone Tumors. Springfield, IL, Charles C Thomas, 1986, p 271.
2. Huvos A, Butler A, Bretsky S: Osteogenic sarcoma associated with Paget's disease of bone. Cancer 52:1489–1495, 1983.
3. Price CHG, Goldie W: Paget's sarcoma of bone: A study of 80 cases from the Bristol and the Leeds Bone Tumour Registries. J Bone Joint Surg 51B:205–224, 1969.
4. Huvos AG: Osteogenic sarcoma of bones and soft tissues in older persons. Cancer 57:1442–1449, 1986.
5. Sordillo PP, Hajdu SI, Magill GB, et al: Extraosseous osteogenic sarcoma. Cancer 51:727–734, 1983.
6. Clark JL, Unni KK, Dahlin DC, et al: Osteosarcoma of the jaw. Cancer 51:2311–2316, 1983.
7. Mirra J: Bone Tumors. Philadelphia, Lea & Febiger, 1989.
8. Weatherby RP, Dahlin DC, Ivins JC: Postradiation sarcoma of bone. Mayo Clin Proc 56:294–306, 1981.
9. Huvos AG, Woodard HQ, Cahan WG, et al: Postradiation osteogenic sarcoma of bone and soft tissues. Cancer 55:1244–1255, 1985.
10. Brooks S, Starkie CM, Clarke NMP: Osteosarcoma after the fourth decade. Arch Orthop Trauma Surg 104:100–105, 1985.
11. Siegel RD, Ryan LM, Antman KH: Osteosarcoma in adults. Clin Orthop 240:261–269, 1989.
12. Gill M, Murrells T, McCarthy M, et al: Chemotherapy for the primary treatment of osteosarcoma: Population effectiveness over 20 years. Lancet 1:689–692, 1988.
13. Rosenberg SA, Flye MW, Conkle D, et al: Treatment of osteogenic sarcoma. II. Aggressive resection of pulmonary metastases. Cancer Treat Rep 63:753–756, 1979.
14. Jaffe N, Smith E, Abelson HE, et al: Osteogenic sarcoma. Alterations in the pattern of pulmonary metastases with adjuvant chemotherapy. J Clin Oncol 1:252–254, 1983.
15. Huvos AG: Bone Tumors. Philadelphia, WB Saunders, 1979, p 206.
16. Capanna R, Bertoni F, Bettelli G, et al: Dedifferentiated chondrosarcoma. J Bone Joint Surg 70A:60–69, 1988.
17. Dahlin DC, Beabout JW: Dedifferentiation of low-grade chondrosarcomas. Cancer 28:461–466, 1971.
18. Sanerkin NG: The diagnosis and grading of chondrosarcoma of bone. A combined cytologic and histologic approach. Cancer 45:582–594, 1980.
19. Huvos AG, Rosen G, Dabska M, et al: Mesenchymal chondrosarcoma. Cancer 51:1230–1237, 1983.
20. Weiner M, Sedlis M, Johnston AD, et al: Adjuvant chemotherapy of malignant fibrous histiocytoma of bone. Cancer 51:25–29, 1983.
21. Urban C, Rosen G, Huvos AG, et al: Chemotherapy of malignant fibrous histiocytoma of bone. Cancer 51:795–802, 1983.
22. den Heeten GR, Koops HR, Kamps WA, et al: Treatment of malignant fibrous histiocytoma of bone: A plea for primary chemotherapy. Cancer 56:37–40, 1985.
23. Capanna R, Bertoni F, Bacchini P, et al: Malignant fibrous histiocytoma. Cancer 54:177–187, 1984.
24. Chawla SP, Benjamin RS, Abdul-Karim FW, et al: Adjuvant chemotherapy of primary malignant fibrous

histiocytoma of bone—prolongation of disease-free and overall survival. Adjuvant Ther Cancer 4:621–629, 1984.
25. Dahlin DC, Unni KK: Bone Tumors. Springfield, IL, Charles C Thomas, 1986, pp 194–205.
26. Brenning G, Wibell L, Bergstrom R: Serum β2-microglobulin at remission and relapse in patients with multiple myeloma. Eur J Clin Invest 15:242–247, 1985.
27. Alexanian R, Barlogie B, Fritsche H: Beta 2 microglobulin in multiple myeloma. Am J Hematol 20:345–351, 1985.
28. Durie BG, Salmon SE: A clinical staging system for multiple myeloma. Cancer 36:842–852, 1975.
29. Bergsagel DE: Treatment of plasma cell myeloma. Annu Rev Med 30:431, 1979.
30. Case DC, Lee BJ, Clarkson BD: Improved survival times in multiple myeloma treated with melphalan, prednisone, cyclophosphamide, vincristine and BCNU: M-2 protocol. Am J Med 63:897, 1977.
31. Barlogie B, Smith L, Alexanian R: Effective treatment of advanced multiple myeloma refractory to alkylating agents. N Engl J Med 310:1353–1356, 1984.
32. Mandelli F, Tribalto M, Cantonetti M, et al: Recombinant alpha 2B interferon as maintenance therapy in responding multiple myeloma patients (abstract 842). Blood 70(Suppl 1):247a, 1987.
33. Oken MM, Kyle RA, Griepp RP, et al: Chemotherapy plus interferon (rIFN a2) in the treatment of multiple myeloma (abstract 116). Proc ASCO 9:288, 1990.
34. Dalton WS, Durie BG, Salmon SE, et al: Multidrug resistance in multiple myeloma: Detection of *p*-glycoprotein in clinical specimens and reversal of resistance with verapamil (abstract 834). Blood 70(Suppl 1):245a, 1987.
35. Tura S: Bone marrow transplantation in multiple myeloma: Current status and future perspectives. Bone Marrow Transplant 1:17–20, 1986.
36. Barlogie B, Hall R, Zander A, et al: High-dose melphalan with autologous bone marrow transplantation for multiple myeloma. Blood 67:1298–1301, 1986.
37. Chak LY, Cox RS, Bostwick DG, et al: Solitary plasmacytoma of bone: Treatment, progression and survival. J Clin Oncol 5:1811–1815, 1987.
38. Crowin J, Lindberg RD: Solitary plasmacytoma of bone vs. extramedullary plasmacytoma and their relationship to multiple myeloma. Cancer 43:1007–1013, 1979.
39. Dosoretz E, Raymond AK, Murphy GF, et al: Primary lymphoma of bone. The relationship of morphologic diversity to clinical behavior. Cancer 50:1009–1014, 1982.
40. Reimer RR, Chabner BA, Young RC, et al: Lymphoma presenting in bone. Ann Intern Med 87:50–55, 1977.
41. Ostrowski ML, Unni KK, Banks PM, et al: Malignant lymphoma of bone. Cancer 58:2646–2655, 1986.
42. Dolan PA: Reticulum cell sarcoma of bone. Am J Roentgenol 87:121–127, 1962.
43. Bacci G, Jaffe N, Emiliani E, et al: Therapy for primary non-Hodgkin's lymphoma of bone and a comparison of results with Ewing's sarcoma. Cancer 57:1468–1472, 1986.
44. Bunn PA, Schechter GP, Jaffe E, et al: Clinical course of retrovirus-associated adult T-cell lymphoma in the United States. N Engl J Med 309:257–264, 1983.
45. Mindell ER: Current concept review. Chordoma. J Bone Joint Surg 63A:501–505, 1981.
46. Gray SW, Singhabhandhu B, Smith RA, et al: Sacrococcygeal chordoma. Report on a case and review of the literature. Surgery 78:573, 1975.
47. Localio AS, Eng K, Ranson JHC: Abdominosacral approach for retrorectal tumors. Am Surg 179:555–560, 1980.
48. Amendola BE, Amendola MA, Oliver E, et al: Chordoma: Role of radiation therapy. Radiology 158:839–843, 1986.
49. Johnston AD: Pathology of metastatic tumors in bone. Clin Orthop 73:8, 1970.
50. Fidler IG, Gersten DM, Hart IR: The biology of cancer invasion and metastasis. Adv Cancer Res 4:237, 1978.
51. Blair RJ, McAfee JG: Radiological detection of skeletal metastases: radiographs versus scans. Int J Radiat Oncol Biol Phys 1:1199, 1976.
52. McNeil BJ: Value of bone scanning in neoplastic disease. Semin Nucl Med 14:277–286, 1984.
53. Daffner RH, Lupetin AR, Dash N, et al: MRI in the detection of malignant infiltration of the bone marrow. AJR 146:353–358, 1986.
54. Zegel HG, Turner M, Velchik MG, et al: Percutaneous osseous needle aspiration biopsy with nuclear medicine guidance. Clin Nucl Med 9:89–91, 1984.
55. Gillespie PJ, Alexander JL, Edelstyn GA: Changes in 87m-Sr concentrations in skeletal metastases in patients responding to cyclical combination chemotherapy for advanced breast cancer. J Nucl Med 16:191, 1975.
56. Rosen G, Marcove RC, Caparros B, et al: Primary osteogenic sarcoma: The rationale for preoperative chemotherapy and delayed surgery. Cancer 43:2163–2177, 1979.
57. Galasko CSB: Skeletal metastases and mammary cancer. Ann R Coll Surg Engl 50:3, 1972.
58. Meissner W, Warren S: Distribution of metastases in 4012 cancer patients. *In* Anderson WAD (ed): Pathology, Vol 1, 6th ed. St Louis, CV Mosby, 1971, p 538.
59. Sherry MM, Greco FA, Johnson DH, et al: Breast cancer with skeletal metastases at initial diagnosis: Distinctive clinical characteristics and favorable prognosis. Cancer 58:178–182, 1986.
60. Legha SS, Davis, HL, Muggia FM: Hormonal therapy of breast cancer: New approaches and concepts. Ann Intern Med 88:69, 1978.
61. Henderson IC: Endocrine therapy of metastatic breast cancer. *In* Harris JR, Hellman S, Henderson IC, Kinne DW (eds): Breast Diseases. Philadelphia, JB Lippincott, 1987, pp 398–428.
62. Kiang DT, Kennedy BJ: Tamoxifen (antiestrogen) therapy in advanced breast cancer. Ann Intern Med 87:687, 1977.
63. Hortobagyi GN, Buzdar AU, Frye D, et al: Oral medroxyprogesterone acetate in the treatment of metastatic breast cancer. Breast Cancer Res Treat 5:321–326, 1985.
64. Brambilla C, Escobedo A, Artioli R, et al: Medical castration with goserelin: A conservative approach to premenopausal breast cancer (abstract 107). Proc ASCO 9:29, 1990.
65. Harvey HA, Lipton A, Max DT, et al: Medical castration produced by the GnRH analogue leuprolide to treat metastatic breast cancer. J Clin Oncol 3:1068–1072, 1985.
66. Lipton A, Santen R: Medical adrenalectomy using aminoglutethimide and dexamethasone in advanced breast cancer. Cancer 33:503, 1974.

67. Henderson IC: Chemotherapy for advanced disease. *In* Harris JR, Hellman S, Henderson IC, Kinne DW (eds): Breast Diseases. Philadelphia, JB Lippincott, 1987, pp 428–479.
68. Canellos GP, DeVita V, Gold GL, et al: Cyclical combination chemotherapy for advanced breast cancer. Br Med J 1:218–220, 1974.
69. Cooper RG: Combination chemotherapy in hormone resistant breast cancer. Proc AACR 10:15, 1969.
70. Smalley R, Carpenter J, Bartolucci A, et al: A comparison of cyclophosphamide, Adriamycin, 5-fluorouracil (CAF) and cyclophosphamide, methotrexate, 5-flourouracil, vincristine, prednisone (CMFVP) in patients with metastatic breast cancer. Cancer 40:625–632, 1977.
71. Jones RB, Holland JF, Bhardwaj S, et al: A phase I-II study of intensive dose Adriamycin for advanced breast cancer. J Clin Oncol 5:172–177, 1987.
72. Perloff M, Hart RD, Holland JF: Vinblastine, Adriamycin, thiotepa and halotestin (VATH) therapy for advanced breast cancer refractory to prior chemotherapy. Cancer 42:2534, 1978.
73. Cadman E, Bertino JR: Chemotherapy of skeletal metastases. Int J Radiat Oncol Biol Phys 1:1211, 1976.
74. Grayhack JT, Keeler TC, Kozlowski JM: Carcinoma of the prostate: Hormonal therapy. Cancer 60:589–601, 1987.
75. Crawford ED, Eisenberger MA, McLeod DG, et al: A controlled trial of leuprolide with and without flutamide in prostatic carcinoma. N Engl J Med 321:419–424, 1989.
76. Schmidt JD, Scott WW, Gibbons R, et al: Chemotherapy programs of the National Prostatic Cancer Project (NPCP). Cancer 45:1937, 1980.
77. Torti FM: Prostatic cancer chemotherapy: Recent results. Cancer Res 85:58–69, 1983.
78. Myers CE, LaRocca R, Stein C, et al: Treatment of hormonally refractory prostate cancer with suramin (abstract 517). Proc ASCO 9:133, 1990.
79. Napoli LD, Hansen HH, Muggia FM, et al: The incidence of osseous involvement in lung cancer, with special reference to the development of osteoblastic changes. Radiology 108:17–21, 1973.
80. Evans WK, Shepherd FA, Feld R, et al: VP-16 and cisplatin as first-line therapy for small-cell lung cancer. J Clin Oncol 3:65–71, 1985.
81. Feld R, Evans WK, DeBoer G, et al: Combined modality induction therapy without maintenance chemotherapy for small cell carcinoma of the lung. J Clin Oncol 2:294–304, 1984.
82. O'Dea MJ, Zincke H, Utz DC, et al: The treatment of renal cell carcinoma with solitary metastasis. J Urol 120:542–549, 1978.
83. Rosenberg SA, Lotze MT, Muul LM, et al: A progress report on the treatment of 157 patients with advanced cancer using lymphohokine-activated killer cells and interleukin-2 or high dose interleukin-2 alone. N Engl J Med 31:889, 1987.
84. McCormack KR: Bone metastates from thyroid carcinoma. Cancer 19:181–184, 1966.
85. Pochin EE: Prospects from the treatment of thyroid carcinoma with radioiodine. Clin Radiol 18:113, 1967.
86. Gottlieb JA, Hill C: Chemotherapy of thyroid cancer with Adriamycin. N Engl J Med 290:193, 1974.
87. Bukowski RM, Brown L, Weick JK: Combination chemotherapy of metastatic thyroid cancer. Am J Clin Oncol 6:579, 1983.
88. Sokal M, Harmar GI: Chemotherapy for anaplastic carcinoma of the thyroid. Clin Oncol 4:3, 1978.
89. Shimaoka K, Schoenfeld DA, DeWys WD, et al: A randomized trial of doxorubicin versus doxorubicin plus cisplatin in patients with advanced thyroid carcinoma. Cancer 56:2155, 1985.
90. Stewart WR, Gelerman RH, Harrelson JM, et al: Skeletal metastases of melanoma. J Bone Joint Surg 60A:645–649, 1978.
91. Bonnheim DC, Petrelli NJ, Herrera L, et al: Osseous metastases from colorectal carcinoma. Am J Surg 151:457–459, 1986.
92. Cancer Statistics. CA 39:12–13, 1989.
93. Laskin WB, Silverman TA, Enzinger FM: Postradiation soft tissue sarcomas: An analysis of 53 cases. Cancer 62:2330–2340, 1988.
94. Hardell L, Sandstrom A: Case-control study: Soft tissue sarcomas and exposure to phenoxyacetic acids or chlorophenols. Br J Cancer 39:711–717, 1979.
95. Hoar S, Blair A, Homes F, et al: Agricultural herbicide use and risk of lymphoma and soft-tissue sarcoma. JAMA 256:1141–1147, 1985.
96. Sarma P, Jacobs J: Thoracic soft-tissue sarcomas in Vietnam veterans exposed to Agent Orange. N Engl J Med 306:1109, 1986.
97. Greenwald P, Kovaszay B, Collins DN, et al: Sarcomas of soft tissues after Vietnam service. J Natl Cancer Inst 73:1107–1109, 1984.
98. Kang H, Enzinger FM, Breslin P, et al: Soft tissue sarcoma and military service in Vietnam: A case-control study. J Natl Cancer Inst 79:693–699, 1987.
99. Brand KG: Foreign body induced sarcomas. *In* Becker FF (ed): Cancer. New York, Plenum Press, 1975, pp 485–511.
100. Stein RG, Longo DL: Clinical, biologic and therapeutic aspects of malignancies associated with the acquired immunodeficiency syndrome. Ann Allergy 60:310–323, 1988.
101. Woodward AH, Ivins JC, Soule EH: Lymphangiosarcoma arising in chronic lymphedematous extremities. Cancer 30:562–572, 1972.
102. Sorensen SA, Mulvihill JJ, Nielsen A: Long-term follow-up of von Recklinghausen neurofibromatosis: Survival and malignant neoplasms. N Engl J Med 314:1010–1015, 1986.
103. Ducatman BS, Scheithauer BW, Piepgras DG, et al: Malignant peripheral nerve sheath tumors. Cancer 57:2006–2021, 1986.
104. Heard G: Malignant disease in von Recklinghausen's neurofibromatosis. Proc R Soc Lond 56:502–503, 1963.
105. Fraumeni JF Jr, Vogel CL, Easton JM: Sarcomas and multiple polyposis in a kindred. A genetic variety of hereditary polyposis. Arch Intern Med 121:57–61, 1968.
106. Turc-Carel C, Dalcin D, Limon J: Translocation x:18 in synovial sarcoma. Cancer Genet Cytogenet 22:93–94, 1986.
107. Turc-Carel C, Lizard-Nacol S, Justrabs E, et al: Consistent chromosomal translocation in alveolar rhabdomyosarcoma. Cancer Genet Cytogenet 19:361–362, 1986.
108. Limon J, Turc-Carel C, Dalcin P, et al: Recurrent chromosome changes in liposarcoma. Cancer Genet Cytogenet 22:93–94, 1986.
109. Coindre JM, Trojani M, Contesso G, et al: Reproducibility of a histopathologic grading system for adult soft tissue sarcoma. Cancer 58:306–309, 1986.
110. Lawrence W Jr, Donegan WL, Nachimuth N, et al: Adult soft tissue sarcomas. A pattern of care survey of the American College of Surgeons. Ann Surg 205:349–359, 1987.

111. Beahrs OH, Henson DG, Hutter RV, Myers MH (eds): Manual for Staging of Cancer, 3rd ed. Philadelphia, JB Lippincott, 1988.
112. Costa J, Wesley RA, Glatstein E, et al: The grading of soft tissue sarcomas. Results of a clinicohistopathologic correlation in a series of 163 cases. Cancer 53:530–541, 1984.
113. Russell WO, Cohen J, Edmonson JH, et al: Staging system for soft tissue sarcoma. Semin Oncol 8:156–159, 1981.
114. Enneking WF, Spainer SS, Goodman MA: The surgical staging of muscoloskeletal sarcoma. J Bone Joint Surg 62A:1027–1030, 1980.
115. Heise HW, Myers MH, Russell WO, et al: Recurrence-free survival time for surgically treated soft tissue sarcoma patients. Cancer 57:172–177, 1986.
116. Enzinger FM, Winslow DJ: Liposarcoma: A study of 103 cases. Virchows Arch (Pathol Anat) 335:367, 1962.
117. Enzinger FM, Smith BH: Hemangiopericytoma. An analysis of 106 cases. Hum Pathol 7:61, 1976.
118. Blum RH: An overview of studies in Adriamycin (NSC-123127) in the United States. Cancer Chemother Rep 6:247–251, 1975.
119. O'Bryan RM, Luce JK, Talley RW, et al: Phase II evaluation of Adriamycin in human neoplasia. Cancer 32:1–8, 1973.
120. Benjamin RS, Wiernik PH, Bachur NR: Adriamycin: A new effective agent in the therapy of disseminated sarcomas. Med Pediatr Oncol 1:63–76, 1975.
121. O'Bryan RM, Baker LH, Gottlieb JE, et al: Dose response evaluation of Adriamycin in human neoplasia. Cancer 39:1940–1948, 1977.
122. Henderson IC, Frei E. Adriamycin cardiotoxicity. Am Heart J 99:671–674, 1980.
123. Lefrak EA, Pitha J, Rosenheim S, et al: A clinicopathologic analysis of Adriamycin cardiotoxicity. Cancer 32:302–314, 1973.
124. Unverferth DV, Magorien RD, Leier CV, et al: Doxorubicin cardiotoxicity. Cancer Treat Rev 9:149–164, 1982.
125. Samuels BL, Vogelzang NJ, Ruone M, et al: Continuous venous infusion of doxorubicin in advanced sarcomas. Cancer Treat Rep 71:971–972, 1987.
126. Legha S, Benjamin RS, MacKay B, et al: Reduction of doxorubicin cardiotoxicity by prolonged continuous infusion. Ann Intern Med 96:133–139, 1982.
127. Cohen M, Kronzon I, Lebowitz A: Reversible doxorubicin-induced congestive heart failure. Arch Intern Med 142:1570–1571, 1982.
128. Saini J, Rich MW, Lyss AP: Reversibility of severe left ventricular dysfunction due to doxorubicin cardiotoxicity. Ann Intern Med 106:814–816, 1987.
129. Speyer JL, Green MD, Kramer E, et al: Protective effect of the bispiperazinedione ICRF-187 against doxorubicin-induced cardiac toxicity in women with advanced breast cancer. N Engl J Med 319:745–752, 1988.
130. Chevallier B, Montcuquet P, Faschini T, et al: Phase II study of epirubicin in advanced soft tissue sarcoma (abstract 1256). Proc ASCO 8:323, 1989.
131. Mouridsen HT, Bastholt L, Somers R, et al: Adriamycin versus epirubicin in advanced soft tissue sarcomas. A randomized phase II/III study of the EORTC Soft Tissue and Bone Sarcoma Group. Eur J Cancer Clin Oncol 23:1477–1483, 1987.
132. Zalupski M, Baker LH: Ifosfamide. J Natl Cancer Inst 80:556–566, 1988.
133. Bramwell VH, Mouridsen HT, Santoro A, et al: Cyclophosphamide versus ifosfamide. Final report of a randomized phase II trial in adult soft tissue sarcomas. Eur J Cancer Clin Oncol 3:311–321, 1987.
134. Antman KH, Montella D, Rosenbaum C, et al: Phase II trial of ifosfamide with mesna in previously treated metastatic sarcoma. Cancer Treat Rep 69:499–504, 1985.
135. Scheulen ME, Niederle N, Bremer K, et al: Efficacy of ifosfamide in refractory malignant diseases and uroprotection by mesna: Results of a clinical phase II study with 151 patients. Cancer Treat Rev 10(Suppl A):93–101, 1983.
136. Stuart-Harris RC, Harper PG, Parsons CA, et al: High dose alkylation therapy using ifosfamide with mesna in the treatment of adult advanced soft tissue sarcoma. Cancer Chemother Pharmacol 11:69–72, 1983.
137. Zalupski M, Baker LH. Ifosfamide. J Natl Cancer Inst 80:556–566, 1988.
138. Gottlieb JA, Benjamin RS, Baker LH, et al: The role of DTIC (NSC-45388) in the chemotherapy of sarcomas. Cancer Treat Rep 60:199–293, 1976.
139. Bergsagel DE, Levin WC: A preclusive clinical trial of cyclophosphamide. Cancer Chemother Rep 8:120–134, 1960.
140. Korst DR, Johnson D, Frenkel EP, et al: Preliminary evaluation of the effect of cyclophosphamide on the course of human neoplasms. Cancer Chemother Rep 7:1–12, 1960.
141. Sordillo PP, Magill GB, Brenner J, et al: Cisplatin: A phase II trial in previously untreated patients with soft tissue sarcomas. Cancer 59:884–886, 1987.
142. Brenner J, Magill GB, Sordillo PP, et al: Phase II trial of cisplatin (CPDD) in previously treated patients with advanced soft tissue sarcoma. Cancer 50:2031–2033, 1982.
143. Samson MK, Baker LH, Benjamin RS, et al: Cisdichlorodiammine-platinum (II) in advanced soft tissue and bony sarcomas: A Southwest Oncology Group study. Cancer Treat Rep 63:2027–2029, 1979.
144. van-Oosterom AT, Santoro A, Bramwell V, et al: Mitomycin C (MCC) in advanced soft tissue sarcoma: A phase II study of the EORTC Soft Tissue and Bone Sarcoma Group. Eur J Cancer Clin Oncol 4:459–461, 1985.
145. Selawry OS, Holland JF, Wolman LJ: Effect of vincristine (NSC-67574) on malignant tumors in children. Cancer Chemother Rep 52:497–499, 1968.
146. Golbey R, Li MC, Kaufman RF: Actinomycin in the treatment of soft part sarcomas (abstract). James Ewing Society Scientific Program, 1968.
147. Amato DA, Borden EC, Shiraki M, et al: Evaluation of bleomycin, chlorozoticin, MGBG, and bruceantin in patients with advanced soft tissue sarcoma, bone sarcoma or mesothelioma. Invest New Drugs 3:397–401, 1985.
148. Radice PA, Bunn PA Jr, Ihde DC: Therapeutic trials with VP-16 and VM26. Cancer Treat Rep 63:1231–1239, 1979.
149. Karakousis CP, Rau U, Carlson M: High-dose methotrexate as secondary chemotherapy in metastatic soft-tissue sarcomas. Cancer 46:1345–1348, 1980.
150. Subramanian S, Wiltshaw E: Chemotherapy of sarcoma–a comparison of three regimens. Lancet 1:683–686, 1978.
151. Buesa JM, Mouridsen HT, Santoro A, et al: Treatment of advanced soft tissue sarcomas with low-dose methotrexate: A phase II trial by the European Organization for Research and Treatment of Cancer (EORTC) Soft Tissue and Bone Sarcoma Group. Cancer Treat Rep 68:683–694, 1984.

152. Harris JE, Das Gupta TK, Vogelzang N, et al: Treatment of soft tissue sarcoma with fibroblast interferon—American Cancer Society/Illinois Cancer Council study. Cancer Treat Rep 70:293–294, 1986.
153. Rosenberg SA, Lottze MT, Muul LM, et al: A progress report on the treatment of 157 patients with advanced cancer using lymphokine-activated killer cells and interleukin-2 or high dose interleukin-2 alone. N Engl J Med 316:890–897, 1987.
154. Gottlieb JA, Baker LH, Quagliana JM, et al: Chemotherapy of sarcomas with a combination of Adriamycin and dimethyl triazeno imidazole carboxamide. Cancer 30:1632–1638, 1972.
155. Borden EC, Amato D, Rosenbaum C, et al: Randomized comparison of three Adriamycin regimens for metastatic soft tissue sarcomas. J Clin Oncol 5:840–850, 1987.
156. Yap BS, Baker LH, Sinkovics JG, et al: Cyclophosphamide, vincristine, Adriamycin and DTIC (CyVADIC) combination chemotherapy for the treatment of advanced sarcomas. Cancer Treat Rep 64:93–98, 1980.
157. Gottlieb JA, Baker LH, O'Bryan RM, et al: Adriamycin (NSC-123127) used alone and in combination for soft tissue and bony sarcomas. Cancer Chemother Rep 6:271–282, 1975.
158. Baker LH, Frank J, Fine G, et al: Combination chemotherapy using Adriamycin, DTIC, cyclophosphamide and actinomycin D for advanced soft tissue sarcomas: A randomized comparative trial. A phase III, Southwest Oncology Group Study (7613). J Clin Oncol 5:851–861, 1987.
159. Schoenfeld D, Rosenbaum C, Horton J, et al: A comparison of Adriamycin versus vincristine and Adriamycin, and cyclophosphamide versus vincristine, actinomycin-D, and cyclophosphamide for advanced sarcoma. Cancer 50:2757–2762, 1982.
160. Elias AD, Antman KH: Doxorubicin, ifosfamide and dacarbazine (AID) with mesna uroprotection for advanced untreated sarcoma: A phase I study. Cancer Treat Rep 70:827–833, 1986.
161. Elias AD, Ryan L, Aisner J, et al: Doxorubicin, ifosfamide and DTIC (AID) for advanced untreated sarcomas (abstract 524). Proc ASCO 6:134, 1987.
162. Loehrer PJ Sr, Sledge GW Jr, Nicaise C, et al: Ifosfamide plus doxorubicin in metastatic adult sarcomas: A multi-institutional phase II trial. J Clin Oncol 7:1655–1659, 1989.
163. Santoro A, Rouesse J, Steward W, et al: A randomized EORTC study in advanced soft tissue sarcomas (STS) (abstract 1196). Proc ASCO 9:309, 1990.
164. Antman KS, Griffin JD, Elias A, et al: Effect of recombinant human granulocyte-macrophage colony stimulating factor on chemotherapy-induced myelosuppression. N Engl J Med 319:593–598, 1988.
165. Gerlach JH, Bell DR, Karakousis C, et al: P-glycoprotein in human sarcoma: Evidence for multidrug resistance. J Clin Oncol 5:1452–1460, 1987.
166. Gherlinzoni F, Bacci G, Picci P, et al: A randomized trial for the treatment of high-grade soft-tissue sarcomas of the extremities: Preliminary observations. J Clin Oncol 4:552–558, 1986.
167. Rosenberg SA, Tepper J, Glatstein E, et al: The treatment of soft-tissue sarcomas of the extremities. Ann Surg 196:305–315, 1982.
168. Rosenberg SA, Tepper J, Glatstein E, et al: Prospective randomized evaluation of adjuvant chemotherapy in adults with soft tissue sarcomas of the extremities. Cancer 52:424–434, 1983.
169. Potter DA, Kinsella T, Glatstein E, et al: High grade soft tissue sarcomas of the extremities. Cancer 58:190–205, 1986.
170. Chang AE, Kinsella T, Glatstein E, et al: Adjuvant chemotherapy for patients with high-grade soft-tissue sarcomas of the extremity. J Clin Oncol 6:1491–1500, 1988.
171. Lindberg R, Murphy W, Benjamin R, et al: Adjuvant chemotherapy in the treatment of primary soft tissue sarcomas. A preliminary report. *In* Management of Primary Bone and Soft Tissue Tumors. Chicago, Year Book Medical Publishers, 1977, pp 343–352.
172. Benjamin RS, Terjanian TO, Fenoglio CJ, et al: The importance of combination chemotherapy for adjuvant treatment of high-risk patients with soft-tissue sarcomas of the extremities. *In* Salmon S (ed): Adjuvant Therapy of Cancer V. Orlando, FL, Grune & Stratton, 1987, pp 735–744.
173. Bramwell V, Rouesse J, Steward W, et al: European experience of adjuvant chemotherapy for soft tissue sarcoma: Interim report of a randomized trial of CyVADIC versus control. *In* Ryan J, Baker L (eds): Recent Concepts in Sarcoma Treatment. Dordrecht, Netherlands, Kluwer Academic, 1988, pp 157–164.
174. Bui NB, Maree D, Coindre JM, et al: First results of a prospective randomized study of CyVADIC adjuvant chemotherapy in adults with operable high risk soft tissue sarcoma (abstract 1236). Proc ASCO 8:318, 1989.
175. Antman K, Amato D, Pilepich M, et al: A preliminary analysis of a randomized intergroup (SWOG, ECOG, CALGB, NCOG) trial of adjuvant doxorubicin for soft tissue sarcomas. *In* Salmon S (ed): Adjuvant Therapy of Cancer V. Orlando, FL, Grune & Stratton, 1987, pp 725–734.
176. Antman K, Suit H, Amato D, et al: Preliminary results of a randomized trial of adjuvant doxorubicin for sarcomas: Lack of apparent difference between treatment groups. J Clin Oncol 2:601–608, 1984.
177. Antman K, Amato D, Lerner H, et al: Adjuvant doxorubicin for sarcoma: Data from the ECOG and DFCI/MGH studies. Cancer Treat Symp 3:109–115, 1985.
178. Lerner HJ, Amato DA, Savlov ED, et al: Eastern Cooperative Oncology Group: A comparison of adjuvant doxorubicin and observation for patients with localized soft tissue sarcoma. J Clin Oncol 5:613–617, 1987.
179. Alvegard TA: Adjuvant chemotherapy with Adriamycin in high grade malignant soft tissue sarcoma—a Scandanavian randomized study (abstract 485). Proc ASCO 5:125, 1986.
180. Eilber FR, Giuliano AE, Huth JF, et al: Postoperative adjuvant chemotherapy (Adriamycin) in high grade extemity soft tissue sarcoma: A randomized prospective trial. *In* Salmon S (ed): Adjuvant Therapy of Cancer V. Orlando, FL, Grune & Stratton, 1987, pp 719–724.
181. Edmonson JH, Fleming TR, Ivins JC, et al: Randomized study of systemic chemotherapy following complete excision of nonosseous sarcomas. J Clin Oncol 2:1390–1396, 1984.
182. Jablons D, Steinberg SM, Roth J, et al: Metastatectomy for soft tissue sarcoma. J Thorac Cardiovasc Surg 97:695–705, 1989.

CHAPTER 7

Radiation Therapy in the Treatment of Bone and Soft Tissue Sarcomas

SHALOM KALNICKI
WILLIAM D. BLOOMER

William Conrad Roentgen described x-rays in 1895[180]; Henri Becquerel and the Curies discovered natural radioactivity a year later.[17] It was soon recognized that cell damage and death were among the biologic effects of these newly discovered radiations; those properties were soon applied in the treatment of malignant neoplasms, with the first tumor regressions being described before the turn of the century.

Basics of Radiology

Ionizing radiation causes cell death by the formation of highly reactive intracellular free radicals that in turn produce nuclear DNA damage.[59] For nonproliferating cells, such as those of muscle and nerve, radiation may lead to loss of a specific cell function. For high-turnover cell renewal systems, such as those of the gastrointestinal tract or the bone marrow, radiation damage is manifested as the loss of the ability to reproduce. Although some cells may undergo several mitoses after exposure to radiation, if they ultimately lose their potential to divide indefinitely, they may be considered killed; this is commonly known as clonogenic death.[20]

Survival curves for cultured cells exposed to single-hit, conventional, low linear energy transfer (LET) radiation have two components—an initial bending or "shoulder" region at low doses followed by a linear region at higher dose levels.[86, 171] The shoulder region, where incremental dosage increases result in little additional damage, reflects the capacity of cells to repair sublethal radiation damage; the size of the shoulder varies widely.[60]

The straight-line portion of the survival curve at higher doses represents exponential cell killing; linearity implies that there is no repair of radiation damage in this region.[20] The slope of the straight-line portion of the survival curve is a measure of cellular radiosensitivity. The therapeutic ratio of radiation is based, at least to some extent, on the assumption that normal cells repair sublethal or potentially lethal damage better than neoplastic cells do.[172]

The sensitivity of individual cells to radiation also varies with their position in the cell cycle, being greatest at mitosis and early synthesis.[84] After a single exposure to ionizing radiation, those cells in the most sensitive phases of the cell cycle are differentially killed, and the population is partially cycle synchronized temporarily. Within tumor masses containing hypoxic centers, decreases in tumor cell numbers may lead to reoxygenation of cells that were otherwise not cycling, recruiting them into active cycling again. Reoxygenation and repopulation form part of the biologic rationale on which the utilization of multiple fractions in clinical radiotherapy regimens is based.[106]

The radiosensitivity of most biologic systems can be enhanced as much as threefold in the presence of oxygen.[80] The free radicals generated during the intracellular ionization events undergo an irreversible reaction with oxygen, referred to as oxygen fixation.[5] Under hypoxic conditions, repair of radiation damage proceeds more easily and radiosensitivity is consequently reduced.[32] The ratio of the doses necessary to achieve the same biologic effect is called the oxygen enhancement ratio (OER). There is a steep rise in the OER as oxygen tension increases from 0 to 33 mm Hg, beyond which the OER is constant at about 3, regardless of oxygen tension.[85]

Thomlinson and Gray described the histologic pattern of hypoxia in malignant tumors: cords of healthy tumor cells surrounded necrotic-appearing cells and central areas of overt necrosis.[210] As tumor cells outgrow their blood supply, central hypoxic areas (with relatively radioresistant cells) develop in many large solid tumors.[47] Central tumor hypoxia is a major limiting factor for radiocurability. It can be difficult to cure bulky tumor masses utilizing clinically tolerable doses of irradiation, whereas the same doses can be extremely effective for sterilization of microscopic, well-oxygenated tumor deposits in a surgical field, after debulking has been performed.[66, 67]

As early as 1934, Coutard recognized that fractionated radiation therapy regimens led to better tumor control and lower complication rates.[38] With the use of small daily doses of radiation in protracted treatment regimens, reoxygenation of previously hypoxic tumor tissue may occur, with increased cell killing. Experimental proof was provided with RIF-1 sarcomas in which almost 100% of surviving tumor cells were hypoxic immediately after a single dose of 1.5 Gy, but only 50% remained hypoxic within 1 hour after irradiation.[51]

Substantial experimental evidence supports the relevance of the oxygen effect in sarcomas. OERs for KHT sarcoma cells were estimated at 2.4, 2.6, and 2.5 for the G_1, S, and G_2-M phases of the cell cycle, respectively[193]; the proportion of hypoxic cells in these tumors was estimated to be about 10%.[196] Anesthesia-induced hypotension and hypoxia have radioprotective effects in RIF-1 sarcomas.[39] Other clinical evidence for the importance of hypoxia has been established for carcinomas of the uterine cervix and other sites.[93, 218]

The hypoxic cell fraction of a tumor mass is directly affected by circulatory patterns; this tumor bed effect (TBE) influences response to radiation and chemotherapy.[101] Murine fibrosarcomas become less sensitive to irradiation after being transplanted into previously irradiated, poorly oxygenated tissues.[139, 141] Radiation-induced injury to the tumor bed stroma can play an important role in radiocurability, with carcinomas being more affected by radiation-induced injury than sarcomas.[142]

The dose of radiation absorbed in tissue is measured in grays (Gy), defined as one joule of absorbed energy per kilogram of tissue. The gray has replaced the rad and equals 100 rads; for convenience, the term centigray (cGy) is widely used because 1 cGy equals 1 rad. The biologic effect of a fractionated radiation therapy regimen depends not only on the total dose delivered, but also on the number and size of each individual fraction and on the total treatment time.[61] This time-dose relationship is one of the cornerstones of clinical radiation therapy, affecting tumor control as well as normal tissue tolerance. Mathematical formulas have been derived for comparing the effectiveness of different treatment schedules, the most commonly used being the "time-dose factor" (TDF) of Orton and Ellis.[62, 153]

Protracted treatment regimens strive to use daily doses that are within the shoulder or repair region of normal tissues while in the exponential killing region for tumor cells; reoxygenation of hypoxic tumor cells and recruitment into active cycling increase tumor cell killing in multiple-fraction regimens. Radiation-induced cell division delay and cycling synchronization are other biologic attributes of protracted schedules.[6] Care must be taken that tumor repopulation does not exceed radiation-induced cell killing if treatment regimens become too protracted. In most clinical settings, daily doses in clinical radiation therapy range from 1.5 to 2 Gy, delivering 9 to 10 Gy per week.

When irradiated cells are prevented from progressing through the cell cycle, their surviving fraction increases; this is due to repair of "potentially lethal damage."[163] This phenomenon can be particularly important in clinical situations in which tumor bed conditions affect cell cycling times. Osteosarcoma cell lines show a significantly smaller amount of potentially lethal damage repair than normal fibroblasts do.[131] Relatively radioresistant tumors may contain a higher proportion of cells that can effectively repair potentially lethal damage; survival curve analysis of cultured tumor cells may lead to response-predictive assays.[162, 221, 222]

Radiation Response Modifiers

The characterization of radiation-induced nuclear damage as a chemical reaction prompted the search for substances that act as radiation response modifiers. Oxygen was the obvious first choice, in the form of hyperbaric oxygen breathing. Milas reported increased radiosensitivity of murine fibrosarcomas by a factor of 1.13 when animals were exposed to hyperbaric oxygen.[141] In clinical settings, some beneficial effects were reported in advanced head and neck and uterine cervix cancers, but in general, the results were not encouraging. The use of hyperbaric oxygen is cumbersome, the bulky chambers interfering with daily treatment. Normal tissue reactions were also enhanced. Furthermore, the inhalation of hyperbaric oxygen does not always translate into a decreased tumor hypoxic cell fraction.[92]

Emphasis has recently shifted to chemical modifiers of radiation response. Electron-affinic radiosensitizing compounds such as metronidazole (Flagyl) and misonidazole have been extensively tested, but with little clinical impact, because of dose-limiting neurotoxicity.[64, 165] Other nitroimidazole derivatives, RO-03-8799[95] and RSU-1069,[219] showed some therapeutic advantage, the latter in BP-8 murine sarcoma cells. Flutarabine phosphate has also shown sensitizing effects in murine fibrosarcoma,[109] but clinical testing is not available. Most radioprotectors are sulfhydryl compounds. One example, WR-2721, was shown to reduce experimental radiation injury to normal lung and colonic mucosa.[102, 214]

Chemotherapeutic agents have also shown substantial radiosensitizing effects. Pyrimidine analogues have radiomimetic mechanisms of action. Bromodeoxyuracil (BUDR) and iododeoxyuridine (IUDR) are subjects of intensive investigation, the latter showing less systemic toxicity, higher arterial levels, and up to 70% tumor incorporation in phase I soft tissue sarcoma studies.[114] Studies with nitrosoureas (lomustine [CCNU] and carmustine [BCNU]), alone or combined with misonidazole,[193, 194] cyclophosphamide,[127] doxorubicin (Adriamycin),[176] actinomycin D,[34] and cisplatin,[36, 48] have shown reduced hypoxic cell fractions and increased tumor response to irradiation.

At the National Cancer Institute, Kinsella and Glatstein reviewed 29 patients with unresectable sarcomas treated with the radiosensitizers misonidazole and IUDR[111]; local control was achieved in 11 of 15 patients with localized disease. Some large tumors showed little IUDR shrinkage but were found to be sterilized in posttherapy biopsy specimens.

The interaction of biologic response modifiers and radiation is currently under investigation. Radioresponsiveness can be increased by pretreatment of tumor cells with tumor necrosis factor, while a protective effect on normal bone marrow cells is maintained. Ongoing studies are addressing the simultaneous use of interferon and radiation.[146, 186]

The use of heat as an antineoplastic agent can be traced to early in the twentieth century when fever was induced by injected bacterial toxins and produced tumor regressions. The development of sophisticated heat delivery and thermometry equipment, allied with the recognition of the chemical nature of radiation-induced cell killing, led to research combining the two modalities. Hyperthermia primarily affects hypoxic cells in the S phase of the cell cycle, when they are most radioresistant. Heat causes greater cell cycle delay than does ionizing radiation, further affecting the cell population distribution.[46] Malignant cells seem to be more sensitive to thermal damage than normal tissues are. Temperatures between 42° and 43° C provide the highest tumor cell killing and are still within the range of normal tissue tolerance.[75]

The optimal sequence for combining hyperthermia and radiation was studied in RIF-1 murine sarcomas. When both were delivered within 1 hour, 67% of the tumors were cured; if given 72 hours apart, only 20% of the lesions were eradicated. There were no cures with either modality alone.[145] Thermal enhancement ratios of 3.4 to 3.9 were reported with interstitial implantation of iridium-192 and hyperthermia.[147] Best results in soft tissue sarcomas were obtained with temperatures of 42° C applied for 1 hour twice weekly within 30 to 60 minutes of irradiation.[123]

Radiation responses and normal tissue tolerance can also be modified by altering therapy fractionation. Most treatment schedules call for one treatment session a day, 5 days per week (conventional fractionation). Alternatively, large weekly doses (hypofractionation) or several fractions a day (hyperfractionation) can be administered. There was no improvement in response rates with large weekly fractions in sarcomas.[8] Hyperfractionated regimens yielded some therapeutic gain in advanced head and neck cancers.[220] Preliminary studies in soft tissue sarcomas are encouraging, although no randomized data are currently available.[129]

Basics of Radiation Physics

Radiation therapy can be delivered by means of external beams such as cobalt-60 (teletherapy) or linear accelerators, as well as by the placement of radioactive sources into the tumor or tumor bed (brachytherapy). External beams of photon radiation have different energies, ranging from orthovoltage (100 to 300 kV) to megavoltage irradiation from linear accelerators (generally 4 to 25 MV). Advantages of high-energy irradiation include greater-percentage depth dose (better penetration into deep tissues), skin-sparing effects (maximal energy deposition at depths between 0.5 and 5 cm below the skin), and precise beam definition with minimal scatter of radiation outside the desired treatment field.

High-energy electron beams can be produced by linear accelerators. Because electrons are physically stopped in tissue, they provide sparing of deep-seated structures and are particularly useful for scar boosts and for treatment of superficial tumors. Their use is currently under investigation for intraoperative treatment of retroperitoneal disease and for use in some extremity tumors.[115, 178] Although early results are promising, prospective randomized trials are needed.

Neutrons are densely ionizing particles that have higher LET than do x-rays or photons. The OER for neutrons decreases from 3 to 1, one explanation being direct formation of molecular oxygen from neutron-induced radiolysis of water.[16] Lower numerical doses of neutron radiation are given because neutrons have a higher relative biologic effectiveness (RBE). In a review of the literature, Cohen and colleagues concluded that local control with neutrons alone is comparable to or better than with high-energy x-rays, but at the expense of significantly higher complication rates.[30] Mixed beams of photons and neutrons show marginally better local control than conventional photon irradiation does, and complications can be kept at acceptable levels. The greatest benefit of neutron irradiation was observed in sarcomas and melanomas. Owing to the relatively poor neutron depth dose distribution, the most severe complications were seen when deep-seated tumors were treated.[15] Local control rates for neutron-treated sarcomas throughout the world were estimated at 58% for bone and 60% for soft tissue lesions.

In the Fermilab neutron project, patients with bone and soft tissue sarcomas were treated twice weekly to total doses of 18 to 26 neutron Gy; long-term local control was achieved in 24 of 51 patients (47%).[31] At the Hammersmith Hospital Cyclotron Unit in England, local control rates were 94% for adjuvant irradiation and 52% with gross tumor present[166]; German studies reported 15% recurrence rates in patients treated with adjuvant postoperative neutron therapy to doses averaging 10 neutron Gy.[55]

There is increasing concern regarding late morbidity of neutron irradiation. In the Edinburgh trial, an unusually high 50% complication rate was reported in 30 patients treated exclusively with neutrons.[53] The German group, utilizing neutron boosts after conventional courses of photon therapy, lowered the morbidity to 15% while maintaining local control rates comparable with those achieved with a full neutron treatment regimen.[185] In the Hamburg study, severe local reactions were limited to 10% of irradiated patients when total doses were kept below 15.6 Gy in four weeks.[69] Patients submitted to compartmental resections before neutron irradiation seem to be especially prone to severe late tissue damage.[76]

The role of neutron therapy in the treatment of musculoskeletal malignancies is not yet established; there are no randomized studies comparing local control and survival rates obtained with neutron and photon irradiation. Further technique refinements are necessary to reduce morbidity.

Heavy charged particles, such as pions (pi-mesons), alpha particles, and protons, are characterized by high LET, high RBE, and low OER. Their energy is preferentially deposited at a certain depth in their path, the Bragg peak, allowing for better normal tissue sparing than with neutrons. The depth of the Bragg peak is a function of the energy of the particle; its width can be customized by utilizing mixed energy particle beams.

Negative pions are being evaluated at facilities in Los Alamos (United States), Vancouver (Canada), and Villigen (Switzerland). The Swiss experience showed one local failure in ten retroperitoneal sarcomas treated with 30 Gy, with acceptable bowel morbidity.[211] Equally encouraging results were obtained by the Harvard cyclotron group, with 78% actuarial local control.[9] At the Lawrence Berkeley Laboratories, Saunders and associates delivered alpha particle doses equivalent to 80 Gy of conventional irradiation to chordomas, meningiomas, and low-grade chondrosarcomas of the cervical spine and base of skull. Outside of the Bragg peak distribution, there was a precipitous fall in dose toward the adjacent central nervous system, where tolerance is 45 to 50 Gy; tumors in 9 of 11 patients were controlled locally.[177, 184]

External beam irradiation for bone and soft tissue sarcomas can be given preoperatively or postoperatively, or as the sole treatment modality. In most cases, relatively high doses of 55 to 70 Gy in 5 to 8 weeks are utilized. With the addition of interstitial or intraoperative boosts, total doses in excess of 80 Gy can be delivered with acceptable normal tissue changes.[118]

Intraoperative external beam irradiation with high-energy electron beams has enjoyed recent interest as part of the treatment regimen for retroperitoneal sarcomas. In this situation, the low tolerance of small bowel and kidneys to irradiation can be circumvented by surgically displacing these sensitive organs from the treatment field. Single doses of 15 to 20 Gy are generally applied as a boost for subsequently delivered, more generously applied external beam irradiation.

Treatment planning for external beam irradiation starts with close interaction among the surgeon, the diagnostic radiologist, the pathologist, and the radiation oncologist. In a team effort, the target volume is identified; this includes the tumor or tumor bed, with all potential areas of soft tissue and bone spread. It is essential that scars be included in the target volume. Data are obtained from clinical examination, x-ray films, computed tomography (CT) scans, and magnetic resonance imaging (MRI). Treatment volume is defined as the target volume plus a margin of safety.

The radiation oncologist, the physicist, and the dosimetrist then proceed to study the appropriate radiation field arrangement to treat the target volume, with maximal sparing of normal tissue. This is done with the aid of a simulator, a fluoroscopic unit that mimics all movements and characteristics of a linear accelerator or cobalt-60 teletherapy unit. Multiple portals are often utilized to minimize irradiation of normal tissue.

Treatment devices are custom built for each patient set-up. These include extremity immobilization supports for precise day-to-day positioning, wedge filters and tissue compensators to homogenize the dose along irregular surfaces such as sloping edges on extremities and joints, and custom lead-alloy blocks to shape the beams in any form needed to cover the target volume while preventing unnecessary irradiation of critical structures. Precise immobilization and optimal treatment reproduction are mandatory.

Precise calculation of dose delivery from each treatment portal is then performed, utilizing treatment planning computers in which all beam data for the therapy unit have been entered.[158] These provide accurate dose mapping throughout the treatment field and precise setting of the linear accelerator monitor unit counter to provide the desired daily dose.

Verification x-ray films (or portal films) are then obtained on the treatment unit and are compared with simulator films to assure precise beam reproduction. Linear accelerators typically deliver 2.5 to 5 Gy per minute in air, so daily fractions of 1.8 to 2 Gy can be delivered in seconds, minimizing the possibility of significant patient motion.

Interstitial implantation of radioactive isotopes can deliver high doses of radiation to a small target volume. The commonly utilized isotopes are iridium-192 and iodine-125. Owing to the physical characteristics of these and other interstitially applied radionuclides, the radiation levels fall off rapidly at the edge of the implant volume, with normal tissues being spared. Afterloading techniques permit placement of hollow guide catheters and radiographic documentation of positioning before actually loading the radioactive material. Computer calculations of dose delivery determine the duration of radiation exposure for the implant.

Brachytherapy implants are utilized to deliver radiation boosts to small treatment volumes such as areas of gross residual disease or tight resection margins. They can be performed after external irradiation or at the time of initial surgical resection. In the latter setting, hollow guide catheters are inserted during the operative procedure and loaded with the radioisotopes after the patient's condition has stabilized in the postoperative period.[190] Brachytherapy can also be utilized in pediatric patients, with good tolerance and excellent local results.[40]

Side Effects

The most common acute side effect of radiation for bone and soft tissue sarcomas is skin reaction. Large areas of irradiated skin and glancing fields over sloped surfaces tend to increase the risk of radiation-induced skin damage. The initial erythema may develop into dry and, later, moist desquamation. Decreasing the daily fraction size may be all that is necessary to minimize skin reactions. On the other hand, rest periods may be required for healing if moist desquamation develops. Care must be taken not to extend rest periods beyond a few days, so as not to decrease the therapeutic regimen's biologic effectiveness.

Healing of the skin reaction takes place by repopulation conducted by epithelial stem cells coming from nonirradiated peripheral skin or from surviving epithelial islands within the treatment field.[37] Treatment plans that minimize permanent skin damage are especially important in preoperative irradiation regimens.[128] The combination of irradiation with cytotoxic agents, such as doxorubicin (Adriamycin) or actinomycin D, may significantly increase skin toxicity.[42]

Acute radiation enteritis has been observed with doses lower than 30 Gy. On the other hand, normal mobility of bowel loops and good regenerative capacity make it possible to deliver doses up to 50 Gy to the pelvis without significant long-term morbidity. The threat of radiation enteropathy is real in retroperitoneal sarcomas, in which large bowel volumes have to be irradiated, or in postoperative treatment of pelvic tumors, when loops of bowel may be adherent in the pelvis. Bowel displacement from the irradiated field can be achieved by placement of absorbable mesh during the surgical procedure.[168]

Additional acute side effects may include mild fatigue, anorexia, and, in cases in which bowel or bladder is included in the radiation portals, diarrhea and urinary frequency. Xerostomia, xerophthalmia, dysphagia, and alopecia may be seen during treatment of head and neck sarcomas.

Late effects of radiation therapy of extremity lesions are mostly due to lymphatic and vascular obstruction, both of which may occur at doses in excess of 45 Gy. It is important to spare a peripheral strip of normal tissue to prevent lymphatic obstruction. Lower extremities are more prone to radiation-induced edema than are upper extremities.[121] If joints are included in the treatment fields, appropriate physical therapy should be instituted after irradiation to prevent stiffness and loss of function. Epilation and mild subcutaneous fibrosis are common late sequelae of treatment of soft tissue sarcomas and bone tumors.

Osteonecrosis is a rare complication in patients treated with megavoltage radiation. It generally occurs at doses in excess of 50 to 60 Gy,[97] no evidence of osteocyte death being found with doses less than 40 Gy.[103] The widespread use of megavoltage beams, which lack the preferential bone absorption of orthovoltage x-rays, resulted in a marked decrease in the incidence of this complication.[200] On the other hand, irradiated bones are more prone to fractures, and their healing may be delayed.[201] The differential diagnosis between radiation necrosis and sarcoma arising in irradiated bone may be difficult. Both have long latency periods and may contain calcifications. The absence of a soft tissue mass and a lack of progression of the lesion on serial imaging studies favors a diagnosis of osteoradionecrosis.[43]

When large fields close to the scrotal area are treated, as in thigh sarcomas, radiation scatter to the testis may lead to gonadal dysfunction. Special lead shielding devices can reduce the testicular dose to less than 1% of the prescribed dose, i.e., 0.5 Gy from a typical 50-Gy treatment course.[68] Testicular injury is dose dependent and is detected by increasing serum concentrations of follicle-stimulating and luteinizing hormones; a peak is observed at 6 months after treatment, followed by a gradual decrease. With gonadal doses of 0.5 Gy or less, complete recovery can be seen at 12 months; in patients receiving greater than 2 Gy, changes persist up to 30 months after completion of treatment.[187]

Bone growth retardation is a major concern in pediatric patients.[3] It is greater in younger patients and with high total radiation doses.[41, 78] Sequential measurements of irradiated and nonirradiated limbs show that there is a temporary but marked decrease in growth rate shortly after treatment; recovery usually occurs, and 2 years after therapy irradiated and nonirradiated bone grow at similar rates. When growing vertebral bodies are irradiated, both pedicles should be included in the treatment portals to avoid severe spinal curvatures.[149] In the case of permanent deformities, reconstructive surgery has been used with good functional results, especially in the chest wall.[157] Slipped femoral head epiphyses may occur as a result of pelvic irradiation in children; selectively blocking the femoral heads should prevent this complication.[197] There is experimental evidence that multiple daily treatments (hyperfractionation) may increase the growing bone's tolerance to radiation therapy.[56, 88]

Fromm reported on late effects in 20 children treated for soft tissue sarcomas of the head and neck, most of them with combined radiotherapy and chemotherapy.[71] Findings included xerophthalmia, cataracts, hearing loss, dental caries and maleruption, hypopituitarism, and craniofacial bone deformities. Attentive follow-up is necessary for prompt recognition and therapy of treatable abnormalities.

Radiation-induced sarcomas have been described in heavily irradiated tissues of long-term survivors. Although extremely rare, they are almost always diagnosed at advanced stages and high grade and beyond surgical resectability; their prognosis is generally poor and only early detection may improve patient's survival.[100, 179] Up to 52% of all radiation-induced neoplasms are sarcomas.[65] They have been recognized after therapy of retinoblastomas,[2] Hodgkin's and non-Hodgkin's lymphomas,[18, 199] several central nervous system tumors,[26, 148, 156, 188] breast cancer,[89, 119, 120] and other primary tumors. A 4% incidence of second primary tumors has been reported in children followed for 25 years after irradiation.[90] Associated chemotherapy increases the chance of developing sarcomas in previously irradiated areas.[83, 216]

Postirradiation soft tissue sarcomas are of various histologic types. In a review of 53 such cases, Laskin and colleagues found 68% malignant fibrous histiocytomas, 13% extraskeletal osteosarcomas, 11% fibrosarcomas, 4% malignant schwannomas, one extraskeletal chondrosarcoma, and one angiosarcoma.[122]

Huvos and Woodard reviewed 59 patients with osteogenic sarcomas and 20 patients with malignant fibrous histiocytomas arising in irradiated areas.[99] The mean radiation dose was 60.4 Gy and the mean latency period was 16.4 years. Disease-free survivals were 58% at 3 years for malignant fibrous histiocytomas and only 17% at 5 years for osteosarcomas. There were no second malignancies seen at doses less than 20 Gy. Most of the osteosarcomas arose in pelvic and shoulder girdle bones.[100]

Specific Applications

OSTEOGENIC SARCOMA

Studies addressing the role of radiation in osteogenic sarcomas are rare, because the natural history of the disease shows that the majority of treatment failures are due to distant metastases. Radiation therapy can palliate pain arising from a local recurrence and prevent the need for amputation in patients who present with metastatic disease.[206]

Osteogenic sarcoma is classically regarded as a relatively radioresistant tumor. Weichselbaum, however, studying *in vitro* survival curves of seven human osteosarcoma cell lines, found that the data did not predict radioresistance, as values obtained were similar to those for four Ewing's sarcoma cell lines, which are thought to be more radiosensitive.[223] Gaitan-Yanguas analyzed the surgical specimens of 18 patients submitted to irradiation followed by amputation 6 months later, concluding that doses greater than 32 Gy in 10 days or 80 Gy in 60 to 70 days resulted in tumor sterilization.[73] Side effects were tolerable with the prolonged fractionation, and radionecrosis was present only in patients treated with 80 Gy in less than 20 days.

In an attempt to prevent unnecessary amputations, Cade proposed initial irradiation (70 to 80 Gy) followed by a 4 to 6 months' wait and amputation in patients who did not present with metastatic disease during the observation period. Local control and function were reasonable, but 5-year survival was only 22%.[23] Phillips and Sheline obtained similar results utilizing higher dose levels.[164]

Trials of preoperative neutron irradiation for locally advanced lesions are being conducted in Japan. In one study, 66% of 36 preoperatively treated patients showed no histologic evidence of tumor at surgery; 3- and 5-year survival rates were 68% and 63%, respectively.[215] Takada and associates reported on 38 patients with unresectable lesions.[205] All but three had resectable tumors and underwent limb salvage procedures; only one patient had a local recurrence, with follow-up ranging from 9 to 120 months.

Another novel approach for improving resectability is the use of radiosensitizers. Martinez reported local control in seven of nine patients treated with hypofractionated irradiation and BUDR infusions[134]; pulmonary metastasis, however, developed in six and severe normal tissue complications occurred in five patients. New approaches in radiosensitization, with IUDR or cisplatin, concurrently with new fractionation schemes may improve these results.

The European Organization for Research on Treatment of Cancer (EORTC) is conducting several trials including radiation therapy as part of a multimodality treatment regimen. In one EORTC study, the primary tumor was treated with radiation in 37 patients, 23 of whom (62%) had local control; unfortunately, only three retained normal limb function.[22] Severe extremity abnormalities were observed in eight patients (all treated with chemotherapy and radiation), three of whom required amputation; ten patients sustained mild functional impairment. The recent development of customized expandable bone prosthesis allows for limb-sparing therapy of the primary tumor, usually with better functional results than those obtained with high-dose irradiation.[124]

Because of chemotherapy's potential efficacy against micrometastases, so-called neoadjuvant chemotherapy has replaced preoperative radiation in most American treatment protocols. The concept was introduced by Rosen and associates,[181] utilizing high-dose methotrexate with citrovorum factor rescue, combined with several other agents; initial 4-year disease-free survival was 80%.

Several trials have studied the role of bilateral pulmonary irradiation combined with multiagent chemotherapy. At the Mayo Clinic, Rab and associates found no difference between patients who received 15 Gy and those who received no lung irradiation[174]; Newton and Barrett obtained favorable results by increasing the dose to 19.5 Gy.[150] Weichselbaum and coworkers reported on ten patients with lung metastases treated with high-dose methotrexate and bilateral whole lung radiation (15 Gy) followed by booster doses to individual metastatic lesions (additional 20 to 40 Gy); only two patients remained continuously disease free at 2 years.[224]

In the EORTC 03 study, bilateral lung irradiation to 20 Gy had the same effect on pulmonary metastasis as did adjuvant chemotherapy[22]; radiation, however, was less toxic, and successful surgical resection of residual lung lesions could be carried out more frequently in the irradiated group. The ability to resect pulmonary nodules remaining after therapy may have significant prognostic implications.[132] In the French Bone Tumor Study Group, prophylactic bilateral lung irradiation was given simultaneously with two alternating drug combinations[70]; 16 of 41 patients developed metastasis and died within 60 months. Although the role of prophylactic lung irradiation remains unclear and is unaccepted in the United States, it may warrant prospective randomized studies, especially if it can be safely combined with effective chemotherapeutic regimens.

CHONDROSARCOMA

Chondrosarcomas often occur as large lesions in sites where surgical resection is not feasible. Conventional irradiation regimens can increase symptom-free survival for patients with these lesions; innovative approaches utilizing hyperfractionation, radiation sensitizers, particle beams, and chemotherapy, by either systemic or intraarterial infusion, may hold better promise for these patients.

Krochak and coworkers, at the Princess Margaret Hospital, reported on 38 irradiated patients, 9 of whom had concomitant chemotherapy.[117] Minimum radiation doses of 40 Gy were utilized; 5- and 10-year survival rates were 41 and 36%, respectively, with 13 of 25 patients in the group with favorable histologic findings remaining progression free at 10 years. Of the nine patients treated with Cyclophosphamide, vincristine, doxorubicin (Adriamycin), and dacarbazine (DTIC), only one of seven with favorable histologic findings had disease progression. They concluded that chondrosarcoma is not radioresistant and that radiation therapy is a viable alternative for patients with unresectable disease, as well as for those in whom surgery would cause unacceptable morbidity.

Particle beam studies show encouraging results. In 20 patients with unresectable tumors treated by McNaney and colleagues with a combination of neutrons and photons (40 to 70 Gy), the 5-year survival rate was 65%[137]; two patients with recurrent disease were salvaged by surgery. Austin-Seymour and associates reported on 68 patients with chondrosarcomas or chordomas of the skull base treated with the proton beam, achieving an 82% actuarial 5-year local control, while complications were kept at very low levels.[10]

EWING'S SARCOMA

Until two decades ago, disease-free survival for patients with Ewing's sarcoma was dismal, as most patients had undetected metastatic disease at presentation. The advent of effective chemotherapeutic regimens has significantly increased disease-free survival.[217] With improved results for control of metastatic disease, the issue of local control of the primary lesion acquired a new perspective, as local treatment failures and complications after primary irradiation became increasingly evident.[160]

The ability of Ewing's sarcoma to extend throughout the marrow cavity and into the adjacent soft tissue compartments makes the delineation of radiotherapy portals a complex problem. Most authors recommend the inclusion of the whole affected bone and soft tissue compartments, sparing only uninvolved epiphyseal areas (if at all possible) and a strip of soft tissue away from the primary tumor. Shrinking field technique treatment programs have to be carefully planned to avoid marginal recurrences.[170] Delineation of marrow involvement patterns by CT numbers, as well as special attention to areas of soft tissue extension, are requirements for precise treatment planning.[13] It is feasible to deliver postoperative irradiation with bone prosthesis, even expandable ones, as long as the radiation scatter characteristics of the prosthetic material are known.

Ewing's sarcoma is regarded as a radiosensitive tumor; *in vitro* studies by Kinsella and coworkers showed no repair of potentially lethal damage after 4.5 Gy in plateau-phase Ewing's sarcoma cells.[113] Well-tolerated doses of radiation therapy could sterilize areas of potential microscopic spread, such as soft tissue margins and the marrow cavity of long bones. Doses in excess of 60 Gy are likely to produce severe late morbidity without improving local control; lesions greater than 10 cm were almost never sterilized by irradiation alone, regardless of the dose delivered.[21]

In the Intergroup Ewing's Sarcoma Study I (IESS-I), patients were treated with radiation therapy to the primary bone lesion as well as both lungs (15 to 18 Gy to the latter) and randomized into two chemotherapy groups. Results showed increased survival rates for patients who received a four-drug regimen (VACA, vincristine, actinomycin D, cyclophosphamide, and doxorubicin [Adriamycin]) and a much worse prognosis for those with primary pelvic lesions.[161] Evans and associates reviewed the records of 62 patients with pelvic primary tumors entered in the IESS-I protocol[63]; local recurrence developed in 27% of these, and there was no dose-response curve above 46 Gy. On the basis of these results, the IESS-II study separated pelvic and long bone primary tumors, delivering more intensive upfront chemotherapy to the former. Radiation doses were 45 Gy to the whole bone with two cone-down field boosts of 5 Gy each to the lesion with its soft tissue extension.

The St. Jude's Children's Research Hospital evaluated 18 patients with metastatic Ewing's sarcoma treated with chemotherapy and lower doses of radiation (30 to 35 Gy)[91]; only one of six children with tumors smaller than 8 cm developed a local failure, whereas 7 of 12 patients with larger tumors have experienced recurrence.

At the Instituto Ortopedico Rizzoli, Italy, higher dose levels of 35 to 45 Gy were given after surgical resection of the primary tumor; patients with unresectable lesions or those who refused surgery were treated with radiation alone (60 Gy).[12] Local recurrences were 8% in the operated group and 36% for the ones treated with radiation only; this difference translated into better disease-free survival rates (60 and 28%, respectively). The authors recommended that all patients be evaluated for surgical resection of the primary tumor, especially if it is in expendable bone. The radiation dose effectively controlled microscopic disease in patients who underwent resection, while yielding acceptable functional results.

Several multimodality regimens, which include surgical resection of the primary tumor, are currently being evaluated. The German Cooperative Ewing's Sarcoma Study compared patients treated by amputation, conservative surgery followed by irradiation (36 Gy), and radiation therapy alone (36 Gy whole bone plus 10 to 24 Gy cone-down irradiation to the tumor with a 2-cm margin). Of 29 patients irradiated after resection, nine (31%) experienced recurrence, while 18 of 32 patients (56%) treated with radiation alone demonstrated local treatment failure; there was no significant difference in local control between 46 and 60 Gy; review of treatment techniques revealed that poor tumor localization was responsible for a large proportion of local recurrences.[105] In the follow-up German study, Dunst and colleagues reported excellent (92%) local control rates utilizing postoperative split-course hyperfractionated irradiation to a total dose of 46 Gy, combined with chemotherapy.[54]

In a review of 140 patients treated at the Mayo Clinic, Wilkins described major radiation-induced complications in 11%, including differences in limb length greater than 4 cm and severe joint contractures that required surgical correction; one patient required amputation.[225] In an attempt to decrease radiation-induced morbidity, the Pediatric Oncology Group is currently studying the effectiveness of "tailored ports" that include the primary tumor (as defined by CT and MRI scanning) with a 2-cm margin; results are not yet available.[50]

Marcus studied the effectiveness of hyperfractionation in reducing radiation-induced morbidity, delivering 1.2 Gy twice daily (50.4 to 60 Gy total dose), with 1 of 11 standard-risk patients experiencing local relapse and no patients demonstrating severe reactions; total body irradiation (TBI), 8 Gy in two fractions, followed by autologous bone marrow transplantation was utilized for poor-risk patients, with nine of ten patients being relapse free at median follow-up of 22 months.[133] At the National Cancer Institute, high-risk patients (with pelvic primary tumors or metastatic disease at diagnosis) were submitted to the same intense regimen; 10 of 21 patients have thus far relapsed.[144] Because of their systemic failure rates, high-risk Ewing's sarcoma patients, such as those presenting with metastatic disease, central axis lesions, or proximal extremity localized lesions are being entered into protocols combining intensive chemotherapy, TBI, and bone marrow transplantation[167]; results of these studies are forthcoming.

At the Mount Sinai Medical Center, the authors treated 25 patients with neoadjuvant chemotherapy and limb-preserving surgery followed by irradiation and maintenance chemotherapy. The whole bone was irradiated with 36 Gy, and a boost of an additional 9 Gy was delivered to the tumor bed with 5-cm margins. Treatment volumes were defined with the aid of CT scans, MRI images, and arteriograms. Special attention was paid to the bone marrow CT numbers that define the volume of intramedullary tumor involvement and to areas of soft tissue extension. In cases in which expandable bone prostheses were implanted, the metal scatter pattern was determined before surgery using a radiation beam scanner so that appropriate dose corrections and custom-made radiation blocks could be prepared. Only one local recurrence was observed with follow-up ranging from 6 months to 4 years.

One of the most complex technical challenges in radiation therapy is the delivery of high tumoricidal doses to lesions of the hands and the feet while preserving normal function. Kinsella treated seven patients with such Ewing's sarcomas with 50 Gy, utilizing elaborate treatment techniques; five remain disease free and with excellent motor and sensory function.[112] Head and neck bone primary tumors, although rare, carry an excellent prognosis; in a review of ten patients, 80% survived for 3 years and no recurrences were noted beyond 5 years' follow-up.[192]

SOFT TISSUE SARCOMAS

Soft tissue sarcomas have been traditionally classified as radioresistant, radical surgery being considered the sole modality of curative treatment. With the utilization of modern surgical limb preservation techniques, the problem of local recurrence has become relevant.[24, 203] Although high-grade lesions commonly have systemic spread, local recurrence is generally associated with decreased survival[33]; several multimodality regimens including preoperative and postoperative radiation are currently being evaluated.[45, 58]

The advantages of preoperative radiation include the treatment of smaller target volumes (as muscle planes have not been violated by the surgical procedure), the inactivation of a large number of peripheral tumor cells (with reduced chance of contamination in the operative field), histologic evaluation of radiation effect in the surgical specimen, and the conversion of patients with inoperable disease into candidates for limb-preserving procedures.[226]

Barkley and colleagues reported on 114 patients treated preoperatively with 50 Gy in 5 weeks[14]; there were 11 local failures, 4 occurring simultaneously with distant metastases. Failures were correlated with anaplastic histologic features and tumor size greater than 15 cm. Complications occurred in 14% of patients; these were mainly edema and soft tissue necrosis. Distant metastases were the main cause of failure, appearing in 35 patients (30%).

At the Massachusetts General Hospital, Suit and associates treated 60 patients with preoperative doses of 60 Gy, six (10%) of whom experienced local failure.[204] The major complication was delayed wound healing in 17 patients; nine healed conservatively, seven required skin grafting, and one required amputation. In an attempt to decrease surgical complications, Tepper and Suit modified the regimen to 50 Gy preoperative irradiation, followed by limb-sparing resection and a postoperative or intraoperative boost dose of 14 Gy[207]; in 60 patients so treated, local control was 84% and the 5-year survival rate was 69%; there were no major wound healing delays.

A group at UCLA studied the combination of preoperative radiation therapy (35 Gy in ten fractions) and intraarterial doxorubicin (Adriamycin), immediately followed by conservative resection.[57] There were three local recurrences in 96 patients (3.1%). High complication rates, however, required reduction of the total radiation dose to 17.5 Gy. Other groups reported similarly high local control rates with intraarterial chemotherapy and radiation, with good functional and cosmetic results in 84 to 94% of patients with unresectable high-grade lesions.[79, 94, 130]

The histologic response of soft tissue sarcomas to hyperfractionated preoperative radiation was studied by Willett and colleagues.[226] Patients were treated with 47.7 Gy in two daily fractions of 1.8 Gy each, given 4 hours apart. Six patients with lesions larger than 10 cm exhibited a marked histologic response, whereas only three of seven patients treated once a day exhibited the same degree of necrosis. Twice-a-day fractionation could be an effective method for the treatment of large lesions that would otherwise require amputation.

The degree to which a sarcoma responds to preoperative therapy can be of prognostic value. Huth and associates correlated survival rates with histologic response, finding 82 and 55% 4-year survival rates for good and poor responders, respectively.[98]

Postoperative radiation therapy allows for histologic evaluation of the entire specimen and does not interfere with typing and grading. There is no delay in surgery, and wound healing is not affected.[7] The actual tumor margins can be assessed and outlined with radiopaque clips. At the National Cancer Institute, patients were assigned randomly to amputation or limb-sparing procedures followed by radiation therapy, with no difference in survival between the two groups.[169] Suit and associates utilized elaborate multiportal techniques for the irradiation of 110 patients who received 50 Gy to a wide field, encompassing the muscle compartment, followed by boosts with shrinking fields to the minimal total dose of 60 Gy to the tumor bed[204]; local control was 84% for grossly resected lesions, with good functional results.

At the Roswell Park Memorial Institute, 82 patients with extremity lesions were initially submitted to limb-sparing surgical procedures; no further therapy was given if margins were greater than 2 cm; the 5-year local recurrence rate was 17%. When margins were closer than 2 cm, patients received postoperative radiation as described by Suit and associates,[204] yielding a 7% 5-year recurrence rate. Histologic grade had no impact on local control, although survival was significantly better for well-differentiated lesions.[107]

In France, Abbatucci conducted a trial of "sandwich" preoperative and postoperative radiation[1]; 113 patients received 6.5 Gy in two sessions, followed by surgery after 48 hours, and more radiation (minimum 41.5 Gy), bringing the total dose to 50 to 60 Gy. The local recurrence rate was 13.6% for the entire group but only 1.9% in patients who underwent gross complete resection. Five-year survival rates were 65.6% for the entire group and 75% for the 85 patients treated with curative intent.

Results with conventional radiation therapy alone were reported by Tepper and Suit[208]; having received 64 Gy through multiportal techniques, 11 of 51 patients were alive and disease free after 5 years' minimal follow-up; lesions in 43.5% of patients were controlled locally. Pickering and colleagues studied the effect of fast neutron therapy on 50 unresectable sarcomas, reporting a 68% complete regression rate and 52% local control.[166] Although fast neutron therapy yielded lower recurrence rates than those observed in conventional photon irradiation studies, skin and soft tissue complications were more frequent and severe.

Radiation treatment techniques for soft tissue sarcomas remain somewhat controversial; some investigators advocate treating the tumor with a "safety margin," whereas others irradiate the entire muscle compartment. A few principles, however, appear to be universally adopted:

1. The sparing of a strip of normal tissue along the irradiated extremity to minimize postirradiation edema
2. The utilization of shrinking field techniques, with doses of about 50 Gy to large volumes and 55 to 65 Gy to smaller or "final" target volumes, all delivered at the rate of 9 to 10 Gy per week
3. Precise immobilization techniques for daily treatment reproduction
4. Multiportal arrangements
5. The utilization of custom field shaping and computerized treatment planning whenever feasible.[35]

Retroperitoneal sarcomas remain a therapeutic challenge, owing to their advanced stage at diagnosis and the difficulties of irradiating a target area containing large volumes of small bowel, kidney, and spinal cord.[227] In a review of the Yale University experience, Harrison and associates established that local control and survival were dose dependent[87]; among ten patients irradiated after biopsy only, the four who received an average dose of 44 Gy survived 1 year, compared with no survivors at 1 year among the six patients who received an average dose of 27 Gy. The Massachusetts General Hospital group recommended preoperative irradiation for unresectable lesions (40 to 50 Gy), followed by an attempt at surgical resection; postoperative treatment of resectable disease should aim to deliver similar doses, although tolerance becomes a problem with conventional therapy methods.[209]

At the National Cancer Institute, Kinsella and coworkers randomly assigned 35 adults with resectable retroperitoneal soft tissue sarcomas to two treatment groups: intraoperative therapy (20 Gy with electrons plus 35 to 40 Gy external irradiation) and standard therapy (50 to 55 Gy)[115]; 40% of all patients were alive at 5 years, with 20% disease free, and there was no significant survival difference between the two groups. Adjuvant chemotherapy did not seem to improve survival but significantly increased morbidity.[77]

The conservative treatment of sarcomas of the hands and the feet is challenging to the radiation oncology team; meticulous positioning and treatment planning are required to avoid severe complications; nail beds should be excluded from the beams whenever possible.[110] Okuneieff and associates reviewed 17 patients treated at the Massachusetts General Hospital, with 87% local control and near-normal hand function.[152] Amputation has yielded 68% local control rates in similar situations.[155] Head and neck primary tumors can be effectively treated by postoperative irradiation, a 45-Gy wide field with 15 to 18 Gy cone-down doses, at low daily dose rates to avoid intense acute mucosal reactions; 10 of 16 patients so treated were disease free with median follow-up time of 43 months; local control was 75%.[136]

Interstitial implantation of iridium-192 is utilized for tumor bed irradiation of popliteal and antecubital lesions at Memorial Sloan-Kettering Cancer Center; external beam irradiation of these areas can induce severe changes in the underlying joint spaces, which can be spared by implants owing to the rapid fall-off of iridium-192 radiation. Treatment takes only 5 days and is completed before the patient is discharged from the hospital for the original surgical procedure. Local control is almost universal, with eight of ten patients alive and disease free beyond 4 years.[190, 191]

The value of complex multimodality regimens combining chemotherapy, radiation therapy, and surgical resection is now well established in pediatric sarcomas; despite increased early local reactions and chemotherapy toxicity, survival results are much improved.[49, 229] Impressive results, with up to 93% 5-year survival in early-stage disease, were obtained by the Intergroup Rhabdomyosarcoma Study I.[135] Pelvic lesions in adolescents and young adults have a particularly poor prognosis; in a review of 23 such patients, Stea and coworkers achieved universal local control with combined intensive chemotherapy and radiation[202]; the seven patients with metastasis all died of disease shortly thereafter.

Synovial sarcomas of childhood also carry a poor prognosis; Horowitz and colleagues,[96] reviewing the experience at the St. Jude's Children's Research Hospital, found only 1 survivor among 26 patients with incompletely resected tumors, even when the patients underwent aggressive multimodality therapy regimens.[96] Malignant fibrous histiocytomas have patterns of spread and prognosis similar to those of pediatric rhabdomyosarcomas; in a review of seven children treated at the Children's Hospital of Philadelphia, three of five with residual disease after surgery experienced a complete response to doses ranging from 15 to 55 Gy.[175] Peripheral neuroepitheliomas, being small round cell tumors, can resemble Ewing's sarcoma in histologic pattern and behavior; multimodal regimens, including radiation, yield 94% complete remission and 68% actuarial 5-year survival.[143]

Some unusual soft tissue sarcomas benefit from therapeutic irradiation. In a review of 14 hemangiopericytomas treated at the M. D. Anderson Hospital and Tumor Institute, there were no local recurrences, and nine patients were disease free from 3.5 to 20 years after irradiation.[104] Although their regression after radiotherapy can be slow, these tumors should not be regarded as radioresistant. Desmoid tumors, or aggressive fibromatoses, also respond slowly to irradiation; 17 such patients were irradiated at the Massachusetts General Hospital; lesions in eight of ten treated with radiation alone achieved stabilization; the regression rate of the whole group was 76%; latent periods up to 27 months were required to observe complete responses.[108] Good local results were also observed in epithelioid sarcomas and low-grade synovial sarcomas[25, 189]; the frequency of metastatic disease in high-grade or proximal lesions calls for the study of integrated radiotherapeutic and chemotherapeutic regimens.

Accumulating evidence suggests that limb-preserving surgery with adjuvant chemotherapy and radiation therapy yields the highest cure and local control rates as well as the best quality of life for patients with soft tissue sarcoma. The development of the ideal regimen, however, still remains a challenge for the multidisciplinary team.

OTHER BONE NEOPLASMS

Non-Hodgkin's Lymphoma of Bone

Although most non-Hodgkin's lymphomas present as systemic disease, localized bone lesions can be effectively eradicated with radiation alone, with local recurrence rates ranging from 14 to 47%.[52] At the Mayo Clinic, Ostrowski and coworkers delivered 40 Gy to the entire bone, followed by a boost of 5 to 10 Gy to the tumor, and reported a 53% survival rate at 10 years.[154] The primary site was a major prognostic factor, with mandibular lymphomas presenting a much higher local recurrence rate, and pelvic primary tumors having an increased incidence of systemic involvement (24% 5-year survival). The addition of intensive chemotherapy regimens has improved disease-free survival to 88% at 5 years, with almost no local recurrences seen with radiation doses between 40 and 50 Gy.[11]

Patients with aggressive lymphomas who present with stage IV disease may benefit from prophylactic central nervous system irradiation or from TBI before autologous bone marrow transplantation.[27]

Loeffler and colleagues reviewed the Harvard Joint Center for Radiation Therapy experience with primary lymphoma of bone in 11 pediatric patients[126]; treatment consisted of 40 Gy of whole bone irradiation followed by a boost of 10 Gy to the primary lesion (total tumor dose 50 Gy), concomitantly with doxorubicin (Adriamycin), prednisone, and vincristine (Oncovin) chemotherapy; prophylactic brain irradiation therapy was part of the treatment program. There were no local relapses at 8 years' follow-up; two patients, however, developed second primary tumors in the radiation field, raising the question of the carcinogenicity of the regimen.

Plasmacytoma

Solitary plasmacytomas can be found in bone or soft tissues; although local results with radiation therapy can be equally good for both entities, bone lesions tend to progress to multiple myeloma and carry a less favorable prognosis.[28, 81] Doses in the range of 40 to 50 Gy are recommended,[116] with 40 Gy curing approximately 94% of recorded patients.[138]

Multiple Myeloma

Pain relief is the goal of radiation therapy in multiple myeloma, a systemic disease in which only chemotherapy has an impact on survival. Effective palliation is usually achieved by utilizing doses between 20 and 24 Gy in relatively rapid fractionation schedules.[151] Patients are usually subjected to multiple courses of palliative radiation for symptomatic bone lesions during the progression of their disease. Portals should include the entire affected bone.

Attempts at half body irradiation (HBI), given either sequentially or to the most symptomatic half, resulted in good palliative effects; bone marrow and lung toxicity, however, limit the usefulness of these regimens.[173, 182] Tobias and coworkers delivered single fractions of 7.5 Gy for upper hemibody and 10 Gy for lower hemibody irradiation; 11 of 13 patients had significant reduction in pain medicine requirements and tolerated treatment better, with only 2 patients requiring transfusion.[212] TBI followed by bone marrow transplantation is currently under investigation for refractory myelomas.[228]

Giant Cell Tumor of Bone

With the refinement in surgical techniques, the use of radiation therapy in this relatively benign but locally aggressive entity is diminishing, being currently reserved for unresectable lesions, or for the histologically aggressive ones after undergoing partial excision. Doses in excess of 40 Gy are required.[29, 44]

Histiocytosis X

Although the syndromes constituting histiocytosis X were originally categorized as neoplasms, their indolent nature lends them to conservative management.[125] Radiation therapy is employed in the treatment of localized bone lesions or when bone deformities, pathologic fractures, ocular compression, and cranial nerve dysfunction are present; diabetes insipidus, characteristic of many of these syndromes, can be effectively controlled by pituitary irradiation. Radiation doses range between 5 and 15 Gy at conventional fractionation, depending on the size and location of the target lesion.[82, 198]

Bone Metastases

Palliation of symptomatic bone metastasis is one of the most frequently encountered problems in oncology. It is estimated that more than 30% of metastatic bone sites require radiation therapy.[72] Lesions in weight-bearing areas with greater than 50% cortical destruction should initially undergo surgical treatment in an attempt to prevent pathologic fracture; postoperative radiotherapy should be given to prevent tumor regrowth and the necessity for prosthetic displacement.[74]

Multiple treatment regimens have been studied for the treatment of bone metastasis, ranging from single doses of 8 to 10 Gy to 50 Gy in 5 weeks.[159] The Radiation Therapy Oncology Group conducted a prospective randomized trial of multiple-dose schedules, initially concluding that short courses were as effective as the more protracted ones[213]; analysis of long-term palliation data from the same study suggested that 30 Gy in ten sessions provided the best results, with lasting pain relief being obtained in 80% of patients so treated.[19] For patients with terminal disease, 10 Gy in one or two fractions can provide excellent short-term palliation.[4]

HBI can be utilized for patients with extensive disease with multiple painful sites. In the Radiation Therapy Oncology Group study, single doses of 6 Gy of upper HBI and 8 Gy of lower HBI were followed by pain relief within 48 hours in 80% of 168 treated patients, with 30% not needing any additional pain treatment measures.[183]

References

1. Abbatucci JS, Boulier N, Ranieri J, et al: Local control and survival in soft tissue sarcomas of the limbs, trunk walls and head and neck: A study of 113 cases. Int J Radiat Oncol Biol Phys 12:579–586, 1986.
2. Abramson DH, Ellsworth RM, Kitchin FD, Tung G: Second nonocular tumors in retinoblastoma survivors. Are they radiation-induced? Ophthalmology 91:1351–1355, 1984.
3. Ackman JD, Rouse L, Johnston CE: Radiation induced physeal injury. Orthopedics 11:343–349, 1988.
4. Allen KL, Johnson TW, Hibbs GG: Effective bone palliation as related to various treatment regimens. Cancer 37:984–987, 1976.
5. Alper T, Howard-Flanders P: Role of oxygen in modifying the radiosensitivity of *E. coli* B. Nature 178:978–979, 1956.
6. Ang KK, Thames HD, Jones SD, et al: Proliferation kinetics of a murine fibrosarcoma during fractionated irradiation. Radiat Res 116:327–336, 1988.
7. Arbeit JM, Hilaris BS, Brennan MF: Wound complications in the multimodality treatment of extremity and superficial truncal sarcomas. J Clin Oncol 5:480–488, 1987.
8. Ashby MA, Ago CT, Harmer CL: Hypofractionated radiotherapy for sarcomas. Int J Radiat Oncol Biol Phys 12:13–17, 1986.
9. Austin-Seymour MM, Munzenrider JE, Goitein M, et al: Progress in low-LET heavy particle therapy: Intracranial and paracranial tumors and uveal melanomas. Radiat Res 104(Suppl):S219–226, 1985.
10. Austin-Seymour M, Munzenrider J, Goitein M, et al: Fractionated proton radiation therapy of chordoma and low-grade chondrosarcoma of the base of skull. J Neurosurg 70:13–17, 1989.
11. Bacci G, Jaffe N, Emiliani E, et al: Therapy for primary non-Hodgkin's lymphoma of bone and a comparison of results with Ewing's sarcoma. Cancer 57:1468–1472, 1986.
12. Bacci G, Toni A, Avella M, et al: Long term results in 144 localized Ewing's sarcoma patients treated with combined therapy. Cancer 63:1477–1486, 1989.
13. Barbieri E, Emiliani E, Zini G, et al: Computed tomography in diagnosis and treatment planning for localized Ewing's sarcoma. Proc Br Inst Radiol 61:743, 1989.
14. Barkley HT, Martin RG, Romsdahl MM, et al: Treatment of soft tissue sarcomas by preoperative irradiation and conservative surgical resection. Int J Radiat Oncol Biol Phys 14:693–699, 1988.
15. Battermann JJ, Mijnheer BJ: The Amsterdam fast neutron therapy project: A final report. Int J Radiat Oncol Biol Phys 12:2093–2099, 1986.
16. Baverstock KF, Burns WG: Primary production of oxygen from irradiated water as an explanation for decreased radiobiological enhancement at high LET. Nature 260:316–318, 1976.
17. Becquerel H, Curie P: Action physiologique des rayons du radium. C R Acad Sci (Paris) 132:1289–1291, 1901.
18. Billman P, Hinkelbein W, Reinwein W: Benign and malignant tumors of the thoracic skeleton after percutaneous radiotherapy of Hodgkin's and non-Hodgkin's lymphomas. Strahlentherapie 161:699–703, 1985.
19. Blitzer P: Reanalysis of the RTOG study of the palliation of symptomatic bone metastasis. Cancer 55:1468–1472, 1985.
20. Bloomer WD, Adelstein SJ: The mammalian radiation survival curve. J Nucl Med 23:259–265, 1982.
21. Brown AP, Fixsen JA, Plowman PN: Local control of Ewing's sarcoma: An analysis of 67 patients. Br J Radiol 60:261–268, 1987.

22. Burgers JMV, Glabbeke MV, Busson A, et al: Osteosarcoma of the limbs: Report of the EORTC-SIOP 03 trial 20781 investigating the value of adjuvant treatment with chemotherapy and/or prophylactic lung irradiation. Cancer 61:1024–1031, 1988.
23. Cade S: Osteogenic sarcoma: A study based in 133 patients. J R Coll Surg Edinb 1:79–111, 1955.
24. Cantin J, McNeer GP, Chu FC, Booker RJ: The problem of local recurrence after treatment of soft tissue sarcoma. Ann Surg 168:47–53, 1968.
25. Carson JH, Harwood AR, Cummings BJ, et al: The place of radiotherapy in the treatment of synovial sarcoma. Int J Radiat Oncol Biol Phys 7:49–53, 1981.
26. Casentini L, Visona A, Colombo F, et al: Osteogenic sarcoma of the calvaria following radiotherapy for cerebellar astrocytoma: Report of a case in childhood. Tumori 71:391–396, 1985.
27. Chadha M, Shank B, Fuks Z, et al: Improved survival of poor prognosis diffuse histiocytic (large cell) lymphoma managed with sequential induction chemotherapy, boost radiation therapy and autologous bone marrow transplantation. Int J Radiat Oncol Biol Phys 14:407–415, 1988.
28. Chak LY, Cox RS, Bostwick DG, Hoppe RT: Solitary plasmacytoma of bone: Treatment, progression and survival. J Clin Oncol 5:1811–1815, 1987.
29. Chen ZX, Gu DZ, Yu ZH, et al: Radiation therapy of giant cell tumor of bone: Analysis of 35 patients. Int J Radiat Oncol Biol Phys 12:329–334, 1986.
30. Cohen L, Hendrickson F, Kurup PD, et al: Clinical evaluation of neutron beam therapy. Current results and prospects. Cancer 55:10–17, 1985.
31. Cohen L, Hendrickson F, Mansell J, et al: Response of sarcomas of bone and soft tissue to neutron beam therapy. Int J Radiat Oncol Biol Phys 10:821–824, 1984.
32. Coleman CN: Hypoxia in tumors: A paradigm for the approach to biochemical and physiologic heterogeneity. J Natl Cancer Inst 80:310–317, 1988.
33. Collin C, Goldbold J, Hadju S, Brennan MF: Localized extremity soft tissue sarcoma: An analysis of factors affecting survival. J Clin Oncol 5:601–612, 1987.
34. Concannon JP, Summers RE, King J, et al: Enhancement of x-ray effects on the small intestinal epithelium of dogs by actinomycin D. Radiology 105:126–134, 1969.
35. Consensus Conference: Limb-sparing treatment of adult soft tissue sarcomas and osteosarcomas. JAMA 254:1791–1794, 1985.
36. Coughlin CT, Richmond RC: Biologic and clinical developments of cisplatin combined with radiation: Concepts, utility, projections for new trials and the emergence of carboplatin. Semin Oncol 16(Suppl 6):31–43, 1989.
37. Coutard H: Roentgen therapy of epitheliomas of the tonsillar fossa, hypopharynx and larynx from 1920 to 1926. Am J Roentgenol 28:313–331, 1932.
38. Coutard H: Principles of x ray therapy of malignant diseases. Lancet 2:1–8, 1934.
39. Cullen BM, Walker HC: The effect of several different anesthetics on the blood pressure and heart rate of the mouse and on the radiation response of the mouse sarcoma RIF-1. Int J Radiat Biol 48:761–771, 1985.
40. Curran WJ Jr, Littman P, Raney RB: Interstitial radiation therapy in the treatment of childhood soft-tissue sarcomas. Int J Radiat Oncol Biol Phys 14:169–174, 1988.
41. D'Angio GJ: The late consequences of successful treatment given children and adolescents. Radiology 114:145, 1975.
42. D'Angio GJ, Farber S, Maddock CL: Potentiation of x-ray effect of actinomycin D. Radiology 73:175–177, 1975.
43. Dalinka MK, Mazzeo VP Jr: Complications of radiation therapy. CRC Crit Rev Diagn Imaging 23:235–267, 1985.
44. Daugaard S, Johansen HF, Barford G, et al: Radiation treatment of giant-cell tumor of bone (osteoclastoma). Acta Radiol (Oncol) 26:41–43, 1987.
45. DeVita VT, Lipman M, Hubbard SM, et al: The effect of combined modality therapy on local control and survival. Int J Radiat Oncol Biol Phys 12:487–501, 1986.
46. Dewey WC, Hopwood LE, Sapareto SA, et al: Cellular responses to combinations of hyperthermia and radiation. Radiology 123:463, 1977.
47. Dewhirst MW, Tso CY, Oliver R, et al: Morphologic and hemodynamic comparison of tumor and healing normal tissue microvasculature. Int J Radiat Oncol Biol Phys 17:91–99, 1989.
48. Dewit L: Combined treatment of radiation and *cis*-diaminedicholoroplatinum (II): A review of experimental and clinical data. Int J Radiat Oncol Biol Phys 13:403–426, 1987.
49. Donaldson SS: The value of adjuvant chemotherapy in the management of sarcomas in children. Cancer 55:2184–2197, 1985.
50. Donaldson SS: Unpublished data.
51. Dorie MJ, Kallman RF: Reoxygenation in the RIF-1 tumor. Int J Radiat Oncol Biol Phys 10:687–693, 1984.
52. Dosoretz DE, Raymond AK, Murphy GF, et al: Primary lymphoma of bone: The relationship of morphological diversity to clinical behavior. Cancer 50:1009–1014, 1982.
53. Duncan W, Arnott SJ, Jack WJ: The Edinburgh experience of treating sarcomas of soft tissue and cone with neutron irradiation. Clin Radiol 37:317–320, 1986.
54. Dunst J, Sauer R, Burgers JM, et al: Radiotherapy in Ewing's sarcoma: Current results of the German Society of Pediatric Oncology studies CESS 81 and CESS 86. Klin Pediatr 200:261–266, 1988.
55. Eichhorn HJ, Dalluge KH: Results of neutron therapy for soft tissue sarcomas. Strahlentherapie 161:801–803, 1985.
56. Eifel PJ: Decreased bone growth arrest in weaning rats with multiple radiation fractions per day. Int J Radiat Oncol Biol Phys 15:141–145, 1988.
57. Eilber FR: Soft tissue sarcomas of the extremity. Curr Probl Cancer 8:3–41, 1984.
58. Eilber FR, Morton DL, Eckhardt J, et al: Limb salvage for skeletal and soft tissue sarcomas: Multidisciplinary preoperative therapy. Cancer 54:2695–2701, 1984.
59. Elkind MM: DNA damage and cell killing: Cause and effect? Cancer 56:2351–2363, 1985.
60. Elkind MM, Sutton H: Radiation response of mammalian cells grown in culture. I. Repair of x-ray damage in surviving Chinese hamster cells. Radiat Res 13:556–593, 1960.
61. Ellis F: Dose, time and fractionation: A clinical hypothesis. Clin Radiol 20:1–7, 1969.
62. Ellis F: Is NSD-TDF useful to radiotherapy? Int J Radiat Oncol Biol Phys 11:1685–1697, 1985.
63. Evans R, Nesbit M, Askin F, et al: Local recurrence, rate and sites of metastases, and time to relapse as a function of treatment regimen, size of primary and

surgical history in 62 patients presenting with nonmetastatic Ewing's sarcoma of pelvic bones. Int J Radiat Oncol Biol Phys 11:129–136, 1985.

64. Fazekas J, Pajak TF, Wasserman T, et al: Failure of misonidazole sensitized radiotherapy to impact upon outcome among stage III–IV squamous cancers of the head and neck. Int J Radiat Oncol Biol Phys 13:1155–1160, 1987.
65. Fietkau R, Diegpen TL, Stehr L, Sauer R: Induction of malignancies by radiotherapy: A retrospective study of 454 tumors. Strahlenther Onkol 164:247–259, 1988.
66. Fletcher GH: Subclinical disease. Cancer 53:1274–1284, 1984.
67. Fletcher GH: Implications of the density of clonogenic infestation in radiotherapy. Int J Radiat Oncol Biol Phys 12:1675–1680, 1986.
68. Fraass BA, Kinsella TJ, Harrington FS, Glatstein E: Peripheral dose to the testis: The design and clinical use of a practical and effective gonadal shield. Int J Radiat Oncol Biol Phys 11:609–615, 1985.
69. Franke HD, Schmidt R: Clinical results with fast neutrons (DT, 14 MV). Radiat Med 3:151–160, 1985.
70. French Bone Tumor Study Group: Age and dose of chemotherapy as a major prognostic factor in a trial of adjuvant therapy of osteosarcoma combining two alternating drug combinations and early prophylactic lung irradiation. Cancer 61:1304–1311, 1988.
71. Fromm M, Littman P, Raney RB, Nelson L, Handler S, Diamond G, Stanley C: Late effects after treatment of twenty children with soft tissue sarcomas of the head and neck. Experience at a single institution with review of the literature. Cancer 57:2070–2076, 1986.
72. Front D, Scheneck SO, Frankel A, et al: Bone metastases and bone pain in breast cancer. JAMA 42:1747–1748, 1979.
73. Gaitan-Yanguas M: A study of the response of osteogenic sarcoma and adjacent normal tissues to irradiation. Int J Radiation Oncol Biol Phys 7:593–595, 1981.
74. Galasko CSB: The management of skeletal metastases. J R Coll Surg Edinb 3:148–151, 1980.
75. Giovanella BC, Stehlin JS, Morgan AC: Selective lethal effect of supranormal temperatures on human neoplastic cells. Cancer Res 36:3944, 1976.
76. Glaholm J, Harmer C: Soft tissue sarcoma: Neutrons versus photons for post-operative irradiation. Br J Radiol 61:829–834, 1988.
77. Glenn J, Sindelar WF, Kinsella TJ, et al: Results of multimodality therapy of resectable soft tissue sarcomas of the retroperitoneum. Surgery 97:316–325, 1985.
78. Gonzalez DG, Breuer K: Clinical data from irradiated growing long bones in children. Int J Radiat Oncol Biol Phys 9:841–846, 1983.
79. Goodnight JE Jr, Bargar WL, Voegeli T, Blaisdell FW: Limb-sparing surgery for extremity sarcomas after preoperative intraarterial doxorubicin and radiation therapy. Am J Surg 150:109–113, 1985.
80. Gray LH, Conger AD, Ebert M, et al: The concentration of oxygen dissolved in tissues at the time of irradiation as a factor in radiotherapy. Br J Radiol 26:638, 1953.
81. Greenberg P, Parker RG, Fu YS, Abemayor E: The treatment of solitary plasmacytoma of bone and extramedullary plasmacytoma. Am J Clin Oncol 10:199–204, 1987.
82. Greenberger JS, Cassady JR, Jaffe N, Wawter G, Crocker A: Radiation therapy in patients with histiocytosis. Management of diabetes insipidus and bone lesions. Int J Radiat Oncol Biol Phys 5:1749, 1979.
83. Griesser GH, Hansmann ML: Soft tissue sarcoma as second malignant lesion after therapy for Hodgkin's disease. Report of two cases and review of the literature. J Cancer Res Clin Oncol 110:238–243, 1985.
84. Hall EJ: Radiosensitivity and cell age in the mitotic cycle. *In* Hall EJ: Radiobiology for the Radiologist, 3rd ed. Philadelphia, JB Lippincott, 1988.
85. Hall EJ: The oxygen effect and reoxygenation. *In* Hall EJ: Radiobiology for the Radiologist, 3rd ed. Philadelphia, JB Lippincott, 1988.
86. Hall EJ: Cell survival curves. *In* Hall EJ: Radiobiology for the Radiologist, 3rd ed. Philadelphia, JB Lippincott, 1988.
87. Harrison LB, Gutierrez E, Fischer JJ: Retroperitoneal sarcomas: The Yale experience and a review of the literature. J Surg Oncol 32:159–164, 1986.
88. Hartsell WF, Hanson WR, Conterato DJ, Hendrickson FR: Hyperfractionation decreases the deleterious effects of conventional radiation fractionation on vertebral growth in animals. Cancer 63:2452–2455, 1989.
89. Hatlinghus S, Rode L, Christense I, Vaage S: Sarcoma following irradiation for breast cancer. Report of three unusual cases including one malignant mesenchymoma of bone. Acta Radiol (Oncol) 25:239–242, 1986.
90. Hawkins MM, Draper GJ, Kingston E: Incidence of second primary tumors among childhood cancer survivors. Br J Cancer 56:339–347, 1987.
91. Hayes FA, Thompson EI, Parvey L, et al: Metastatic Ewing's sarcoma: Remission induction and survival. J Clin Oncol 5:1199–1204, 1987.
92. Henk JM: Does hyperbaric oxygen have a future in radiation therapy? Int J Radiat Oncol Biol Phys 7:1125, 1981.
93. Hirst DG: Anemia: A problem or an opportunity in radiotherapy? Int J Radiat Oncol Biol Phys 12:2009–2017, 1986.
94. Hoekstra HJ, Koops HS, Molenaar WM, et al: A combination of intraarterial chemotherapy, preoperative and postoperative radiotherapy, and surgery as limb-saving treatment of primarily unresectable high-grade soft tissue sarcomas of the extremities. Cancer 63:59–62, 1989.
95. Hofer KG, Lakkis M, Hofer MG: Cytocidal effects of misonidazole, RO-03-8799 and RSU-1164 on euoxic and hypoxic BP-8 murine sarcoma cells at normal and elevated temperatures. Cancer 63:1501–1508, 1989.
96. Horowitz ME, Pratt CB, Webber BL, et al: Therapy for childhood soft-tissue sarcomas other than rhabdomyosarcoma: A review of 62 cases treated at a single institution. J Clin Oncol 4:559–564, 1986.
97. Howland WJ, Loeffler RK, Starchman DE, Johnson RB: Post irradiation atrophic changes of bone and related complications. Radiology 117:677–685, 1975.
98. Huth JF, Mirra JJ, Eilber FR: Assessment of *in vivo* response to preoperative chemotherapy and radiation therapy as a predictor of survival in patients with soft-tissue sarcoma. Am J Clin Oncol 8:497–503, 1985.
99. Huvos AG, Woodard HQ: Postirradiation sarcomas of bone. Health Phys 55:631–636, 1988.
100. Huvos AG, Woodard HQ, Cahan WG, et al: Postirradiation osteogenic sarcoma of bone and soft tissues. A clinicopathologic study of 66 patients. Cancer 55:1244–1255, 1985.

101. Ito H, Barkley T Jr, Peters LJ, Milas L: Modification of tumor response to cyclophosphamide and irradiation by preirradiation of the tumor bed. Prolonged growth delay but reduced curability. Int J Radiat Oncol Biol Phys 11:547–553, 1985.
102. Ito H, Meistrich ML, Barkley T Jr, Thames HD, Milas L: Protection of acute and late radiation damage of the gastrointestinal tract by WR-2721. Int J Radiat Oncol Biol Phys 12:211–219, 1986.
103. Jacobsson M, Kalebo P, Tjellstrom A, Turesson I: Bone cell viability after irradiation. An enzyme histochemical study. Acta Oncol 26:463–465, 1987.
104. Jha N, McNeese M, Barkley HT Jr, Kong J: Does radiotherapy have a role in hemangiopericytoma management? Report on 14 new cases and a review of the literature. Int J Radiat Oncol Biol Phys 13:1399–1402, 1987.
105. Jurgens H, Exner U, Gadner H, et al: Multidisciplinary treatment of primary Ewing's sarcoma of bone. A 6 year experience of a European cooperative trial. Cancer 61:23–32, 1988.
106. Kallman RF: The phenomenon of reoxygenation and its implications for fractionated radiotherapy. Radiology 105:135–142, 1972.
107. Karakousis CP, Emrich LJ, Rao U, Krishnamsetty RM: Feasibility of limb salvage and survival in soft tissue sarcoma. Cancer 57:484–491, 1986.
108. Kiel KD, Suit HD: Radiation therapy in the treatment of aggressive fibromatoses (desmoid tumors). Cancer 54:2051–2055, 1984.
109. Kim JH, Alfieri AA, Kim SH, Fuks Z: The potentiation of radiation response on murine tumor by flutarabine phosphate. Cancer Lett 31:69–76, 1986.
110. Kinsella TJ: Limited surgery and radiation therapy for sarcomas of the hand and foot. Int J Radiat Oncol Biol Phys 12:2045–2046, 1986.
111. Kinsella TJ, Glatstein E: Clinical experience with intravenous radiosensitizers in unresectable sarcomas. Cancer 59:908–915, 1987.
112. Kinsella TJ, Loeffler JS, Fraass BA, Tepper J: Extremity preservation by combined modality therapy in sarcomas of the hand and foot: An analysis of local control, disease free survival and functional results. Int J Radiat Oncol Biol Phys 9:1115–1119, 1983.
113. Kinsella TJ, Mitchell JB, McPherson S, et al: *In vitro* radiation studies on Ewing's sarcoma cell lines and human bone marrow. Application to the clinical use of total body irradiation (TBI). Int J Radiat Oncol Biol Phys 10:1005–1011, 1984.
114. Kinsella TJ, Russo A, Mitchell JB, et al: A phase I study of intravenous iododeoxyuridine as a clinical radiosensitizer. Int J Radiat Oncol Biol Phys 11:1041–1046, 1985.
115. Kinsella TJ, Sindelar WF, Lack E, et al: Preliminary results of a randomized study of adjuvant radiation therapy in resectable adult retroperitoneal soft tissue sarcomas. J Clin Oncol 6:18–25, 1988.
116. Knowling MA, Harwood AR, Bergsagel DE: Comparison of extramedullary plasmacytomas with solitary and multiple plasma cell tumors of bone. J Clin Oncol 1:255, 1983.
117. Krochak R, Harwood AR, Cummings BJ, Quirt IC: Results of radical radiation for chondrosarcoma of bone. Radiother Oncol 1:109–115, 1983.
118. Kumar PP, Good RR, Jones EO: Techniques to deliver high dose localized irradiation for tissue sparing management of sarcomas. Radiat Med 6:171–178, 1988.
119. Kurtz JM, Amalric R, Brandone H, et al: Contralateral breast cancer and other second malignancies in patients treated by breast-conserving therapy with radiation. Int J Radiat Oncol Biol Phys 15:277–284, 1988.
120. Kuten A, Sapir D, Cohen Y, et al: Postirradiation soft tissue sarcoma occurring in breast cancer patients: Report of seven cases and results of combination chemotherapy. J Surg Oncol 28:168–171, 1985.
121. Lampert MH, Gerber LH, Glatstein E, et al: Soft tissue sarcoma: Functional outcome after wide local excision and radiation therapy. Arch Phys Med Rehabil 65:477–480, 1984.
122. Laskin WB, Silverman TA, Enzinger FM: Postirradiation soft tissue sarcomas. An analysis of 53 cases. Cancer 62:2330–2340, 1988.
123. Leopold KA, Harrelson J, Prosnitz L, et al: Preoperative hyperthermia and radiation for soft tissue sarcomas: Advantage of two versus one hyperthermia treatments per week. Int J Radiat Oncol Biol Phys 16:107–115, 1989.
124. Lewis MM: The use of an expandable and adjustable prosthesis in the treatment of childhood malignant bone tumors of the extremity. Cancer 57:499–502, 1986.
125. Lipton JM: The pathogenesis, diagnosis and treatment of histiocytosis syndromes. Pediatr Dermatol 1:112–120, 1983.
126. Loeffler JS, Tarbell NJ, Kozakewich H, et al: Primary lymphoma of bone in children: Analysis of treatment results with Adriamycin, prednisone, Oncovin (APO) and local radiation therapy. J Clin Oncol 4:496–501, 1986.
127. Looney WB, Hopkins HA, Carter WH: Solid tumor models for the assessment of different treatment modalities. XXII. The alternate utilization of radiotherapy and chemotherapy. Cancer 54:416–425, 1984.
128. Luce EA: The irradiated wound. Surg Clin North Am 64:821–829, 1984.
129. Mandell L, Ghavimi F, Exelby P, Fuks Z: Preliminary results of alternating combination chemotherapy (CT) and hyperfractionated radiotherapy (HART) in advanced rhabdomyosarcoma (RMS). Int J Radiat Oncol Biol Phys 15:197–203, 1988.
130. Mantravadi RVP, Trippon MJ, Patel MK, et al: Limb salvage in extremity soft tissue sarcoma: Combined modality therapy. Radiology 152:523–526, 1984.
131. Marchese MJ, Minarik L, Hall EJ, Zaider M: Potentially lethal damage repair in cell lines of radioresistant human tumors and normal skin fibroblasts. Int J Radiat Biol 48:431–439, 1985.
132. Marcove RC, Lewis MM: Prolonged survival in osteogenic sarcoma with multiple pulmonary metastasis. J Bone Joint Surg 55A:1516–1520, 1973.
133. Marcus RB, Graham-Pole JR, Springfield DS, et al: High-risk Ewing's sarcoma: End-intensifications using autologous bone marrow transplantation. Int J Radiat Oncol Biol Phys 15:53–59, 1988.
134. Martinez A, Goffinet DR, Donaldson SS, et al: Intraarterial infusion of radiosensitizer (BUdR) combined with hypofractionated irradiation and chemotherapy for primary treatment of osteogenic sarcoma. Int J Radiat Oncol Biol Phys 11:123–128, 1985.
135. Maurer HM, Beltandady M, Gehan EA, et al: The Intergroup Rhabdomyosarcoma Study—I. A final report. Cancer 61:209–220, 1988.
136. McKenna WG, Barnes MM, Kinsella TJ, et al: Combined modality treatment of adult soft tissue

sarcomas of the head and neck. Int J Radiat Oncol Biol Phys 13:1127–1133, 1987.
137. McNaney D, Lindberg RD, Ayala A, et al: Fifteen year radiotherapy experience with chondrosarcoma of bone. Int J Radiat Oncol Biol Phys 8:187–190, 1982.
138. Mendenhall CM, Thar TL, Million RR: Solitary plasmacytoma of bone and soft tissue. Int J Radiat Oncol Biol Phys 6:1497–1501, 1980.
139. Milas L, Hunter N, Peters LJ: The tumor bed effect: Dependence of tumor take, growth rate and metastasis on the time interval between irradiation and tumor cell transplantation. Int J Radiat Oncol Biol Phys 13:379–383, 1987.
140. Milas L, Hunter N, Peters LJ: Tumor bed effect—induced reduction of tumor radiocurability through the increased ion hypoxic cell fraction. Int J Radiat Oncol Biol Phys 16:139–142, 1989.
141. Milas L, Hunter NM, Ito H, Brock WA, Peters LJ: Increase in radiosensitivity of lung micrometastases by hyperbaric oxygen. Clin Exp Metastasis 3:21–27, 1985.
142. Milas L, Ito H, Hunter N, Jones S, Peters LJ: Retardation of tumor growth in mice caused by radiation induced injury of tumor bed stroma: Dependency on tumor type. Cancer Res 46:723–727, 1986.
143. Miser JS, Kinsella TJ, Triche TT, et al: Treatment of peripheral neuroepithelioma in children and young adults. J Clin Oncol 5:1752–1758, 1987.
144. Miser JS, Kinsella TJ, Triche TJ, et al: Preliminary results of treatment of Ewing's sarcoma of bone in children and young adults: Six months of intensive combined modality therapy without maintenance. J Clin Oncol 6:484–490, 1988.
145. Mittal B, Emami B, Sapareto SA, et al: Effects of sequencing of the total course of combined hyperthermia and radiation on the RIF-1 murine tumor. Cancer 54:2889–2897, 1984.
146. Miyoshi T, Saito M, Arimizu N, Akiyama S: Modifying effects of interferon on the growth of irradiated sarcoma 180 cells *in vitro*. Nippon Igaku Hoshasen Gakki Zasshi 44:88–92, 1984.
147. Moorthy CR, Hahn EW, Kim JH, et al: Improved response of a murine fibrosarcoma (Meth-A) to interstitial radiation when combined with hyperthermia. Int J Radiat Oncol Biol Phys 10:2145–2148, 1984.
148. Nagatani M, Ikeda T, Otsuki H, et al: Sellar fibrosarcoma following radiotherapy for prolactinoma. No Shinkei Geka 12:339–346, 1984.
149. Neuhauser EBD, Wittenborg MH, Bergman CZ, Cohen J: Irradiation effects of roentgen therapy in the growing spine. Radiology 59:637–650, 1952.
150. Newton KA, Barrett A: Prophylactic lung irradiation in the treatment of osteogenic sarcoma. Clin Radiol 29:493–495, 1978.
151. Nill WB, Griffith R: The role of radiation therapy in the management of plasma cell tumors. Cancer 45:647, 1980.
152. Okuneieff P, Suit HD, Proppe KH: Extremity preservation by combined modality treatment of sarcomas of the hand and wrist. Int J Radiat Oncol Biol Phys 12:1923–1929, 1986.
153. Orton CG, Ellis F: A simplification in the use of the NSD concept in practical radiotherapy. Br J Radiol 46:529–537, 1973.
154. Ostrowski ML, Unni KK, Banks PM, et al: Malignant lymphoma of bone. Cancer 58:2646–2655, 1986.
155. Owens JC, Shiu MH, Smith R, Hadju SI: Soft tissue sarcomas of the hand and foot. Cancer 55:2010–2018, 1985.
156. Pages A, Pages M, Ramos J, Benezech J: Radiation induced intracranial fibrochondrosarcoma. J Neurol 233:309–310, 1986.
157. Pairolero PC, Arnold PG: Thoracic wall defects: Surgical management of 205 consecutive patients. Mayo Clin Proc 61:557–563, 1986.
158. Parker RG, Selch MT, Eilber F, Kobe L: Radiation treatment planning for soft tissue sarcomas. Front Radiat Ther Oncol 21:247–255, 1987.
159. Penn CRH: Single dose and fractionated palliative irradiation for osseous metastasis. Clin Radiol 27:405–408, 1976.
160. Perez CA, Teft M, Nesbit M, et al: The role of radiation therapy in the management of non metastatic Ewing's sarcoma of bone: Report of the Intergroup Ewing's Sarcoma Study. Int J Radiat Oncol Biol Phys 7:141–149, 1981.
161. Perez CA, Teft M, Nesbit ME, et al: Radiation therapy in the multimodal management of Ewing's sarcoma: Report of the Intergroup Ewing's Sarcoma Study. Natl Cancer Inst Monogr 56:263–271, 1981.
162. Peters LJ, Brock WA, Johnson T, et al: Potential methods for predicting tumor radiocurability. Int J Radiat Oncol Biol Phys 12:459–467, 1986.
163. Phillips TL, Rolmach RJ: Repair of potentially lethal damage in x-irradiated HeLa cells. Radiat Res 29:413, 1966.
164. Phillips TL, Sheline GE: Radiation therapy of malignant bone tumors. Radiology 92:1537–1545, 1969.
165. Phillips TL, Wasserman TH, Johnson RJ, et al: Final report on the United States Phase I trial of the hypoxic cell radiosensitizer misonidazole. Cancer 48:1697, 1981.
166. Pickering DG, Stewart JS, Rampling R, et al: Fast neutron therapy for soft tissue sarcoma. Int J Radiat Oncol Biol Phys 13:1489–1495, 1987.
167. Pilepich MV, Vietti TJ, Nesbit ME, et al: Ewing's sarcoma of the vertebral column. Int J Radiat Oncol Biol Phys 7:27–31, 1981.
168. Plowman PN, Shand WS, Jackson DB: Use of absorbable mesh to displace bowel and avoid radiation enteropathy during therapy of pelvic Ewing's sarcoma. Hum Toxicol 3:229–237, 1984.
169. Potter DA, Kinsella TJ, Glatstein E, et al: High-grade soft tissue sarcomas of extremities. Cancer 58:190–205, 1986.
170. Prindull G, Jurgens H, Jentsch F, et al: Radiotherapy of nonmetastatic Ewing's sarcoma. J Cancer Res Clin Oncol 110:127–130, 1985.
171. Puck TT, Marcus PI: Action of x-rays on mammalian cells. J Exp Med 103:653, 1956.
172. Puck TT, Morkovin D, Marcus PI, et al: Action of x-rays on mammalian cells. II. Survival curves of cells from normal human tissues. J Exp Med 106:483–500, 1957.
173. Qasim MM: Techniques and results of half body irradiation (HBI) in metastatic carcinomas and myelomas. Clin Oncol 5:65, 1979.
174. Rab GT, Ivins JC, Childs DS Jr, et al: Elective whole lung irradiation in the treatment of osteogenic sarcoma. Cancer 38:939–942, 1976.
175. Raney RB, Allen A, O'Neill J, et al: Malignant fibrous histiocytoma of soft tissue in childhood. Cancer 57:2198–2201, 1986.
176. Redpath JL, Colman M: The effect of Adriamycin and actinomycin D on radiation-induced skin reactions in mouse feet. Int J Radiat Oncol Biol Phys 5:483–486, 1979.

177. Reimewrs M, Castro JR, Linsradt D, et al: Heavy charged particle therapy of bone and soft tissue sarcoma. A phase I–II trial of the University of California Lawrence Berkeley Laboratory and the Northern California Oncology Group. Am J Clin Oncol 9:488–493, 1986.
178. Rich TA: Intraoperative radiotherapy. Radiother Oncol 6:207–221, 1986.
179. Robinson E, Neugut AI, Wylie P: Clinical aspects of postirradiation sarcomas. J Natl Cancer Inst 80:233–240, 1988.
180. Roentgen WC: On a new kind of rays (preliminary communication). Physikalische-medicinischen Gesellshaft of Wurzburg, December 28, 1895.
181. Rosen G, Marcove RC, Caparros B, et al: Primary osteogenic sarcoma: The rationale for preoperative chemotherapy and delayed surgery. Cancer 43:2163–2177, 1979.
182. Rostom AY, O'Cathail SM, Folkes A: Systemic irradiation in multiple myeloma: A report on 19 cases. Br J Haematol 58:423–431, 1984.
183. Salazar OM, Rubin P, Hendrickson FR, et al: Single-dose half-body irradiation for palliation of multiple bone metastases from solid tumor. Final Radiation Therapy Oncology Group Report. Cancer 58:29–36, 1986.
184. Saunders WM, Chen GT, Austin-Seymour M, et al: Precision high dose radiotherapy. II. Helium ion treatment of tumors adjacent to critical central nervous system structures. Int J Radiat Oncol Biol Phys 11:1339–1347, 1985.
185. Schmitt G, Scherer E, von Essen CF: Neutron and neutron boost irradiation of soft tissue sarcomas. Strahlentherapie 161:784–786, 1985.
186. Sersa G, Willingham V, Milas L: Anti-tumor effects of tumor necrosis factor alone or combined with radiotherapy. Int J Cancer 42:129–134, 1988.
187. Shapiro E, Kinsella TJ, Makuch RW, et al: Effect of fractionated irradiation on endocrine aspects of testicular function. J Clin Oncol 3:1232–1239, 1985.
188. Shi T, Farrell MA, Kaufmann JC: Fibrosarcoma complicating irradiated pituitary adenoma. Surg Neurol 22:277–284, 1984.
189. Shimm DS, Suit HD: Radiation therapy of epithelioid sarcoma. Cancer 52:1022–1025, 1983.
190. Shiu MH, Collin C, Hilaris BS, et al: Limb preservation and tumor control in the treatment of popliteal and antecubital soft tissue sarcomas. Cancer 57:1632–1639, 1986.
191. Shiu MH, Turnbull AD, Nori D, et al: Control of locally advanced extremity soft tissue sarcomas by function-saving resection and brachytherapy. Cancer 53:1385–1392, 1984.
192. Siegal GP, Oliver WR, Reinus WR, et al: Primary Ewing's sarcoma involving the bones of the head and neck. Cancer 60:2829–2840, 1987.
193. Siemann DW, Alliet KL: Combinations of CCNU, MISO and fractionated radiotherapy. Int J Radiat Oncol Biol Phys 12:1379–1382, 1986.
194. Siemann DW, Hill SA: Enhanced tumor responses through therapies combining CCNU, misonidazole and radiation. Int J Radiat Oncol Biol Phys 10:1623–1626, 1984.
195. Siemann DW, Keng PC: *In situ* radiation response and oxygen enhancement ratio of KHT sarcoma cells in various phases of the cell cycle. Br J Radiol 57:823–827, 1984.
196. Siemann DW, Keng PC: Characterization of radiation resistant hypoxic cell subpopulations in KHT sarcomas. I. Centrifugal elutriation. Br J Cancer 55:33–36, 1987.
197. Silverman CL, Thomas PRM, McAllister WH, et al: Slipped femoral capital epiphyses in irradiated children: Dose, volume and age relationships. Int J Radiat Oncol Biol Phys 7:1357–1363, 1981.
198. Smith DS, Nesbit ME, D'Angio GJ, Levitt SH: Histiocytosis X: Role of radiation therapy in management with special reference to dose levels employed. Radiology 106:419, 1973.
199. Smith J: Postradiation sarcoma of bone in Hodgkin's disease. Skeletal Radiol 16:524–532, 1987.
200. Spiers FW: A review of the theoretical and experimental methods of determining radiation dose in bone. Br J Radiol 39:216–221, 1966.
201. Springfield DS, Pagliarullo C: Fractures of long bones previously treated for Ewing's sarcoma. J Bone Joint Surg 67A:477–481, 1985.
202. Stea B, Kinsella TJ, Triche TJ, et al: Treatment of pelvic sarcomas in adolescents and young adults with intensive combined modality therapy. Int J Radiat Oncol Biol Phys 13:1797–1805, 1987.
203. Suit HD, Tepper JE: Impact of improved local control on survival in patients with soft tissue sarcoma. Int J Radiat Oncol Biol Phys 12:699–700, 1986.
204. Suit HD, Mankin HJ, Wood WC, Proppe KH: Preoperative, intraoperative and postoperative radiation in the treatment of soft tissue sarcoma. Cancer 55:2659–2667, 1985.
205. Takada N, Hodaka E, Umeda T, Hayashi H: Fast neutron radiotherapy and limb-salvage surgery in patients with osteosarcoma. Gan To Kagaku Ryoho 145:1405–1411, 1987.
206. Tefft M, Chabora BM, Rosen G: Radiation in bone sarcomas: A re-evaluation in the era of intensive systemic chemotherapy. Cancer 39:806–816, 1977.
207. Tepper JE, Suit HD: Radiation therapy for soft tissue sarcomas. Cancer 55:2273–2277, 1985.
208. Tepper JE, Suit HD: Radiation therapy alone for sarcoma of soft tissue. Cancer 56:475–479, 1985.
209. Tepper JE, Suit HD, Wood WC, et al: Radiation therapy of retroperitoneal soft tissue sarcomas. Int J Radiat Oncol Biol Phys 10:825–830, 1984.
210. Thomlinson RH, Gray LH: The histological structure of some human lung cancers and the possible implications for radiotherapy. Br J Cancer 9:539–549, 1955.
211. Thum P, Greiner R, Blattman H, et al: Pion radiotherapy of unresectable soft tissue sarcomas at the Swiss Institute of Nuclear Research. Strahlenther Onkol 1464:714–723, 1988.
212. Tobias JS, Richards JD, Blackman GM, et al: Hemibody irradiation in multiple myeloma. Radiother Oncol 3:11–16, 1985.
213. Tong D, Gillick L, Hendrickson FR: The palliation of symptomatic osseous metastases—final results of the study by the Radiation Therapy Oncology Group. Cancer 50:893–899, 1982.
214. Travis EL, Meistrich ML, Finch-Neimeyer M, et al: Protection by WR-2721 of late functional and biochemical changes in mouse lung after irradiation. Radiat Res 103:219–231, 1983.
215. Tsunemoto H, Arai T, Morita S, et al: Japanese experience with clinical trials of fast neutrons. Int J Radiat Oncol Biol Phys 8:2169–2172, 1982.
216. Tucker MA, D'Angio GJ, Boice JD Jr, et al: Bone sarcomas linked to radiotherapy and chemotherapy in children. N Engl J Med 317:588–593, 1987.
217. Vietti T, Gehan E, Nesbit M, et al: Multimodal therapy in metastatic Ewing's sarcoma: An intergroup study. Natl Cancer Inst Monogr 56:279–284, 1978.

218. Vuigario G, Kurohara SS, George FW: Association of hemoglobin levels before and during radiotherapy with prognosis in uterine cervix cancer. Radiology 106:649–652, 1973.
219. Walton MI, Workman P: Pharmacokinetics and metabolism of the mixed-function hypoxic cell sensitizer prototype RSU 1069 in mice. Cancer Chemother Pharmacol 22:275–281, 1988.
220. Wang CC, Blitzer PH, Suit HD: Twice-a-day radiation therapy for cancer of the head and neck. Cancer 55:2100, 1985.
221. Weichselbaum RR: Radioresistant and repair proficient cells may determine radiocurability in human tumors. Int J Radiat Oncol Biol Phys 12:637–691, 1986.
222. Weichselbaum RR, Beckett M: The maximum recovery potential of human tumor cells may predict clinical outcome in radiotherapy. Int J Radiat Oncol Biol Phys 13:709–713, 1987.
223. Weichselbaum RR, Beckett MA, Simon MA, et al: *In vitro* radiobiological parameters of human sarcoma cell lines. Int J Radiat Oncol Biol Phys 15:937–942, 1988.
224. Weichselbaum RR, Cassady JR, Jaffe N, et al: Preliminary results of aggressive multimodality therapy for metastatic osteosarcoma. Cancer 40:78–83, 1977.
225. Wilkins RM, Pritchard DJ, Burgert EO, Unni KK: Ewing's sarcoma of bone: Experience with 140 patients. Cancer 58:2551–2555, 1986.
226. Willett CG, Schiller AL, Suit HD, et al: The histologic response of soft tissue sarcoma to radiation therapy. Cancer 60:1500–1504, 1987.
227. Willett CG, Tepper JE, Orlow EL, Shipley WU: Renal complications secondary to radiation treatment of upper abdominal malignancies. Int J Radiat Oncol Biol Phys 12:1601–1604, 1986.
228. Wolff SN, McCurley TL, Giannone L: High dose chemoradiotherapy with syngeneic bone marrow transplantation for multiple myeloma: Case report and literature review. Am J Hematol 26:191–198, 1987.
229. Young MM, Kinsella TJ, Miser JS, et al: Treatment of sarcomas of the chest wall using intensive combined modality therapy. Int J Radiat Oncol Biol Phys 16:49–57, 1989.

CHAPTER 8

The Geriatric Patient

ROBERT N. BUTLER

Demographics of Aging

The population of the United States is aging. Since the start of the twentieth century, industrialized nations have seen an unprecedented increase in the absolute number and relative proportion of older people. In 1900, an American, on average, lived to age 47 years; those older than age 65 years made up only 4% of the population. Today's average life expectancy, however, is 75 years, and 12.2% of Americans are older than 65 years. This 28-year gain in average life expectancy is remarkable, nearly equaling that from the Bronze Age (approximately 3000 BC) to 1900. Furthermore, the average life expectancy is increasing at a rapid pace. Between 1900 and 1960, life expectancy after age 65 years increased by 2.4 years. Yet, between 1960 and 1986—a period of just 26 years—it increased by 2.6 years.

This gain in average life expectancy is a social achievement, not a result of biologic evolution. It is a function not only of medical science but also of socioeconomic progress, better sanitation, and improved nutrition. Marked reductions in maternal, childhood, and infant mortality rates account for approximately 80% of this gain in average life expectancy. The other 20% that has been achieved from a base age 65 years is a result of effective prevention, management, or control of acute diseases and of chronic diseases such as hypertension and diabetes.

This increase in the number and proportion of older persons is only partially explained by a rise in longevity. An increased birth rate in the 1920s and after World War II, the aging of those born before 1920, and the decline in birth rates in the mid-1960s have all contributed to an increased proportion of elderly and a rise in the median age of the US population (Fig. 8–1).

If current fertility and immigration levels remain constant, the age group older than 55 years will be the only group to experience significant growth in the twenty-first century. This will most likely occur in two stages. Until the turn of the century, the proportion of those 55 years and older will be approximately one in five, staying relatively stable. However, when the baby boomers (those born between 1946 and 1964) move into old age in the year 2011, this proportion will rise dramatically: More than one fourth of the US population will be 55 years and older. One of every seven people will be at least age 65 years. When the number of these baby boomers reaches a peak between the years 2020 and 2030, one third of

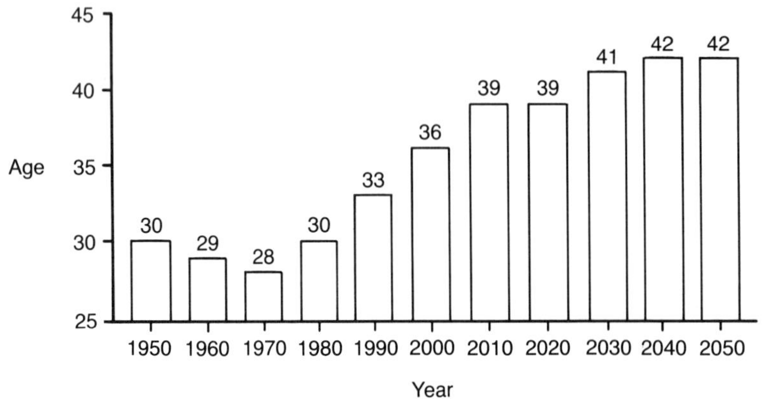

FIGURE 8–1. Estimates and projections of median age of the US population, 1950 to 2050. (From U.S. Bureau of the Census: Projections of the population of the United States by age, sex, and race, 1963 to 2080. Current Population Reports Series P-25, No. 952 [May] 1984.)

the US population will be 55 years and older, while 20%—some 51 to 65 million people—will be at least 65 years old.

After the huge baby boomer population, the 85 years and older age group is growing most rapidly. Since 1960, life expectancy at age 85 has grown by 24%. In addition, the number of centenarians is increasing. Between 1980 and 1986, the number rose from 15,000 to 25,000. One consequence of this increase in the very old is the likelihood that the elderly themselves will have at least one surviving parent, making four- and five-generation families more and more common and increasing the number of caregivers providing unpaid assistance to noninstitutionalized older disabled persons.

There is a sharp difference in life expectancy rates between the sexes. On average, women live 7.3 years longer than men. The proportion of women to men increases with age. In 1986, 34.5 million females were younger than age 20 years, compared with 36.1 males. The 30 to 34 year old age group had an equal number of females and males (10.4 million). The group older than 65 years, however, had 17.4 million women and just 11.8 million men. Among those older than 65 years, even more marked differences were seen relative to age: in the 65 to 69 year age group, there were 83 men for every 100 women; in the 85 years and older group, there were only 40 males for every 100 women (Fig. 8–2).

Approximately 75% of this distinction between the sexes is due to disease and accidents. The higher male mortality rate is a consequence of the higher incidence of men of coronary artery disease; lung cancer; emphysema associated with tobacco intake, industrial accidents, and exposure to toxic chemicals; automobile and other accidents; suicide; and cirrhosis of the liver. Further research is needed to determine to what extent the other 25% is affected by differences in life style, stress, hormonal status, immune function, genetic make-up, and other factors.

The difference in mortality between the sexes accounts for widows' outnumbering widowers three to one. Older women are more likely to live alone for a longer period of time; they are the ones who especially must confront the challenge of aging.

From 1900 to 1902, male and female survival rates were about equal. Race, rather than sex, was the dominant factor in life expectancy. Only two of every ten blacks lived to age 65 years compared with four of every ten whites. At that time, there was a 14.1-year difference in life expectancy at birth between white and black men and a 15.2-year difference between white and black women. Today, whites still

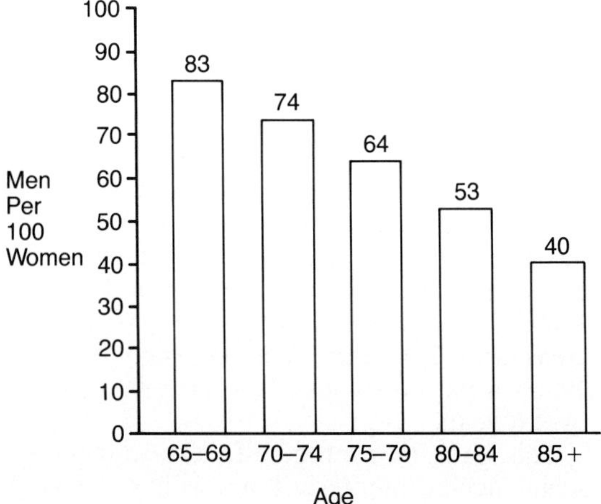

FIGURE 8–2. Number of men per 100 women by elderly age group, 1986. (From U.S. Bureau of the Census: Estimates of the population of the United States by age, sex, and race, 1980–1986. Current Population Reports Series P-25, No. 1000 [February] 1987.)

live longer, but the gap is narrowing, with only a 6.5-year difference in life expectancy at birth between white and black men and a 5-year difference between white and black women.

Growing Body of Knowledge in Geriatrics

This great demographic shift is apt to have a significant impact not only on personal lives, but also on social, political, and economic institutions and medical care. It will be necessary for all primary and specialty care physicians (with the possible exception of pediatricians) to adapt to the new longevity.

Current demographic trends are also reflected in the development of geriatrics, which is less advanced in the United States than in Great Britain and Scandinavia, in particular, and, to some extent, in Japan. There is a growing body of knowledge concerning the basic biology of aging. Greater attention is being paid to the diseases of old age. This follows the addition of the National Institute of Aging (NIA) to the National Institutes of Health. In turn, the creation of the NIA has helped further expand this rapidly increasing knowledge. Currently, the National Academy of Sciences is involved in developing a National Research Agenda on Aging. Rising health care costs have led to health care reforms; changes in methods of physician payment; new research, such as in Alzheimer's disease; and development of preventive interventions, such as in osteoporosis.

In addition, great strides are being made in medical education initiated by the NIA, the Institute of Medicine, the Association of American Medical Colleges, and various organizations in the field of aging. Reforms have been instituted in medical curricula and in support of new leaders in the geriatrics field.

Attitudes Toward the Geriatric Patient

Specific knowledge about old age, especially about healthy old age, is still limited. Despite the trends in demographics and geriatrics, physicians continue to attribute their older patients' symptoms to advanced age. They may think that there is little time left for these patients and that their problems are irreversible, unexciting, and unprofitable. Alternatively, physicians may become anxious about having to confront the reality of aging, disability, and death. As a result, they are not as invested in their older patients and spend less time with them. In this manner, physicians are engaging in a subtle form of ageism.

As a result of this medical ageism, elderly patients may have negative feelings about growing older and, consequently, may accept deterioration fatalistically, either making light of or underreporting their symptoms.

Epidemiology of Aging

During the past century, there have been changes in the ranking of causes of death, particularly a reduction in deaths from infectious diseases and an increase in those attributable to chronic diseases. For example, not until 1950 did cancer become the third leading cause of death.

National Cancer Institute data reveal that the incidence of primary tumors in the musculoskeletal system of older patients is modest, usually peaking before age 65 years. The median age at which these tumors occur in all races is 56 years for males and 58 years for females.

Musculoskeletal cancer among the geriatric population is exceedingly rare, except for myeloma. Of 556 patients with solitary plasmacytoma studied by Dahlin and Unni, 106, 166, 163, and 80 were in their 50s, 60s, 70s, and 80s, respectively. In addition, the majority of another 2376 patients with myeloma diagnosed on the basis of bone marrow aspiration ranged in age from 50 to 75 years.

Metastases to the bone are common, on average five times more prevalent than primary bone sarcoma—and even more so in the elderly population. More than 80% of secondary tumors in bone originate from the prostate, the breast, the lungs, the kidney, or the thyroid. Any malignancy may spread to the bone, causing considerable pain and disability. Persons with localized skeletal symptoms, together with a history of malignant epithelial tumors, or those with unexplained radiodense or radiolucent bone lesions should be strongly suspected of having metastases. In addition, metastatic carcinoma should also be considered in hip fractures and compression fractures of the spine.

In the twenty-first century, the oncologist will be confronted with an even greater increase in the number and proportion of older persons. Eighty percent of all cancer, regardless of source, occurs in patients older than 50 years (and some 50% in those older than 65 years). This age-related incidence of malignancies, coupled with the increasingly aging population, will have a dramatic effect on the practice of oncologists. Because of this increased cancer incidence and the multiplicity of treatment modalities (e.g., medications), special consideration and unique cautions must be applied in both diagnostic examination and the effective care of the older patient.

Special Diagnostic and Treatment Considerations

The geriatric patient tends to be 75 years and older. He or she usually has acute and chronic, complex, interacting psychosocial and physical pathologic conditions.

In the diagnostic examination of an older patient, one must be sensitive to the possibilities of muscle and bone tumors, because problems of mobility and ambulation are common in old age. When examining such patients, the physician must consider the whole range of possible reasons for such problems, including tumors and polypharmacy. Older people are often taking numerous medications at one time—perhaps as many as five or six. This can not only obscure the character of disease but also create confusion and depression.

A geriatric patient may leave the hospital with improvement of an acute condition; however, he or she may have lost overall functional capacity. To provide comprehensive care, the oncologist must work with a health care team—a nurse, a social worker, and perhaps a physical medicine expert, a psychiatrist, and/or a neuropsychologist, among others—to help the patient restore and maintain function. A comprehensive assessment of an older patient goes beyond the traditional medical model. It includes evaluation (and eventual treatment and follow-up) of social, economic, emotional, and psychologic problems. An interdisciplinary approach is critical.

The National Institutes of Health Consensus Conference on Geriatric Assessment stressed the value of the emphasis on function. An older patient's multiple problems, resources, strengths, and need for services are all uncovered, described, and explained through geriatric assessment. A coordinated care plan is devised, with a focus on possible interventions.

A collaborative relationship must also be fostered between physician and patient. Older patients are especially concerned with being able to maintain some control over their lives for as long as they can. Thus, the physician should develop a partnership with patients, with the ultimate goal being to help them contribute to their own care. This includes instruction in health promotion and disease prevention techniques so that patients can take responsibility for self-care.

Because of the number and complexity of conditions affecting older patients, treatment is often complicated by the concurrent multiplicity of therapy, including polypharmacy. When prescribing medication, a physician should initially prescribe a low dosage and increase the dosage slowly. If additional medications are necessary, only one should be prescribed at a time, if possible. Careful evaluation should be made at each step. Readable labeling of medications is extremely important to ensure that the patient can understand the directions. Clear oral instructions should also be given.

Patients should be told of possible side effects that a drug may have. Too often older patients fail to ask their physicians about the side effects of prescribed drugs. Many physicians believe that knowing the side effects causes patients not to take their medication; however, this is not a solution to the problem. If a drug causes a patient to feel dizzy, for example, he or she will stop taking it anyway.

Conclusion

Primary and secondary musculoskeletal tumors (metastases) in older patients require special attention because of the likely concurrence of multiple conditions, polypharmacy, and psychosocial problems. Therefore, evaluation must be comprehensive and go beyond the traditional medical examination. Working with a team is of particular value, both in evaluation and in treatment.

References

Aging Alone: Profiles and Projections. Report of The Commonwealth Fund Commission on Elderly People Living Alone, Baltimore, 1988.

Butler RN: Geriatrics and internal medicine. Ann Intern Med 91:903–908, 1979.

Butler RN: The longevity revolution. Mt Sinai J Med 54:5–8, 1987.

Dahlin DC, Unni KK: Bone Tumors: General Aspects and Data on 8,542 Cases, 4th Ed. Springfield, Illinois, CC Thomas, 1986.

Einhorn TA, Lewis M, Klein MJ: Organ system geriatrics: Musculoskeletal disorders. *In* Abrams WB, Berkow R (eds): The Merck Manual of Geriatrics. Rahway, NJ, Merck, Sharp & Dohme Research Laboratories, Division of Merck & Co., Inc., 1990.

National Institutes of Health Consensus Development Panel: National Institutes of Health Consensus Development Conference Statement: Geriatric assessment methods for clinical decision-making. J Am Geriatr Soc 36:342–347, 1988.

SEER Program, National Cancer Institute, National Institutes of Health, 1980–1986. Unpublished raw data.

US Senate Special Committee on Aging, American Association of Retired Persons, the Federal Council on the Aging, and the US Administration on Aging: Aging America: Trends and Projections, 1987–1988. U.S. Dept. of Health and Human Services, Washington, DC.

CHAPTER 9

Osteochondral Allografts and Bone Banking

GARY E. FRIEDLAENDER
HENRY J. MANKIN

The field of musculoskeletal oncology has significantly advanced in knowledge and technique associated with diagnosis, staging, and treatment. The general understanding of the pathophysiology of malignancies of bone and cartilage as well as understanding of the metastatic process has also improved. Molecular biology, materials science, and innovative surgical approaches have all contributed to this current level of sophistication and efficacy. Few of these new directions, however, have proved more practical, effective, or reliable than osteochondral allograft reconstruction after limb-sparing tumor resection. With a century of evolving surgical technique, improved understanding of the biologic and immunobiologic features of allograft incorporation, and development of appropriate tissue banking methods, bone transplantation has emerged as a gratifying and dependable choice for selected patients.[25] Furthermore, this approach has proved useful in other circumstances requiring skeletal reconstruction, especially total joint arthroplasty.

The concept of bone or limb transplantation has a lengthy, indeed ancient, history. The current approach, however, began with the observations made and reported by Ollier[50] in the midnineteenth century. He recognized the osteogenic potential of periosteum as well as the ability to preserve this activity by refrigerated storage. Macewen established the clinical technique by utilizing tibial wedges, which were removed in the course of corrective osteotomies, as graft material in unrelated patients. In 1881, he described in great detail the multistaged reconstruction of an entire diaphyseal defect of the humerus in a young child.[42] The bone loss, caused by osteomyelitis, responded to a series of grafting procedures using allogeneic bone. Although today an infected wound would represent a relative contraindication, the youth of the patient, perhaps careful débridement, and most probably an element of good fortune combined to initiate a sequence of clinical investigations that have culminated in the present approach. Lexer, another important contributor to the early clinical science, used massive osteochondral allografts to replace all or part of the knee joint, generally subsequent to trauma, and judged this approach successful in approximately half his patients.[39, 40]

A major advance occurred in the 1950s when Herndon, Chase, Curtiss, and colleagues[9, 32] demonstrated that the much feared (but rarely observed) immune response, which appeared to be associated with implantation of fresh allograft and was thought to impede graft incorporation,[7, 24] could be significantly reduced by freezing of the tissue. Consequently, preservation by deep-freezing became the cornerstone of contemporary bone and cartilage allograft storage. This, in turn, proved to be an important factor in the evolution of the current clinical programs.[44, 45]

Armed with these favorable methods and, perhaps more importantly, the capacity to store physically unaltered bones under sterile conditions in a freezer, a number of clinical investigators, in several countries, were responsible for major advances. Parrish[52, 53] in the United States, Ottolenghi[51] in Argentina, Koskinen[37] in Finland, and Volkov[66] in the Soviet Union all began using massive osseous and osteochondral allografts, usually frozen, to replace deficits caused by tumor resections or trauma. Grafts were acquired from cadaveric sources using aseptic technique and most commonly were stored at −20C until implanted. Each of these innovative clinicians met these reconstructive challenges by independently developing surgical techniques and, to a limited degree, bone banking methods. Their careful follow-up reports, particularly that of Parrish,[53] provided both guidance and incentive for contemporary transplantation activities.

Parallel to these clinical endeavors was the establishment of bone banks and appropriate methods to ensure a supply of safe and useful graft material. The use of fresh allografts posed problems in storage of parts and precluded thorough evaluation of these tissues and their donors for the purpose of minimizing the transmission of disease to recipients. Inclan[34] in Cuba and Wilson[71] in the United States were among the first to describe their approaches, followed by Hyatt and associates at the United States Naval Tissue Bank in Bethesda.[33, 38] The Navy's program responded to the perceived needs of the military to provide bone, cartilage, and skin for combat casualties incurred during the Korean War. An approach was developed and implemented for the sterile retrieval of bone followed by lyophilization (freeze-drying).[18, 33, 38] The method proved helpful in reducing the immune response to grafts and was clearly effective for long-term preservation at room temperature, without requiring an elaborate storage system.[18] The process of freezing and drying, however, was also known to alter significantly the physical state of the graft and thereby to diminish the mechanical properties essential to structural integrity of the skeleton.[54, 55] Although the freeze-drying of bone was useful in massive allogeneic segmental replacement, its application was problematic and the outcome was somewhat unpredictable.

Biology

Incorporation of bone graft, whether autogenous or allogeneic, reflects a sequence of biologic events characterized initially by hemorrhage and bone necrosis and ending with remodeling of the implanted graft. The histologic aspects of the repair process were described in detail by Burchardt, Enneking, and associates[4, 5, 16] for cortical grafts and by Heiple and colleagues[31] for cancellous tissues. More recently, the understanding of the complex cascade of biologic activity at the molecular level of the graft has improved, but much remains unknown or unclear.

AUTOGRAFTS

Using fresh autograft as a prototype, without the benefit of immediate vascular reanastomosis, the general nature of graft incorporation can be appreciated as a partnership between the host bed and the implanted bone.[21] The graft itself is initially devoid of a blood supply, and only those cells at or near the bony surface have an opportunity to survive by diffusion. The primary contributions of the graft are its passive physical structure and active inductive properties. The recipient site provides new blood vessels, and the host, through this neoangiogenesis, is the source of cells required to resorb preexisting matrix and form new bone.

After implantation, the graft is surrounded by a hematoma, which, over 1 to 3 weeks, gradually transforms into fibrovascular tissue. Necrosis of the graft, even though autogenous, evokes a nonspecific inflammatory reaction. As the graft is invaded by a new blood supply, recruitment of committed cells that resorb old matrix occurs, followed by new osteoblastic cellular activity. The passive nature of the graft, through which this cellular response permeates, is termed osteoconduction. It is also clear that molecular messengers associated with the matrix actively stimulate the host response. This osteoinductive nature is widely attributed to bone morphogenetic proteins, which Urist and colleagues traced to a 14 to 19 K matrix molecule.[64, 65] There is undoubtedly a cascade of humoral messengers, mitogens, and differentiation factors involved in the biology of bone repair and remodeling, but understanding in this area remains superficial and incomplete.

After the recruitment of cells, cortical grafts undergo substantial osteoclast-mediated resorption along their periphery and within preexisting vascular channels. This necessitates a period of relative mechanical weakness, lasting until sufficient new bone is laid down within these resorption sites.[16] In the dog, this process may take 1 to 2 years before the original mechanical integrity is restored to a cortical graft and, in the human, appears to take twice this time.

Cancellous tissues are revascularized more rapidly than cortical bone, reflecting their more porous structure. Preexisting trabeculae, devoid of viable cells, serve as a trellis for the deposition of new osteoid followed by mineralization. Alternating resorption and formation activity causes the graft to remodel, generally resulting in its complete incorporation. This is in contrast to cortical bone grafts, which tend to plateau their repair after approximately half the matrix has been remodeled.

Immediate reanastomosis of blood supply to a graft precludes the need for a lengthy incorporation process. Instead, these bones maintain their cellularity and remodeling activity and need only repair at their osteosynthesis sites by a process analogous to fracture healing.[70] This is a relatively rapid and predictably successful process and is of particular value in a compromised recipient site, such as an irradiated bed.[69] Disadvantages of vascularized bone grafts include their technical demands in terms of the surgical procedure, their restriction to autogenous sources, and the limited size and shape constraints imposed by the fibula, rib, and iliac crest donor sites.

Limitations of bone autografts have driven development of alternatives. Autografts require sacrifice of normal structures, are associated with increased postoperative morbidity and pain, and are limited in quantity and shapes. Allografts circumvent these disadvantages but present their own set of concerns. These include the quality of their biologic repair, the potential to transfer disease from donor to recipient, and the consequences of immune responses after implantation of foreign tissue. Each of these issues has been evaluated in substantial detail, and none has precluded the clinical efficacy or safety of this approach.[25]

ALLOGRAFTS

The histologic sequence of bone allograft incorporation, confirmed in several animal models, parallels events noted with autogenous tissues.[4, 7, 31] Differences exist, including slower and less complete incorporation and a more intense inflammatory reaction with allografts, and these alterations can be correlated with the degree of genetic disparity between donor and recipient as well as methods of graft treatment and preservation before implantation.[7, 30, 60]

The major approaches used for long-term preservation of bone allografts include freezing, freeze-drying, and demineralization in combination with lyophilization. Substantial clinical experience supports the biologic usefulness of grafts treated in each of these manners,[25] but data also demonstrate characteristic changes in graft biomechanics and immunogenicity.[19] For example, freeze-drying, demineralization, and the use of megavoltage doses of irradiation for sterilization all cause structural changes in bone that reduce its initial mechanical strength at the outset of surgical implantation.[54, 55]

These changes are important in planning surgical procedures using grafts, particularly in terms of defining the necessary internal fixation and postoperative care. However, the ultimate biologic potential of the graft is crucial. Despite important transient changes in mechanical behavior, the completeness of the repair process and the time schedule for this activity determine the usefulness of the reconstructive approach. Deep-freezing is the authors' preferred method of long-term preservation, in great measure because it permits the viable storage of articular cartilage.[61] Freeze-drying and demineralization of bone also have strong support, justified on the basis of substantial clinical success.

IMMUNOGENICITY

Unquestionably, bone allografts, in a similar manner to all fresh allogeneic transplants, evoke immunologic responses.[7, 19, 20, 26, 27] There are, however, much controversy and little data pertaining to the significance of these host reactions.[22] Immune responses can be heterogeneous in timing, intensity, precise nature, and biologic significance. Not all responses by immunocompetent cells, for example, are harmful.

Bone is a composite tissue, and potential sources of immunogenicity include matrix proteins, collagen, and, most notably, cells. Many investigators, using a variety of animal models and assay techniques during the past 30 to 40 years, have evaluated graft-evoked responses.[19] Whether based on plain histologic features, examination of draining lymph nodes, or sophisticated *in vitro* isotope-release approaches, and regardless of whether assessed in rats, cats, rabbits, or dogs, fresh bone allografts were found to be immunogenic. Also found with relative uniformity were that the use of deep-freezing reduces the observed production of humoral antibody or cell-mediated immunity, and that lyophilization renders these responses less intense or undetectable.[26] Similar patterns were confirmed in humans.[20]

What remains enigmatic is the relationship between the production of immunologic responses and the biologic nature of the bone graft. Burchardt and colleagues, in canine studies, identified three patterns of repair by both radiography and histologic examination.[5] Type I repair was uncomplicated and characteristic of the anticipated autogenous response. Type III repair represented histologic failure with x-ray evidence of nonunion, fracture, and even dissolution of the graft. Type II was intermediate, abnormal, but at least partially successful in histologic repair and plagued by only a modest incidence of fracture and nonunion by x-ray evaluation. It was hypothesized that type I repair would be characteristic of autograft; type II would indicate a minor immunologic mismatch; and type III would be reflective of a major histoincompatibility. In fact, 20% of autografts underwent a type II response, and 20% of allografts were repaired in a type I fashion, indistinguishable from the pattern of repair observed with the majority of autografts evaluated by this approach. Another 20% of allografts underwent type III repair, and the 60% balance was of the type II variety. The relationship, therefore, between histocompatibility differences and graft biologic features was inconsistent and unclear.

Of more clinical relevance, as many as 80 to 85% of patients receiving massive, preserved osteochondral allografts demonstrate detectable antibody to graft-specific HLA specifities.[20, 22, 58] A similar high percentage of these patients have a satisfactory clinical course,[45] but the members of these subgroups are not synonymous, reemphasizing the incomplete understanding of the biologic significance of sensitization. More recent observations suggest that presensitized individuals, including those with prior pregnancy or previous blood transfusions, are more likely to have a poor clinical result than nonsensitized recipients.[22]

INFLUENCE OF CHEMOTHERAPY

Chemotherapeutic agents interfere with normal cellular metabolism and, thereby, protein synthesis. The degree to which cell function is impaired depends on the specific drug, its dose, and the susceptibility of a selected cell population to the antimetabolite. Both methotrexate and doxorubicin have profound suppressive effects on intact bone turnover in the rat, on fracture repair in the rat, and on graft incorporation in the dog.[6, 28] Bone formation rates were reduced by more than 50% with each of these drugs, and their adverse influence on osteoblasts was more substantial than that on osteoclasts, resulting in a net loss of bone during short-term administration. Recent clinical observations by Gebhardt and colleagues support the adverse consequences of chemotherapy, but it was of insufficient magnitude to prevent satisfactory results.[29]

Bone Banking

The primary purpose of bone banks is to provide safe and effective graft material and to do so in a timely fashion. These goals are accomplished by careful attention to donor selection criteria, tissue recovery techniques, and preservation methods, as well as storage, distribution, and record-keeping approaches. Each of these areas represents an important contribution to the overall process, which has evolved from the casual use of household freezers in the 1940s and 1950s to rigorously controlled and scientifically sound practices used widely today. The guidelines and standards of the American Association of Tissue Banks reflect the sophistication of this evolving technology and the importance of quality control.[1, 23, 63]

DONOR SELECTION

It is critical that the medical history of prospective donors be carefully reviewed to eliminate the transmission of disorders and diseases capable of causing harm to the recipient. Infection is of particular concern because it is associated with a high rate of graft failure.

Besides bacterial contamination, fungal and viral diseases must also be screened out. The human immunodeficiency virus, responsible for acquired immunodeficiency syndrome (AIDS), can be detected with a high degree of sensitivity and selectivity by assays directed at antibody. Because there is a delay between infection and detectable antibody production of 3 months or longer, retesting of live donors at least 90 days after tissue recovery is mandatory to minimize risk of transmitting this fatal disease.[56] Laboratory tests for syphilis and hepatitis are also routinely obtained.

Other areas of concern in donor screening include the existence of a malignancy of bone or other tumors with a propensity to metastasize to the skeleton, metabolic bone disease, harmful diseases of unknown causes, and the presence of toxic substances in significant amounts. It should also be kept in mind that individuals receiving artificial respiration for more than 3 to 4 days have a high incidence of septicemia and that the chronic use of steroids likewise is associated with microabscesses or other forms of occult infection.

Some programs also place age limits on potential donors, usually accepting individuals from skeletal maturity (approximately 15 to 18 years) through age 50 or 55 years. The lower age limit is important only if massive osteochondral allografts are going to be acquired and used intact because an open physis can slip during the incorporation process. Advancing age is associated with articular cartilage degeneration as well as occult disease, particularly malignancies. Bone from older individuals retains its osteoinductive nature and, if properly screened and not used for structural purposes, remains biomechanically satisfactory.

Both living and cadaveric donors are useful sources of graft material. Live donors, of course, are limited to providing those tissues normally acquired and discarded in the course of an operative procedure, most often the femoral head after fracture or arthroplasty. Regardless of the status of the donor, careful attention to selection criteria must be pursued.

The consent of the donor or the next of kin is necessary for removing tissues for transplantation. In the United States, traditional voluntary consent[59] has been revised to include "routine inquiry" or "required request." Although the decision remains with the donor, health care institutions must establish mechanisms to identify potential donors and develop procedures leading to the request for organ and tissue donation when appropriate. This change in consent approach reflects an insufficient supply of grafts, causing unmet needs. It is not yet clear to what degree required request legislation has reduced the deficit, but a greater opportunity to recover tissues, and to a lesser degree organs, is anticipated.

TISSUE RECOVERY

Two general approaches to tissue recovery have been successfully used for decades. First, bone may be removed in a clean but nonsterile fashion, and the tissue must then be secondarily sterilized by chemicals (e.g., ethylene oxide) or megavoltage irradiation. Whatever sterilization method is chosen, it must be safe to the recipient, leave the tissue biologically useful, and produce only tolerable changes in biomechanical properties. Alternatively, grafts may be recovered in a sterile environment and kept free from contamination throughout the remainder of the processing and storage approaches. This method places emphasis on donor selection criteria and a careful set of laboratory screening procedures. Although more time consuming, it is compatible with cryopreservation of articular cartilage and avoids the introduction of biologic and biomechanical changes caused by secondary sterilants.

Any bone of potential clinical usefulness can be removed from cadaveric sources, generally through longitudinal incisions and subperiosteal dissection. Ligament and capsule are retained at joint surfaces to aid in reconstruction after implantation.

PROCESSING AND STORAGE

Numerous approaches to long-term preservation of bone grafts are available, but deep-freezing, freeze-drying, and demineralizing coupled with freeze-drying are most common. Deep-freezing offers several advantages. It is relatively simple and inexpensive, is widely available, and is compatible with preservation of articular cartilage.[61] If temperatures in the −70 to −80C range are maintained, grafts can be stored for several years.[14] Furthermore, freezing does not change biomechanical properties[54] but does result in a reduced immunogenicity.[19] Freeze-drying requires more expensive and time-consuming technology. It is also incompatible with viable articular cartilage and may diminish the strength of bone.

On the other hand, freeze-dried bone can be stored indefinitely at room temperature in vacuum-sealed containers, and transportation of grafts is convenient. The major advantage of demineralized lyophilized bone is its highly inductive nature; however, it has little structural integrity.[57, 64, 65]

RECORD-KEEPING

Bone banks must keep accurate records of donor screening procedures; laboratory tests, including bacteriologic tests; preservation techniques; and any adverse reactions recognized in the recipient after implantation. This is crucial for optimal safety of the public and opportunities to enhance efficacy.

Grafts are most conveniently catalogued by their x-ray appearance, reflecting their size and shape. Fit at the articular surface is clearly important, as is joint stability, but routine radiographs offer as much information as can be addressed at the present time. More sophisticated computerized analysis and storage of this geometric information has been developed but has not yet proved useful given the limited numbers, sizes, and shapes of available grafts for selected patients.

Clinical Experience

In 1971, shortly after Parrish's monumental article appeared in the Journal of Bone and Joint Surgery,[52] the Orthopaedic Oncology Unit at the Massachusetts General Hospital in Boston began to investigate the use of allogeneic osteochondral grafts in the management of patients with bone tumors. Since that time, more than 550 allograft transplantation procedures have been performed, mostly for aggressive or malignant disease. Although the experiences of this group and those of other investigators have not been uniformly satisfactory, sufficient success has been achieved to encourage continued use, evaluation, and improvement of the system. The approach, in fact, may provide a valuable technique in the management of patients in whom a significant portion of the bony framework must be removed for nonneoplastic disorders.[11, 35, 43–49]

CONSIDERATIONS IN ALLOGRAFT TRANSPLANTATION

Advantages. The experience gained during the past 19 years at the orthopedic service at the Massachusetts General Hospital and other clinical units with large series of patients led to several key considerations focusing on the advantages of this system as compared with alternative means of compensating for a lost osseous fragment. Current information suggests that the alloimplants have merit in such a setting for the following reasons:

1. Allografts are available in appropriate sizes and shapes, and if a bone bank has a large enough inventory, nearly any part can be replaced with a segment almost anatomically equivalent to the lost part.[62]
2. It is possible to perform joint reconstructions with allograft segments covered with articular cartilage so that the function of a part can be restored without the necessity of introducing complicated custom mechanical devices.[35, 45–47]
3. Allografts can be retrieved so that attachment sites for detached or resected muscles and joint stabilizers are included with the part, thus allowing restoration of soft tissue stability and increasing the potential for more normal function.[62]
4. If an allograft is to be used, the patient has no donor site morbidity or potential compromise of the opposite normal part.
5. On the basis of the type of experience and knowledge cited above, it is hoped that over time the host tissues will invade the donor part and convert it to at least partially "autogenous" tissue.[7, 10, 24]
6. If the allograft fails by virtue of fracture, nonunion, joint instability, or even infection, more options are available with which to recoup.

Disadvantages. On the other hand, there are currently some significant disadvantages of the use of allografts. Although these issues are in part surmountable, they remain major obstacles in the minds of many clinicians and have curtailed the use of these materials for skeletal reconstruction. These factors include the following:

1. One can only expect about 80% excellent or good results.[11, 35, 43–48] This is certainly better than the 50 or 60% rates published in early series but not yet in a range that is acceptable to the orthopedist treating nonmalignant states.
2. The published rates of infection, fracture, and nonunion are disturbingly high.[2, 12, 41, 49] Any procedure in which infection occurs in as many as 10% of cases must be viewed with

concern, even with the extensive exposure often required to remove a tumor. The rate has been reduced from previously higher levels, principally by use of improved techniques for filling dead space with viable muscle flaps. The fracture rate, although high (approximately 18%), is more acceptable because it does not signify a failure of the system. With appropriate treatment, fractures usually progress to union.

3. The implanted bones do not incorporate or remodel completely, so that one cannot remove hardware or rely on solid fracture healing (although about 15% of them heal spontaneously!).[2] This factor makes the requirements for a more exacting surgical approach and technique of fixation sometimes formidable, if not overburdening after a major resection of a part.

4. Even with large bone banks, sizing is still a significant problem.[13, 62] There is little doubt that a banking network is essential to developing a better technology for allograft replacement. No single bank can support the inventory necessary to supply all those who need replacement of a part.

5. Virus transmission with the graft is a major worry for the patient and the physician. Although only one case has been reported to date,[67] it is quite evident that AIDS can be transmitted with the allograft. Although earlier studies suggested that a screening test would eliminate contaminated parts, the 3- to 6-month "window" is a concern.[3, 56, 68] Furthermore, contrary to prior expectations, radiation of the graft does not guarantee sterilization.[8, 72]

6. Recovering, storing, sizing, shaping, and attaching the graft and restoring the ligamentous and tendinous structures are often technically difficult and sometimes place strenuous demands on the caretaking team. Allograft replacement is not an "off the shelf" procedure!

TECHNICAL ASPECTS

The currently accepted approach to retrieving and processing alloimplants is based on an understanding of the biologic attributes of grafts (see above).[7, 10, 24] There seems to be little doubt that the parts are less acceptable to the host than autograft and that, despite freezing of the bone, an immune response interferes with and retards the incorporation of the graft into the host tissues. This delay in revascularization and the "walling off" of the graft as a result of the host immune reaction is believed to render the part more susceptible to infection (as a *locus minoris resistentiae*) as well as to fracture, because often incomplete and asymmetric vascularization coupled with poor placement of the hardware may produce areas of increased strain and major stress risers. Thus, as emphasized above, the tissue recovery process must be meticulous, the implantation must be well planned and executed, and the patient must be cautiously protected postoperatively in a manner that may appear overly conservative to some surgeons who perform reconstructive procedures.

The ablative surgery includes usually either wide or limited margins, depending on the nature of the tumor and the anatomic site from which the segment is resected. After removal of the lesion, the appropriate graft is selected on the basis of radiographic sizing. It is shaped to fit the defect and then fixed in place, usually with screws and plates or, less commonly, intramedullary rods. It is essential to maintain the best possible soft tissue bed for graft incorporation, and transfer of muscle for coverage has now become routine. For lower extremities, gastrocnemius, soleus, or rectus flaps are used to fill dead space and to cover the graft with viable tissue; for upper extremities, the latissimus or pectoralis flap is equally valuable. The authors have occasionally performed a free flap for complicated cases to be certain that the soft tissue coverage is adequate.

The wounds are drained via suction for several days during the initial postoperative period to minimize hematoma formation or a dead space, both of which may predispose to infection. For most patients with transplants in the lower extremity, anticoagulants are used for several weeks to several months to reduce the likelihood of thrombosis and pulmonary embolism. Intravenous antibiotics are given in the immediate postoperative period, and their administration is maintained longer than is usual for a standard orthopedic procedure. Oral antibiotics were administered in prior years when the patient was discharged from the hospital. The authors have since abandoned that practice but continue to prescribe tetracycline for many patients not only to provide a modest bacteriostatic effect but also to label new bone in the graft.

The limb is placed in a cast for a period ranging from 4 to 8 weeks, depending on the anatomic site and the stability of the reconstructed joint. Joints and host-donor junction sites are braced, usually for several months, in polypropylene cast-type orthotic devices. These are usually not removed until the joints are stable and the osteosynthesis sites are healed. The procedure is described in considerable detail in a number of publications from the Massachusetts General Hospital Orthopaedic Oncology Unit and the Bone Bank.[35, 44–47]

CLINICAL SERIES

Between November 24, 1971 and February 26, 1990, 554 orthotopically placed frozen cadaveric allografts were implanted by surgeons on the Orthopaedic Oncology Unit of the Massachusetts General Hospital. Included in this number are a group of 34 patients who received hemipelvis grafts, whose reconstructive problems are unique and are therefore excluded from the analysis described below. Deleting the pelvic grafts leaves a series of 520 consecutively performed operations on patients followed for an average duration of 51 months (range 1 to 219 months). Two hundred thirty-nine (46%) of the patients were males and 281 (54%) were females, with a mean age for the series of 32.6 years (range 4 to 80 years). Patient records are maintained in a computer file, which is updated with each visit. End results, tumor complications (recurrence, metastasis, and death), and allograft complications (infection, fracture, nonunion, and unstable joint) are recorded. End results are defined by an evaluation system first introduced for the authors' patients[44] and not unlike that subsequently proposed by Enneking[15] or more recently modified by Johnson and colleagues.[36] All of these systems are dependent on functional evaluation of the part. Results are classified as *excellent* if patients are restored to virtually full function, have no pain, have no limitations, require no braces or supports, and are free of local tumor. A *good* result is one in which the patient is free from pain, has no evident recurrence, and needs no braces or supports, but accepts some limitations, particularly for sports activities. With a *fair* result, the patient is markedly limited in activity, has pain, or is unable to function without a brace or support. A patient who has a local recurrence, whose graft must be resected, or who requires an amputation is considered to represent a treatment *failure*.

This study included a variety of types of grafts and anatomic sites into which they were implanted. The anatomic sites for the 520 procedures are shown in Table 9–1. As can be noted, 288 included not only a shaft of a bone but also an adjacent articular surface and are thus considered to be *osteoarticular* (Fig. 9–1). Most of these grafts were inserted about the knee, the shoulder, the hip, or the wrist. The *intercalary* category (bone alone) (Fig. 9–2) included 112 patients, with the majority of the grafts replacing the shafts of the femur, the tibia, or the humerus. In 66 of the patients, the allograft was combined with a prosthesis *(alloprosthesis)* (Fig. 9–3), and as can be noted, these devices were inserted almost exclusively about the hip and the knee. In 54 of the patients, an allograft was used to achieve an arthrodesis *(alloarthrodesis)* of the knee (27 patients), the shoulder (21), the hip (3), the ankle (2), or the wrist (1) (Table 9–1).

TABLE 9–1

Anatomic Sites for Allograft Transplantation*

Osteoarticular	
Distal femur	129
Proximal tibia	68
Proximal humerus	29
Proximal femur	24
Distal radius	21
Distal humerus	11
Proximal ulna	3
Distal tibia	3
Total	288
Intercalary	
Tibia	35
Femur	49
Humerus	22
Ulna	2
Radius	4
Total	112
Allograft-Prosthesis	
Proximal femur	45
Distal femur	13
Proximal tibia	4
Entire femur	3
Entire humerus	1
Total	66
Allograft-Arthrodesis	
Distal femur	24
Proximal tibia	3
Proximal humerus	21
Proximal femur	3
Distal tibia	2
Distal radius	1
Total	54

*520 procedures performed between November 24, 1971 and February 26, 1990.

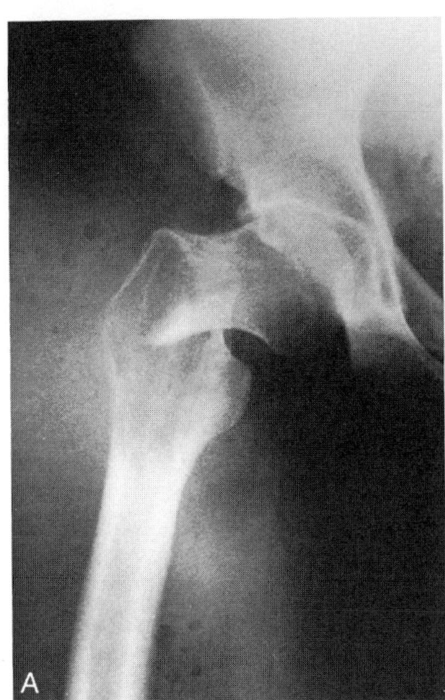

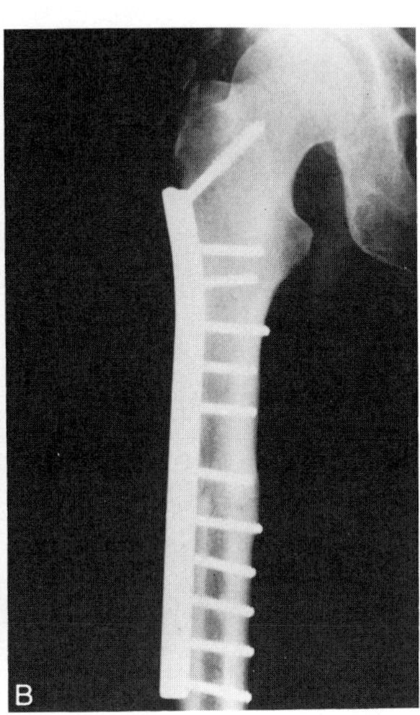

FIGURE 9–1. Osteoarticular allograft. *A,* A 44-year-old man with a non-Hodgkin's lymphoma was seen in January 1983. A resection was performed and a proximal femoral allograft was implanted. The fit of the donor head in the host acetabulum seemed excellent, and restoration of function was accomplished by suturing the gluteal muscles and the iliopsoas muscle to the tendinous attachment sites on the graft. *B,* Anteroposterior radiograph taken 6 years after the surgery. The patient walks with a slight limp but without aids and has no pain. He remains disease free.

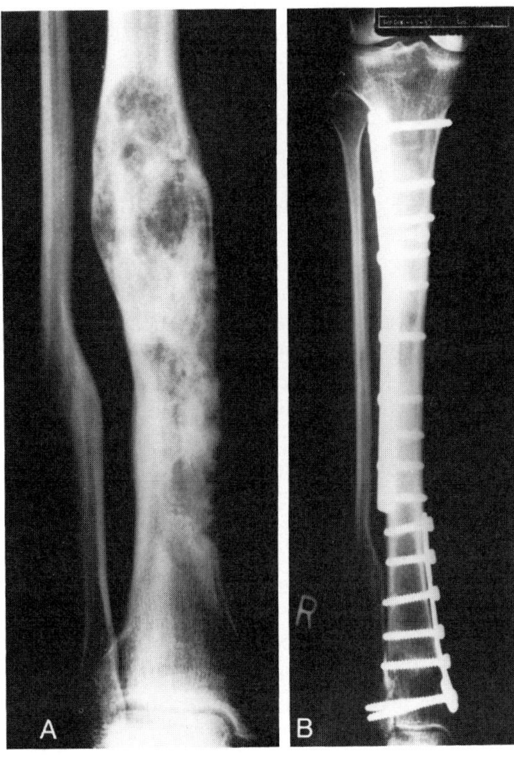

FIGURE 9–2. Intercalary allograft. *A,* Radiograph of the tibia of a 21-year-old woman who had two previous attempts to eradicate an adamantinoma. In May 1975, she had a resection of the tibial shaft and introduction of an intercalary allograft. *B,* Radiograph taken more than 10 years later discloses that both host-donor junction sites are healed. The patient has no evidence of recurrence of the tumor and has no symptoms related to the tibia graft.

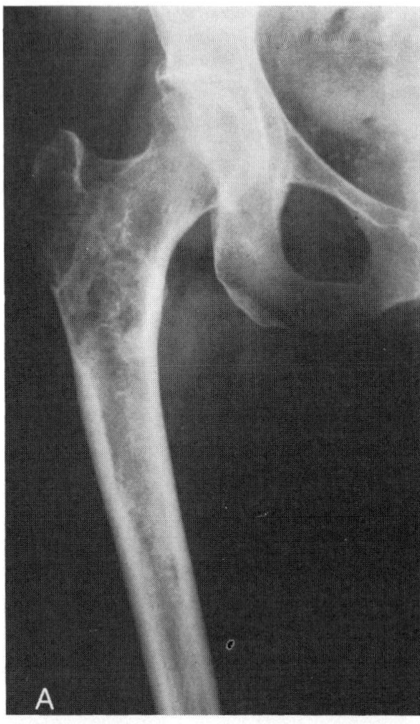

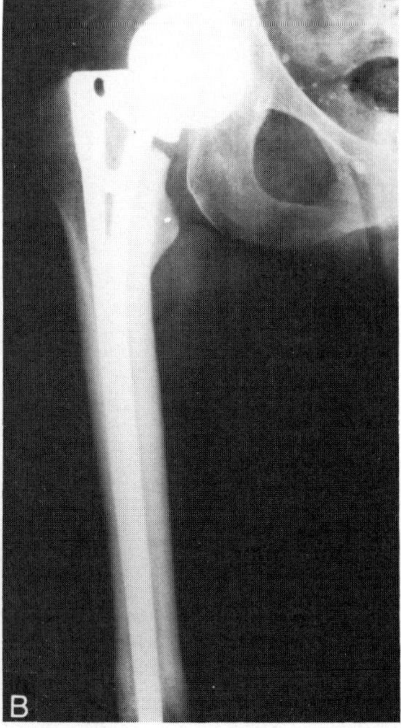

FIGURE 9–3. Alloprosthesis. *A,* A 58-year-old woman was first seen in December 1978 with complaints of pain about the right hip. A diagnosis of high-grade chondrosarcoma was established by biopsy. *B,* The proximal femur was resected and replaced by an allograft with a long-stemmed Austin-Moore device. More than 12 years following the surgery the patient has no recurrence and minimal complaints referable to the hip. She does not use walking aids.

The diagnoses for the 520 patients are shown in Table 9–2. In terms of the stage of the lesions for which the patients were treated, 19% of the cases were stage 0; 48%, stage IA or IB; and the remainder (33%), stage IIA, IIB, or III (using the staging system described by Enneking and associates).[17] As to specific diagnoses, giant cell tumor (120 cases) was commonly found early in the study but was a much less frequently encountered diagnosis in the past few years, in view of the apparent success of cementation in preventing recurrence. The next most frequent diagnoses in the series were central osteosarcoma (87 cases), chondrosarcoma (76), and parosteal osteosarcoma (27). Twenty-two of the patients had malignant fibrous histiocytoma or fibrosarcoma, and 14 each had either an adamantinoma or Ewing's sarcoma.

RESULTS AND COMPLICATIONS

Four hundred fourteen of the patients in the series were followed for 2 years or longer (with a mean duration of follow-up of 45 months). These patients constitute the group for which the end results and complication rates were assessed. It should be noted that 284 of these 414 patients have been continuously followed since their surgery. Of the remaining 130, 35 were lost to the series as a result of death of the patient from malignant disease; an additional 89 patients were dropped because of failure of the graft (but are not lost to follow-up; more than half of these have received new grafts and been reentered into the series as new cases). Only 6 of the 414 patients were truly lost to follow-up. The demographic data and the distribution of sites and diagnoses of the 284 patient subset did not materially differ from those for the overall series (see text and Tables 9–1 and 9–2).

Table 9–3 shows the results for the patients in the series as determined by the grading system described above. As can be readily noted, the results varied according to the type of graft, with the best outcomes noted for intercalary grafts (more than 88% excellent or good) and the poorest for the allograft arthrodeses (only 4% excellent and 64% good). These variations in end result, however, are not statistically significant. Overall analysis of the results for all the patients shows that 77% are currently graded as excellent or good; and if the 23 tumor failures in the series are excluded, the percentage of satisfactory results rises to more than 81%.

The complications of the procedure are shown in Table 9–4, and it should be evident that they are of considerable significance in terms of influencing the end result. Of the 414 patients, more than half showed one or several tumor or allograft complications, and these in many cases led to failure.

Although most of the patients (318 of 414)

TABLE 9–2

Diagnoses in Allograft Transplantation*

Tumors	
Giant cell tumor	120
Chondrosarcoma	77
Central osteosarcoma	87
Parosteal osteosarcoma	27
Fibrosarcoma or malignant fibrous histiocytoma	22
Adamantinoma	14
Ewing's sarcoma	14
Osteoblastoma	9
Metastatic carcinoma	13
Chondroblastoma	7
Soft tissue tumors	5
Desmoplastic fibroma	6
Angiosarcoma	4
Lymphoma	3
Chondromyxoid fibroma	2
Aneurysmal bone cyst	2
Myeloma	2
Osteochondroma	2
Ossifying fibroma	2
Leiomyosarcoma	3
Osteoid osteoma	1
Liposarcoma	2
Nontumorous Conditions	
Failed allograft or total joint replacement	48
Traumatic loss	13
Massive osteonecrosis	19
Fibrous dysplasia	8
Gaucher's disease	4
Villonodular synovitis	2
Paget's disease	1
Eosinophilic granuloma	1

*520 patients seen between November 24, 1971 and February 26, 1990.

were treated for bone tumors, the tumor complications were assessed only in the 127 patients at highest risk because their lesions were classified as high grade (stages IIA, IIB, or III). Thirty-five (28%) of these patients died, 51 (40%) developed metastases, and 15 (12%) experienced a local recurrence. These values do not materially differ from those reported by other investigators for high-grade tumors treated with this or other techniques, nor are they significantly different from those for patients treated by the authors' group with techniques other than allograft implantation.

In terms of the complications associated with the allograft procedure, only infection, fracture, nonunion, and joint instability appeared to be consistent problems; these were assessed in all 414 patients in the series. As can be noted in Table 9–4, infection was and is the most serious of these, occurring in slightly more than 10%. Fracture was not nearly as devastating to outcome; nevertheless, it occurred in more than 18% of the patients and accounted for much of the reoperation rate. Nonunion was declared to exist if the host-donor junction site or sites were not healed at 12 months, and this complication occurred in 14%. The percentage of unstable joints was surprisingly less than 7%.

Kaplan-Meier plots and Cox regression analyses were performed on the entire series of patients and showed that if one analyzed for failure of the graft (end result equals fair or poor), infection, recurrence, stage, site, and fracture had an effect on the outcome (all at $P < 0.0001$) (Fig. 9–4). Furthermore, almost all of the failures occurred during the first 3 years; nearly all of the infections were manifest by 7 months (Fig. 9–5), and the fractures by 3 years (Fig. 9–6). After that time, the patients were remarkably trouble free to more than 17.5 years. The data for the effects of stage of the lesion and recurrence on outcome are shown in Figures 9–7 and 9–8. Although not considered sufficiently independent to appear as significant on the Cox regression equation, the use of chemotherapy appears to have an adverse effect (Fig. 9–9) whereas age, type of lesion, sex, and whether the graft was a total replacement of articular surface or circumference of a shaft or a hemigraft (Fig. 9–10) seemed not to have a significant influence on outcome.

DISCUSSION

Limb-sparing surgery has now become a major component of the treatment protocols for aggressive and malignant tumors of the skeletal system, and almost every center engaged in therapy for orthopedic oncologic lesions has introduced the practices and disciplines required to utilize this rather demanding type of therapy. Virtually every center fully determines the stage of lesions in their patients, treats the patients (when indicated) with adjuvant and neoadjuvant radiation and chemotherapy, and extirpates the tumor with appropriate intralesional, marginal, or wide resection. All units do virtually the same studies in the same way, and there exists a rather remarkable similarity of the treatment rendered to patients throughout the world. This seeming homogeneity of approach, however, fails to hold up when it comes to the manner of reconstructing the part after resection, and

TABLE 9–3

Results of Allograft Transplantation*

Type of Graft (number)	Results			
	Excellent	*Good*	*Fair*	*Failure*
Osteoarticular (236)	89 38%	85 36%	4 2%	58 25%
Intercalary (83)	59 71%	14 17%	0 0%	10 12%
Alloprosthesis (50)	22 44%	18 36%	1 2%	9 18%
Alloarthrodesis (45)	2 4%	29 64%	1 2%	13 29%
TOTAL (414)	172 42%	146 35%	6 1%	90 22%
If Tumor Failures (23) Are Deleted				
TOTAL (391)	172 44%	146 37%	6 2%	23 17%

*414 patients seen between November 24, 1971 and February 27, 1988 and followed for 2 years or longer.

it is in this major area that most of the differences arise among the surgical oncologists and their programs. Vascularized or nonvascularized autografts, cemented metallic implants, cementless systems, expandable devices, turnabouts, and massive frozen allografts all have their advocates, who speak to the indications, the complications, and the end results. None is trouble free, and no one technique stands out as superior to all others. The authors have also utilized other systems, but it should be evident from the data presented that the authors have made a major investment in clinical care and research using allograft and banking technology.

The biologic and immunologic data presented above are the foundation for the clinical series. Although not all of the issues are clear, it is evident from the studies presented that, with the use of the current banking and clinical technology, it is possible to introduce allografts with a high expectation of success. Furthermore, it is evident from observations of the series that the patients have most of their complications early in the course and that, after the 3-year mark is reached, the system stabilizes and patients continue to do well for years. It is the authors' hypothesis, supported by evolving knowledge from experimental studies, that the reason for this success and improvement over time is the invasion and incorporation of the donor bone by the host connective tissue, leading eventually to a living system.

The difficulties with the system are the obvious need to eliminate the complications of infection and fracture, both of which almost invariably occur before the 3-year mark and may have a disastrous outcome. In the authors' series, all but 15% of the patients in whom infection developed were classified as treatment failures and ultimately lost their graft (see Fig. 9–5). Currently, infection is considered to have such a dismal outlook that, except in superficial infections or those associated with a skin slough, early management includes

Text continued on page 193

TABLE 9–4

Complications of Allograft Transplantation*

Tumor complications in 127 patients with high-grade tumors	
Death	35 (28%)
Metastasis	51 (40%)
Recurrence	15 (12%)
Allograft complications for all 414 procedures	
Infection	42 (10%)
Fracture	76 (18%)
Nonunion	58 (14%)
Unstable joint	20 (7%)†

*414 patients seen between November 24, 1971 and February 27, 1988 and followed for 2 years or longer. It should be noted that some of the patients had more than one complication, so that the numbers displayed above are not additive. In fact, 201 patients (49%) had neither tumor nor allograft complications.

†Only patients with osteoarticular grafts and alloprostheses are at risk for joint instability.

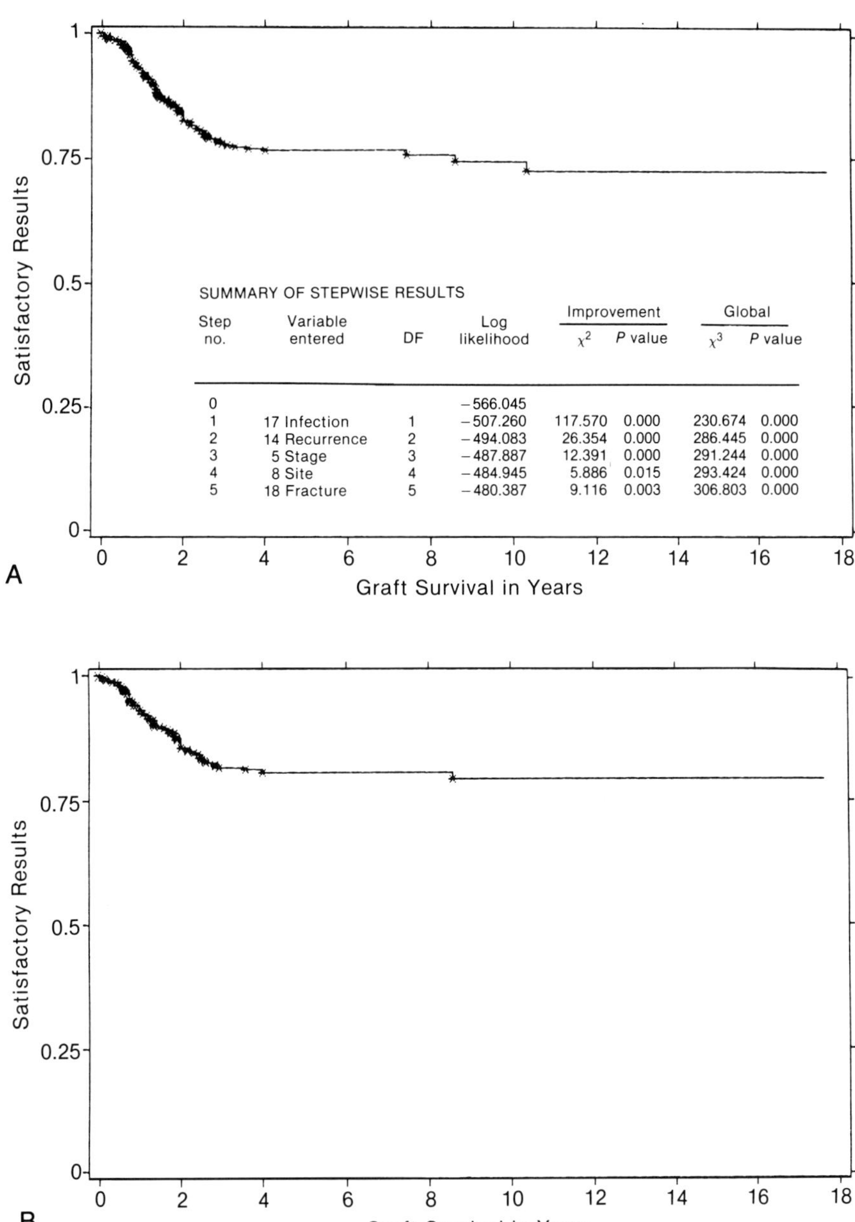

SUMMARY OF STEPWISE RESULTS

Step no.	Variable entered	DF	Log likelihood	Improvement χ^2	Improvement *P* value	Global χ^3	Global *P* value
0			−566.045				
1	17 Infection	1	−507.260	117.570	0.000	230.674	0.000
2	14 Recurrence	2	−494.083	26.354	0.000	286.445	0.000
3	5 Stage	3	−487.887	12.391	0.000	291.244	0.000
4	8 Site	4	−484.945	5.886	0.015	293.424	0.000
5	18 Fracture	5	−480.387	9.116	0.003	306.803	0.000

FIGURE 9–4. Life table for allograft transplantation showing graft survival. *A*, The Kaplan-Meier plot for the authors' series of 414 patients undergoing allograft transplantation. The Cox regression data are shown. *B*, The same plot when the 23 tumor failures are excluded. The mean for the series is excellent or good results in more than 80%, and the majority of the failures occurred in the first 3 years.

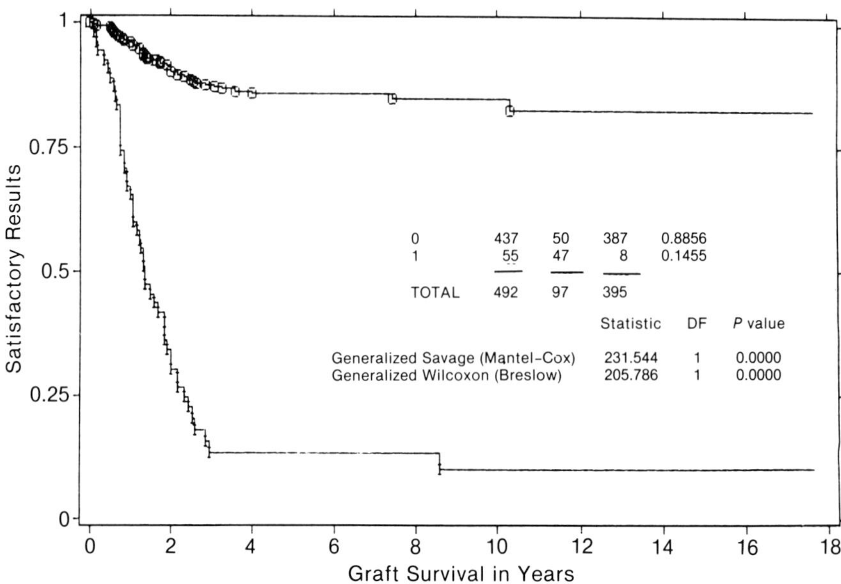

FIGURE 9–5. Life table for allograft transplantation showing the effect of infection on graft survival. Kaplan-Meier plot defining the devastating effect of infection. Only 15% of the infected cases ended with satisfactory results. 0, no infection; 1, infection.

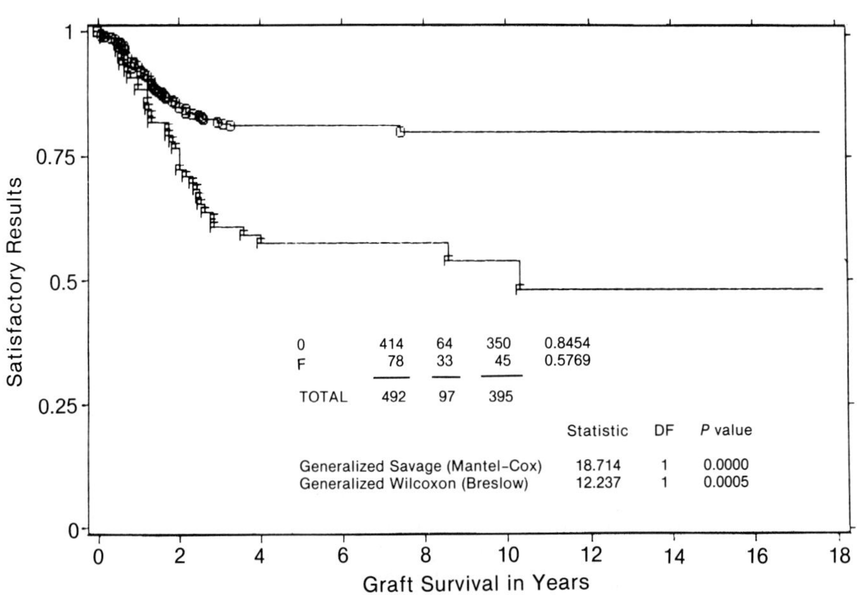

FIGURE 9–6. Life table for allograft transplantation showing the effect of allograft fracture on graft survival. Almost 60% of the grafts in patients with fractures were salvaged. 0, no fracture; F, fracture.

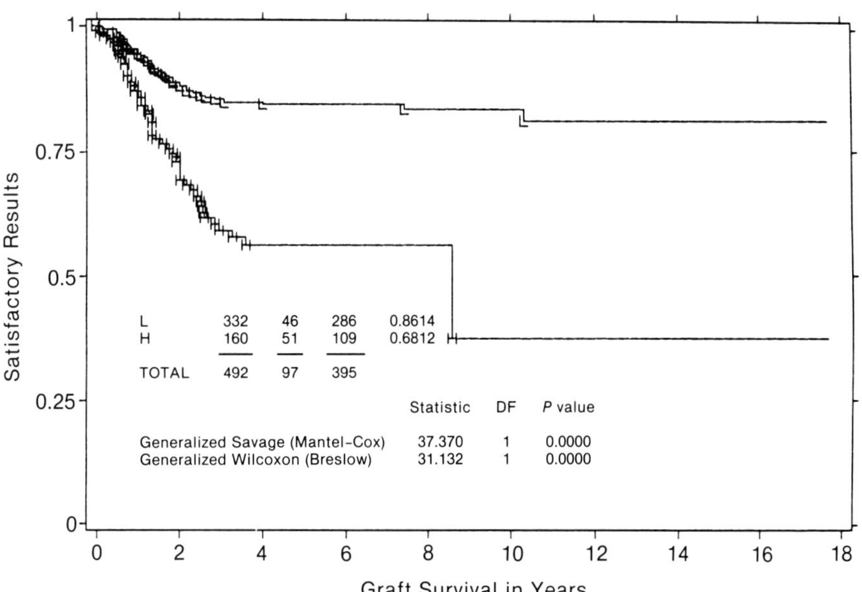

FIGURE 9–7. The stage of the lesion had an effect on outcome. Grafts in those with high-grade lesions (stages IIA, IIB, or III) were less satisfactory than grafts in patients with stage 0, IA, or IB lesions. L, low-grade lesion; H, high-grade lesion.

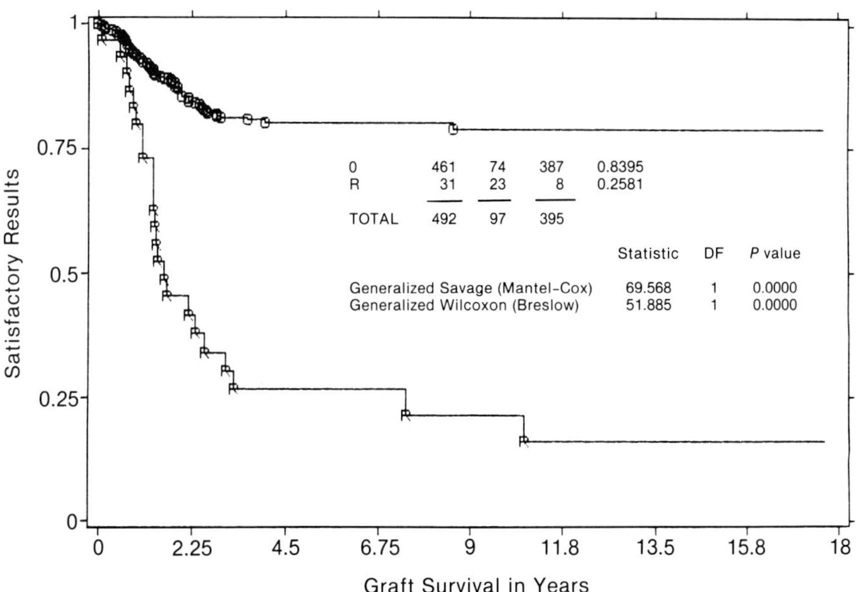

FIGURE 9–8. Life table for allograft transplantation showing that tumor recurrence affected graft survival and was clearly a major determinant of outcome. In the group experiencing recurrence, less than 25% of the grafts were salvaged. 0, no recurrence; R, recurrence.

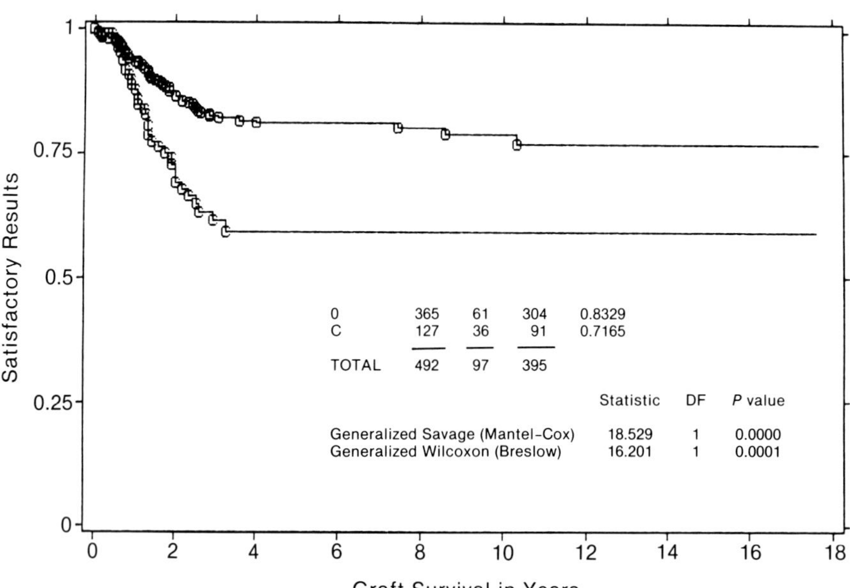

FIGURE 9–9. Chemotherapy affected outcome, as shown in this Kaplan-Meier plot. Its effect was not considered independent of that of other factors (such as stage of the lesion), and hence chemotherapy did not appear as a principal determinant in the Cox regressions shown in Figure 9–4*A*. 0, no chemotherapy; C, chemotherapy.

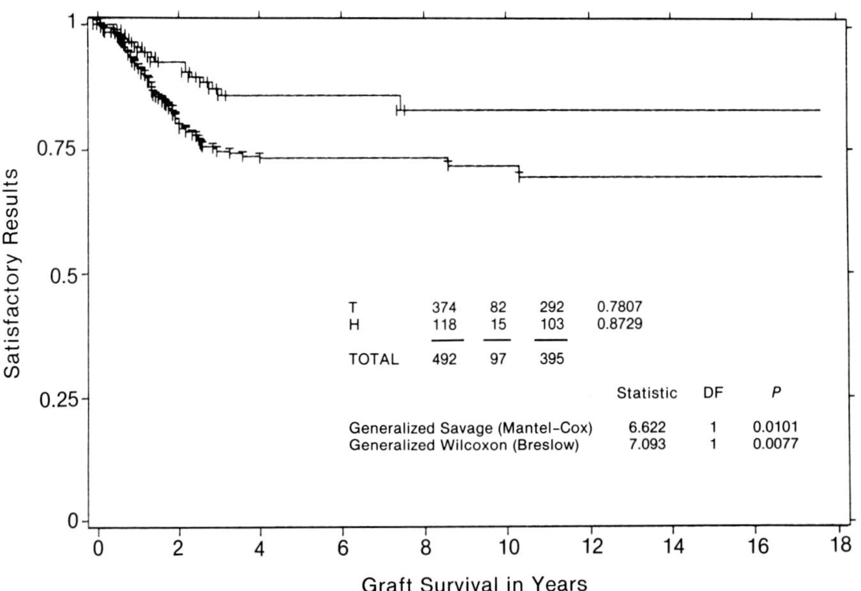

FIGURE 9–10. Hemiallografts are intercalary or osteoarticular grafts in which the host bone was not circumferentially removed. The implication is a more benign diagnosis. a broader healing surface, and less extensive surgery. Thus, hemiallografts should have considerably better results. Surprisingly, as shown in this Kaplan-Meier plot, hemigrafts and total grafts did not materially differ in outcome. H, hemigrafts; T, total grafts.

resection of the graft, implantation of a polymethyl methacrylate spacer (impregnated with suitable antibiotics), systemic antibiotic administration, and then another allograft transplant.[41]

With respect to the patients in whom a fracture occurs, it is clear from examination of the data presented in Figure 9–6 that such an event adversely influences the end result, although not as profoundly as does an infection. It is evident that 42% of the patients experiencing graft fracture proceed to an unsatisfactory result (fair or failure), and this is significantly different from those that do not experience fracture ($P < 0.0001$, Mantel-Cox). Evaluation of the ultimate outcome after this complication by Berrey and colleagues[2] showed that with immobilization alone, rearrangement of the internal fixation and autografting, introduction of a conventional total joint replacement, or replacement of the graft, well over 80% of the patients eventually are restored to useful and often surprisingly competent function.[46, 47]

Nonunion is a common problem, 58 of the 414 patients experienced nonunion at one host-donor osteosynthesis site at 1 year. As could be clearly anticipated, a positive correlation for the incidence of this complication exists with the use of chemotherapy and/or radiation to the bed.[29] Evidence for this statement lies in the statistics for the 8 patients with Ewing's sarcoma followed for 2 years or longer, all of whom were treated with radiation and chemotherapy before resection. Five of this group (62.5%) experienced nonunion. Of interest, however, was the relative ease with which this complication was corrected by surgical intervention. Specifically, for 51 patients whose only complication was nonunion, the ultimate outcome after rearrangement of hardware and addition of autograft judged excellent or good in 76.5%.

Another less common but probably almost unavoidable complication of the procedure is joint instability. For patients with osteoarticular allograft or allograft-prosthesis, the complication occurred in less than 7%. Much of the problem in this group was mechanical, in that the donor distal femur or proximal tibia did not fit the opposing host part; or insufficient soft tissues were left with the donor part to reconstruct resected ligaments. In only one patient who had extensive chemotherapy for the primary osteosarcoma as well as for a pulmonary relapse, there appeared to be some degree of impairment of collagen synthesis and a resultant ligamentous laxity, affecting not only the donor proximal tibia but other joints as well.

RESEARCH

Allograft transplantation has some role in skeletal reconstruction after massive bone loss. The impediments to more widespread use principally consist of the complexity of the procedure, the difficulties of obtaining suitable parts, and the currently unacceptable complication rate. The latter may be tolerable if one considers amputation or a custom metallic device as the alternative, but it is still necessary to improve the system. Work proceeds in several laboratories and, although not the subject of this chapter, it seems logical to briefly describe some of the current research protocols that in the not-too-distant future may result in improved systems for allograft utilization and a more predictable outcome.

The laboratories and clinics with which the authors are associated and several other units in the country continue to study the rates and patterns of revascularization. It seems essential to define the effect of the immune system not only on the processes of graft revascularization and incorporation, but also on the susceptibility to infection (is the graft really a *locus minoris resistentiae* for transient organisms, and for how long?) and the patterns of fractures (is the cause of fracture really asymmetric revascularization?). The authors, like investigators at several other laboratories, are continuing to study the survival of joint structures with allograft transplantation. Is cryopreservation essential, and if so, what is the optimal method for reducing the crystal burden in and on the cell with freezing and thawing? The search for improvements in surgical technique should continue, particularly in relation to avoidance of infection, improvements in internal fixation, and optimal suturing technique for soft tissue repairs of joints. One of the major changes in surgical technique in recent years is the more frequent use of muscle flaps to cover the graft and to decrease the likelihood of skin slough. Gastrocnemius, rectus, soleus, latissimus, and pectoral muscle flaps have all been used to aid primary wound healing over the graft and to reduce the infection rate, achieving the all-time low for the authors' series of less than 10% (which is comparable to that reported by other investigators using metallic devices).

One of the most important projects involves a correlation of long-term results of allografts with a retrospective HLA match between the donor and the recipient. There are suggestions that class II matches are important in this regard and may in the future allow preselection of the immunologically correct frozen donor part for the patient (provided the bank inventory is large enough). Another crucial developmental area is to continue to strive for improved methods of tissue retrieval and more frequent donation rates to maintain a large and safe bone bank. It seems essential that the assessment of donors is broadened and extended to be certain that the grafts are free from transmissible disease. Similarly, the grafts must be more fully evaluated to be certain that they will be predictably effective in terms of structure and mechanical properties. Networking of selected banks will help guarantee an appropriate host-donor fit. The process may become even more important if partially matching the HLA characteristics of the graft to the host becomes an integral part of the system. The most important breakthrough, however, is yet to occur—the discovery of methods of specific reduction of immunogenicity of the graft for a particular host, or possibly altering the host response in a safe fashion to reduce the reaction to the graft. If some of these research objectives can be accomplished, the outcome of the procedure should be more assured, and the results can be sufficiently predictable to warrant application to a broader panel of disorders than bone tumors.

References

1. American Association of Tissue Banks: Standards for Tissue Banking, 1987. Arlington, VA, American Association of Tissue Banks, 1987.
2. Berrey WH Jr, Lord CF, Gebhardt MC, Mankin HJ: Fractures of allografts. Frequency, treatment, and end-results. J Bone Joint Surg 72A:825–833, 1990.
3. Buck RE, Malinin TI, Brown MD: Bone transplantation and human immunodeficiency virus. An estimate of risk of acquired immunodeficiency syndrome (AIDS). Clin Orthop 240:129–136, 1989.
4. Burchardt H: Biology of bone transplantation. Orthop Clin North Am 18:187–196, 1987.
5. Burchardt H, Glowczewskie FP, Enneking W: Allogeneic segmental fibular transplants in azathioprine immunosuppressed dogs. J Bone Joint Surg 59A:881–894, 1977.
6. Burchardt H, Glowczewskie FP Jr, Enneking WF: The effect of Adriamycin and methotrexate on the repair of segmental cortical autografts in dogs. J Bone Joint Surg 65A:103–108, 1983.
7. Burwell RG: The fate of bone grafts. *In* Apley AG (ed): Recent Advances in Orthopaedics. London, Churchill Livingstone, 1969, pp 115–207.
8. Conway B, Tomford WW, Hirsch MS, Schooley RT, Mankin HJ: Effects of gamma irradiation on HIV-1 in a bone allograft model. Trans Orthop Res Soc 15:225, 1990.
9. Curtiss PH, Powell AE, Herndon CH: Immunological factors in homogeneous bone transplantation. III. The inability of homogeneous rabbit bone to induce circulating antibodies in rabbits. J Bone Joint Surg 41A:1482–1488, 1959.
10. Czitrom AA, Langer F, McKee N, Gross AE: Bone and cartilage allotransplantation. A review of 14 years of research and clinical studies. Clin Orthop 208:141–145, 1986.
11. Delloye C, DeNayer P, Allington N, Munting E, Coutelier L, Vincent A: Massive bone allografts in large skeletal defects after tumor surgery: A clinical and microradiographic evaluation. Arch Orthop Trauma Surg 107:31–41, 1988.
12. Dick HM, Malinin TI, Mnaymneh WA: Massive allograft implantation following radical resection of high-grade tumors requiring adjuvant chemotherapy treatment. Clin Orthop 197:88–95, 1985.
13. Doppelt SH, Tomford WW, Lucas A, Mankin HJ: Operational and financial aspects of a hospital bone bank. J Bone Joint Surg 63A:1472–1479, 1981.
14. Ehrlich MG, Lorenz J, Tomford WW, Mankin HJ: Collagenase activity in banked bone. Trans Orthop Res Soc 8:166, 1983.
15. Enneking WF: A system for evaluation of the surgical management of musculoskeletal tumors. *In* Enneking WF (ed): Limb Salvage in Musculoskeletal Oncology. New York, Churchill Livingstone, 1987, pp 145–150.
16. Enneking WF, Burchardt H, Puhl JJ, Pistrowski G: Physical and biological aspects of repair in dog cortical bone transplants. J Bone Joint Surg 57A:237–252, 1975.
17. Enneking WF, Spanier SS, Goodman MA: Current concepts review: The surgical staging of musculoskeletal sarcoma. J Bone Joint Surg 62A:1027–1030, 1980.
18. Flosdorf EW, Hyatt GW: The preservation of bone grafts by freeze drying. Surgery 31:716–719, 1952.
19. Friedlaender GE: Immune responses to osteochondral allografts: Current knowledge and future directions. Clin Orthop 174:58–68, 1983.
20. Friedlaender GE: Immune responses to preserved bone allografts in humans. *In* Friedlaender GE, Mankin HJ, Sell KW (eds): Osteochondral Allografts: Biology, Banking and Clinical Applications. Boston, Little, Brown, 1983, pp 159–164.
21. Friedlaender GE: Bone grafts: The basic science rationale for clinical applications. J Bone Joint Surg 69A:786–790, 1987.
22. Friedlaender GE: Morphologic and immunologic responses to bone allografts in humans: A preliminary report. *In* Enneking WF (ed): Limb Salvage in Musculoskeletal Oncology. New York, Churchill Livingstone, 1987, pp 562–566.
23. Friedlaender GE, Mankin HJ: Bone banking: Current methods and suggested guidelines. *In* Murray DG (ed): AAOS Instructional Course Lectures, Vol 30. St Louis, CV Mosby, 1981, pp 36–55.
24. Friedlaender GE, Mankin HJ, Langer F: Immunology of osteochondral allografts: Background and general considerations. *In* Friedlaender GE, Mankin HJ, Sell KW (eds): Osteochondral Allografts: Biology, Banking and Clinical Applications. Boston, Little, Brown, 1983, pp 133–140.
25. Friedlaender GE, Mankin HJ, Sell KW (eds): Osteo-

chondral Allografts: Biology, Banking and Clinical Applications. Boston, Little, Brown, 1983.
26. Friedlaender GE, Strong DM, Sell KW: Studies on the antigenicity of bone. I. Freeze-dried and deep-frozen bone allograft in rabbits. J Bone Joint Surg 58A:854–858, 1976.
27. Friedlaender GE, Strong DM, Sell KW: Studies on the antigenicity of bone. II: Donor-specific anti-HLA antibodies in human recipients of freeze-dried allografts. J Bone Joint Surg 66A:107–112, 1984.
28. Friedlaender GE, Tross RB, Doganis AC, Kirkwood JM, Baron R: Effects of chemotherapy on bone. I. Short-term methotrexate and doxorubicin (Adriamycin) treatment in rat model. J Bone Joint Surg 66A:602–606, 1984.
29. Gebhardt MC, Lord F, Friedlaender GE, Mankin HJ: The effect of chemotherapy on the clinical results of allograft transplantation in the treatment of malignant tumors of bone. (in manuscript).
30. Goldberg VM, Powell A, Schaffer JW, Zika J, Bos GD, Heiple KG: Bone grafting. Role of histocompatibility in transplantation. J Orthop Res 3:389–404, 1985.
31. Heiple KG, Chase SW, Herndon CH: A comparative study of the healing process following different types of bone transplantation. J Bone Joint Surg 45A:1593–1616, 1963.
32. Herndon CH, Chase SW: The fate of massive autogenous and homogenous bone grafts including articular surfaces. Surg Gynecol Obstet 98:273–290, 1954.
33. Hyatt GW, Butler MC: Bone grafting: The procurement, storage and clinical use of bone homografts. *In* AAOS Instructional Course Lectures, Vol 14. Ann Arbor, MI, JW Edwards, 1957, pp 343–373.
34. Inclan A: Use of preserved bone graft in orthopaedic surgery. J Bone Joint Surg 24(1):81–96, 1942.
35. Jofe MH, Gebhardt MC, Tomford WW, Mankin HJ: Osteoarticular allografts and allografts plus prosthesis in the management of malignant tumors of the proximal femur. J Bone Joint Surg 70A:507–516, 1988.
36. Johnson ME, Tomford WW, Mankin HJ, Butterfield L: Reconstruction of the hip and knee with allograft-endoprosthesis composites. Presentation at the 57th Annual Meeting of the American Academy of Orthopaedic Surgeons, New Orleans, LA, February 10, 1990.
37. Koskinen E: Wide resection of primary tumors of bone and replacement with massive bone grafts. Clin Orthop 134:302–319, 1978.
38. Kruez FP, Hyatt GW, Turner TC, Bassett CAL: The preservation and clinical use of freeze-dried bone. J Bone Joint Surg 33A:863–872, 1951.
39. Lexer E: Die verwendung der freien knochenplastik nebst versuchen uber gelenkversteifung und gelenktransplantation. Arch f Klin Chir 86:939–954, 1908.
40. Lexer E: Joint transplantation and arthroplasty. Surg Gynecol Obstet 40:782–809, 1925.
41. Lord CF, Gebhardt MC, Tomford WW, Mankin HJ: The incidence, nature and treatment of allograft infections. J Bone Joint Surg 70A:369–376, 1988.
42. Macewen W: Observations concerning transplantation of bones: Illustrated by a case of inter-human osseous transplantation, whereby over two-thirds of the shaft of a humerus was restored. Proc Roy Soc London 32:232–234, 1881.
43. Makley JT: The use of allografts to reconstruct intercalary defects of long bones. Clin Orthop 197:58–75, 1985.
44. Mankin HJ, Doppelt SH, Sullivan TR, Tomford WW: Osteoarticular and intercalary allograft transplantation in the management of malignant tumors of bone. Cancer 50:613–630, 1982.
45. Mankin HJ, Doppelt SH, Tomford WW: Clinical experience with allograft implantation. The first ten years. Clin Orthop 174:69–86, 1983.
46. Mankin HJ, Gebhardt MC, Tomford WW: The use of frozen cadaveric allografts in the management of patients with bone tumors of the extremities. Orthop Clin North Am 18:275–289, 1987.
47. Mankin HJ, Gebhardt MC, Tomford WW: The use of frozen cadaveric osteoarticular allografts in the treatment of benign and malignant tumors about the knee. *In* Enneking WF (ed): Limb Salvage in Musculoskeletal Oncology. New York, Churchill Livingstone, 1987, pp 354–363.
48. Mnaymneh W, Malinin T: Massive allografts in surgery of bone tumors. Orthop Clin North Am 20:455–467, 1989.
49. Mnaymneh W, Malinin TI, Makley JT, Dick HM: Massive osteoarticular allografts in the reconstruction of extremities following resection of tumors not requiring chemotherapy and radiation. Clin Orthop 227:666–677, 1986.
50. Ollier L: Traite Experimental et Clinique de la Regeneration des Os et de la Production Artificelle du Tissue Osseux. Paris, Masson, 1867.
51. Ottolenghi CE: Massive osteoarticular bone grafts. J Bone Joint Surg 48B:646–659, 1966.
52. Parrish FF: Treatment of bone tumors by total excision and replacement with massive autologous and homologous grafts. J Bone Joint Surg 48A:968–990, 1966.
53. Parrish FF: Allograft replacement of part of the end of a long bone following excision of a tumor: Report of twenty-one cases. J Bone Joint Surg 55A:1–22, 1973.
54. Pelker RR, Friedlaender GE: Biomechanical aspects of bone autografts and allografts. Orthop Clin North Am 18:235–241, 1987.
55. Pelker RR, Friedlaender GE, Markham TC, Panjabi MM, Moen CJ: The effects of freezing and freeze-drying on the biomechanical properties of rat bone. J Orthop Res 1:405–411, 1984.
56. Ranki A, Krohn M, Allain J-P, Franchi G, Valle S-L, Leuther M, Krohn K: Long latency precedes overt seroconversion in sexually transmitted human immunodeficiency virus infection. Lancet 2:589–593, 1987.
57. Reddi AH, Weintraub S, Muthikumaran N: Biologic principles of bone induction. Orthop Clin North Am 18:207–212, 1987.
58. Rodrigo JJ, Fuller TC, Mankin HJ: Cytotoxic HLA antibodies in patients with bone and cartilage allografts. Trans Orthop Res Soc 1:131, 1978.
59. Sadler AM Jr, Sadler BL, Stason EB, Stickel DL: Transplantation—a case for consent. N Engl J Med 280:862–867, 1969.
60. Stevenson S: The immune response to osteochondral allografts in dogs. J Bone Joint Surg 69A:573–582, 1987.
61. Tomford WW: Cryopreservation of articular cartilage. *In* Friedlaender GE, Mankin HJ, Sell KW (eds): Osteochondral Allografts: Biology, Banking and Clinical Applications. Boston, Little, Brown, 1983, pp 215–218.
62. Tomford WW, Doppelt SH, Mankin HJ: Organization, legal aspects and problems of bone banking in a large orthopaedic center. *In* Aebi M, Regazzoni P (eds): Bone Transplantation. Berlin, Springer-Verlag, 1989, pp 145–150.
63. Tomford WW, Mankin HJ, Friedlaender GE, Doppelt

SH, Gebhardt MC: Methods of banking bone and cartilage for allograft transplantation. Orthop Clin North Am 18:241–248, 1987.

64. Urist MR, Masiarz FR, Barr PJ, Kiefer M, Bathurst I, Finerman GAM: Recombinant bone morphogenetic protein by a yeast expression system. Trans Orthop Res Soc 15:68, 1990.
65. Urist MR, Silverman BG, Buring K, Dubuc FL, Rosenberg JM: The bone induction principle. Clin Orthop 53:279–280, 1967.
66. Volkov M: Allotransplantation of joints. J Bone Joint Surg 52B:49–53, 1970.
67. Transmission of HIV through bone transplantation: Case report and public health recommendations. MMWR 37:597–599, 1988.
68. Ward JW, Holmberg SD, Allen JR, Cohn DL, Critchley SE, Kleinman SH, Lenes BA, Ravenholdt O, Davis JR, Quinn MG, Jaffe HW: Transmission of human immuno-deficiency virus (HIV) by blood transfusions screened as negative for HIV antibody. N Engl J Med 318:473–478, 1988.
69. Weiland AJ: Vascularized free bone transplantation: Current concept review. J Bone Joint Surg 63A:166–169, 1981.
70. Weiland AJ, Daniel RK: Microvascular anastomoses for bone grafts in the treatment of massive defects in bone. J Bone Joint Surg 61A:98–104, 1979.
71. Wilson PD: Follow-up study of the use of refrigerated homogeneous bone transplants in orthopaedic operations. J Bone Joint Surg 33A:307–323, 1951.
72. Withrow SJ, Oulton SA, Suto TL, Wilkins RM, Straw RC, Rose BJ, Gasper PW: Evaluation of the antiretroviral effect of various methods of sterilizing/preserving corticocancellous bone. Trans Orthop Res Soc 15:226, 1990.

CHAPTER 10

Osseous Lesions of the Vertebral Axis and Tumors of the Cervical Spine

MARTIN B. CAMINS
BRUCE ROSENBLUM
MICHAEL J. HARRISON

Neoplastic lesions of the vertebral axis may either be symptomatic or be incidentally discovered on a routine radiograph. Histopathologic characteristics reveal a spectrum of changes, varying from benignity to frank malignancy. Definitive diagnosis and appropriate management require a team approach by a neurosurgeon, an orthopedist, a neuroradiologist, a pathologist, and an oncologist to characterize the lesion and guide the choice of appropriate therapeutic procedures.

DIAGNOSIS

Tumors of the spinal axis may displace or replace normal bone and spread to adjacent paraspinous soft tissues and the spinal canal. The clinical presentation usually correlates with the anatomic location of a primary or a metastatic tumor. Pain is the most common symptom. The age and sex of the patient and the anatomic location of the lesion (Table 10–1) help in formulating a differential diagnosis. For example, myeloma and metastatic tumor are more common in an older population, whereas histiocytosis X, Ewing's sarcoma, neuroblastoma metastatic to bone, and bone cysts are more frequently found in a younger age group.

A detailed neurologic examination is essential to identify the anatomic spinal levels of a lesion. Radicular distribution is important in localizing the lesion. Associated soft tissue tumor extension may cause mechanical limitation of motion, paraspinous muscle spasms, local heat, or tenderness. Upper motor neuron lesions may result from lesions of the cervical and thoracic vertebral bodies, whereas lesions in the lumbosacral region produce sphincteric and sexual dysfunction and other lower motor neuron deficits.

The examination of the patient should proceed with systematic laboratory and roentgenographic studies. The basic tests include a complete blood count, erythrocyte sedimentation rate, and determination of serum calcium, phosphorus, alkaline phosphatase, and total protein levels. A urinary vanillylmandelic acid measurement is helpful in the diagnosis of neuroblastoma, whereas an elevated prostatic acid phosphatase concentration is found with metastatic prostatic carcinoma. Routine radiographs should include the standard anteroposterior, lateral, and oblique projections. An effective skeletal survey may be obtained with a technetium bone scan. A gallium bone scan is helpful in searching for an inflammatory process or malignant lymphoma. Computed tomography (CT) and magnetic resonance im-

TABLE 10–1

Incidence of Vertebral Lesions by Anatomic Location

Cervical
Chordoma
Thoracic
Osteochondroma
Sarcoidosis
Hemangioma (lower thoracic)
Histiocytosis X
Metastatic carcinoma (breast/lung)
Lumbar
Osteochondroma
Osteosarcoma
Hemangioma
Metastatic carcinoma (prostate)
Sacrum
Chordoma
Ewing's sarcoma
Lipoma/liposarcoma
Giant cell tumor
Coccyx
Glomus tumor
Chordoma
Equally throughout spinal axis
Chondrosarcomas

aging (MRI) are routinely used to evaluate osseous lesions of the vertebral axis as well as their paraspinous and intraspinal components. Myelography reveals the extent of epidural spinal cord compression, whereas angiography demonstrates lesion vascularity. Embolization at the time of angiography may be essential in some cases to decrease the blood supply to highly vascular lesions to allow surgical resection.

Most portions of the spine are accessible for either open or closed biopsy. Unfortunately, some needle biopsies may not provide representative tissue for diagnosis. In addition, a biopsy should be planned so as not to interfere with later, more definitive surgery. Accurate histologic diagnosis provides significant information on the radiosensitivity of the tumor and is important in planning definitive therapy.[13]

TREATMENT

Surgical resection of a vertebral axis tumor should be considered when there is significant or intractable pain, spinal deformity or instability, and clinical phenomena representing progressive epidural spinal cord compression. Surgical results are now enhanced by radical decompression followed by spinal column stabilization. Guidelines in resecting bone tumors of the vertebral axis should include an anterior approach for lesions of the vertebral body and a posterior or lateral approach for lesions of the pedicle, the lamina, or the spinous process. In some instances, a combined one-stage anterior and posterior approach can be used. After resection of the tumor, stabilization with various internal fixation devices (rods, plates, screws, and acrylic and bone grafts) should be performed.[68]

In patients who are not surgical candidates, steroids and radiation remain effective alternatives for relieving pain and reversing progressive neurologic compromise. Unfortunately, the majority of statistical information on treating patients for spinal cord compression is based on surgical procedures (such as posterior decompression) alone.[56] With more aggressive surgical procedures, the administration of newly developed oncologic agents, and adjuvant therapy, the life expectancy of this group of patients has been extended significantly. Adjuvant interstitial brachytherapy with implanted iodine-125 sources is another form of therapy. In these patients, radiation sources are implanted into the tumor bed at the time of the primary resection as an internal boost to conventional teletherapy.[23] If a patient has received conventional teletherapy and the plan is to augment radiotherapy, the spinal cord can be protected with 0.762-nm-thick platinum foil molded to the contour of the cord and inserted into the epidural space.

Primary Bone Tumors

BENIGN BONE-FORMING TUMORS

Osteoid Osteoma

Osteoid osteomas are benign bone-forming tumors characterized by a well-defined nidus. They are common lesions, representing 11% of benign bone tumors.[26] There is a male preponderance and the mean age at occurrence is 19 years. Pain is the principal symptom; it is aggravated by activity and is more intense at night. The response of the pain to a trial dose of salicylates is variable and not a totally reliable sign. The inflammatory features of the lesion have been correlated with high levels of prostaglandin metabolites present in the tumor, which suggests that prostaglandins may play an important role in the mediation of osteoid osteoma pain.[46] White blood cell counts, erythrocyte sedimentation rates, and alkaline phosphatase levels are routinely normal.

Although the occurrence of these tumors in the spine is unusual, the characteristic clinical and radiologic features are usually diagnostic. From 10 to 18% of the cases occur in the spine and have a predilection for the posterior elements, especially the facet joints. They are usually less than 1.5 cm. A lesion can produce a clinically painful scoliosis. The diagnosis of spinal osteoid osteomas includes bone scanning and CT imaging, because routine radiographs may fail to reveal any abnormality. The characteristic radiographic appearance is sclerosis around a lucent nidus (Fig. 10–1).

The treatment of choice is complete surgical excision. Fusion of the spine after resection of an osteoid osteoma should be considered only if instability is apparent. A simple technique that confirms that the nidus has been excised at surgery is intraoperative tetracycline-fluorescence demonstration of the nidus. The patient receives 750 to 4000 mg of tetracycline preoperatively. Surgically removed specimens are immediately examined under an ultraviolet light, which demonstrates fluorescence of the nidus. Some surgeons favor intraoperative localization of osteoid osteomas by a radionuclide scintillation probe. These two techniques allow prompt localization of the tumor and minimize the amount of bone resection.

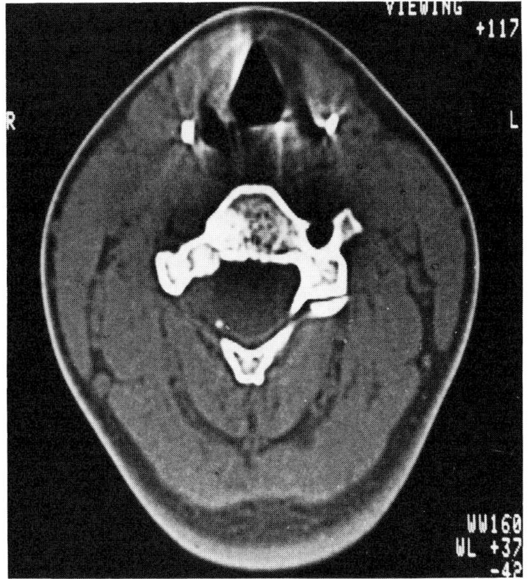

FIGURE 10–1. Osteoid osteoma. Computed tomography (CT) scan with bone windows demonstrates a faintly irregular, sclerotic and blastic lesion involving the pedicle and the adjacent vertebral body.

Osteoblastoma

Although osteoblastoma is less common (1% of all bone tumors) than osteoid osteoma, the two have certain resemblances,[26] including similar age and sex distributions. The appearance of histological osteoblastoma is closely related to that of an osteoid osteoma, but it can be differentiated primarily by its size and progressive history. The pain is a persistent dull ache and is less localized than the severe nocturnal pain of the osteoid osteoma. Scoliosis and back stiffness are present with the majority of osteoblastomas of the lumbar spine.[35] In view of the milder symptoms, its clinical course may be longer than that of osteoid osteomas. Approximately 35% of the cases involve the spine. When the vertebral axis is involved, both radicular and myelopathic components may be present. Anatomically, the transverse and spinous processes and the posterior elements are involved, while the vertebral body is spared.

Radiographic characteristics are those of an expansile mass with an intact rim of bone. A central lytic area (greater than 2 cm) is surrounded by a rim of sclerosis. Bone scans demonstrate an intense uptake, and CT and MRI are essential in planning for surgical resection (Figs. 10–2 to 10–4).

Marginal resections of these tumors can be curative, but in aggressive lesions with destruction of the body, pedicle, and transverse process, it may be impossible to completely resect the tumor. Radiation therapy is rarely recommended for treatment of osteoblastomas because the response to radiation has been poor.

MALIGNANT BONE-FORMING TUMORS

Osteogenic Sarcoma

Osteogenic sarcoma is the second most common primary malignant bone tumor. Males are affected more frequently than females, with the majority of cases presenting between ages 15 and 20 years.[3, 40] A second peak of occurrence is in later life (60 to 80 years) and is associated with Paget's disease and fibrous dysplasia. It rarely originates in the spine; the

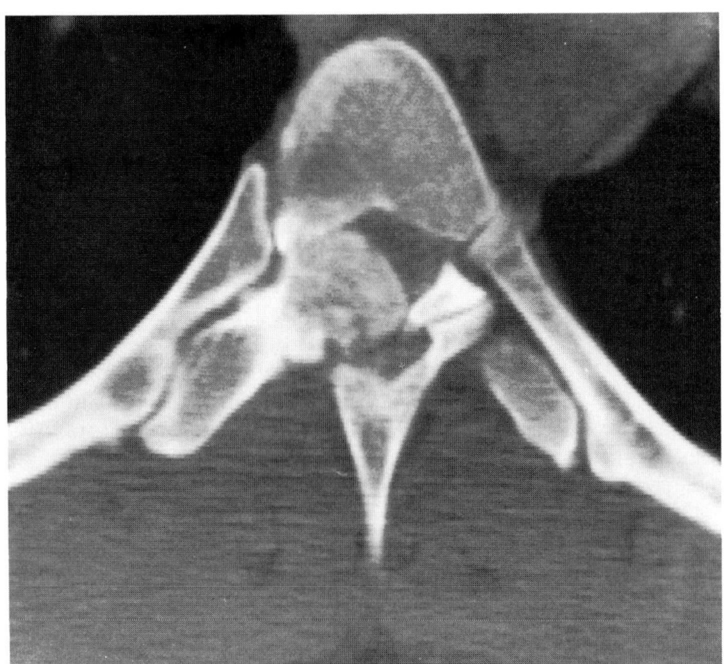

FIGURE 10–2. Osteoblastoma. A round osseous mass arises from the facet joint, replacing the pedicle and impinging on the spinal canal. A CT scan shows the mass to be isodense with surrounding normal osseous structures.

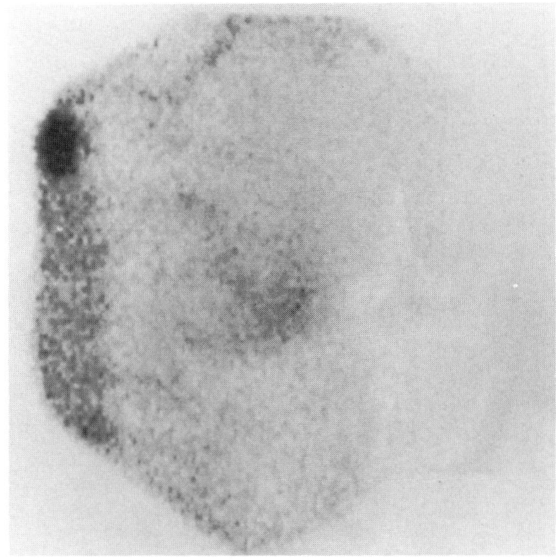

FIGURE 10–3. Same patient as in Figure 10–2. The mass appears as an area of increased radioactivity on total body bone scan performed with technetium Tc-99m hydroxydiphosphonate.

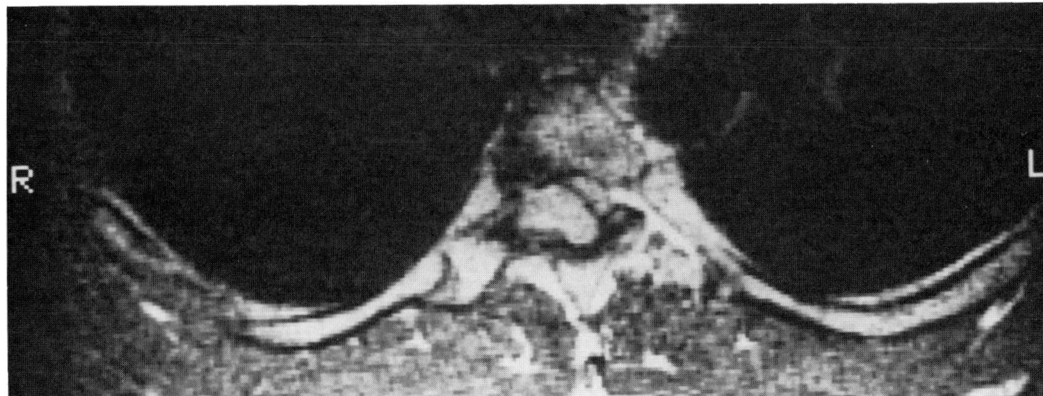

FIGURE 10–4. Same patient as in Figure 10–2. T2-weighted image of a transverse magnetic resonance imaging (MRI) scan shows the hyperintense mass projecting from the pedicle, as a smooth, finger-like extension, into the spinal canal.

appendicular skeleton is more commonly involved. It arises in areas with the largest number of active osteoblastic cells. Multiple metastatic lesions in the vertebral column are more common than primary osteosarcoma. In spinal osteosarcoma, pain is usually the initial symptom. The majority of reported lesions occur in the lumbar spine and are associated with cauda equina symptoms.[2] Although long-term survival of patients with osteogenic sarcoma of the spine is rare, there are cases in which staged anterior and posterior intralesional resections allow longer survival. Enhanced survival rates may be attributed to earlier diagnosis, preoperative and postoperative chemotherapy, and more radical resection followed by staged stabilization procedures.

Most osteogenic sarcomas have high-grade aggressive malignant features and a significant mitotic rate. Histologically, they can be divided into chondroblastic, osteoblastic, fibroblastic, telangiectatic, and small cell types. Secondary osteogenic sarcomas may develop after radiation therapy, in association with Paget's disease, or in preexisting benign conditions, such as bone infarctions and fibrous dysplasia. Metastasis is common to the lung and lymph nodes as well as other bones.

On routine radiographs of the spine, there may be lytic or blastic changes, depending on the amount of tumor matrix production and its degree of calcification (Figs. 10–5, 10–6). CT or MRI may demonstrate paraspinous extension with a soft tissue component (Fig. 10–7). Angiography may be valuable in demonstrating the vascularity of the tumor, as well as in planning the appropriate operative procedure. A bone scan should be performed to determine if metastasis is already present. Laboratory studies may assist in the diagnosis and treatment; for example, an elevated alkaline phosphatase level usually decreases during chemotherapy and can be used to judge the success of the treatment.

BENIGN CARTILAGE-FORMING TUMORS

Osteochondromas

One of the most common benign tumors of bone is osteochondroma. It may be solitary, but the majority of cases occur in association with hereditary multiple exostosis. Osteochondromas are more common in men and clinically manifest during the second or third decade of life. These tumors have a sessile or pedunculated bone base with a cartilage cap that develops from progressive endochondral ossification of aberrant growth plate cartilage. Significantly, 1% of solitary and 10% of multiple osteochondromas may undergo chondrosarcomatous degeneration.[34] Solitary osteochondromas causing spinal cord compression affect the thoracic and lumbar vertebrae. They may involve any part of the vertebral body but are most commonly associated with the spinous process or the neural arch. They are usually asymptomatic masses but may cause nerve root or spinal cord compression during adolescence as rapid growth occurs. Multiple osteochondromatosis also manifests during this growth period. CT is essential to demonstrate the site of origin, allowing visualization of the tumor's relationship to the cord. No treatment is warranted unless the lesion becomes clinically symptomatic. There is no tendency for these

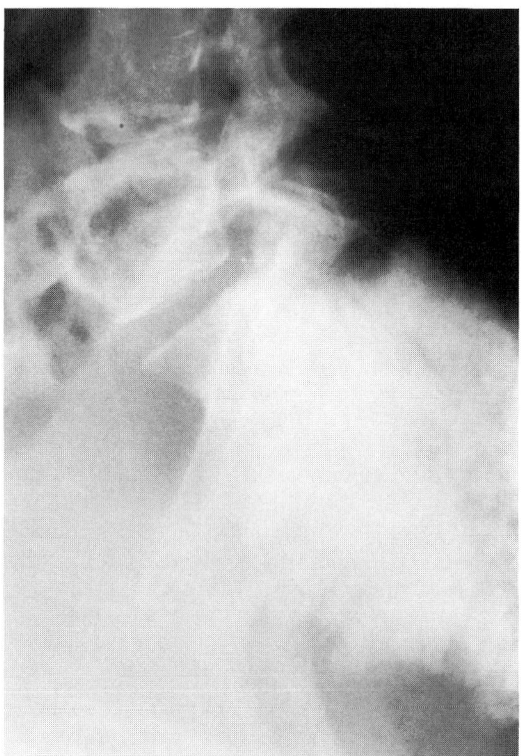

FIGURE 10–5. Osteogenic sarcoma. Plain lateral radiograph demonstrates loss of cortical margins and anatomic detail of the sacrum. A large, expansile lesion arises from the region.

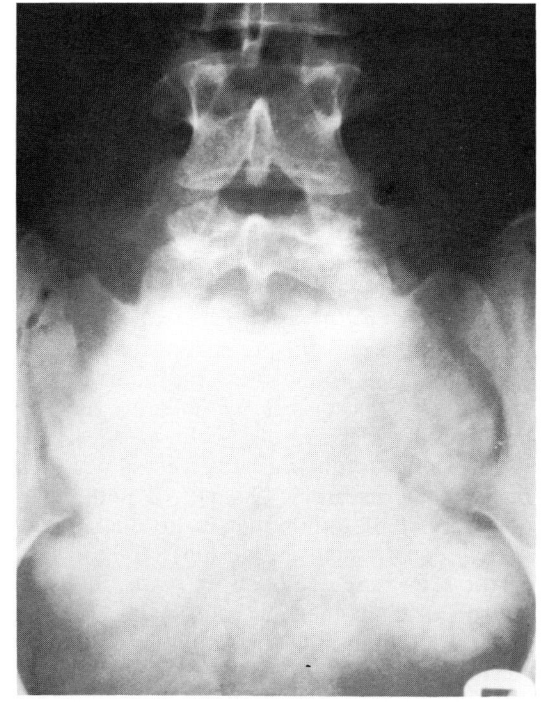

FIGURE 10–6. Same patient as in Figure 10–5. Anteroposterior radiograph of the pelvis reveals that the sacrum has been replaced by an irregular, radiodense, and fluffy-appearing mass.

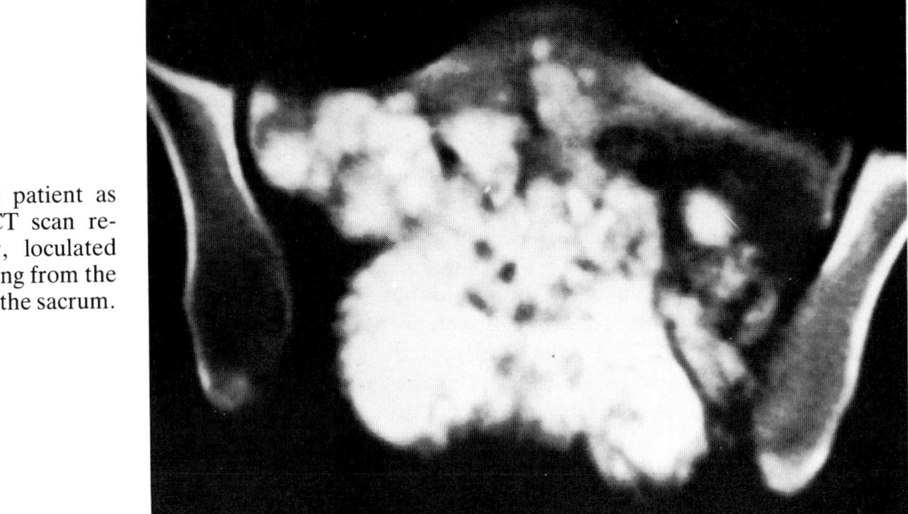

FIGURE 10–7. Same patient as in Figure 10–5. CT scan reveals an irregular, loculated fuzzy mass projecting from the posterior aspect of the sacrum.

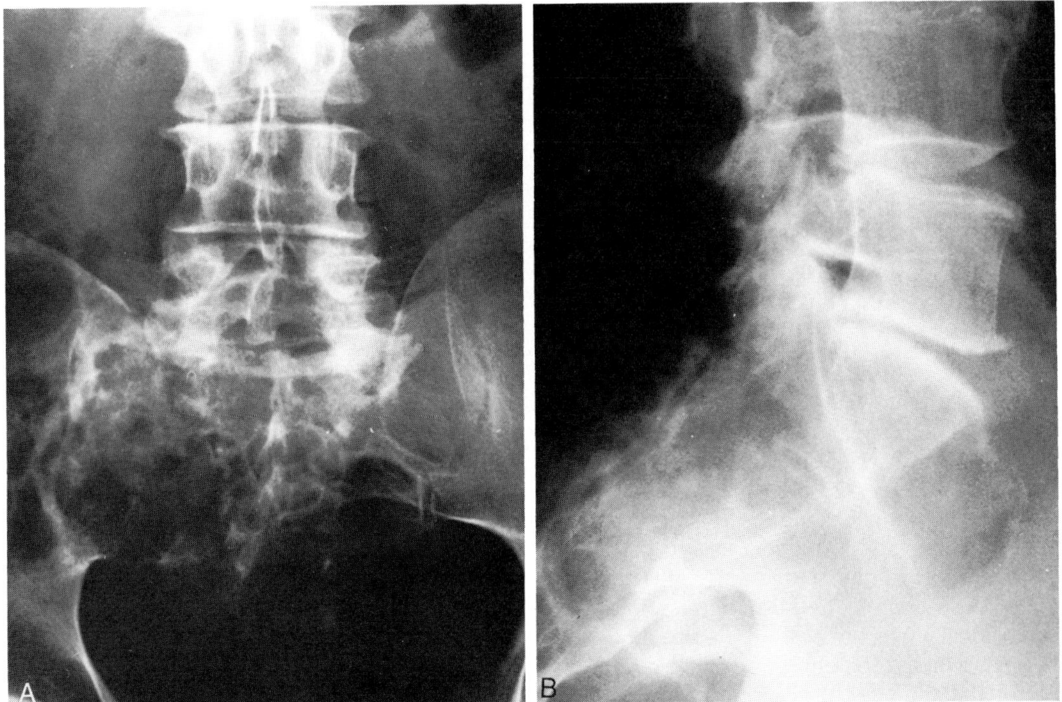

FIGURE 10–8. Chondrosarcoma. *A,* Anteroposterior radiograph of the lower lumbar spine and the pelvis demonstrates a large sacral tumor that extended beyond the sacroiliac joint with involvement of the ilium. There are large areas of radiolucency intertwined with irregular radiopacities owing to calcification or bone metaplasia. *B,* Lateral radiograph demonstrates the extent of tumor involvement.

tumors to recur after they have been surgically resected.

MALIGNANT CARTILAGE-FORMING TUMORS

Chondrosarcoma

Chondrosarcoma is the most common primary malignant bone tumor, excluding myeloma. Involvement of the spine by chondrosarcoma is rare. Recent reports reviewed its grading, prevalence, surgical treatment, and oncologic therapy.[5, 37] It may appear in the neural arches along the spinal axis but is found more commonly in the centra. The tumor frequently extends from one level to another. Although this tumor can be found in any bone with cartilaginous origin, approximately 6% are along the vertebral axis.[5, 27] The tumor appears to be evenly distributed throughout the spinal axis.

Histologic grading criteria depend on the morphologic features of the nuclei, the size of the cells, and the presence of mitosis. There are three classic histologic grades: grade I tumors have cellular atypia, doubled nuclei, and enlarged lacunae; grade II tumors have marked atypia and multiple nuclei; and grade III tumors have dramatic atypia, mitotic figures, and the presence of spindle cell elements. The differentiation of a grade I tumor from enchondromas is difficult. Matrix formation and chromosomal characteristics of chondroid tumors have been compared. Chondrosarcomas with a normal RNA content (diploid) were associated with a higher 10-year survival rate than those with abnormal chromosome content per cell.[37] Patients with the low-grade chondrosarcomas have a 5-year survival rate of 65 to 85%, whereas in those with the highest-grade tumors, the 5-year rate may only be 15%. Low-grade lesions infrequently metastasize, whereas high-grade lesions spread to the lungs or other areas of the body. Soft tissue extension is the rule and hematogenous spread is due to local invasion of veins. Cytophotomatrix DNA measurement may prove a potent tool for the clinician in determining the malignancy of cartilage tumors and whether malignant tumors are high or low grade.

The age distribution of patients with chondrosarcomas is broad, ranging from 30 to 60 years. Patients initially have mild local discomfort. As the tumors grow, there may be local or referred pain with extension into the thorax, the pelvis, or the abdomen as well as extradural compression of the spinal cord.

Roentgenographic features include irregular lobular radiopacities due to calcification or bone metaplasia in the cartilage (Figs. 10–8, 10–9). Large areas of radiolucency may also be present and the osteolytic areas have a sclerotic margin. Axial and sagittal CT and MRI reconstruction techniques identify cortical breakthrough, the presence and size of soft tissue masses, and the proximity to important vascular structures (Fig. 10–10). Angiography should be considered in most cases.

Chondrosarcoma of the vertebral column may present as masses in the neck, the thorax, or the abdomen, with symptoms reflecting progressive compression of the dural sac. Treatment depends on the histologic grade and the tumor location. However, radiation therapy is palliative at best and the response to chemotherapy is poor. Recent laboratory work described the use of the vitamin A analogue retinoic acid to enhance lysosomal enzyme release, which results in chondrocyte death.[37] Its clinical value in the treatment of chondro-

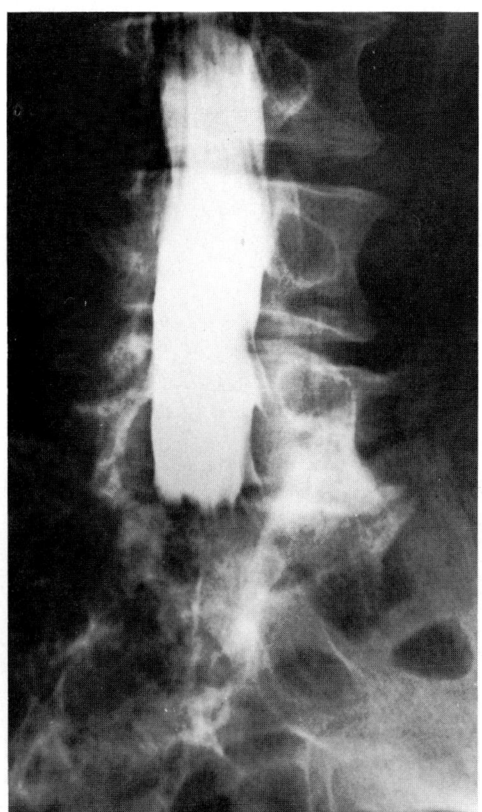

FIGURE 10–9. Lumbar myelogram of the patient in Figure 10–8 demonstrates a complete epidural block at the inferior aspect of L5.

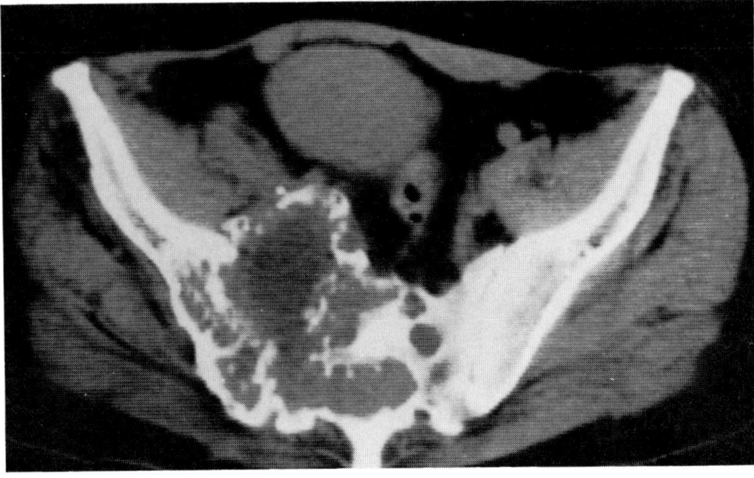

FIGURE 10–10. CT scan of the patient in Figures 10–8 and 10–9, confirming the findings seen in Figure 10–8. There is cortical breakthrough of the anterior sacrum, extending into the pelvic cavity.

sarcoma can only be speculated. Surgical ablation is therefore the treatment of choice. Radical *en bloc* extirpation is difficult and at times impossible in spinal surgery. Repetitive local debulking procedures may be necessary and can be effective in controlling tumor growth. It is important to perform spinal stabilization and fusion early in the treatment of this tumor because local recurrence is probable. In a composite series of spinal chondrosarcoma (19 cases), a 21% 5-year survival was found.[5]

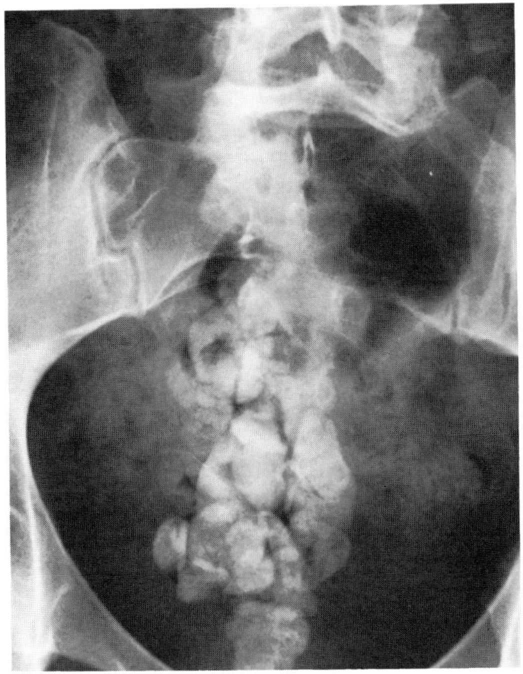

FIGURE 10–11. Giant cell tumor. Plain radiograph of the pelvis shows destruction of the sacral ala on one side with disappearance of the arcuate lines. The boundaries of the pathologic region are sharply defined.

Giant Cell Tumors

Giant cell tumors of the vertebral axis are a complex management problem because they are not amenable to complete surgical resection. Huvos found an 8% incidence of giant cell tumors in the vertebral axis, primarily in the lumbosacral region.[33] Most series report a female preponderance, with 70 to 80% of tumors developing between the ages of 20 and 40 years.[14, 15] Pain is the most frequent symptom. In spite of their size, sacral lesions rarely produce bowel, bladder, or sexual dysfunction.

Giant cell tumor is a primary bone neoplasm composed of varying numbers of multinucleated giant cells dispersed throughout a stroma of mononuclear cells that coalesce to form the giant cells.[14] Giant cell tumor appears as a lytic lesion that lacks stippling or calcifications. Periosteal reaction is absent. Campanacci and colleagues developed a staging system for giant cell tumors, which is based on the degree of increased histologic stromal atypia and radiographic features.[7] A more aggressive surgical approach is necessary for the more aggressive lesion. When present along the spinal axis, giant cell tumors have a predilection for the vertebral body with spread into the pedicles. There is a high propensity for local recurrence, as well as the potential to metastasize.

On routine films, this tumor appears as a slow-growing solitary lesion in the spine associated with cystic rarefaction and ill-defined margins that may progress to vertebral collapse. Sacral tumors are eccentric, in contrast to chordomas, which are central. They may abut the sacroiliac joint (Fig. 10–11). Their anterior location is in contrast to that of osteoblastomas and aneurysmal bone cysts, which routinely involve the posterior elements. A

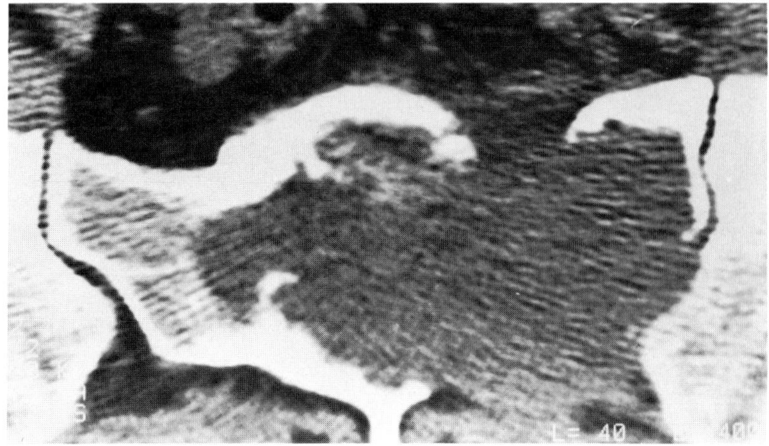

FIGURE 10–12. Same patient as in Figure 10–11. CT scan demonstrates a homogeneous soft tissue mass, which destroyed half of the sacrum and filled the spinal canal. The sacroiliac articulation was partially violated on the affected side. Although the cavitated sacrum has mostly sharp borders, the ventral wall of the sacrum was completely destroyed in a particularly ragged area.

technetium-99m bone scan can rule out multicentricity, whereas CT and MRI are essential in determining the intraosseous and extraosseous extent of the lesion (Fig. 10–12). Because the lesion may be vascular, angiography and embolization are beneficial before surgery (Figs. 10–13, 10–14).

The goal of complete eradication of these vertebral tumors is formidable. Local curettage or, if feasible, *en bloc* resection followed by stabilization with a bone graft or rods is the best form of treatment. Alternative methods include liquid nitrogen cryotherapy, phenol and alcohol cautery, and heat cauterization with polymethyl methacrylate. These techniques, unfortunately, cannot be used if the tumor is in juxtaposition to nervous tissue.

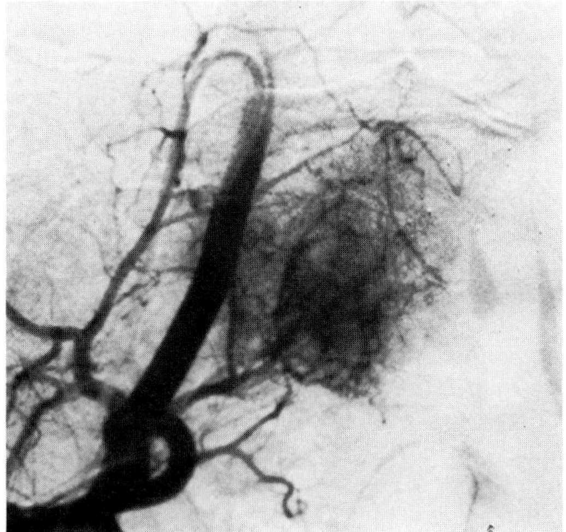

FIGURE 10–13. Same patient as in Figure 10–11. Angiography reveals an extensive blush with prominent tumor neovascularity. The blood supply was from branches of both internal iliac arteries and one of the L4 lumbar arteries.

Local recurrence of vertebral tumors is common and repeated curettage and bone grafting may be necessary. Radiation therapy can play a primary role in the management of giant cell tumors that cannot be adequately resected.[3, 11, 15, 33] Patients treated with radiation must be followed closely, for there is a 10 to 20% incidence of postirradiation sarcomas.

MALIGNANT BONE MARROW TUMORS

Multiple Myeloma

Multiple myeloma is the most common primary malignant bone tumor. It frequently involves the spine, producing destructive lesions of the vertebral body with ill-defined margins. The vertebrae collapse *in toto,* usually with preservation of the disk space. Destruction of the pedicles and the neural arches is more frequently seen in metastatic lesions and is less common in primary myeloma.

Multiple myeloma and solitary plasmocytoma are part of the continuum of B cell lymphoproliferative diseases.[20] The peak incidence of the diseases is between the ages of 60 and 70 years, and it is more common in men than in women. Pain is the initial symptom and is followed by weight loss and lethargy. Characteristically, the pain is exacerbated by activity and is relieved by rest.

Classic laboratory studies include serum and urine protein electrophoresis and immunoelectrophoresis, which confirm the diagnosis. The majority of patients demonstrate a monoclonal spike and loss of the normal polyclonal distribution. In addition, there is a reversal of the albumin/globulin ratio, as well as anemia with a normal white blood cell count. The erythro-

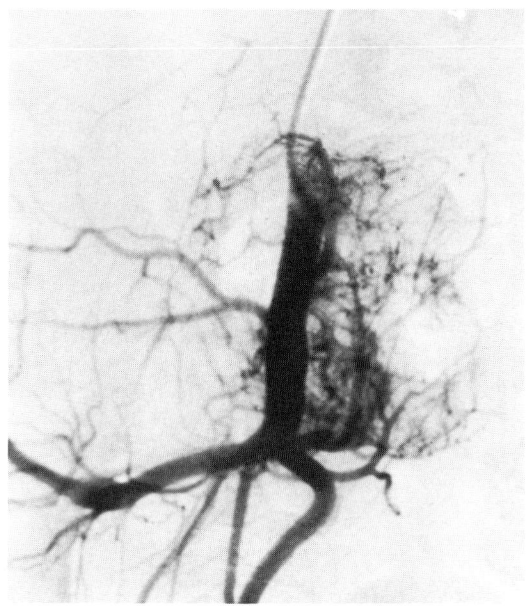

FIGURE 10–14. Same patient as in Figure 10–11. Subsequent angiography after selective embolization with ethyl alcohol and polyvinyl alcohol particles. The former has excellent tumor penetration and causes extensive tumor necrosis. The fine-vessel neovascularity has been largely obliterated.

cyte sedimentation rate is frequently elevated. Urinalysis reveals the presence of Bence Jones proteins. Bone marrow studies should be carried out to evaluate the extent of plasmacytosis. In cases in which there is widespread destruction of bone, hypercalcemia may develop.

Routine radiographs usually demonstrate the classic lytic punched-out lesions in the ribs, the clavicle, the sternum, or the proximal long bones without significant new bone formation or sclerosis. Classically, the vertebral bodies collapse (Fig. 10–15). CT or MRI further assess the extent of extramedullary spread of myeloma as well as demonstrate the degree of spinal cord compression.

Multiple myeloma of the spine should be treated by local radiation therapy combined with systemic chemotherapy. Current therapies include administration of melphalan or cyclophosphamide in combination with corticosteroids. Patients who subsequently have cord compression should have a laminectomy or anterior decompression in conjunction with stabilization and fusion to prevent further complications of instability.

Ewing's Sarcoma

Ewing's sarcoma is a primary malignant bone tumor that usually presents between the ages of 5 and 30 years.[50] Although the most usual sites of origin are the long tubular bones of the extremities, it may originate in the spine. Kornberg's review of the literature found a 3.5% incidence of primary spine involvement.[36] The most frequent site is the sacrum. The differentiating clinical factors are swelling and unremitting pain that is not relieved by bed rest. An elevated erythrocyte sedimentation rate, leukocytosis, and low-grade fever are frequently seen. Ewing's sarcoma lesions are destructive lesions of the vertebral body with associated compression fractures and significant paravertebral soft tissue masses. Extension into the pedicles may be seen. The tumors may be primary or may represent a metastasis from other skeletal sites.

Routine spine radiographs demonstrate a destructive lesion with moth-eaten appearance. On initial routine radiograph, it may be difficult to distinguish Ewing's sarcoma from an infectious process (such as osteomyelitis), a lymphoma, or metastatic disease. Surgical biopsy, either fine needle aspiration or open biopsy, is necessary to confirm the diagnosis and allow staging protocols. Histopathologically, these tumors are classified using special stains to visualize anaplastic sheets of small round cells and the presence of glycogen granules in the cells. The marrow stem cell, the reticulum, is believed to be the parent cell of Ewing's tumor.

After a diagnostic biopsy, induction chemotherapy is administered to decrease the size of the primary tumor. If surgical resection with fusion and stabilization is deemed possible, it should be performed and followed by radiation. This combination of chemotherapy and irradiation raised the survival rates to greater than 75%.[61] Razek and associates found 100% local control and 86% disease-free survival for lesions in the spine (other than the sacrococcygeal segments).[58] This confirms the more aggressive nature of tumors arising in the coccyx and the sacrum. For lesions of the sacrum and the coccyx, local control was achieved in only 62.5%. Pulmonary metastasis is not as frequent as bony metastasis.

Primary Reticulum Cell Sarcoma

Reticulum cell sarcoma of the vertebral axis is extremely rare, and this diagnosis should be considered only after more common pathologic entities. It usually presents in young adults (20 to 30 years), with pain as the most frequent initial symptom. Characteristically, it involves

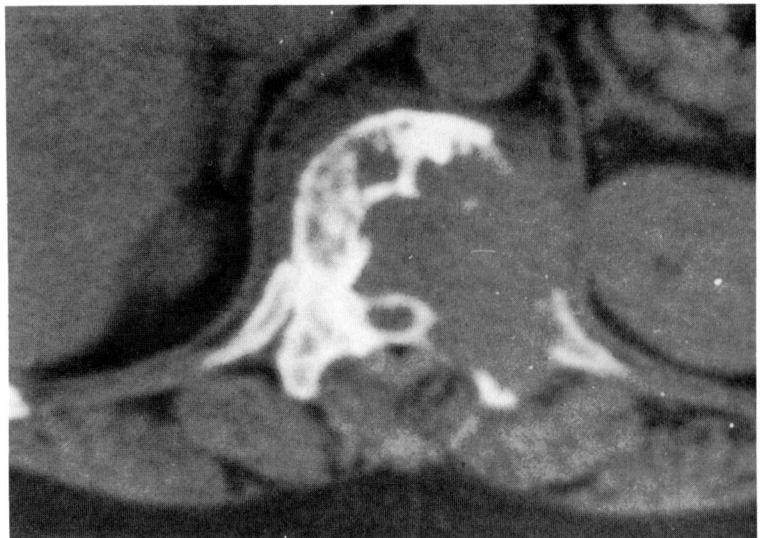

FIGURE 10–15. Multiple myeloma. A soft tissue mass replaced the body, the pedicle, the transverse process, and the lamina on one side of the vertebral body. The mass both extends ventrally into the paraspinal space and flattens the column of subarachnoid metrizamide within the spinal canal. CT scan with bone window settings is ideal for revealing tumor infiltration of the remainder of the body.

a single osseous site but may metastasize to regional lymph nodes.

On routine radiographs and CT scans, the destructive process involves the body of the vertebra with partial or total collapse. Histologic confirmation and differentiation from Ewing's sarcoma is essential because reticulum cell sarcoma is a highly radiosensitive lesion. On histologic examination, there is a proliferation of anaplastic reticulum cells with a variable number of lymphoblasts and lymphocytes. Five-year survival rates of greater than 50% in one patient group have been reported.[17] Adjuvant chemotherapy may enhance the overall survival statistics, especially if there is associated disseminated disease.

Lymphoma

Spinal lymphoma with invasion of the epidural space and cord compression occurs in 0.5 to 15% of patients with lymphoma.[29] Invasion of the spine occurs only late in the disease when the lesion is widely disseminated.

Although the location of metastatic disease of the spine can frequently be determined on the basis of bone destruction on plain films, lymphomas have a notoriously permeative growth pattern and may not demonstrate bone destruction despite widespread infiltration.[29, 54] Radionuclide studies are far better for determining involvement of the spinal column by lymphoma. CT is best for paraspinal infiltration, whereas myelography and MRI have been the most helpful in determining intraspinal involvement.[29] Lymphomas frequently invade through the neural foramina and are best demonstrated in this location by surface coil MRI.

Patients with lymphomatous involvement of the spine typically have localized pain, tenderness, and signs of compressive myelopathy. Compared with other metastatic lesions, lymphomas are quite responsive to multimodality therapy, including conventional radiation and surgical decompression in certain cases of acute compression.

Metastatic Tumors

Metastatic lesions constitute the majority of tumors of the spine.[41, 56] The skeleton is the third most frequent site for distant metastases.[49] The spine is the most common site for skeletal metastases. More than 70% of patients who die from cancer have vertebral metastases on postmortem examination.[25] Of vertebral metastases, 75% originate from the breast, the lung, the prostate, the kidney, or the thyroid. Carcinoma of the breast or the lung commonly spreads to the thoracic area, whereas prostatic carcinoma typically spreads to the lumbar spine and the sacrum. The frequency of secondary tumors in the spine is attributed to hematogenous spread of neoplastic cells through Batson's vertebral plexus. There is an equal sex distribution, but the metastatic lesions to the spine almost exclusively affect those in the fourth to sixth decades of life.[63]

Vertebral metastases are generally asymptomatic until the development of localized pain and myelopathy owing to a paravertebral mass, compression of nerve roots, pathologic fractures, spinal instability, or compression of the spinal cord.[25] The pain is progressive and is often worse at night. Radicular pain may precede myelopathic features by weeks or months. Those with rapidly progressive neurologic deficits more frequently have lesions of the thoracic spine, which carry a poorer prognosis.[25] Although the lumbar region is the most common site of metastases, lesions in the thoracic spine most frequently result in spinal cord compromise and neurologic deficit.[25] It is thought that vascular compression and thrombosis of adjacent spinal vessels result in progression of neurologic deficit.[63]

Although the findings of multiple spinal lesions on radionuclide bone scans is diagnostic of metastases, there is a high false-positive rate for solitary lesions, even in patients with known carcinoma.[24] Plain films are useful for demonstrating bone destruction. Between 30 and 50% of a vertebral body must be destroyed before any changes can be recognized on plain film. Although the posterior elements are involved only one seventh as frequently as the vertebral body, destruction of a pedicle is seen more commonly on plain radiographs as evidence of metastatic disease. Plain radiographic findings may lag 3 to 18 months behind abnormal bone scan appearance.[53] Involved vertebral bodies, including those that are destroyed and collapsed, more frequently demonstrate lytic rather than blastic metastatic lesions. If extension to the epidural space is suspected, myelography should be performed via a C1-2 puncture with follow-up CT. MRI may further define paravertebral extension, although it is associated with poorer results for the definition of osseous involvement and destruction.

Operation for vertebral metastases is indicated for a pathologic fracture causing anterior spinal compression if the causative tumor is radioresistant, if the maximal radiation dose has already been given, or if a patient's condition continues to deteriorate despite conservative therapy.[16] Fine needle biopsy may be used if the primary tumor is not known, although this may only confirm the presence of tumor and not reveal the primary site. Decompression by laminectomy alone results in improvement in only 30% of cases because most tumors involve the anterior column. Radiotherapy for compressive lesions of the vertebral column results in improvement in 50% of cases.[50] More direct approaches with anterior resection of the involved vertebral body and stabilization with prosthetic devices and methyl methacrylate result in equal or better recovery rates.[16, 25] Embolization during preoperative angiography may make these procedures less formidable.

Immediate outcome most closely correlates with the rate and extent of neurologic deterioration. Overall prognosis is dependent on the nature of the metastatic tumor and its propensity to recur.[16]

Primary Benign Vascular Tumors

Hemangioma

Hemangiomas of the spine are benign tumors arising from newly formed blood vessels. In large autopsy series, they occur in approximately 10% of cases.[21, 28, 42, 70] In the majority of cases, they are asymptomatic and are found only incidentally on roentgenograms. Females are more commonly affected than males. Clinically, they have been estimated to constitute 2 to 3% of all spinal tumors.

Although usually asymptomatic, these telangiectasias may occur as part of a syndrome of diffuse skeletal and metameric hemangiomatosis, which carries a poor prognosis or may result in neural compression.[11, 22] The latter results from subperiosteal expansion of the tumor into the epidural space, spinal canal narrowing due to vertebral enlargement, epidural hemorrhage from the lesion, or pathologic fracture of the involved vertebra.

Radiographically, the tumors present a classic honeycomb or wheelspoke pattern of parallel, coarse, vertically oriented trabeculations surrounding dilated vascular spaces (Figs. 10–16, 10–17). The involved vertebrae contain expansile and well-defined regions of alternating sclerosis and osteolysis.[11, 59] Typically, the body is involved and the disk space is spared, although extension into the lamina, the pedicle, the transverse and spinous processes, and the ribs has been described.[21] Clinical symptoms occur when the involved vertebra expands toward the spinal canal, resulting in subacute cord compression. Predilection for the lower thoracic and lumbar spines has been well demonstrated.[22, 28, 59] Although hemangiomas are usually isolated lesions, approximately one third of involved spines have up to five vertebrae affected.

Pathologically, the tumors are blue, firm, honeycombed masses with interspersed bony trabeculae.[11] The microscopic appearance is that of cavernous channels embedded in a connective tissue matrix. The classification of

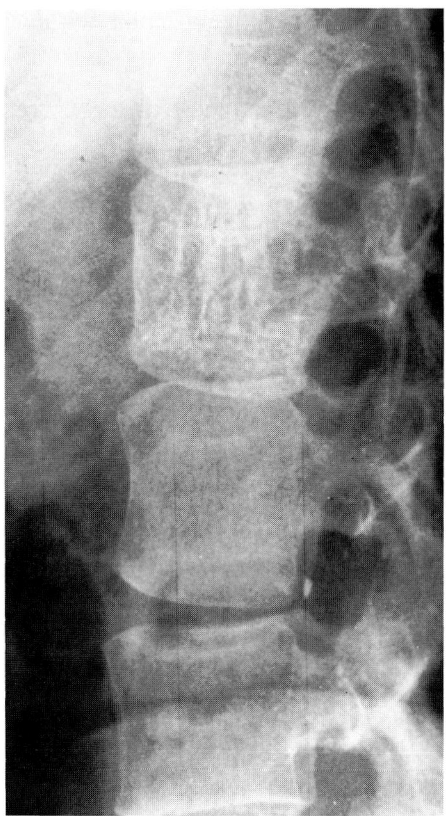

FIGURE 10–16. Hemangioma. Plain lateral radiograph of the thoracic spine shows characteristic pattern of vertical striations traversing the vertebral body.

hemangiomas as capillary, cavernous, venous, or mixed type depends on the predominant vascular structure present. Pathologic fractures are rare.

Although the incidental lesion needs no treatment, painful tumors have traditionally been irradiated.[11] Lesions resulting in neurologic deficit, especially partial or complete spinal blocks, should be aggressively approached. Advances in preoperative angiography and embolization and spinal stabilization procedures have permitted radical excision of these vascular tumors.[21]

Lymphangioma

Lymphangioma is an unusual tumor of the spinal column. The spine is the sixth most common site for this tumor, but lymphangioma may coexist with the more prevalent spinal hemangioma. Classically, it occurs twice as frequently in males, generally between the first and third decades.[59] It most frequently presents as a painful swelling after a pathologic fracture. It is associated with soft tissue and visceral abnormalities, lymphedema, and chylous pleural effusions. Lymphangiomas appear radiographically as solitary or multiple zones of rarefaction surrounded by well-defined sclerosis. The pathologic appearance is that of dilated lymph vessels or cystic endothelium-lined channels containing red blood cells.

Angiosarcoma

Angiosarcomas, also known as hemangioendotheliomas or hemangiosarcomas, vary from debatably malignant capillary and cavernous proliferations to highly lethal tumors. These exceedingly rare neoplasms demonstrate a slight male preponderance and occur in all age groups.[11, 59] Those with a multifocal disposition occur in a younger age group.

The roentgenographic appearance of osteolysis without new bone formation is pathognomonic. The thinned, expanded cortex becomes less well demarcated with more aggressive lesions. The more malignant variants also lose the normal trabeculations, which persist in low-grade lesions. Destruction may extend over more than one vertebral body.

The tumor is hemorrhagic and necrotic and demonstrates irregular, anastomosing channels composed of atypical endothelial cells. Intravascular tufts of plump, proliferating cells display rare mitoses. Treatment consists of surgical excision plus radiation.

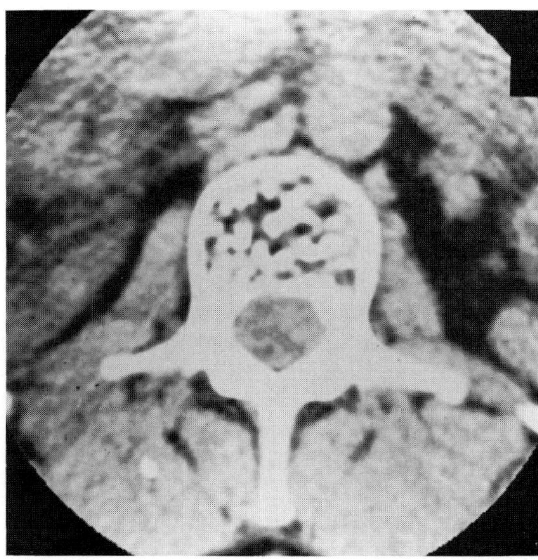

FIGURE 10–17. Same patient as in Figure 10–16. CT scan demonstrates the trabeculation of the vertebral body, which is pathognomonic of hemangioma.

Glomus Tumor

Angioglomoid tumors are rare benign lesions associated with vascular structures derived from neuromyoarterial arteriovenous anastomoses.[55, 59] Most occur in the fourth to fifth decades. Multiple lesions are usually asymptomatic. The solitary tumors cause a burning and lancinating pain. These lytic lesions are tiny, well-encapsulated tumors composed of vascular spaces surrounded by a single layer of endothelial cells and associated glomus cells.

Their occurrence at the tip of the coccyx can cause coccydynia.[55, 70] Resection of the tip of the coccyx, with particular attention to removal of pericoccygeal soft tissues, results in complete relief of pain.

Connective Tissue Tumors

Fibrosarcoma

Fibrosarcoma of bone occurs between the third and sixth decades of life with an equal sex distribution.[11, 59] Secondary fibrosarcomas are the most common form, arising in the spine and generally developing at sites of giant cell tumors, previous irradiation, or Paget's disease. Pain and swelling of short duration are the usual presenting features of fibrosarcoma;[11, 59] neurologic manifestations appear early.[19]

A moth-eaten pattern of radiolucency is more common than bone destruction surrounded by periosteal reaction and new bone formation. The tumor margins are always indistinct and solitary foci are more common. Vertebral localizations are frequent in multicentric or metastatic Paget's sarcoma.

The tumor appears as a firm, whitish mass that may be well circumscribed. Microscopically, poorly differentiated fibrous tissue with malignant characteristics and foci of hemorrhage, necrosis, and calcium predominate. The absence of malignant bone or osteoid serves to differentiate the tumor from primary osteosarcoma.

Optimal therapy consists of complete *en bloc* resection of the tumor followed by local radiotherapy.[19] Low-grade fibrosarcomas carry a better prognosis than do osteosarcomas. Generally, a 5% or less 5-year survival is anticipated, despite aggressive therapy.[19]

Lipoma and Liposarcoma

These fatty tumors are rare primary tumors of the vertebral axis. Intraspinal lipomatous neoplasms constitute 1% of the total number of spinal axis tumors and frequently account for changes such as vertebral body sclerosis in the spine.[62, 69] Involvement of the epidural space and even the intradural elements makes neurologic deterioration the most frequent presentation of the spinal lipomas and liposarcomas. Infiltration of a vertebra by lipomatous neoplasms occurs less commonly. The tumors occur with an equal male/female ratio in all decades of life.[11, 59]

Radiographically, these fatty masses appear as radiolucent lesions with sclerotic borders, occasionally with vertical trabeculations. The sacrum is notably involved. The tumors arise from the bone marrow and appear microscopically as yellow and brown soft, amorphous masses. Microscopically, the lipoma contains large differentiated adipocytes, which become poorly differentiated in the liposarcomas.

Microsurgical resection of the fatty elements, with particular care to preserve neural elements, has yielded good results.

Other Tumors and Tumor-like Lesions

Chordoma

Chordomas are slow-growing, locally invasive tumors that arise from the notochord, a midline structure in the developing spine that regresses by the seventh week of embryonic life.[52, 59] They constitute between 1 and 4% of all primary bone tumors.[11, 31, 65] Chordomas are the most common primary neoplasm of the sacrum.[32, 65] Slightly more than half of the chordomas are sacral, with approximately 15% occupying other areas of the spine. The remainder are situated at the base of the skull.[38, 60] The cervical spine is the site of most chordomas not arising at either the sacrococcygeal or the basicranial extremities of the vertebral column. Although this tumor may be noted at any age, its occurrence clusters about the fifth to seventh decades of life and may demonstrate a slight male preponderance.[65]

Back pain, bowel dysfunction, and the finding of a mass on rectal or cutaneous examination have all been described as common presenting signs and symptoms. Vertebral tumors may result in neural compression, neck masses, and the development of retropharyngeal or retroperitoneal tumors. Sacral chordomas always demonstrate sacral destruction, usually below S2, and occasionally enlargement of the neural foramina. The sacrum is usually expanded, with preserved cortical margins, and pieces of destroyed sacrum are present at the periphery of the tumor. A ballooning soft tissue mass, out of proportion to the osseous destruction, in a presacral or postsacral location is commonly demonstrated. Chordomas of the vertebrae most often involve the body, followed in order of decreasing frequency by the pedicle, the lamina, and the spinous process. Late osteosclerosis of the disk space and loss of disk height may be demonstrated. Commonly, ivory vertebrae and vertebral body collapse may be present (Figs 10–18 and 10–19).[38]

Grossly, the tumor is gray, soft, and lobulated and is confined by a pseudocapsule and an intact periosteum. The latter generally serves to isolate the tumor from the intraabdominal contents before any surgical intervention. Microscopically, the tumor demonstrates the classic physaliphorous cell that is reminiscent of primitive notochord. The vacuolated cells contain mucin and are arranged in sheets or cords separated by dense, fibrous septae. The chondroid chordoma, which contains cartilage-forming elements, is generally considered to carry a better prognosis.[52] Metastases to lung, bone, soft tissue, and liver have been demonstrated in up to 40% of cases, generally

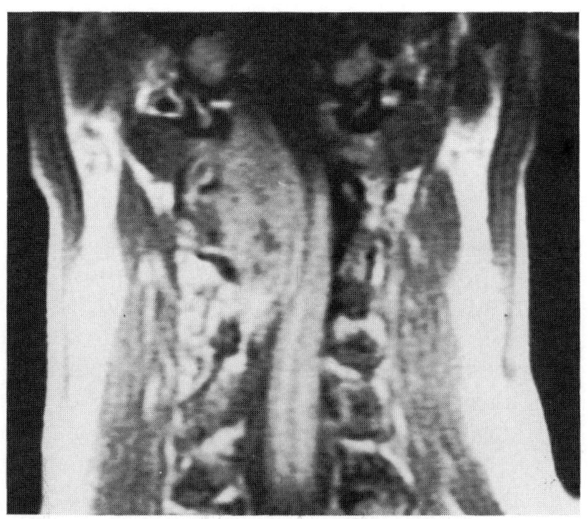

FIGURE 10–18. Chordoma. Coronal MRI with T1-weighted imaging reveals a mass of mottled signal intensity replacing the right articular pillars from C2 through C4. It fills the epidural space and displaces the cervical spinal cord to the left.

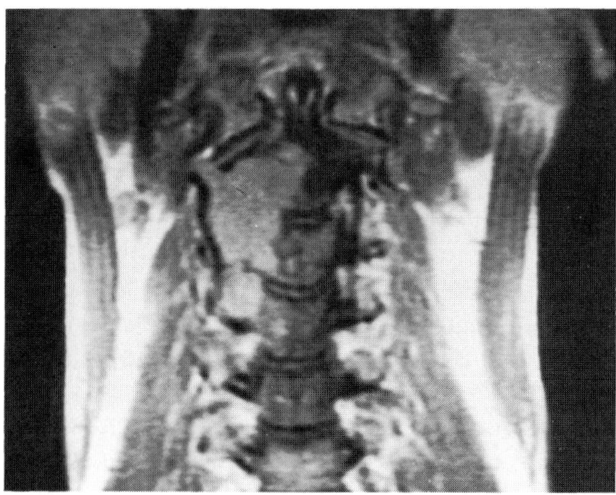

FIGURE 10–19. Same patient as in Figure 10–18. A more ventral coronal section demonstrates the mass arising from the right side of the body of the axis. It replaces the bone of the vertebral bodies with smooth borders. The mass appears predominantly hyperintense.

late in the course of the disease after surgical intervention.[60, 65]

Radical surgical excision followed by high-dose radiotherapy, sometimes in doses exceeding 50 Gy, offers the best chance of local control and survival. Surgical approaches have included radical sacrectomy combined with abdominal and sacral resections.[32, 60, 65] Despite increasingly aggressive strategies, recurrences occur in up to 85% of patients[52] and repetition of local debulking procedures is often necessary. Mortality remains high and has prompted the development of alternative chemotherapeutic regimens, proton beam therapy, and hyperthermia.

Epidermoid Cysts

Epidermoid cysts are slow-growing, tumor-like expansile lesions, which generally occur between the second and fourth decades. Frequently associated with previous trauma, they have been identified in the lumbar spine after the introduction of epidermoid elements via lumbar puncture.[59]

There may be pain and soft tissue swelling. Radiographs demonstrate osteolytic defects, which are expansile and displace adjacent soft tissue. They are sharply defined by sclerosis. The squamous epithelium in bone contains a pearly mass of inspissated keratin and cholesterol.

Treatment is usually by conservative surgical curettage.

Aneurysmal Bone Cysts

Aneurysmal bone cysts are benign destructive lesions of bone, which occur most frequently in children and are seldom found in patients older than 30 years. There is a slight predilection for females. The long bones are most frequently involved but the vertebral axis is involved approximately 12% of the time.[6] Cystic expansion confined by a thin rim of peripheral bone is common. These lesions can produce radicular pain or spinal cord compression resulting from collapse of the vertebral body.

Radiographic features confirm osteolysis and destruction of the vertebral body or the posterior arch. The lesion is radiolucent, with associated cortical erosion that is surrounded by a shell of reactive bone. In the more aggressive lesions, adjacent vertebrae and ribs can be involved. Additional tests should include CT or MRI, angiography, and possibly embolization of the tumor mass (Figs. 10–20, 10–21).

Depending on the site of the lesion, surgical curettage and stabilization should be considered (Fig. 10–22). Unfortunately, it may be impossible to obtain a satisfactory resection because of the size of the tumor, bleeding, or the site of the tumor. Radiation is considered only in surgically inaccessible cases. Relatively small doses of radiation therapy (20 to 30 Gy)

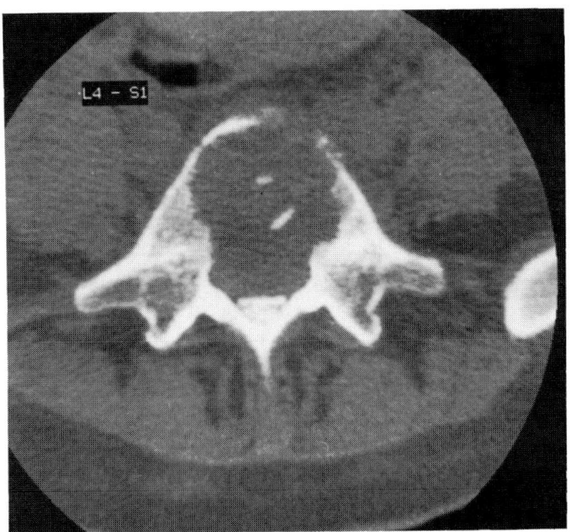

FIGURE 10–20. Aneurysmal bone cyst. The lesion smoothly expanded and eroded the L5 vertebral body. The majority of the cortex was preserved. Several shards of bone are demonstrated within the lesion on the CT scan. The ventral wall of the spinal canal was destroyed, but the column of subarachnoid contrast is intact.

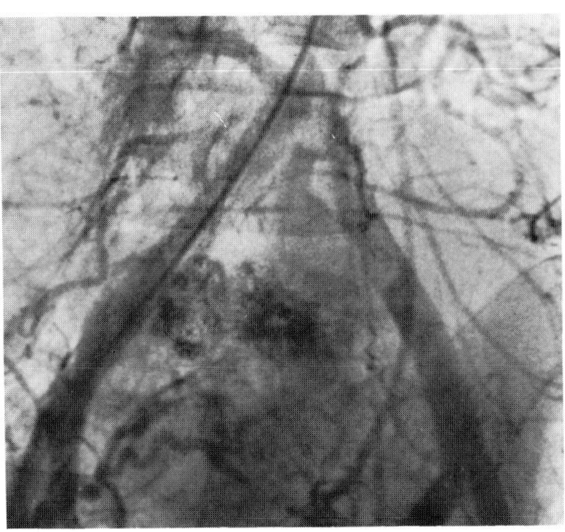

FIGURE 10–21. Same patient as in Figure 10–20. Angiography reveals pooling of contrast within the cyst and several dilated, tortuous vessels near the lesion.

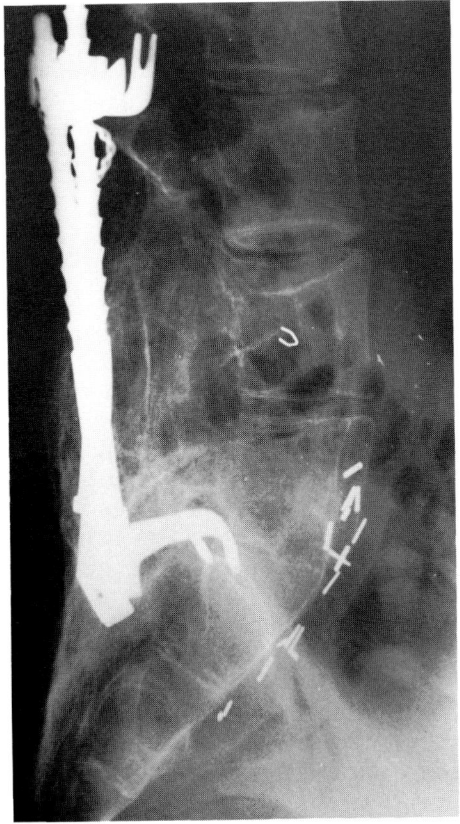

FIGURE 10–22. Same patient as in Figure 10–20. Postoperative lateral radiograph after combined anterior and posterior approach for removal of the cyst. Surgical clips are on the presacral pelvic plexus of veins. Stabilization was accomplished with Harrington rod placement.

are necessary. Recurrences occur even after radiation therapy.

Granulomatous and Histiocytic Tumor-like Processes

SARCOIDOSIS

Sarcoidosis, a multisystem disease, commonly causes hilar adenopathy, skin and eye lesions, and pulmonary infiltration. Vertebral involvement is rare, although multiple vertebral lesions may occur. The thoracic area is most commonly involved. Spinal lesions present with nonradicular focal back pain that occurs with activity but is not relieved by rest.[4] Rarely is there complete vertebral collapse and neurologic impairment. Significant laboratory study results include an elevated erythrocyte sedimentation rate, hypergammaglobulinemia, reduced serum albumin level, and hypercalcemia.

The classic radiographic picture demonstrates an intact disk space with lytic destruction of the vertebral body. There may be a sclerotic rim or the lesion may be sclerotic. Biopsy of the lesion is essential to demonstrate the typical noncaseating granulomas. A fusion should be considered if the spine is unstable after a decompressive procedure.

HISTIOCYTOSIS

Solitary eosinophilic granuloma of the spine (vertebra plana, Calvé's disease) is a variant of the systemic illness histocytosis X, an uncommon disorder of the reticuloendothelial system. Its cause remains unknown. Although eosinophilic granuloma of the spine is rare, it is one of the two commonest lesions of the spinal column in children.[47, 66] Lesions may be solitary or polyostotic. The pain is constant and it may be focal or radicular. It is not relieved by rest or aspirin. The mean age is 7 years and the sex distribution is equal.

Radiographically, the tumor most commonly involves the vertebral bodies, usually of the thoracic spine. Compere described the typical radiographic appearance; the compression may be so severe that the lesion is vertebra plana with lytic involvement of the vertebral body.[8] Even if there is collapse of the vertebral body, the proximal and distal disk space may be intact. Significant collapse can occur without neurologic compromise. Rarely, the lesions involve the pedicles and are associated with paraspinal and intraspinal soft tissue masses.[66] The erythrocyte sedimentation rate is usually low or normal.

The lesion consists of gray-pink soft tissue. Microscopically, there is a background of histiocytes infiltrated by eosinophils. Lymphocytes, plasma cells, and multinucleated giant cells may also be seen.[18]

In the majority of cases, the diagnosis is unclear, and a biopsy is necessary to differentiate eosinophilic granuloma from infection or other tumors. Most lesions of the vertebra heal after simple curettage. Adjuvant low-dose radiation (in the range of 5 to 10 Gy) should be considered in the majority of cases of lesions of the spine.

RHEUMATOID ARTHRITIS

Rheumatoid arthritis is a systematic inflammatory process; the spinal column is involved in approximately 25 to 30% of cases, although sporadic reports claim as high as a 50% incidence.[9, 10, 43, 67] The majority of patients are 50 years or older and usually have a long-standing history.[9, 10, 67] Patients with rheumatoid arthritis affecting the spinal column are generally seropositive for rheumatoid factor.[10]

Individuals are commonly asymptomatic, and the lesion is detected incidentally on radiographs (Fig. 10–23). Patients with a significant myelopathy experience rapid progression of disease and generally die from their illness if surgical intervention is not carried out. The most prominent symptoms of spinal rheumatoid arthritis are pain and occipital neuralgia, which generally precede weakness and paresthesias. Patients whose lesions involve upward movement of the odontoid process may demonstrate syndromes involving the brain stem.

The most commonly affected spinal joint is the atlantoaxial articulation. Although monitored flexion-extension films of the cervical spine provide excellent information regarding the stability of the rheumatoid spine, MRI of the cervicomedullary junction and the upper cervical spine provides excellent details of the osseous, ligamentous, and soft tissue elements of the disease.

The role of pannus formation about the odontoid process and the soft tissue mass produced by the inflammatory process at the craniocervical junction has been underemphasized in the past. The transverse ligament at the atlantoaxial joint may be damaged by riding over the eroded surface of the odontoid peg. Soft pink tissue and oily fluid form the majority of the pannus. Microscopically, it is composed of chronically inflamed synovial tissue with inflammatory cell infiltrates, granulation tissue, and giant cells.

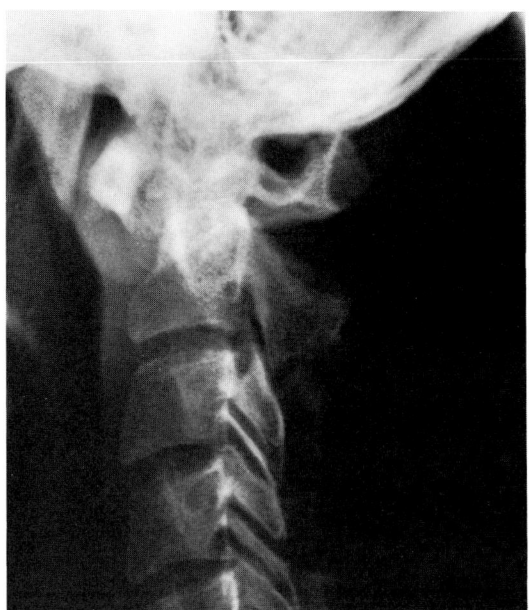

FIGURE 10–23. Rheumatoid arthritis. Plain lateral film of the cervical spine. There is an increased predental space with a C1-2 subluxation. (The C1 spinolaminar line is ventral to its normal position.) There is an extensive soft tissue mass ventral to the dens. This is consistent with the granulation tissue known as pannus, which is seen in rheumatoid arthritis.

In addition to those patients who demonstrate neurologic deficit due to increased mobility at the atlantoaxial joint, patients with greater than 8 mm of predental space (frequently filled with soft tissue pannus) and those with upward migration of the odontoid process should undergo surgical stabilization[43] (Fig. 10–24). Although the majority of patients benefit from simple posterior cervical stabilization after appropriate alignment, a number of other procedures have been advocated. Because some investigators noted significant worsening, including respiratory compromise, after posterior fusion, transoral approaches through the posterior pharyngeal wall with resection of the anterior arch of C1, involved odontoid peg, and pannus have been suggested.[9, 10] The use of nasotracheal intubation with the patient awake and intraoperative evoked potential monitoring have significantly decreased operative morbidity and mortality.

SYPHILIS

Neuroarthropathy is one of the sequlae of tertiary syphilis. One tenth of patients with tabes dorsalis manifest neuropathic joints, with the spinal column being frequently affected.[48]

The spinal disease resembles degenerative disease of the spine and most frequently affects the lumbar spine, with the dorsal spine being the second most common site of the lesion. Dense sclerosis of the vertebral bodies with bridging osteophytes but a lack of ligamentous calcification is the hallmark of the disease.[57] The earliest radiologic change is sclerosis of the opposing vertebral surfaces. The disease is generally localized to one or two vertebral levels but progresses rapidly. Enlargement of the vertebral body (attributable to serpentine sclerosis and microfractures) and facet hypertrophy lead to canal and foraminal stenosis.[48, 57]

The features of the enlarged spinal elements are due to osteitis and periostitis. Loss of articular cartilage and loss of subchondral bone occur with subsequent destruction, reparative osteitis, and new bone formation.

Many patients are asymptomatic until late in the disease. Some recover from their painful syndromes with conservative treatment. It is controversial whether decompression of the enlarged, sclerotic vertebral elements leads to improvement.

TUBERCULOSIS

Skeletal tuberculosis most commonly affects the vertebral column. Pott's disease has as-

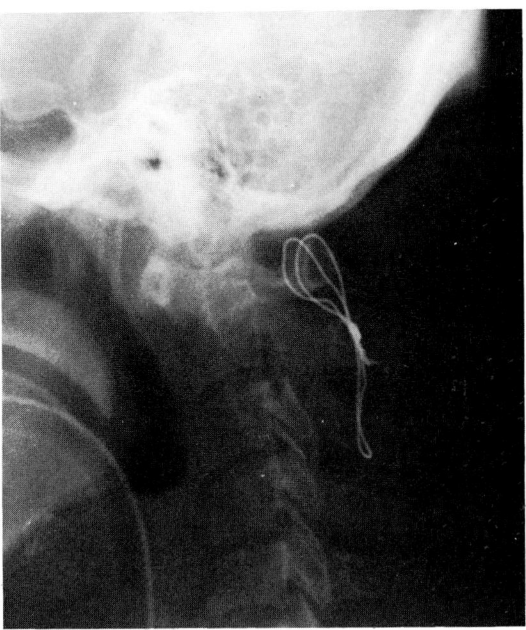

FIGURE 10–24. Same patient as in Figure 10–23. Postoperative lateral radiograph of the cervical spine. A C1 through C3 fusion has been performed using 18-gauge stainless steel wire and methyl methacrylate to prevent further subluxation and progressive neurologic deficit.

sumed increasing importance with its resurgence in the HIV-afflicted population. Involvement of the cervical spine is relatively uncommon, occurring in only 3 to 5% of cases. The average number of involved vertebral bodies is two. In more than 98% of cases, the body of the vertebra is involved adjacent to the disk, with other parts of the vertebra and the epidural space rarely being involved. Subligamentous spread and paraspinal extension from adjacent involved vertebral bodies and their disk spaces is common. Bilateral abscesses with floccular calcification are pathognomonic of tuberculosis. Healing in tuberculous spondylitis can lead to spontaneous fusion of adjacent vertebral bodies. The plain radiographic appearance consists of irregularity of the end plates, decreased height of the intervertebral disk, sclerosis of the surrounding bone, and late anterior wedging or fusion (Fig. 10–25).

CT scan demonstrates paraspinal abscesses with a clear low-density center. MRI in T2-weighted images is particularly well suited for the demonstration of paraspinal abscesses as a high-signal intensity region.[12] Inflammatory tissue enhances with the intravenous injection of gadolinium-diethylenetriaminepentaacetic acid (DTPA) during MRI and indicates active disk space infection.[12]

The myriad antituberculous drugs are the mainstay of therapy for tuberculous spondylitis.[30, 44] If the diagnosis is in doubt, skinny needle biopsy of a related abscess may provide useful information. A portion of the material thus obtained should *always* be sent for acid-fast culture. Anterior approaches for excision of involved bone, granulomatous tissue, and purulence are the most common approaches, combined with either anterior bone grafting at a second stage or posterior fusion. Definitive surgery for therapeutic purposes should be reserved for patients with severe neurologic deficits, those who fail to respond to medical management, or those who demonstrate spinal instability. Surgery should also be immediately performed if the lesion involves the upper cervical spine or the cervicothoracic junction or if there is marked kyphosis with active disease. Posterior spinal tuberculosis, although rare, is notorious for causing early spinal compression, and affected patients should be operated on if an extradural component is suspected.

Even patients with Pott's paraplegia or tetraplegia have a good prognosis for functional recovery if they are treated early in the course of their disease.[12, 30, 39, 44]

Conclusion

Although primary osseous lesions of the spine are uncommon, similar principles can be adapted to treating these problems as are used in treating metastatic lesions. Good surgical results depend on a thorough resection followed by vertebral stabilization. The timing and dosage of adjuvant modalities such as chemotherapy and radiation therapy should be coordinated with oncologists and radiologists. If physicians utilize these recommendations, it is hoped that patients will obtain significant relief of pain, reversal of neurologic deficits,

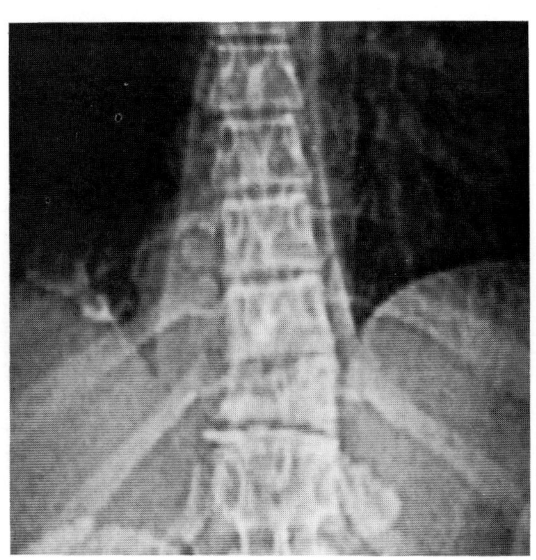

FIGURE 10–25. Tuberculosis. Unilateral collapse of the involved thoracic vertebral body with disappearance of the involved pedicle is seen on a plain film. The disk space above is narrowed. The ipsilateral paraspinal soft tissue shadow is widened.

stabilization of the vertebral axis, and early mobilization.

References

1. Ayala AG, Murray JA, Erling MA, Raymond AK: Osteoid osteoma: Intraoperative tetracycline—fluorescence demonstration of the nidus. J Bone Joint Surg 68A:747–751, 1986.
2. Barwick KW, Huvos AG, Smith J: Primary osteogenic sarcoma of the vertebral column. Cancer 46:595–604, 1980.
3. Boland P, Lane JM, Sundaresan N: Tumors of the lumbar spine. *In* Camins MB, O'Leary PF (eds): The Lumbar Spine. New York, Raven Press, 1987, pp 223–241.
4. Bundens DA, Rechtine GR: Sarcoidosis of the spine: Case report and literature review. Spine 11:209–212, 1986.
5. Camins MB, Duncan AW, Smith J, Marcove RC: Chondrosarcoma of the spine. Spine 3:202–209, 1978.
6. Campanacci M, Capanna R, Picci P: Unicameral and aneurysmal bone cysts. Clin Orthop 204:25–36, 1987.
7. Campanacci M, Giunti A, Olmi R: Giant cell tumours of bone. A study of 209 cases with long term follow-up in 130. Ital J Orthop Traumatol 1:249, 1975.
8. Compere EL: Vertebra plana due to eosinophilic granuloma. J Bone Joint Surg 36A:969–1954, 1954.
9. Crockard HA, Essigman WK, Stevens JM, Pozo JL, Ransford AO, Kendall BE: Surgical treatment of cervical cord compression in rheumatoid arthritis. Ann Rheum Dis 44:809–816, 1985.
10. Crockard HA, Pozo JL, Ransford AO, Stevens JM, Kendall BE, Essigman WK: Transoral decompression and posterior fusion for rheumatoid atlanto-axial subluxation. J Bone Joint Surg 68B:350–356, 1986.
11. Dahlin DC: Bone Tumors: General Aspects and Data on 6221 Cases, 3rd ed. Springfield, IL, Charles C Thomas, 1978.
12. De Roos A, van Persijn van Meerten EL, Bloem JL, Bluemm RG: MRI of tuberculous spondylitis. AJR 146:79–82, 1986.
13. Dunn EJ, Davidison RI, Anas PP: Diagnosis and management of tumors of the cervical spine. Cervical Spine Research Society (ed): The Cervical Spine. Philadelphia, JB Lippincott 1983, pp 477–495.
14. Eckardt JJ, Grogan TJ: Giant cell tumor of bone. Clin Orthop 204:45–57, 1986.
15. Enneking WF: Musculoskeletal tumor surgery. New York, Churchill Livingstone, 1983.
16. Fidler MW: Anterior decompression and stabilization of metastatic spinal fractures. J Bone Joint Surg 68B:83–90, 1986.
17. Friedlaender GE, Southwick WO: Tumors of the spine. *In* Rothman RN, Simeone FA (eds): The Spine. Philadelphia, WB Saunders Co, 1982, pp 1022–1041.
18. Gandolfi A: Vertebral histiocytosis-X causing spinal cord compression. Surg Neurol 19:369–372, 1983.
19. Gandolfi A, Brizzi R, Tedeschi F, Cusmano F, Gabrielli M: Fibrosarcoma arising in Paget's disease of the vertebra: Review of the literature. Surg Neurol 19:72–76, 1983.
20. Goodman MA: Plasma cell tumors. Clin Orthop 204:86–91, 1986.
21. Graham JJ, Yang WC: Vertebral hemangioma with compression fracture and paraparesis treated with preoperative embolization and vertebral resection. Spine 9:97–101, 1984.
22. Greenspan A, Klein MJ, Bennett AJ, Lewis MM, Neuwirth M, Camins MB: Hemangioma of the T6 vertebra with a compression fracture, extradural block and spinal cord compression. Skeletal Radiol 10:183–188, 1983.
23. Gutin PH, Leibel SA, Hosobuchi Y, et al: Brachytherapy of recurrent tumors of the skull base and spine with iodine-125 sources. Neurosurgery 20:938–945, 1987.
24. Harbin WP: Metastatic disease and the nonspecific bone scan: Value of spinal computed tomography. Radiology 145:105–107, 1982.
25. Harrington KD: Metastatic disease of the spine. J Bone Joint Surg 68A:1110–1117, 1986.
26. Healey JH, Ghelman B: Osteoid osteoma and osteoblastomas. Clin Orthop 204:76–85, 1986.
27. Healey JH, Lane JM: Chondrosarcoma. Clin Orthop 204:119–129, 1986.
28. Healey M, Herz DA, Pearl L: Spinal hemangiomas. Neurosurgery 13:689–691, 1983.
29. Holtas SL, Kido DK, Simon JH: MR imaging of spinal lymphoma. J Comput Assist Tomogr 10:111–115, 1986.
30. Hsu LCS, Leong JCY: Tuberculosis of the lower cervical spine (C2 to C7). J Bone Joint Surg 66B:1–5, 1984.
31. Hudson TM, Galceran M: Radiology of sacrococcygeal chordoma. Clin Orthop 175:237–242, 1982.
32. Huth JF, Dawson EG, Eilber FR: Abdominosacral resection for malignant tumors of the sacrum. Am J Surg 148:157–161, 1984.
33. Huvos AG: Bone tumors: Diagnosis, Treatment and Prognosis. WB Saunders Co, Philadelphia, 1979.
34. Karian JM, DeFilipp G, Buchheit WA, Bonakdarpour A, Eckhardt W: Vertebral osteochondroma causing spinal cord compression: Case report. Neurosurgery 14:483–484, 1984.
35. Kirwin EOG, Hutton PAN, Pozzo JL, Ransford AO: Osteoid osteomas and benign osteoblastoma of the spine. J Bone Joint Surg 66B:21–26, 1984.
36. Kornberg M: Primary Ewing's sarcoma of the spine: A review and case report. Spine 11:54–57, 1986.
37. Kriecbergs A, Boquist L, Borssen B, Larson S: Prognostic factors in chondrosarcoma. A comparative study of cellular DNA content and clinicopathologic features. Cancer 50:577, 1982.
38. Krol G, Sundaresan N, Deck M: Computed tomography of axial chordomas. J Comput Assist Tomogr 7:286–289, 1983.
39. Kumar K: A clinical study and classification of posterior spinal tuberculosis. Int Orthop 9:147–152, 1985.
40. Lane JM, Hurson B, Boland P, Glasser DB: Osteogenic sarcoma. Clin Orthop 204:93–110, 1986.
41. Lee CK, Rosa R, Fernand R: Surgical treatment of tumors of the spine. Spine 11:201–208, 1986.
42. Leehey P, Naseem M, Every P, Russell E, Sarwar M: Vertebral hemangioma with compression myelopathy: Metrizamide CT demonstration. J Comput Assist Tomogr 9:985–986, 1985.
43. Lesoin F, Duquesnoy B, Destee A, Leys D, Rousseaux M, Carini S, Verier A, Jomin M: Cervical neurological complications of rheumatoid arthritis. Surgical treatment techniques and indications. Acta Neurochir 78:91–97, 1985.
44. Lifeso RM, Weaver P, Harder EH: Tuberculous spondylitis in adults. J Bone Joint Surg 67A:1405–1413, 1985.
45. Lozes G, Fawaz A, Perper H, et al: Chondroma of the cervical spine. J Neurosurg 66:128–130, 1987.

46. Makely JT: Prostaglandins—a mechanism for pain mediation in osteoid osteoma. Orthop Trans 6:72, 1982.
47. Makely JT, Carter JR: Eosinophilic granuloma of bone. Clin Orthop 204:37–44, 1986.
48. Moran SM, Mohr JA: Syphilis and axial arthropathy. South Med J 76:1032–1035, 1983.
49. Nicholls PJ, Jarecky TW: The value of posterior decompression by laminectomy for malignant tumors of the spine. Clin Orthop Rel Res 201:210–213, 1985.
50. Neff JR: Nonmetastatic Ewing's sarcoma of bone: The role of surgical therapy. Clin Orthop 204:111–118, 1986.
51. Nunez C, Bennett T, Bohlman HH: Chondromyxoid fibroma of the thoracic spine. Case report and review of the literature. Spine 7:436–439, 1982.
52. O'Neill P, Bell BA, Miller JD, Jacobson I, Guthrie W: Fifty years of experience with chordomas in southeast Scotland. Neurosurgery 16:166–170, 1985.
53. O'Rourke T, George CB, Redmond J, Davidson H, Cornett P, Fill WL, Spring DB, Sobel D, Dabe IB, Karl RD, Cromwell LD: Spinal computed tomography and computed tomographic metrizamide myelography in the early diagnosis of metastatic disease. J Clin Oncol 4:576–583, 1986.
54. Palacios E, Gorelick PB, Gonzalez CF, Fine M: Malignant lymphoma of the nervous system. J Comput Assist Tomogr 6:689–701, 1982.
55. Pambakian H, Smith MA: Glomus tumors of the coccygeal body associated with coccydynia. J Bone Joint Surg 63B:424–426, 1981.
56. Posner JB: Neurological complications of systemic cancer. Med Clin North Am 55:625–646, 1971.
57. Radhakrishnan K, Vijayan VP, Ashok PP, Sridharan R, Mousa ME: Syphilitic spinal neuroarthropathy with paraplegia. Clin Neurol Neurosurg 87:61–64, 1985.
58. Razek A, Perez CA, Tefft M: Intergroup Ewing's Sarcoma Study: Local control related to radiation dose, volume, and site of primary lesion in Ewing's sarcoma. Cancer 46:516–521, 1980.
59. Resnick D, Niwayama G: Diagnosis of bone and joint disorders. Philadelphia, WB Saunders Co, 1981.
60. Rich TA, Schiller A, Suit HD, Mank HJ: Clinical and pathologic review of 48 cases of chordoma. Cancer 56:182–187, 1985.
61. Rosen G, Caparros B, Nirenberg A: Ewing's sarcoma: Ten-year experience with adjuvant chemotherapy. Cancer 47:2204–2213, 1981.
62. Schecter MS, Collins JD: Epidural lipoma: An unusual cause of a sclerotic vertebral body. Spine 8:804–805, 1983.
63. Shibasaki K, Harper CG, Bedbrook GM, Kakulas BA: Vertebral metastases and spinal cord compression. Paraplegia 21:47–61, 1983.
64. Standefer M, Hardy RW, Marks K, Cosgrove DM: Chondromyxoid fibroma of the cervical spine—a case report with a review of the literature and a description of an operative approach to the lower anterior cervical spine. Neurosurgery 11:288–292, 1982.
65. Sundaresan N: Chordomas. Clin Orthop 204:135–142, 1986.
66. Thommesen P, Bartholdy N, Bünger E: Histiocytosis X simulating tuberculosis. Acta Radiol (Oncol) 22:295–297, 1983.
67. Thompson RC, Meyer TJ: Posterior surgical stabilization for atlantoaxial subluxation in rheumatoid arthritis. Spine 10:597–601, 1985.
68. Tippetts RH, Apfelbaum RI: Anterior cervical fusion with Caspar instrumentation system. Neurosurgery 22:1008–1013, 1988.
69. Von Hanwehr R, Apuzzo MLJ, Ahmadi J, Chang P: Thoracic spinal angiomyolipoma: Case report and review. Neurosurgery 16:406–411, 1985.
70. Wilner D: Radiology of Bone Tumors and Allied Disorders. Philadelphia, WB Saunders Co, 1982.

> "If thou examinest a man having a displacement in a vertebra of his neck whose face is fixed, whose neck cannot turn for him, (and) thou shouldst say to him: 'Look at thy breast (and) thy two shoulders,' (and) he is unable to turn his face that he may look at his breast (and) his two shoulders, thou shouldst say concerning him: 'one having a displacement in a vertebra of his neck. An ailment which I will treat.' "

This earliest record of disease afflicting the cervical spine is found in Egyptian writings from 2700 to 1700 BC.[4] Our fascination with the cervical spine has persisted through the ages, but not until the late 1800s were the anatomic knowledge and technological advances required for spinal surgery clarified. In the 1900s the improvement of anesthetic techniques enabled surgeons to view abnormalities of the craniovertebral junction as correctable conditions rather than anatomic and pathologic curiosities.

Transoral Approach (With Or Without a Mandibular Split) (Table 10–2)

As early as 1919, Kanavel described a transoral approach to the craniocervical junction,[12] but anterior approaches were generally slow to develop. More recently, however, reports of large series of use of the transoral approach with excellent results have been published.[1, 3, 6, 8, 14, 15]

CASE HISTORY

A 63-year-old female painter with a long history of rheumatoid arthritis complained of dysesthesias of all four extremities, most no-

TABLE 10–2.

Indications for Specific Approaches to the Cervical Spine

Transoral Approach/Mandibular Split
Abnormalities of the craniovertebral junction
- Rheumatoid arthritis
- Odontoid dysgenesis
- Clival tumors
- Basilar impressions
- Unfused odontoid
- Klippel-Feil
- Abnormal condyles and occiput
- Traumatic/tumors: dislocation with posterior compression at occiput, C1, C2

Anterior Approach
Midline soft disk herniation
- Anterior intracanalicular lesions
- Lesions of vertebral bodies
- Osteophytic cord compression by vertebral body
- Vertebral body fracture with posteriorly placed fragments
- Access to vertebral artery
- Type II odontoid fractures (anterior screw fixation)

Lateral Approach
C1 and C2 vertebral body lesions where transoral approach is not feasible
- Exposure of vertebral artery
- Extreme lateral disk herniations
- Exposure of vertebral bodies C1 to T1
- Anterior intracanalicular lesions
- Lesions of vertebral bodies

Posterior Approach
Extreme lateral disk herniation
- Transdural approach to herniated disks
- Posterior spinal cord compression
- Atlanto-occipital instability without anterior compression (i.e., Jefferson fracture)
- Posterior fusions (i.e., odontoid fractures)
- Intramedullary spinal cord tumors
- Intradural spinal cord tumors
- Extradural spinal cord tumors

tably in her hands, and difficulties with balance of several months' duration. Physical examination revealed mildly diminished pin prick sensation throughout both hands and bilateral Babinski responses. MRI revealed a large pannus at CI with cord compression (Fig. 10–26). On flexion-extension lateral radiographs, movement at CI-C2 was visualized. Posterior fusion with wire and iliac crest bone was followed by transoral decompression.

SURGICAL TECHNIQUE

With the patient in a supine position, nasotracheal intubation is performed. The head is then placed in three-pin fixation. If a combined anterior and posterior approach is anticipated during one sitting, the patient is placed in the lateral position after the skull clamps have been applied.[8] At this point a radiograph is taken to ensure alignment of the cervical spine. The esophagus is packed to block passage of fluid and surgical debris, and the mouth and pharynx are prepared with povidone iodine. If plans include dural closure with a fascia lata graft or the use of iliac crest bone, the appropriate area should also be prepared. For all transdural procedures a lumbar cerebrospinal fluid (CSF) drain is inserted to decrease CSF pressure and to guard against formation of a CSF fistula. The drain can be left in place for up to 5 days postoperatively.[1, 10] In the past, difficulty in obtaining adequate dural closure has limited the utilization of this exposure for intradural lesions, but recent work with fibrin glue for sealing the dura, two-layer closures, and fat and bone grafts after transoral surgery appear to have alleviated this problem.[8] Ex-

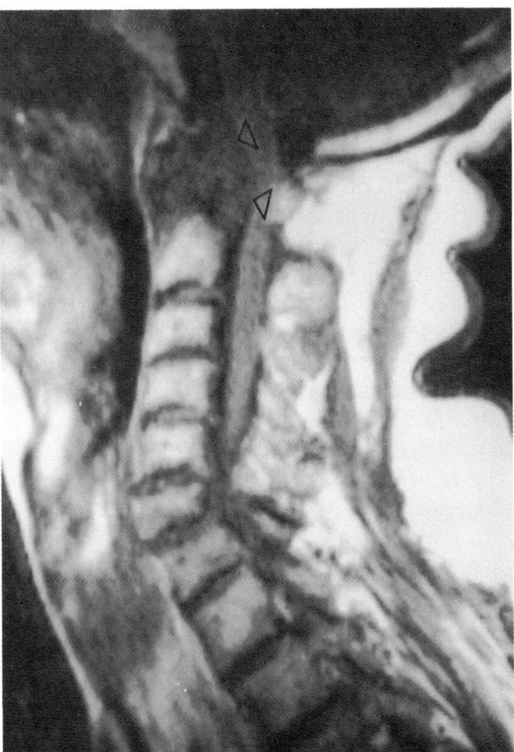

FIGURE 10–26. T1-weighted MRI image of the cervical spine in the sagittal plane reveals an anterior mass at C1-2 with compression of the spinal cord (arrowheads). After transoral resection of the lesion, rheumatoid arthritis pannus was diagnosed. The apparent compression of the spinal cord seen at C5-6 was an artifact of the plane of section.

posure of the pharynx, which is obscured by the soft palate, has also been an impediment with this approach.[1] Crockard has recently developed a retractor that provides for both lateral and midline exposure without requiring incision of the soft palate.[8]

The operating microscope should be used from the beginning of the procedure. In general, the anterior tubercle of C1 is readily palpable and is used as a landmark. A midline pharyngeal incision, extending from the foramen magnum 4 to 5 cm inferiorly to the base of C2, is created. This incision should extend through mucosa and the muscle of the superior and middle constrictors. The tissues are dissected laterally and held with retraction sutures. Deep to the constrictors lie the longus colli muscles, where they insert on the anterior tubercle of C1, and the anterior longitudinal ligament. Once the midline is assured, the anterior longitudinal ligament is incised over the desired area and dissected laterally to complete the exposure. Exposure may be gained from the clivus through C3. A dural exposure extending 2 cm up the clivus and down to C2 can be easily obtained by using an air drill to remove bone of the lower clivus, the anterior arch of C1, and the body of C2. The total exposure should be approximately 5 cm long and just less than 1.5 cm wide.[8] After completion of the procedure, utilization of fibrin glue with a fascial patch (tensor fasciae latae) or autologous fat provides for a watertight dural closure.

If the pathologic process is more extensive, a midline mandibular osteotomy must be used in conjunction with the above procedure to gain access to lower cervical segments. In all cases in which a mandibular split is required, a tracheostomy should be performed.[1, 3, 8, 14] The lower lip is split by a midline incision that is staggered in the crease above the mentum and extends inferiorly in the midline to the level of the hyoid bone. The incision is carried down to the anterior gum margin at the lip and down to bone along the mandible.[3]

With small periosteal elevators the anterior mandibular periosteum is elevated laterally for about 2 cm. An incision is marked out on bone from one of the lower incisors extending inferiorly in a staircase manner to the lower border of the mandible. The lower incisor in line with the bone cut is extracted, and the mandible is divided with either a Gigli saw or an oscillating power saw. A scalpel is used to split the tongue in the midline to the epiglottis; the epiglottis should be preserved and retracted out of the field. With this opening and the use of the Crockard retractor, exposure may be gained from the clivus to the upper portion of C5. The remainder of the opening is performed as described, except that the midline pharyngeal incision may be extended to the top of C5. To reach the vertebral bodies themselves, the prevertebral fascia, longus colli muscles, and anterior periosteum are incised.

At the end of the procedure, Vicryl sutures are used to approximate the floor of the mouth. The muscles are closed with two layers of interrupted sutures, and the mucosa is closed with a single layer of interrupted sutures. The mandible is then reapproximated with two 25-gauge titanium or stainless steel wires passed through the previously placed drill holes. The infralingual mucosa and the subcutaneous tissue of the lip are closed. Care is taken to reattach the orbicularis oris muscle and to realign the vermilion border. Steri-Strip adhesive tape is used to ensure a cosmetically pleasing closure.

Anterior Approach from C3 to T1 (See Table 10–2)

Surgical exposure of the anterior cervical spine evolved in the 1950s.[2, 6, 17] Since then, the approach has remained essentially unchanged, except for some minor modifications during the 1960s.[18]

CASE HISTORY

A 12-year-old male with an unidentified skeletal dysplasia and dwarfism was noted on routine examination to have a spastic gait and Babinski responses. The patient was evaluated with plain cervical radiographs, CT, and MRI (Fig. 10–27). An anterior approach to the lesion was undertaken. A partial vertebrectomy with insertion of a fibular strut bone graft was followed by immobilization in a halo device. Owing to the patient's youth and the potential for growth with dislodgement of an implant, no instrumentation was used.

SURGICAL TECHNIQUE

Advantages exist for either a left- or a right-sided exposure of the spine. A left-sided approach risks injury to the thoracic duct, whereas a right-sided approach carries the pos-

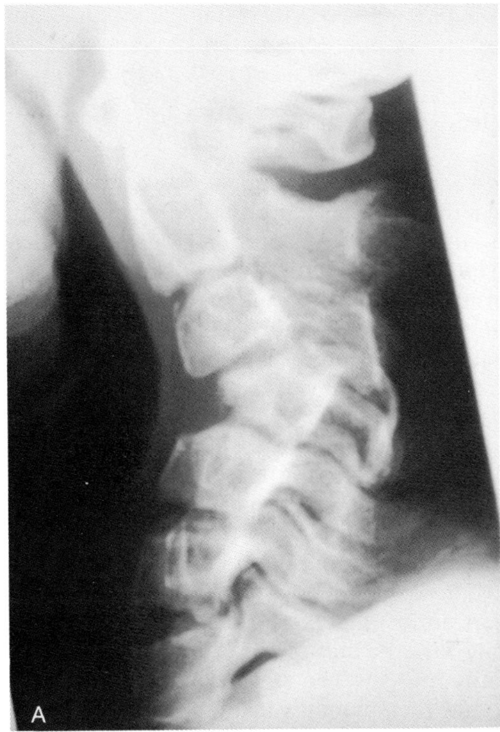

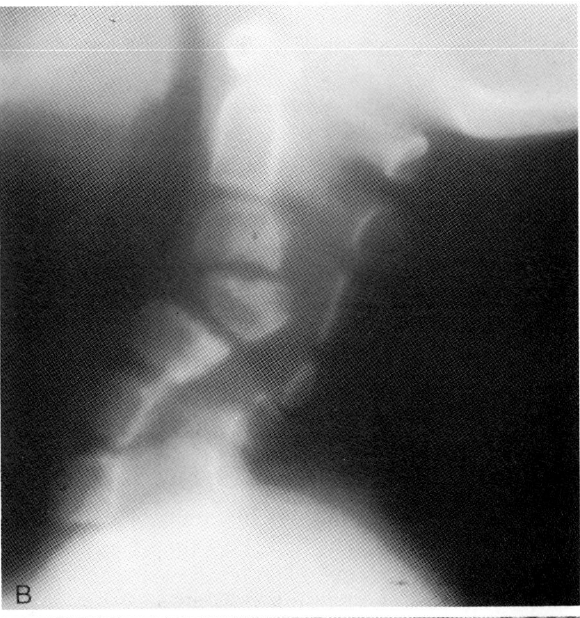

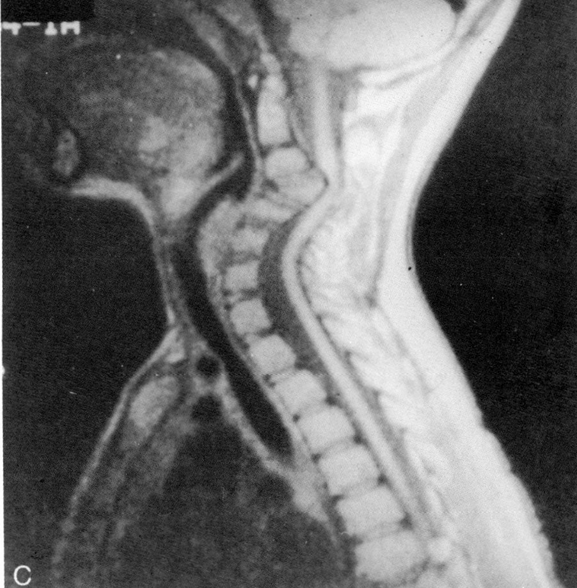

FIGURE 10–27. Lateral radiograph *(A)* and tomogram *(B)* of a 12-year-old child with skeletal dysplasia reveal an abnormal C4 vertebral body with retrolisthesis and marked kyphosis centered around this level. *C*, Sagittal section from a T1-weighted MRI scan reveals spinal cord impingement by the C4 vertebral body.

sibility of injury to the recurrent laryngeal nerve.[2, 6, 13, 17]

If the area to be exposed is at the C3-4 level, an incision should be made just lateral to the midportion of the thyroid cartilage; lesions in the area of C6-7 require an incision at the level of the cricoid cartilage or below. Intraoperative fluoroscopy or a lateral radiograph should be used to confirm the operative level. The initial incision traverses skin and subcutaneous fat down to platysma. The platysma is then carefully divided to prevent damage to the underlying sternocleidomastoid muscle, which would obscure the plane of dissection. The anterior border of the sternocleidomastoid muscle is then clearly visible. A finger is inserted along the plane anterior to the sternocleidomastoid muscle, and the pulsations of the carotid sheath are identified. Medial to the carotid sheath the midcervical fascia is identified and sharply opened. The prevertebral fascia is exposed and the esophagus identified. Self-retaining Cloward retractors are inserted under the longus colli muscle to retract the strap muscles, thyroid, trachea, and esophagus medially and the sternocleidomastoid muscle and carotid sheath laterally. The prevertebral fascia is then incised over the desired area and dissected laterally with a peanut or periosteal elevator to complete the exposure.

To verify the anatomic level, placement of a spinal needle in the disk space should be confirmed radiologically. For lesions lying low in the cervical spine (e.g., C7-T1), it is sometimes necessary to detach the sternocleidomastoid muscle from its origin along the manubrium of the sternum to gain adequate exposure.[10] Occasionally the inferior thyroidal artery prevents adequate exposure of the C7-T1 region. This vessel can usually be retracted, but if necessary it can be ligated without complication. Identification of this artery should alert the surgeon to the proximity of the recurrent laryngeal nerve, particularly during a right-sided approach, where it emerges from the vagus nerve at a higher level than on the left. Closure is achieved by reapproximating the omohyoid muscle and the sternocleidomastoid muscle with interrupted nonabsorbable sutures. The platysma is reapproximated with interrupted 3-0 Vicryl sutures. Subcuticular skin closure with 3-0 or 4-0 Vicryl and Steri-Strips will yield a pleasing cosmetic result.

Lateral Retropharyngeal Approach (See Table 10–1)

Lateral approaches to the cervical vertebrae were pioneered in Ireland during the early 1900s, then later described in detail by Elkin and Harris[9] and Henry.[10] Whitesides and McDonald further developed this exposure for a variety of vertebral lesions extending from the skull base to the thorax.[20]

CASE HISTORY

A 45-year-old male presented with a several-month history of weight loss and severe neck pain. Neurologic examination was unremarkable. Evaluation with plain radiographs, MRI, CT, and vertebral angiography (Fig. 10–28) revealed a neoplastic process involving the C4 and C5 vertebral bodies with encasement of the right vertebral artery and compression of the cord with both anterior and posterior extension. Because neither an anterior nor a posterior approach would adequately expose the tumor, a lateral approach was used. A C4 and C5 partial vertebrectomy was performed, and Steinmann pins and acrylic were used to stabilize the spine. Histopathologic examination revealed an undifferentiated carcinoma.

SURGICAL TECHNIQUE

With the patient in a supine position, nasotracheal intubation is performed. During draping, the ear is retracted anteriorly out of the field or by using a suture. A hockey-stick skin incision is made from the base of the mastoid, below the ear and to the angle of the mandible, where the incision turns inferiorly to run along the anterior border of the sternocleidomastoid muscle. The platysma is then sharply divided and the sternocleidomastoid muscle identified. To protect against injury to the facial nerve and creation of a parotid fistula, the superior limb of the incision must be dissected with great care. At the base of the mastoid an incision is made down to bone dividing the insertion of the sternocleidomastoid muscle along with the mastoid insertion of the splenius capitis muscle. The sternocleidomastoid muscle and the splenius are then retracted posteriorly from the field. At the level of C6, where the omohyoid crosses deep to the sternocleidomastoid muscle and superficial to the internal jugular vein, the tendinous portion of the muscle is severed. Now the sternocleidomastoid muscle complex is completely freed. Next the spinal accessory nerve, which lies 2 to 3 fingerbreadths below the mastoid tip, is defined. The spinal accessory nerve is traced to its exit from the jugular foramen, dissected free of the jugular vein, and retracted posteriorly with the sternocleidomastoid muscle. The transverse process of C1, lying 2 cm inferior and anterior to the mastoid tip, can now be identified.

Beginning just anterior and superior to the transverse process of C1, the prevertebral fascia is incised at an oblique angle posteriorly and inferiorly. The fascia should be opened just medial to the phrenic nerve so that the phrenic nerve will remain undisturbed.[10] An areolar plane is entered between the anterior aspect of the transverse processes and the carotid sheath. This plane is dissected medially until the sagittal partition of Charpy is encountered and divided. By extending this dissection superiorly and inferiorly, a plane extending from C1 to C7 may be created. The carotid sheath is retracted medially with the strap muscles, thyroid, trachea, and esophagus. With this exposure the vertebral bodies may be counted directly. Depending on the proce-

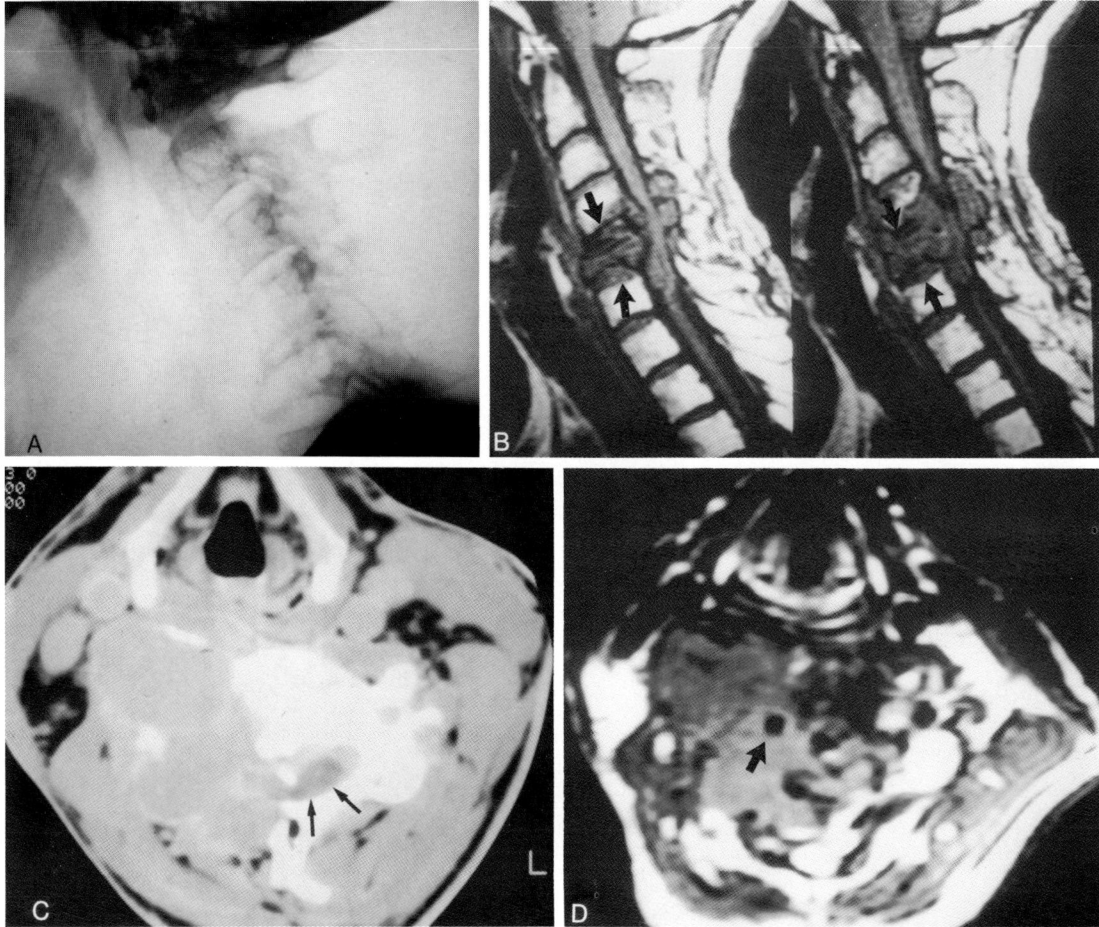

FIGURE 10–28. Subtracted lateral radiograph *(A)* and T1-weighted sagittal sections from MRI *(B)* of the cervical spine reveal destruction of the C5 and C6 vertebral bodies (arrows) with spinal cord compression. CT scan *(C)* and T1-weighted MRI scan in the axial section through the C5-6 region *(D)* reveal encasement of the right vertebral artery (large arrow) and compression of the spinal cord (small arrows).

Illustration continued on following page

dure to be undertaken, the surgeon can proceed with periosteal elevation and the definitive procedure. However, mobilization of the two prevertebral muscles, the longus colli and the longus capitis, is usually required. By detaching the vertical part of the longus colli, both its superior oblique portion and the major portion of the longus capitis may be retracted away from the spine. To expose C1 and C2, the tendinous insertion of the upper oblique portion of the colli must be cut as it inserts into the anterior tubercle of the atlas.

At the completion of the procedure, the longus colli may be reattached to its ligamentous insertion on the anterior tubercle. The two bellies of the omohyoid muscle are rejoined at their tendinous midsection. The mastoid portion of the splenius capitis and the sternocleidomastoid muscles are reapproximated to their tendinous insertion on the mastoid. The platysma is apposed. The skin is closed in a subcuticular fashion, and Steri-Strips are used. Retropharyngeal edema can be anticipated with any extensive procedure, and respiratory embarrassment must be guarded against.

Posterior Approach (See Table 10–1)

Because the posterior aspect of the neck is devoid of major vessels and other vital structures, it is only logical that posterior approaches developed first. Many contributions were made from notable nineteenth-century surgeons,[19] but the first description of a posterior approach for stabilization was published by Church and Eisendrath in 1892.[5]

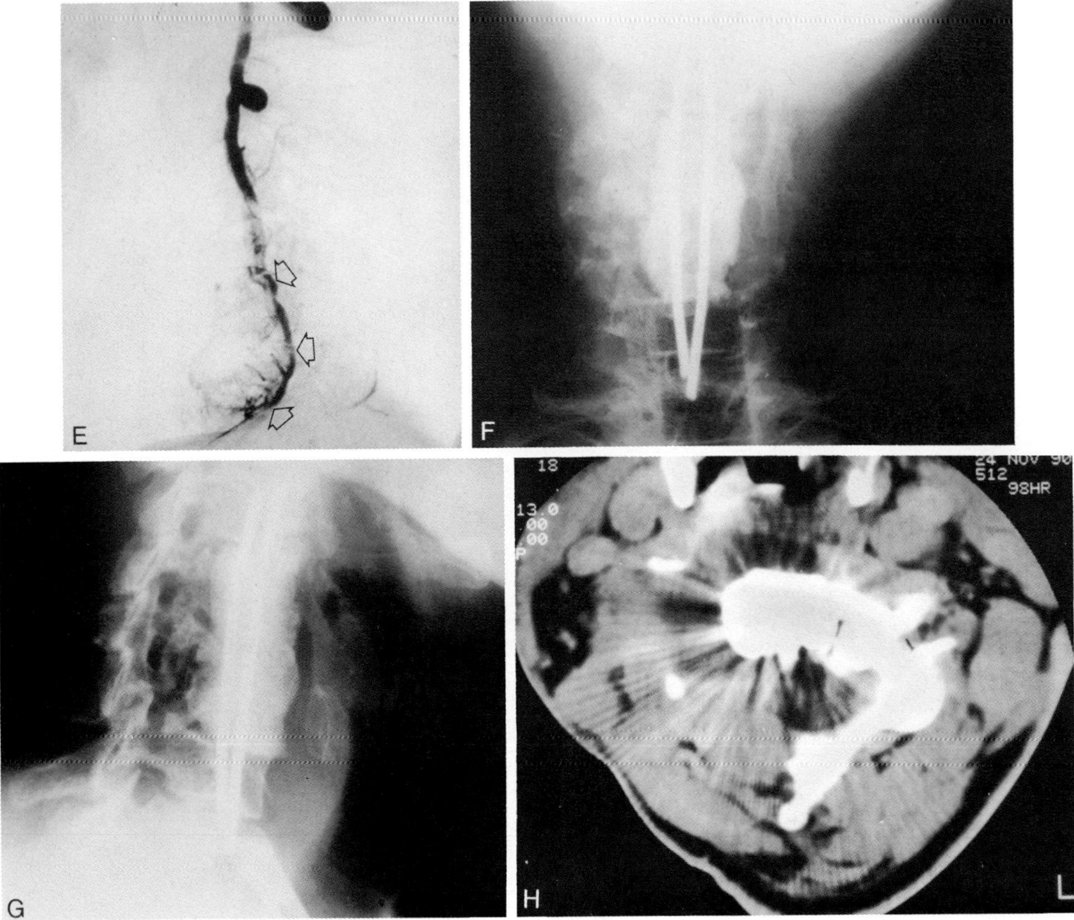

FIGURE 10–28 *Continued. E*, Right vertebral artery angiogram reveals posterior displacement of the artery (arrows) by the mass. Postoperative anteroposterior *(F)* and lateral *(G)* radiographs of the cervical spine as well as an axial CT scan through the C5-6 region *(H)* reveal resection of the tumor and stabilization with Steinmann pins and methyl methacrylate.

CASE HISTORY

A 57-year-old female without a significant past medical history presented with paresthesias in all four extremities. Neurologic examination revealed a spastic gait with hyperreflexia throughout and bilateral, positive Babinski responses. Radiologic work-up, including MRI of the cervical spine with flexion/extension views and myelography, revealed multilevel stenosis (Fig. 10–29). A multilevel laminectomy via the posterior approach was performed for decompression.

SURGICAL TECHNIQUE

For the posterior approach to the cervical spine, numerous positions may be used, including sitting, lateral, three-quarter prone, and prone. If spinal instability is present, the patient is maintained in pin fixation under constant traction, and after positioning, alignment is reconfirmed by an intraoperative radiograph.[7, 11, 16] Newer halo vests allow surgery to be the performed without removing the vest. To monitor spinal cord function before and after surgery, somatosensory evoked potentials are measured. A lateral radiograph with a needle inserted into a spinous process may be used for localization. The opening may be extended from the occiput into the thoracic region. If the suboccipital region must be exposed for a fusion, the incision is simply extended more rostrally. A vertical midline incision extends through skin with its attached superficial fascia and subcutaneous fat. This exposes the deep cervical fascia as it inserts into the nuchal and supraspinous ligaments. Once the spinous processes have been ex-

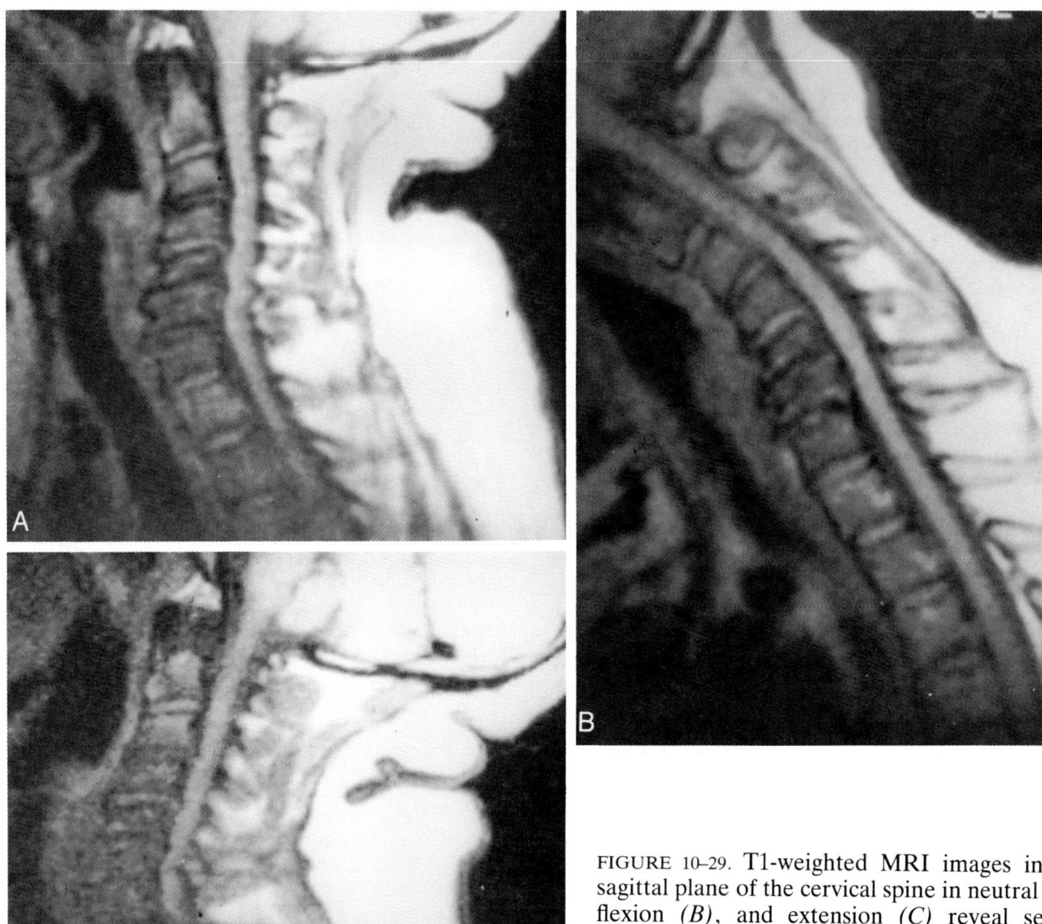

FIGURE 10–29. T1-weighted MRI images in the sagittal plane of the cervical spine in neutral *(A)*, flexion *(B)*, and extension *(C)* reveal severe stenosis from the C2-3 through the C5-6 interspaces.

posed, the remaining muscular insertions are detached and stripped from the spinous processes and lamina. The muscles are stripped lateral to the facets and, if indicated, from the transverse processes. During muscle dissection, self-retaining retractors are used to displace both sets of paraspinal muscles away from the midline, thereby increasing the exposure and aiding the dissection. This must be carried out bilaterally until the spinous processes, lamina, facets, and transverse processes are exposed. While dissecting the transverse processes, great care must be exercised to avoid injury to the exiting nerve roots or to the vertebral artery between the foramina transversaria. In the region of C1, the verebral artery is particularly susceptible to injury as it passes around the lateral masses.

Prior to closure, a drain is placed at the base of the wound. Nonabsorbable 2-0 sutures are used to reapproximate the muscles in the midline, thus closing the dead space. The most critical layer for closure is the deep cervical fascia. Interrupted 3-0 nonabsorbable sutures are placed 3 to 4 mm apart to assure a strong, watertight closure. Next, inverted interrupted 3-0 Vicryl sutures are used in the subcuticular layer. The skin is reapproximated with surgical staples or nonabsorbable 3-0 sutures.

References

1. Appuzzo MLJ, Weiss MH, Heiden J: Transoral exposure of the atlantoaxial region. Neurosurgery 3:201–207, 1978.

2. Bailey RW, Badgley CE: Stabilization of the cervical spine by anterior fusion. J Bone Joint Surg 42A:565–594, 1960.
3. Biller HF, Shugar JMA, Krespi YP: A new technique for wide-field exposure of the base of the skull. Arch Otolaryngol Head Neck Surg 107:698–702, 1981.
4. Breasted JH: The Edwin Smith Surgical Papyrus, Vol 1. Chicago, University of Chicago Press, 1930, pp 333–337.
5. Church A, Eisendrath DW: A contribution to spinal cord surgery. Am J Med Sci 103:395–412, 1892.
6. Cloward RB: The anterior approach for ruptured cervical disc. J Neurosurg 15:602–614, 1958.
7. Collias JC, Robert MP: Posterior operations for cervical disc herniation and spondylytic myelopathy. *In* Schmidek HH, Sweet WH (eds): Operative Neurosurgical Techniques, 2nd ed. New York, Grune and Stratton, 1988, pp 1347–1358.
8. Crockard HA: Anterior approaches to lesions of the upper cervical spine. Clin Neurosurg 34:389–416, 1988.
9. Elkin DC, Harris MH: Arteriovenous aneurysm of the vertebral vessels: Report of ten cases. Ann Surg 124:934–951, 1946.
10. Henry AK: Extensile Exposure, 2nd ed. Edinburgh, E and S Livingston, 1957, pp 47–89.
11. Hoff JT: Cervical disc disease and cervical spondylosis. *In* Wilkins RH, Rengachary SS (eds): Neurosurgery, Vol 3. New York, McGraw-Hill, 1985, pp 2230–2231.
12. Kanavel AB: Bullet located between the atlas and the base of the skull: Technique for removal through the mouth. Surg Clin North Am 1:361–366, 1919.
13. Komisar A, Tabaddor K: Extrapharyngeal (anterolateral) approach to the cervical spine. Head Neck Surg 6:600–604, 1983.
14. Krespi YP, Har-El G: Surgery of the clivus and anterior cervical spine. Arch Otolaryngol Head Neck Surg 114:73–78, 1988.
15. Menezes AH, Van Gilder JC, Graf CJ, McDonnel DE: Craniocervical abnormalities: A comprehensive surgical approach. J Neurosurg 53:444–455, 1980.
16. Murphy MJ, Southwick WO: Posterior approaches and fusions. *In* Cervical Spine Research Society (ed): The Cervical Spine, 2nd ed. Philadelphia, JB Lippincott, 1989, pp 775–791.
17. Robinson RA, Smith G: Anterolateral cervical disk removal and interbody fusion for cervical disk syndrome. Bull Johns Hopkins Hospital 96:223–224, 1955.
18. Verbiest H: A lateral approach to the cervical spine: Technique and indications. J Neurosurg 28:191–203, 1968.
19. Walker AE: Victor Horsley. *In* Haymaker W, Schiller F (eds): The Founders of Neurology, 2nd ed. Springfield, IL, Charles C Thomas, 1970, pp 562–566.
20. Whitesides TE Jr, McDonald AP: Lateral retropharyngeal approach to the upper cervical spine. Orthop Clin North Am 9:1115–1127, 1978.

CHAPTER **11**

Tumors of the Thoracolumbar Spine

ROBERT J. MEISLIN
MICHAEL G. NEUWIRTH
NORMAN D. BLOOM

This chapter formulates a rational plan for the treatment of tumors of the spinal column. A thorough history and physical examination are essential. Relevant laboratory tests, radiographic evaluation, and biopsy are necessary to define the diagnosis and to prepare for appropriate treatment. This chapter examines primary and metastatic tumors of the spinal column and presents guidelines for the selection of appropriate treatment alternatives.

The spinal column allows coordinated movement, it protects the neural elements, and it supports the weight of the trunk. Interference with any of these functions can produce symptoms. Tumor control or ablation, with restoration of normal function, is the primary goal of treatment.

Diagnosis

PATIENT HISTORY

The most common symptom of a tumor of the spinal column is pain. The pain may be localized or radicular and may be due to collapse of bony elements, to neurologic involvement, or to the tumor itself. Tumor pain characteristically worsens at night and is often persistent.

The second most common symptom is spinal deformity. A history of painful scoliosis can, at times, be associated with osteoid osteoma and osteoblastoma.[34] Spinal deformity may also result from either direct bony involvement or secondary fracture, or it can be a postsurgical complication. Sensory and/or motor neurologic dysfunctions are other complaints associated with tumor. If the spinal cord is involved, neurologic involvement may be of upper motor neuron type. Conversely, if the cauda equina or the nerve roots are affected, the neurologic dysfunction is of lower motor neuron type. The prognosis for neurologic involvement is directly linked to the rate of onset of motor weakness. A neurologic deficit that insidiously worsens over several months has a far better prognosis than does weakness that develops suddenly. Acute neurologic compromise is more commonly seen in patients with thoracic metastasis, in whom the ratio of the spinal canal volume to the cord is smallest.[20, 21]

Specific diagnoses are age related. For instance, multiple myeloma is more common in patients ages 40 to 60 years, whereas metastatic disease is more prevalent after the age of 60 years. Ewing's sarcoma and eosinophilic granuloma are more common in younger age groups, as are osteoid osteoma and osteoblastoma. The physician should suspect metastatic spinal disease in any patient with a history of malignant tumor.

PHYSICAL EXAMINATION

The spine is carefully examined for direct bone tenderness, deformity, and range of motion. A careful neurologic examination must be performed, including a rectal examination with assessment of perianal and, in females, perivaginal sensation. The presence of radicular pain, reflex changes, sensory changes, muscle weakness, and muscle atrophy is recorded. Radicular pain may help localize the level of spinal involvement. A sensory deficit is not as specific as a motor deficit in indicating the level of involvement, because a deficit can, at times, be several segments below a myelographically apparent block.[17]

LABORATORY TESTING

After a complete history and physical examination, the following laboratory tests are routinely performed: complete blood count with differential leukocyte count, platelet count, coagulation evaluation, erythrocyte sedimentation rate, and determination of serum calcium, alkaline phosphatase, and acid phosphatase levels.

RADIOGRAPHY

X-ray evaluation of the spine should include anterior, posterior, lateral, and oblique views. Technetium-99m scanning is necessary if primary or metastatic bone tumors are suspected. Because a minimum of 50% destruction of bone is necessary to produce detectable radiographic changes in the vertebral column, a bone scan is an excellent screen for metastatic lesions and is helpful in localizing small lesions, such as an osteoid osteoma. Because a bone scan reflects bone turnover in the presence of vascularity, it may not detect a primarily destructive lesion occurring without associated reactive bone formation, such as multiple myeloma. Bone scan may also fail to demonstrate lesions less than 3 mm in diameter. Single-photon emission computed tomography (SPECT) bone scanning may provide an accurate assessment of smaller lesions.

Computed tomography (CT) with contrast media demonstrates the direction and extent of bone and soft tissue involvement around the spinal canal. CT allows for particularly good visualization of the vertebral bodies and the spinal canal. CT must be used in association with myelography to assess neurologic involvement. Occasionally, there maybe more than one level of vertebral involvement. If a complete block is seen on the myelogram, CT may demonstrate the length of the lesion if a small amount of contrast agent slips by. If not, dye should be introduced above or below the block for proper demonstration.

Cerebrospinal fluid should be analyzed for protein content and for malignant cells after the myelogram.

Magnetic resonance imaging (MRI) is sensitive in indicating paraspinal involvement by tumor, as well as the effects of irradiation on the vertebral elements. It is particularly good for demonstrating cord involvement. Spinal lesions exhibit prolongation of T1 and T2 relaxation times, with decreased signal intensity in T1-weighted studies and increased signal intensity in T2-weighted images. Modic and associates showed that hemangiomas are an exception to the pattern, having short intermediate T1 and long T2.[31] MRI was found to be superior to CT without contrast media, and at least equal to CT with contrast media, in demonstrating anatomic relationships of tumors.[1, 2] As the technique of MRI develops, it will probably become the procedure of choice to demonstrate neurologic involvement. Currently, however, CT is better than MRI in demonstrating the extent of bone involvement. Arteriography may additionally aid the clinician in outlining the borders of a particularly vascular tumor, such as a hemangioma or a metastatic renal cell carcinoma, that has a high risk of hemorrhage. It may also be used for preoperative embolization.

DIFFERENTIAL DIAGNOSIS

The differential diagnosis is made after the history, physical examination, laboratory work-up, and x-ray evaluation.[7] Clinically, localized pain can often be seen in vertebral osteomyelitis.[12] Low back pain and associated radiculopathy are nonspecific indicators of herniated disk and/or spinal stenosis.[38] Patients with herniated disks often obtain relief with bed rest, whereas individuals with spinal tumors frequently have nocturnal pain, with increased pain in the supine position. Syringomyelia, which may be idiopathic or posttraumatic, may also have a picture that is similar to that of a neoplastic lesion.[4] Some of the vertebral tumors are radiographically similar. Osteogenic sarcoma, for example, when it is both lytic and blastic or when it is lytic alone, can be confused with other lytic lesions, including osteoblastoma, hemangioma, myeloma, lymphoma, and metastatic disease. Multiple myeloma, with its diffuse lytic appearance, must also be differentiated from osteoporosis. Furthermore, pathologic fractures of myeloma must be differentiated from pathologic fractures resulting from senile osteoporosis.

After a differential diagnosis is established, the next step is usually biopsy. The final diagnosis depends on evaluation of representative tissue. Prognosis and further medical and/or surgical treatment often depend on this tissue diagnosis.

Types of Spinal Tumors

The typical location of spinal tumors is presented in Table 11–1.

BENIGN PRIMARY BONE TUMORS

Osteoid Osteoma and Osteoblastoma. Osteoid osteoma and osteoblastoma characteristically involve the posterior elements of the spine. Both lesions have a central lytic area surrounded by reactive bone. Osteoblastoma can, however, look more aggressive and can be confused with osteosarcoma. Characteristically, osteoid osteoma and osteoblastoma are differentiated by the size of their central lytic defects, with osteoid osteoma being less than 1.5 cm in diameter. Osteoblastoma can be less sclerotic and more expansile than osteoid osteoma. The two tumors are usually seen in patients younger than 25 years old. Characteristically, osteoid osteoma produces more pain, often nocturnal, which is relieved by aspirin. Because of the small size of the nidus, technetium scanning is often helpful in localizing the lesion (Fig. 11–1*C*). Osteoid osteoma and osteoblastoma are the most common causes of a painful scoliosis in the thoracolumbar spine[34] (Fig. 11–1*D*). It is rare for spinal fusion to be necessary after the excision of an osteoid osteoma. It may be necessary after the excision of an osteoblastoma, which is inherently a larger and more aggressive lesion. The preoperative use of tetracycline and intraoperative evaluation of the specimen with Wood's lamp may help in identifying the tumor at the time of surgery, particularly in the case of osteoid osteoma.

TABLE 11–1

Typical Location of Tumors in the Spinal Column

Anterior Elements: Vertebral Bodies	Posterior Elements: Neural Arch and Transverse Processes
Aneurysmal bone cyst	Aneurysmal bone cyst
Giant cell tumor	Giant cell tumor
Hemangioma	Osteoid osteoma
Eosinophilic granuloma	Osteoblastoma
Ewing's sarcoma	Osteosarcoma
Lymphoma	
Chondrosarcoma	
Osteosarcoma	
Metastatic carcinoma	

Osteochondroma. Osteochondroma has a pathognomonic appearance of an osseous base, which may be pedunculated or sessile, with a cartilage cap. Osteochondromas are the most common benign tumors of bone. In the vertebral column, they are rare and most often occur in association with hereditary multiple exostoses. Solitary occurrences are unusual, but there are cases of solitary osteochondroma with neurologic dysfunction. The treatment is excision.[14, 28]

Aneurysmal Bone Cyst. Aneurysmal bone cyst occurs in children and adolescents and is most commonly found within the vertebral body, although at times it may be found in the posterior elements. This benign tumor is an expansile mass surrounded by a thin rim of reactive bone. Its appearance may be quite aggressive and can be confused with that of a malignant lesion (Fig. 11–2*A* to *D*). Treatment is curettage and bone grafting and, occasionally, stabilization (Fig. 2–11*E*, *F*). Low-dose radiation should be considered only if the tumor has recurred locally, because irradiation may induce sarcomas years later.

Giant Cell Tumor. Giant cell tumor is rare in the spine outside the sacrum. In the thoracic spine, it is often found in the anterior elements, whereas in the lumbar spine, it occurs in the posterior elements. These lesions, although benign, tend to recur, and some have a malignant potential. Treatment is best accomplished by *en bloc* resection and bone

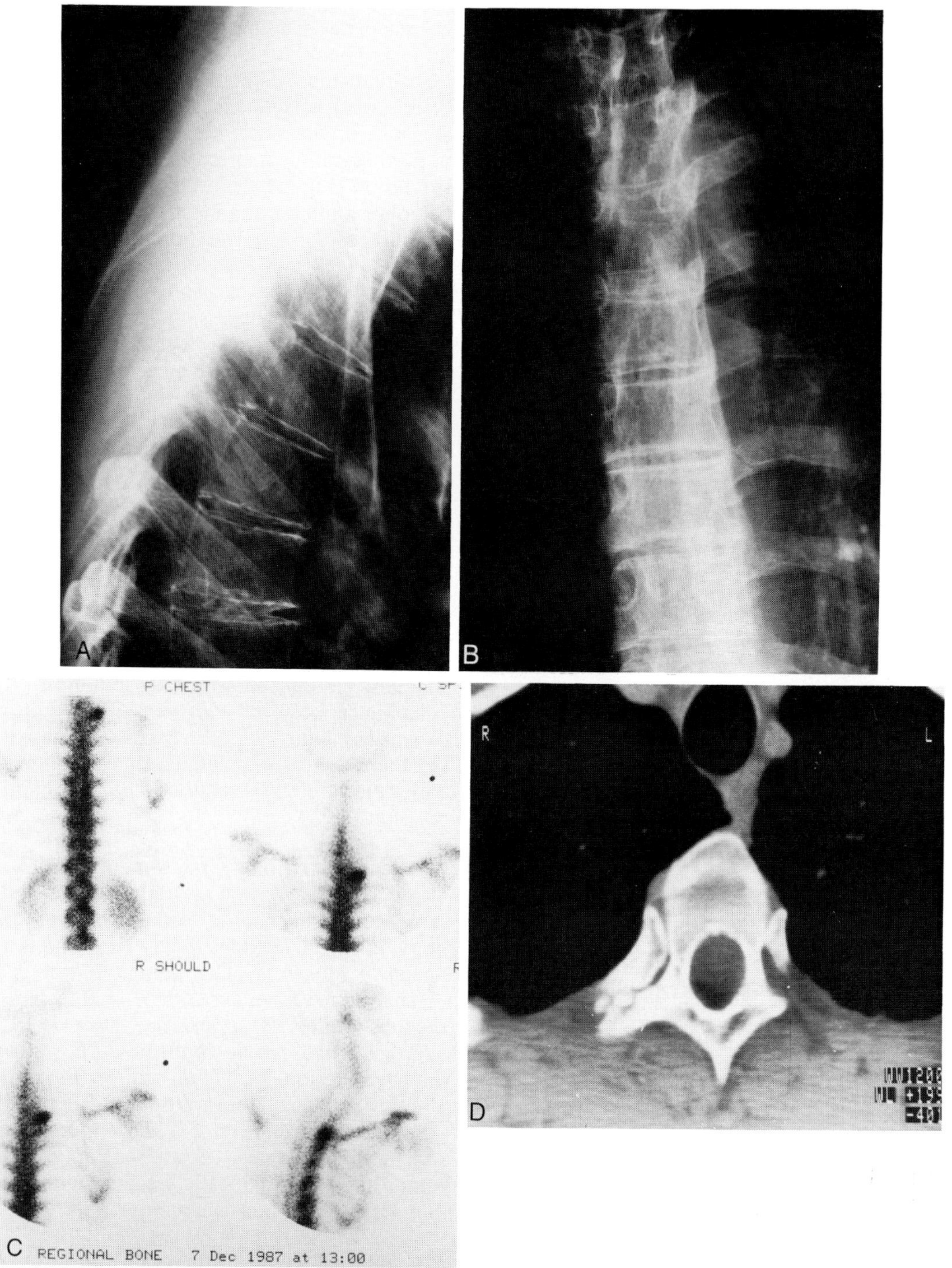

FIGURE 11–1. Osteoid osteoma. A 32-year-old white man with an 18-month history of right upper back pain radiating to the right scapula, which was relieved by aspirin. *A, B,* Normal anteroposterior (AP) and lateral x-ray films of the thoracic spine. *C,* Bone scan with a marked area of increased uptake over the junction of the right fourth rib and the transverse process. *D,* A benign osteoid osteoma between the transverse process and the rib at T4. Resection resulted in complete relief of symptoms. Surgical pathology examination confirmed the diagnosis.

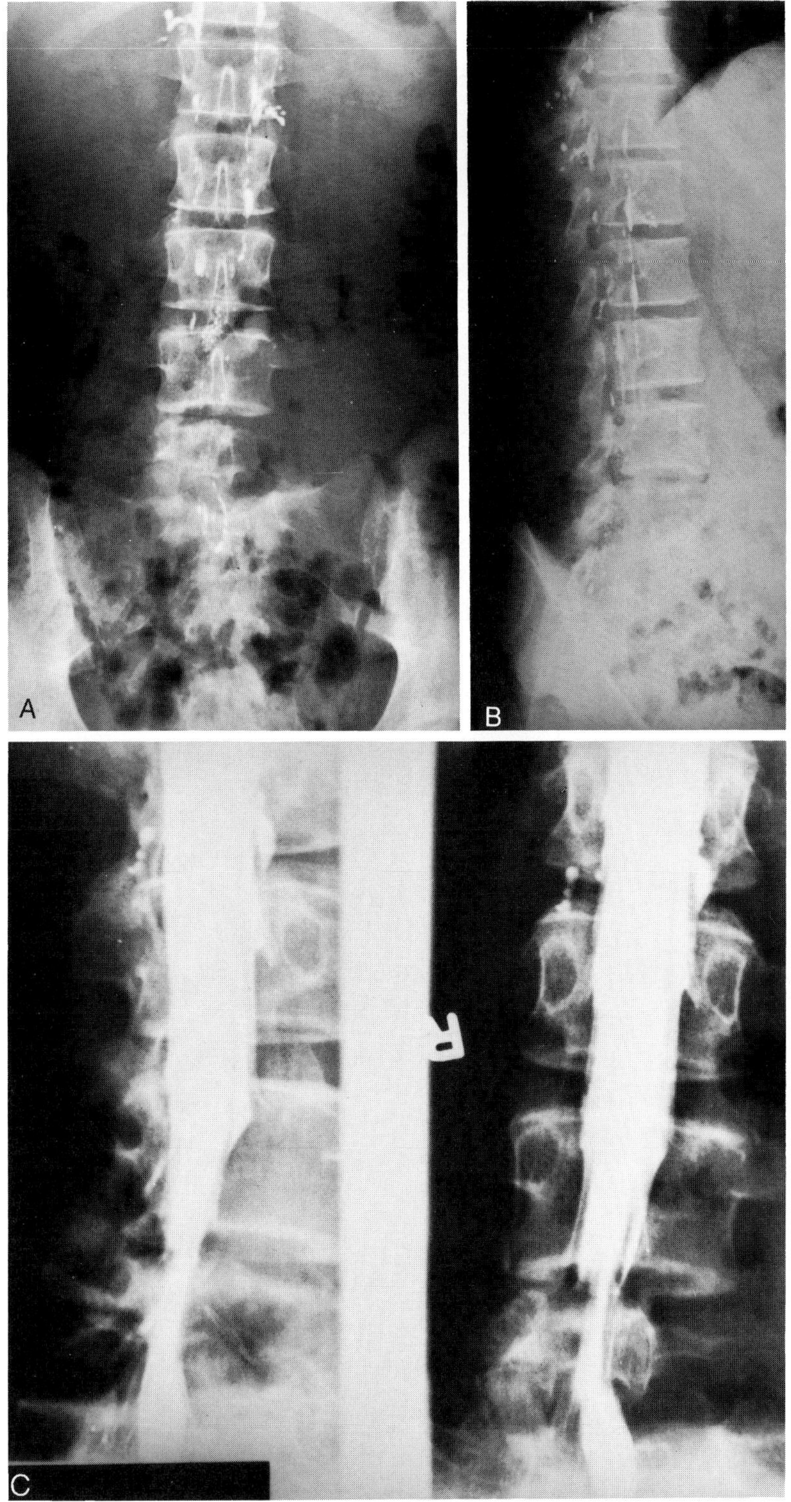

FIGURE 11–2. Aneurysmal bone cyst. A 15-year-old white female adolescent with a 6-month history of back pain radiating to the left lower extremity, associated with progressive weakness in the left lower extremity and a limp. *A, B,* Preoperative AP and oblique x-rays films show marked bone destruction of L5 and a large soft tissue mass extending to the left iliac crest. *C,* Preoperative myelogram shows extensive neural compression.

Illustration continued on following page

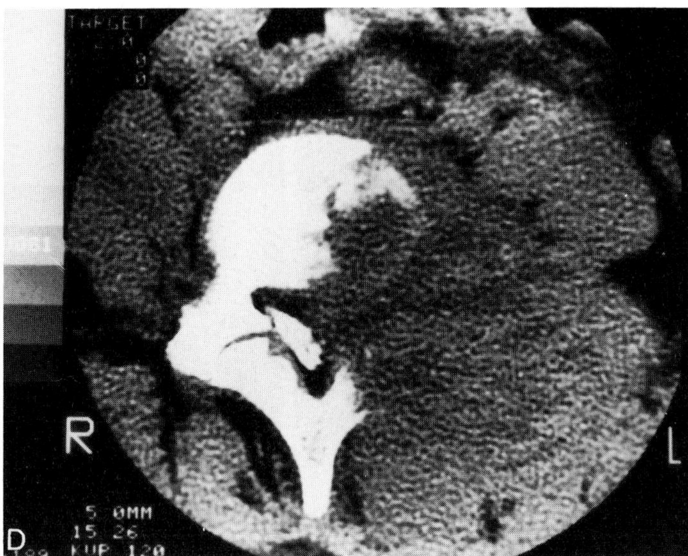

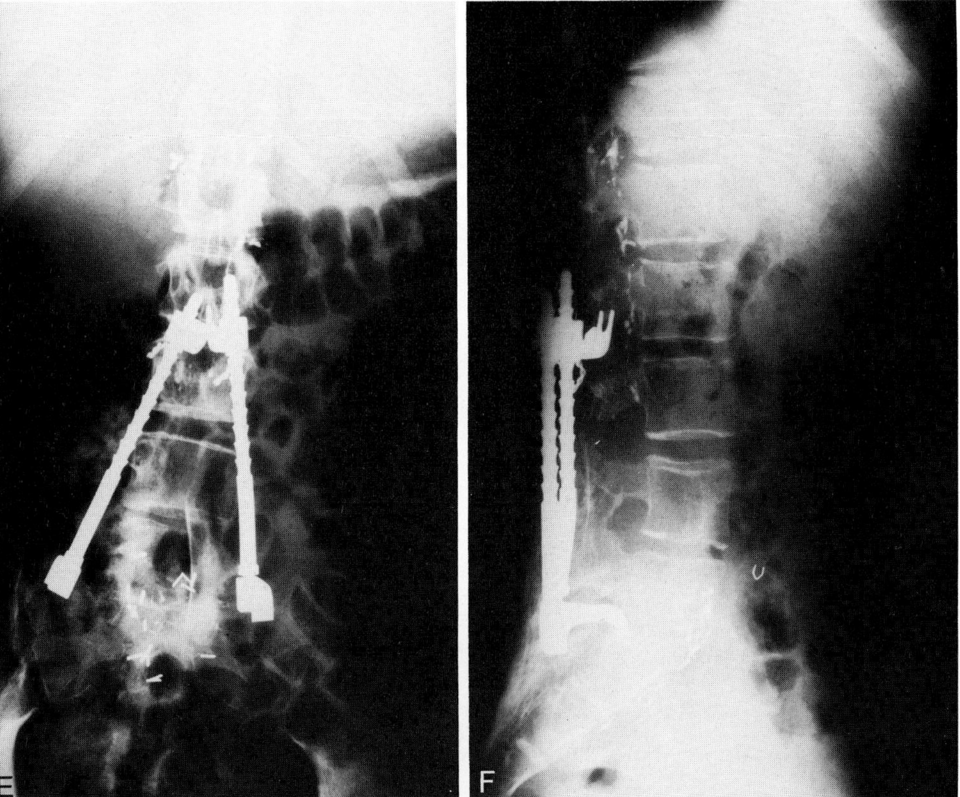

FIGURE 11–2 *Continued D,* Postmyelographic computed tomography (CT) scan shows bone destruction, with a huge soft tissue mass. *E, F,* Postoperative films, after staged anterior and posterior decompression, tumor resection, and spinal stabilization. Surgical pathology findings were consistent with an aneurysmal bone cyst. Six years after treatment, the patient was functioning well, with a solid spinal fusion without any evidence of recurrent disease.

grafting. Local curettage about half the time leads to recurrence.[17]

Eosinophilic Granuloma. Eosinophilic granuloma is found most often in children and adolescents in the vertebral body. Histologically, this tumor consists of eosinophils and histiocytes; anatomically, it may result in complete destruction and flattening of the vertebral body, causing vertebra plana. Eosinophilic granuloma is lytic and the treatment, in general, is observation and support while the lesion is clinically painful. The long-term prognosis is good and, therefore, low-dose radiotherapy should be used only in cases that do not respond to spinal support and appear to be more aggressive than usual.

Hemangioma. Hemangioma is the most common benign tumor of the spine. In the vertebral body, there is a characteristic vertically trabeculated appearance radiographically (Fig. 11–3*A* to *E*). The lesion may occur at any age but has a peak incidence in the 40s. Most hemangiomas are asymptomatic and require no treatment. Occasionally, a painless but progressive paralysis may result from epidural tumor extension. Pathologic fractures with neurologic involvement may also be caused by bony compression of the spinal cord. Treatment is surgical excision, often with preoperative embolization to control intraoperative bleeding (Fig. 11–3*F, G*). Low-dose radiation may also be indicated.[10]

Other Tumors. Giant cells tumors of the synovium (localized nodular synovitis) have been reported, involving the facet joints of the posterior elements. They are histologically related to pigmented villonodular synovitis, and the treatment is wide local excision.[47]

MALIGNANT PRIMARY BONE TUMORS

Multiple Myeloma. Multiple myeloma, the commonest primary malignant bone tumor, primarily affects vertebral bodies, with resulting lytic lesions in multiple levels. Neoplastic plasma cells proliferate, replacing the normal bone marrow. The diagnosis is suggested by an abnormal monoclonal immunoglobulin band and depressed levels of normal immunoglobulin, anemia, and elevated erythrocyte sedimentation rate. It is confirmed by finding replacement of normal marrow sheets of plasma cells on biopsy. Treatment usually includes irradiation and chemotherapy. Rarely, if the disease is localized, surgical decompression and stabilization are necessary.[45]

Ewing's Sarcoma. Ewing's sarcoma histologically presents with glycogen in the cells and copious round cells. It is a rare primary tumor of the spine. Dahlin reported that most cases of Ewing's sarcoma arose in the pelvis and the long bones of the extremities.[6] Radiographically, the lesion is primarily lytic and has a moth-eaten appearance. It occurs commonly in children, and treatment consists primarily of irradiation and chemotherapy.[24, 36]

Lymphoma. Lymphoma involves the vertebral body and radiographically appears lytic. Occasionally, it can produce an ivory or sclerotic appearance. Biopsy is necessary to differentiate it from Ewing's sarcoma or metastatic carcinoma. Treatment is radiotherapy, but chemotherapy is indicated if there is widespread disease. If the spine becomes unstable as a result of bone destruction, surgical stabilization may be indicated.

Osteosarcoma. Osteosarcoma is more commonly seen as a metastatic lesion than as a primary lesion of the spine. When seen in the spine, the tumor may result from Paget's disease, irradiation, or malignant transformation of a benign tumor. This neoplasm is also seen in adolescents. Radiographically, the lesion may be sclerotic, lytic, or mixed.[23] Treatment must be individualized, but wide resection is usually important. Perioperative chemotherapy is often also necessary.[14]

Chondrosarcoma. Chondrosarcoma may involve either the anterior or the posterior elements. It is usually slow growing and may be either primary or secondary. The tumor is seen in adults and often displays soft tissue extension. It is radioresistant and treatment requires *en bloc* excision. Repeated debulking procedures may be necessary.

Chordoma. Chordoma arises from the primitive notocord and is a rare tumor of the spine. It is more commonly seen at the clivus in the base of the skull and in the lumbosacral junction. Radiographically, chordomas form lytic lesions with central calcified prevertebral soft tissue masses. Histologically, they resemble embryonic notochord. Treatment includes irradiation and wide resection.[41]

METASTATIC BONE TUMORS

Metastases to the vertebral column most commonly affect the lumbar vertebrae. However,

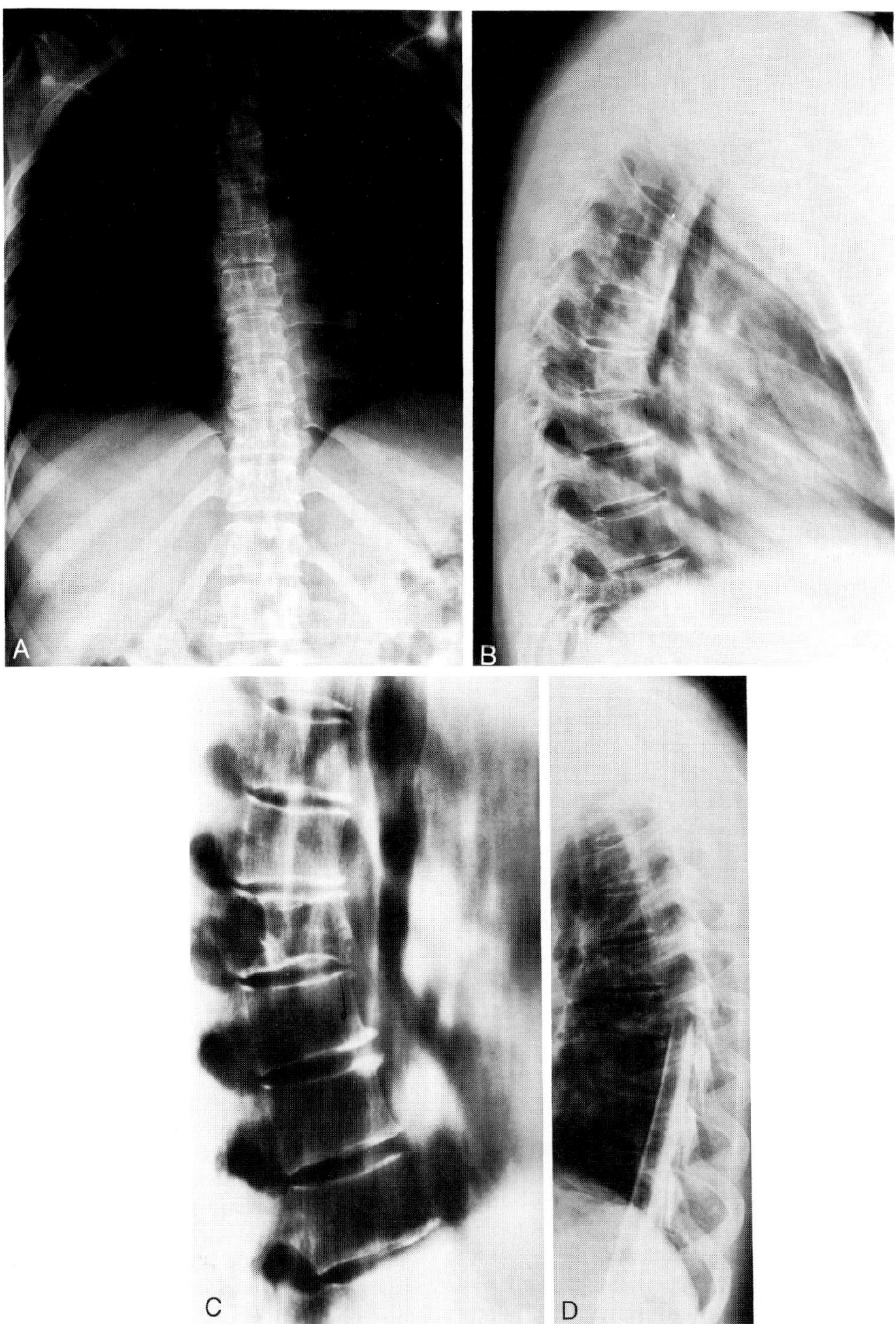

FIGURE 11–3. Hemangioma. A 48-year-old white woman who had upper thoracic back pain and slight weakness in her lower extremities. *A, B,* AP and lateral x-ray films show a small compression fracture of T7 with a slight gibbus deformity. *C,* Lateral tomogram shows a cystic lesion within the body of T7. *D,* Lateral myelogram shows a block at T7.

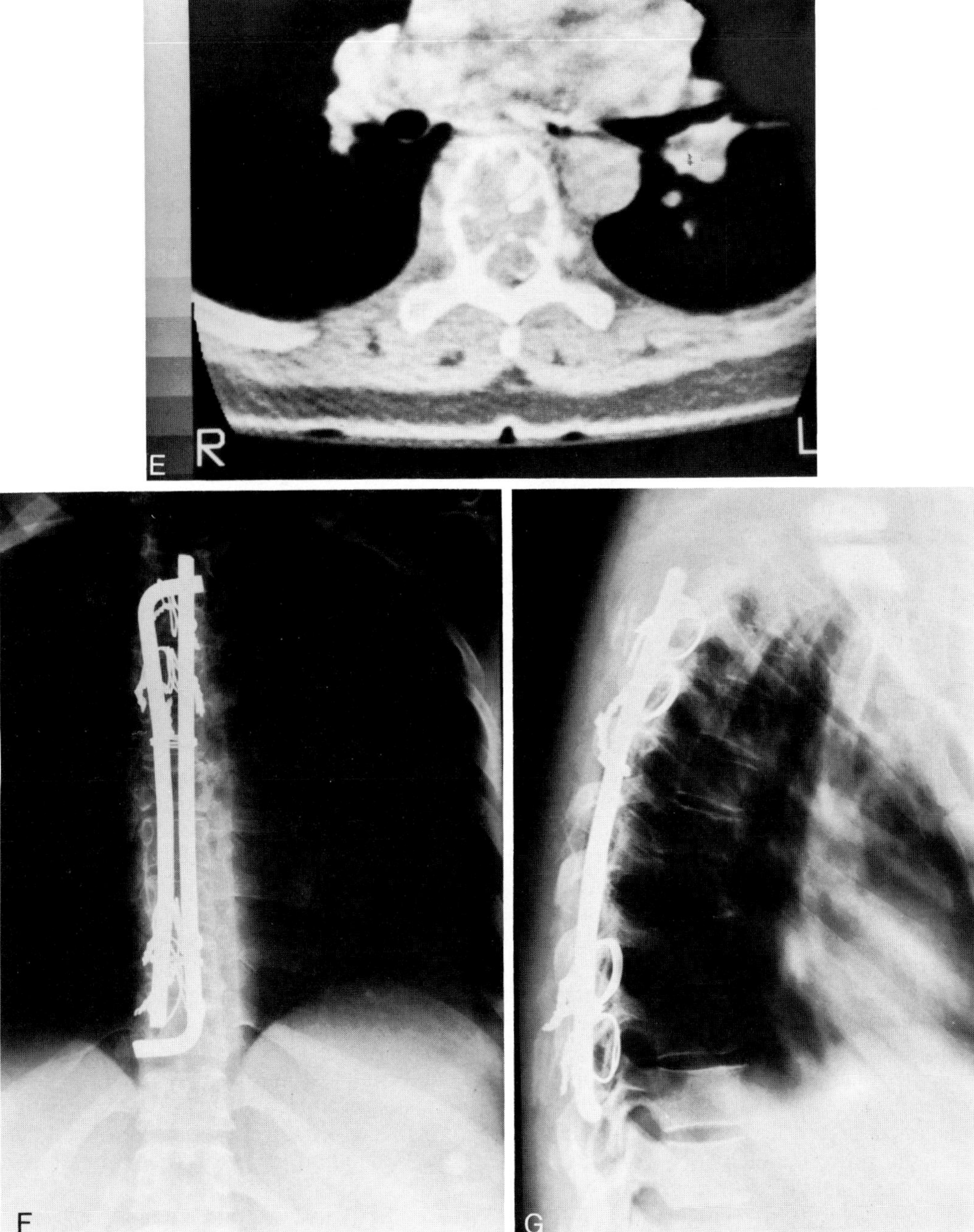

FIGURE 11–3 *Continued. E,* Postmyelographic CT scan reveals a cystic lesion within the body of T7, with epidural tumor within the canal, which (on other sections) revealed extension over three levels. *F, G,* Postoperative AP and lateral x-ray films, after thoracic decompression and stabilization. Pathology examination revealed a benign hemangioma. The patient received low-dose radiation (20 Gy) to supplement her surgical treatment. She is disease free 8 years after treatment.

the thoracic spine, with its smaller canal diameter and more tenuous blood supply, has a greater potential for neurologic compromise. Lung cancer, breast cancer, and lymphoma are the leading primary tumors that metastasize to the spine. Others that metastasize frequently include prostate, renal, thyroid, and gastrointestinal carcimona. The mestastases seed the vertebral body hematogenously, although at times the tumor can extend directly. Batson venous plexus, which lies within the epidural space, is a conduit for tumor spread. While it is in contact with the intercostal and lumbar veins, this valveless system allows metastases from the heart and the prostate through the azygous and the pelvic venous systems, respectively.[3, 13] Five per cent of patients with metastatic disease are said to experience spinal cord fracture (with resulting compression), or intradural metastases. Cancer may seed the spine silently, without symptoms. Bone scans and plain x-ray films may show the first indications of metastatic disease. Radiographically, prostate tumors usually cause blastic lesions; lung tumors are associated with lytic lesions; and breast metastases are mixed. Debate continues over the necessity of open biopsy of metastatic lesions. Harrington believes that open biopsy is rarely indicated, except at the time of surgical stabilization and/or decompression[20, 21] (Fig. 11–4).

Principles of Treatment

In treating both benign and malignant lesions of the spine, the general principles include excision of the tumor if possible, with or without adjuvant therapy. The goal should be control of the individual's pain, prevention and correction of spinal instability and deformity, and reversal of neurologic compromise.

The spine is a weight-bearing structure. Vertebral collapse leads to progressive spinal deformity and progressive cord compromise. Therefore, the spine must be treated in the same manner as any weight-bearing long bone and prophylactically stabilized if there is impending fracture and collapse. Benign lesions require thorough excision. Bone graft may or may not be necessary, depending on the size and location of the lesion. With lesions that involve the posterior elements, complete excision is often possible. Anterior involvement may allow only partial removal. Low-dose irradiation can be considered an alternative therapy or an additive approach for lesions that commonly involve the vertebral body, such as hemangiomas, giant cell tumors, aneurysmal bone cysts, and eosinophilic granulomas. On the other hand, caution must be emphasized in treating patients with adjuvant radiation, because of the risk of secondary malignant transformation.[26] However, most studies that report malignant transformation were done with much higher doses of radiation than would currently be used for such lesions. With benign lesions that are highly aggressive, such as giant cell tumor and osteoblastoma, a more aggressive resection may be necessary. If spinal stability is compromised by either the lesion or surgery, stabilization with fusion may be required. Pettine and Klassen reported that localized spinal fusion was needed after facet resection for osteoid osteoma or osteoblastoma.[34] Usually, however, resection of one facet unilaterally is not an indication for a fusion. Bilateral facet resection, or resection of multiple unilateral facets, is an indication for fusion.

INDICATIONS FOR SURGERY

Indications for surgical management of a primary lesion include unremitting pain not controlled by medical treatment, the presence or imminent probability of neurologic dysfunction, spinal instability, and loss of structural support. For metastatic tumors, the indications have become more clearly defined. DeWald and associates outlined five distinct classes of spinal malignancies and treatment. Class 1 patients have no deformity but moderate pain. With less than 50% destruction of the vertebral body, only radiotherapy and chemotherapy are necessary. With 50% destruction of the anterior elements or greater, or significant pedicle involvement, surgical stabilization is recommended. For class 2 patients, who have moderate deformity and collapse and are immunocompetent, surgical reconstruction is recommended. Class 3 patients who have moderate deformity and collapse, but are immunocompromised, should have surgical decompression and/or stabilization after medical management in an attempt to control the immunocompromised status. Class 4 patients, with marked deformity and paralysis, should have immediate surgical decompression and stabilization. Class 5 patients, with a marked deformity, paralysis, and immunocompromise, have an extremely poor prognosis and, therefore, the oncologist and the spinal surgeon together should decide whether treatment is indeed a viable option at all for these patients.[9]

Harrington divided patients with metastatic disease into five classes.[20] This classification also emphasizes the degree of neurologic involvement and bone destruction. Class 1 patients have no significant neurologic involvement. Class 2 patients have involvement of bone without instability. Patients in these two classes are initially offered chemotherapy, hor-

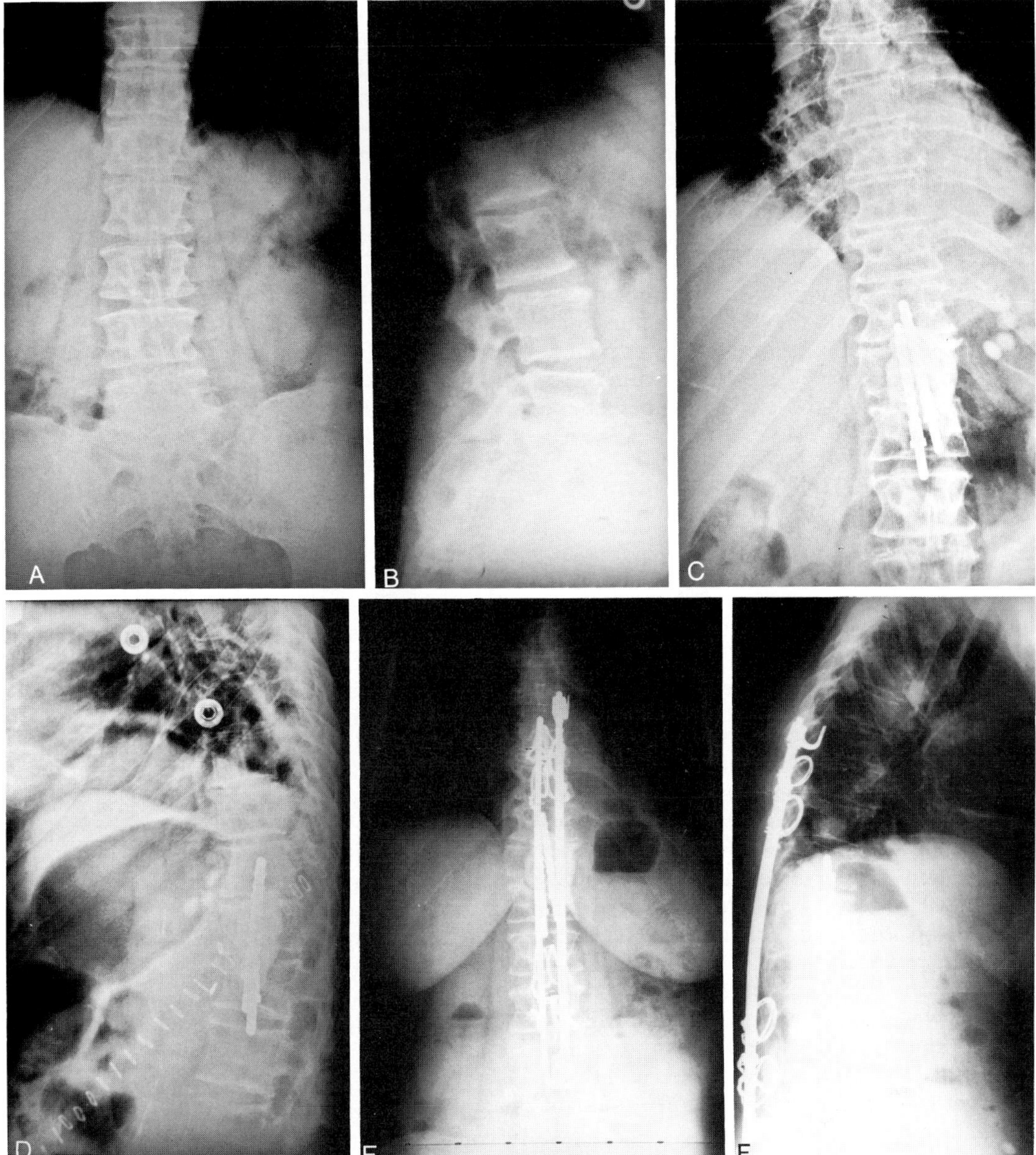

FIGURE 11–4. A 56-year-old white woman with metastatic breast cancer. She was seen 4 months before the initial x-ray films at another institution, with back pain and weakness in her legs. Work-up, at that time, revealed a metastatic lesion of T12 with canal compromise resulting from a pathologic fracture at this level. She underwent a laminectomy, which resulted (predictably) in progressive deformity and increased neurologic compromise. *A, B,* AP and lateral x-ray films after the laminectomy. *C, D,* AP and lateral x-ray films after anterior vertebral resection and stabilization with an acrylic Harrington rod construct. *E, F,* AP and lateral x-ray films after posterior stabilization with Harrington rods and sublaminar wires. Posterior stabilization was necessary because of the prior laminectomy and extensive metastatic disease documented on bone scan.

monal therapy, or local radiation. Class 3 patients have major neurologic dysfunction and no significant involvement of bone. These patients should be treated with irradiation, which alone has been shown to be as effective as decompressive laminectomy.[18] For lesions with acute onset, steroids should be administered. Class 4 patients have vertebral collapse and pain but are neurologically stable, and class 5 patients have collapse and instability with neurologic involvement. Both of the latter classes require surgical decompression and stabilization.[20, 21] Harrington further defined the indications for surgical intervention. Patients with a progressive painful kyphotic deformity, with an intact posterior column, require anterior decompression and stabilization. Patients with a progressive kyphotic deformity and all three columns affected, require anterior and posterior decompression and stabilization. Class 4 and 5 individuals require decompression on the side of the involvement. Other individuals who should be considered candidates for surgery include patients with radioresistant tumors and those who did not respond to radiotherapy.[37]

SURGICAL APPROACH

Historically, metastatic tumors and aggressive primary malignant tumors were treated by radiation alone, posterior laminectomy alone, or laminectomy with adjuvant radiation or chemotherapy. However, because many malignant and metastatic lesions occur primarily anteriorly in the vertebral bodies, a posterior approach may be inadequate to resect the tumor or decompress the spinal canal.[25, 29, 33] Malignant lesions with cord compression must be decompressed anteriorly with the subsequent placement of segmental spinal stabilization. Decompressive laminectomy may, in fact, sacrifice any remaining stability provided by an intact posterior column and is generally contraindicated, except if the lesion is in the epidural space and spinal stabilization will not be compromised. If a posterior approach is chosen, and the spine is destabilized as a result of surgery, immediate stabilization should be added.

Determination of stability is the basis for the spinal surgeon's eventual choice for approach to stabilization. If the anterior spine is involved, an anterior or anterolateral approach is best. If the posterior spine is involved, a posterior approach is required. With extensive involvement, a combined anterior and posterior approach is indicated. A combined approach is probably the most widely implemented because additional posterior stabilization is usually necessary after initial anterior decompression and stabilization.[8, 48]

In the thoracic spine, the rib cage provides additional stability. Because the anterior elements are small at T1 and T2, anterior access is restricted, and a posterior approach is usually preferred.[15] Although an anterior approach to the upper thoracic vertebrae has been described by Sundaresan, the surgery must be individualized and may be performed in one or two stages.[44]

At the time of anterior decompression, the segmental vessels surrounding the vertebral level of the lesion should be ligated. Stabilization can then be carried out in several fashions. Methyl methacrylate has been used successfully alone by several authors after corpectomy for one or more vertebral levels.[19, 37] Radiotherapy may then be carried out postoperatively, as methyl methacrylate has been shown to have no weakening effect from radiation, nor does it interfere with local radiotherapy.[32] Harrington has, in some cases, reinforced methyl methacrylate with Harrington distraction rods anteriorly, and this is preferred when technically possible because it provides a more stable construct.[20] Careful attention is made to remove the vertebral end plates to ensure better cement fixation. For smaller vertebrae in the cervical spine, Rush rods, Kirschner wires, or simply the serrated portion of the Harrington rod can be used. Traditionally, autologous iliac, fibular, and rib grafts have been used to enhance stability. In neoplastic diseases, these strut grafts usually require additional external fixation.

Fusion may not be achieved in the face of postoperative irradiation. Radiotherapy has to be limited to a subtherapeutic dosage of 15 to 20 Gy, compared with a therapeutic dosage of 40 to 50 Gy. In certain cases, stabilization alone, without fusion, is performed when the prognosis is such that it is unclear how long patients will survive. Fusion can always be added, if necessary, if longevity is ensured.

Stener performed spondylectomies and reconstructed the absent vertebral body space with corticocancellous blocks fixed with screws posteriorly.[40] Metallic fixation is added above and below the inserted grafts. In addition to cement and bone for spinal stabilization, metallic devices can be used. Ma and colleagues used a stainless steel prosthetic vertebral body that incorporates bone graft inside and around the prosthesis.[27] Posteriorly, segmental spinal stabilization is the best choice and has been used by Roy-Camille and colleagues,[35] DeWald and associates,[9] Fidler,[15] Harrington,[21] and Flatley and colleagues.[16] Harrington rods alone are not adequate.[42] If life expectancy is longer than 1 year, and stabilization alone has been performed, fusion can be accomplished at a later date. The choice of segmental fixation depends on the specifics of the individual case. Sublaminar wires with a Harrington, Harrington-Luque, or Luque system can be used. Pedicle screws with rods or plates can be used, and Cotrel-Dubousset instruments can be employed. The key, however, in all of these cases, is segmental fixation to prevent failure of fixation and to distribute the forces to the entire length of the spine that is being surgically treated.

COMPLICATIONS

Complications may relate to the disease process, to the choice of treatment, or to unrelated medical or postsurgical complications. Sundaresan and coworkers wrote about postirradiation sarcoma.[43] The latent period for this is usually 5 to 20 years. Irradiation of the spine increases blood loss during surgery and certainly impairs the quality of tissue and bone healing. There are also increased skin problems after radiation and chemotherapy, with a higher incidence of wound diastasis and postoperative infection. Because bone stock is often poor, instrumentation may loosen and dislodge it in the spine. McAfee and colleagues documented complications after the use of methyl methacrylate in stabilization of the vertebral spine after trauma or metastatic disease.[30] Most of the complications reported, however, were in the cervical spine. Thus, the listed complications of loss of fixation and neural deficit and infection may be a problem more specific to the cervical spine than to the spine in general. It is important to remember that methyl methacrylate works only in compression and is of no value to resist torsion or tension.

Late complications, in addition to postirradiation sarcoma, include other sites of spinal cord compression and late collapse resulting from extensive tumor involvement.

SURGICAL TECHNIQUE

The thoracic and/or lumbar spine can be approached through one of three operative procedures depending on the level.[5, 11, 22, 39, 46] For lesions between C7 and T3, a standard left or right thoracotomy incision can be used. The scapula can be lifted from the chest wall and the third rib excised. To improve exposure to a higher level, the second rib may also be excised. Because the scapula covers the defect, no reconstruction is required for multiple rib resections above the fifth rib. Sometimes, this level is best approached by splitting the sternum. For lesions between T4 and T11, the same standard anterolateral thoracotomy can be used, with resection of any single rib, which allows direct access to the lesion to be resected. In young children, unless a rib is required for a graft, a rib resection is not necessary for exposure. For exposure of the T12 to L2 vertebral bodies, the approach described below provided the best exposure with acceptable cosmetic results.

The skin incision is placed directly over the tenth rib and extends through the costal arch onto the anterior abdominal wall. The incision on the abdominal wall is a pararectus incision and can be extended as low as necessary, approximately 3 cm medial to the iliac crest. This incision allows access to the iliac crest if a bone graft is required and is much more cosmetic than the traditional paramedian or midline extensions.

The external oblique fascia is opened, and the muscle is split in the direction of its fibers. The internal oblique and transversus abdominis muscles are divided and the retroperitoneal space is entered. The peritoneal envelope is easily mobilized from the iliac muscle and is reflected medially from the psoas muscle. The attachments of the peritoneum to the undersurface of the diaphragm can then be easily mobilized.

After completing the thoracic incision by dividing the serratus anterior muscle and resecting the tenth rib, the thoracic cavity can be entered. The costal arch is divided, and the diaphragmatic insertion on the undersurface of the tenth rib is detached. The diaphragm can then be incised, leaving a 2-cm cuff for repair. Mobilization of the major vessels from the front of the spine is accomplished by dividing the segmental vessels over the levels to be exposed. After completion of the spinal portion of the operation, closure of the diaphragm is accomplished using 2-0 silk vertical mattress sutures. A chest tube is placed through the resected bed of the tenth rib. The ribs are reapproximated by placing sutures around the upper border of the ninth rib and through holes drilled through the eleventh rib. This prevents entrapment of the eleventh intercostal nerve and a subsequent neuroma.

For lesions of the lower lumbar vertebrae (L2-5), the abdominal portion of the previous incision can be utilized. Extension over the twelfth rib with rib resection can be performed to gain better exposure of the L1-2 interspace.

For exposure of the L4 and L5 vertebral bodies, the iliac vein must be completely mobilized. To accomplish this, the ascending lumbar vein must be divided, and its take-off should be suture ligated. Exposure of the sacrum can be accomplished entirely retroperitoneally. The extraperitoneal rectum is mobilized bluntly from the front of the sacrum. The presacral veins are identified and ligated. Complete mobilization of the iliac vessels is then performed by dividing the multiple small branches from the iliac coursing over the sacrum.

The major complication of the thoracic or thoracoabdominal approaches is postoperative atelactasis and/or pneumonia. This complication occurs in 4% of cases and can be minimized by good preoperative and postoperative pulmonary toilet. Mortality is less than 1%.

Although surgery for tumors of the spinal column, particularly in metastatic disease, has a high complication rate, appropriate spinal surgery can prolong life and improve the quality of life. Emphasis must be placed on educating the entire medical community, particularly oncologists and radiotherapists, as to the indications for earlier surgical intervention. If patients are operated on earlier in the course of their disease, the results will undoubtedly be better and complications less frequent.

References

1. Bale JF, Bell WE, Dunn V, Afifi AK, Menezes A: Magnetic resonance imaging of the spine in children. Arch Neurol 43:1253–1256, 1986.
2. Beltran J, Noto AM, Chakeres DW, Christoforidis AJ: Tumors of the osseous spine: Staging with MR imaging versus CT. Radiology 162:565–569, 1987.
3. Boland PJ, Lane JM, Sundaresan N: Metastatic disease of the spine. Clin Orthop 169:95–102, 1982.
4. Booth RE Jr: Pathogenesis of signs and symptoms in spinal disorders. Instr Course Lect 34:37–54, 1985.
5. Burrington JO, Brown C, Wayne ER, Odom J: Anterior approaches to the thoraco-lumbar spine: Technical considerations. Arch Surg 111:456–463, 1976.
6. Dahlin DC: Bone Tumors: General Aspects and Data on 6221 Cases, 3rd ed. Springfield, IL, Charles C Thomas, 1978.
7. Degesys GE, Miller GA, Newman GE, Cohan RH: Absence of a pedicle in the spine, metastatic disease versus aplasia. Spine 11:76–77, 1986.
8. Denis F: The three-column spine and its significance in the classification of acute thoracolumbar spinal injuries. Spine 8:817–831, 1983.
9. DeWald R, Bridwell KH, Prodromas C, Robts MF: Reconstructive spinal surgery as palliation for metastatic malignancies of the spine. Spine 10:21–26, 1985.
10. DiLorenzo N, Nardi P, Ciappetta P, Fortuna A: Benign tumors and tumorlike conditions of the spine: Radiological features, treatment, and results. Surg Neurol 25:449–456, 1986.
11. Dwyer AF, Newton MC, Sherwood AA: An anterior approach to scoliosis. Clin Orthop 62:192–197, 1969.
12. Eismont FJ, Green BA, Brown MD, Ghandur-Mnaymneh L: Coexistent infection and tumor of the spine. J Bone Joint Surg 69A:452–457, 1987.
13. Emsellem HA: Metastatic disease of the spine: Diagnosis and management. South Med J 79:1405–1412, 1986.
14. Enneking WF: Musculoskeletal Tumor Surgery. New York, Churchill Livingstone, 1983.
15. Fidler MW: Anterior decompression and stabilisation of metastatic spinal fractures. J Bone Joint Surg 68B:83–90, 1986.
16. Flatley TJ, Anderson MH, Anast GT: Spinal instability due to malignant disease. J Bone Joint Surg 66A:47–52, 1984.
17. Friedlaender GE, Southwick WO: Tumors of the spine. *In* Rothman RH, Simeone FA (eds): The Spine, Vol 2. WB Saunders Co, 1982, pp 1022–1040.
18. Gilbert RN, Kim JM, Posner JB: Epidural spinal cord compression from metastatic tumor: Diagnosis and treatment. Ann Neurol 3:40, 1978.
19. Harrington KD: The use of methyl methacrylate for vertebral body replacement and anterior stabilization of pathological fracture-dislocations of the spine due to metastatic malignant disease. J Bone Joint Surg 63A:36–46, 1981.
20. Harrington KD: Current concepts review: Metastatic disease of the spine. J Bone Joint Surg 68A:1110–1115, 1986.
21. Harrington KD: Orthopaedic Management of Metastatic Bone Disease. St Louis, CV Mosby Co, 1988.
22. Hodgson AR, Yau AC: Anterior surgical approaches to the spinal column. *In* Apley AG (ed): Recent Advances in Orthopaedics. Baltimore, Williams & Wilkins, 1969, pp 289–323.
23. Jeanmart L (ed): Radiology of the Spine: Tumors. New York, Springer-Verlag, 1986.
24. Kornberg M: Primary Ewing's sarcoma of the spine. Spine 11:54–57, 1986.
25. Lee CK, Rosa R, Fernand R: Surgical treatment of tumors of the spine. Spine 11:201–208, 1986.
26. Lord CF, Herndon JH: Spinal cord compression secondary to kyphosis associated with radiation therapy for metastatic disease. Clin Orthop 210:120–127, 1986.
27. Ma YZ, Tang HF, Chai BF, Yeh YC, Jiang LP, Zhou SB, Chen WY: The treatment of primary vertebral tumors by radical resection and prosthetic vertebral replacement. Clin Orthop 215:78–90, 1987.
28. Marchand EP, Villemure JG, Rubin J, Robitaille Y, Ethier R: Solitary osteochondroma of the thoracic spine presenting as spinal cord compression. Spine 11:1033–1035, 1986.
29. Martin NS, Williamson J: The role of surgery in the treatment of malignant tumours of the spine. J Bone Joint Surg 52B:227–237, 1970.
30. McAfee PC, Bohlman HH, Ducker T, Eismont BJ: Failure of stabilization of the spine with methyl methacrylate. J Bone Joint Surg 68A:1145–1157, 1986.
31. Modic MT, Masaryk T, Paushter D: Magnetic resonance imaging of the spine. Radiol Clin North Am 24:229–245, 1986.
32. Murray JA, Bruels MC, Lindberg RD: Irradiation of polymethyl methacrylate: *In vitro* gamma radiation effect. J Bone Joint Surg 56A:311–312, 1974.
33. Onimus M, Schraub S, Bertin D, Bosset JF, Guidet M: Surgical treatment of vertebral metastasis. Spine 11:883–891, 1986.

34. Pettine KA, Klassen RA: Osteoid-osteoma and osteoblastoma of the spine. J Bone Joint Surg 68A:354–361, 1986.
35. Roy-Camille R, Saillant G, Mazel C: Internal fixation of the lumbar spine with pedicle screw plating. Clin Orthop 203:7–17, 1986.
36. Russin LA, Robinson MJ, Engle HA, Sonni A: Ewing's sarcoma of the lumbar spine: A case report of long-term survival. Clin Orthop 164:126–129, 1982.
37. Siegal T, Tiqva P, Siegal T: Vertebral body resection for epidural compression by malignant tumors. J Bone Joint Surg 67A:375–382, 1985.
38. Sim FH, Dahlin DC, Stauffer RN, Laws ER: Primary bone tumors simulating lumbar disc syndrome. Spine 2:65–74, 1977.
39. Southwick WO, Robinson A: Surgical approaches to the vertebral bodies in the cervical and lumbar regions. J Bone Joint Surg 39A:631–643, 1957.
40. Stener B: Musculoskeletal tumor surgery in Goteborg. Clin Orthop 191:8–20, 1984.
41. Sundaresan N: Chordomas. Clin Orthop 204:135–142, 1986.
42. Sundaresan N, Galicich JH, Lane JM: Harrington rod stabilization for pathological fractures of the spine. J Neurosurg 60:282–286, 1984.
43. Sundaresan N, Huvos AG, Krol G, Hughes JEO, Cahan WG: Postradiation sarcoma involving the spine. Neurosurgery 18:721–724, 1986.
44. Sundaresan N, Shah J, Foley KM, Rosen G: An anterior surgical approach to the upper thoracic vertebrae. J Neurosurg 61:686–690, 1984.
45. Torma T: Malignant tumors of the spine and spinal extradural space. Acta Chir Scand (Suppl) 225:1–176, 1957.
46. Watkins PG: Surgical Approaches to the Spine. New York, Springer-Verlag, 1983.
47. Weidner N, Challa VR, Bonsib SM, Davis CH, Carroll TJ: Giant cell tumors of synovium (pigmented villonodular synovitis) involving the vertebral column. Cancer 57:2030–2036, 1986.
48. White AA, Panjabi MM: Clinical Biomechanics of the Spine. Philadelphia, JB Lippincott, 1978.

CHAPTER 12

Tumors of the Thoracic Skeleton

NORMAN D. BLOOM

Primary tumors of the chest wall are uncommon malignancies. Of 4277 primary bone tumors identified at the Mayo Clinic, there were 35 benign and 234 malignant lesions arising in either the ribs or the sternum (6.29%).[27] In a similar series of 750 primary bone tumors reported at the Barnes Hospital, 61 (8%) occurred in the chest wall; 58 of the 61 lesions were in the ribs.[34]

Because of the rarity of these lesions, the establishment of an accurate diagnosis is often elusive. Pain and the presence of a mass have been the two most common complaints of patients with chest wall tumors and many patients experience both. Patients often notice a mass several months before seeking a physician's advice, and local trauma frequently calls attention to the lesion.

The location of the mass on clinical examination is sometimes helpful in the differential diagnosis because the majority of rib tumors of cartilaginous origin occur along the costochondral junctions, whereas fibrous dysplasias occur over the posterior chest wall.

The sex distribution of these lesions is a 2:1 male/female ratio, and the age of the patient may suggest the type of tumor that is present (Table 12–1). The average age of patients with benign tumors is 26 years. Eosinophilic granulomas, aneurysmal bone cysts, and osteochondromas occur in a younger population, whereas fibrous dysplasia and bone islands are seen in older individuals.

TABLE 12–1

Age Distribution of Common Neoplasms of the Chest Wall

Type of Tumor	Range (years)	Average Age (years)
Benign		
Eosinophilic granuloma	1–30	15
Aneurysmal bone cyst	10–20	15
Osteochondroma	10–40	20
Fibrous dysplasia	20–70	40
Bone islands	30–60	50
Malignant		
Ewing's sarcoma	10–20	15
Osteogenic sarcoma	5–40	25
Lymphoma	15–50	30
Chondrosarcoma	15–70	45
Plasmacytoma	40–85	55

The average age of patients with primary malignant lesions is approximately 40 years. Ewing's sarcoma is most common in adolescents. Osteosarcoma, lymphoma, chondrosarcoma, and plasmacytoma occur more frequently in subsequent decades. Although metastatic carcinomas to the thoracic skeleton are the commonest malignant tumors, these patients, on average, are in their fifth and sixth decades.

With certain exceptions, laboratory examinations are usually of little help. The erythrocyte sedimentation rate may be elevated in some instances of Ewing's sarcoma and the alkaline phosphatase level is often elevated in osteosarcoma. Electrophoresis of serum proteins may uncover proteins specific for myelomas, although urinary Bence Jones protein has been identified rarely in solitary plasmacytoma.

Radiographic evaluation of the chest wall is helpful in diagnosis and in determination of the extent of disease. A localized abnormality is almost always visible. Most rib lesions, although visualized on posterior and lateral x-rays films, are better defined with oblique views. Standard and computed tomographic technique better delineate the tumor and the extent of its local involvement.

Sharp delineation and intact cortical margins seen on plain radiographs are characteristic of benign tumors, whereas malignant tumors are usually poorly defined and show cortical disruption. Occasionally, old rib fractures, calcified prominent costal cartilages, myositis ossificans, prominent or bifid xyphoids, and osteomyelitis of bony structures in the chest may give misleading pictures that may suggest tumors. Because of this, an accurate histologic diagnosis is essential for the treatment of chest wall tumors. In general, needle biopsy is not recommended, unless there is a strong suspicion of myeloma or metastatic disease. Small tumors (2 cm) should be excised, a procedure that in most cases is curative. For larger tumors, a carefully planned open biopsy should be undertaken to obtain adequate tissue and should be performed so as not to compromise the incision for a future definitive resection.

Rib Tumors

The reported distribution of tumors in several large series is summarized in Table 12–2. The most common benign lesions, in order of frequency, are fibrous dysplasia (34%), osteochondroma (22%), enchondroma (11%), and eosinophilic granuloma (6%). The most common malignant lesions are chondrosarcoma (31%), plasmacytoma (31%), Ewing's sarcoma (12%), and osteogenic sarcoma (10%)[7, 11, 34, 35] (Table 12–3).

TABLE 12–2

Histologic Classification of Benign Chest Wall Neoplasms

Type of Tumor	Number of Patients	Percentage of Total
Fibrous dysplasia	28	34
Osteochondroma	18	23
Enchondroma	11	14
Eosinophilic granuloma	5	7
Osteoblastoma	3	4
Bone islands	3	4
Aneurysmal bone cyst	2	2
Hemangioma	2	2
Xanthoma	2	2
Fibroma	2	2
Fibroxanthoma	1	1
Giant cell	1	1
Lipoma	1	1
Osteoid osteoma	1	1
Angiomatosis	1	1
Chondroblastoma	1	1
TOTAL	82	100

Data from references 7, 11, 34, and 35.

BENIGN RIB TUMORS

Fibrous Dysplasia

The lesions of fibrous dysplasia are usually asymptomatic and are discovered on routine radiographic examination of the chest. The characteristic lesion has a homogeneous gray or ground-glass appearance with a sharply defined edge to the lesion. There is usually a thin sclerotic rim due to a narrow zone of deposition of reactive bone around the fibrous tissue.

Histologically, the major feature is a proliferation of fibroblasts in a dense collagenous matrix that typically contains immature bone trabeculae, which are too small to be resolved radiographically but can be delineated on com-

TABLE 12–3

Histologic Classification of Malignant Chest Wall Neoplasms

Type of Tumor	Number of Patients	Percentage of Total
Chondrosarcoma	29	31
Myeloma	29	31
Ewing's sarcoma	11	12
Osteogenic sarcoma	10	10
Lymphoma	7	8
Other	7	8
TOTAL	93	100

Data from references 7, 11, 34, and 35.

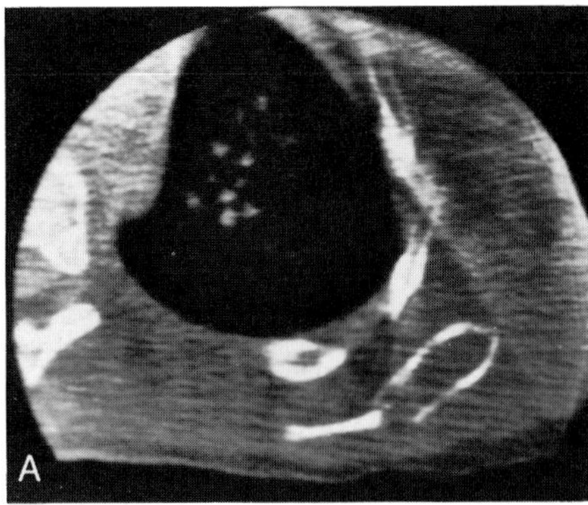
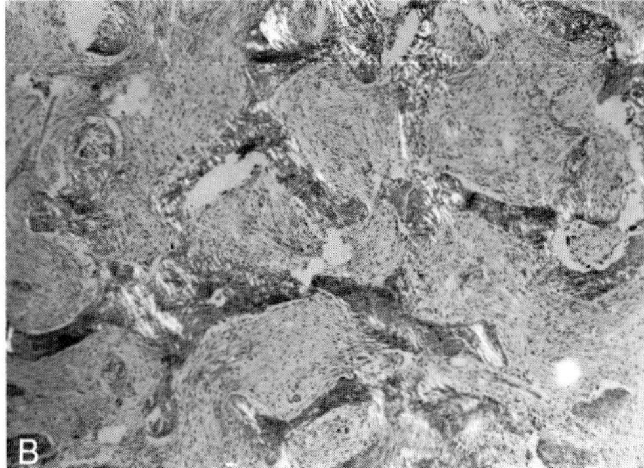

FIGURE 12–1. Fibrous dysplasia. *A,* Computed tomography (CT) scan demonstrates a fibrous dysplasia of the clavicle with some trabeculae of osteoid *B,* Classic pathologic features of a fibrous dysplasia.

puted tomography scans with attenuated values of 20 to 40 H (Fig. 12–1). Fibrous dysplasia typically exhibits intense uptake on bone scan, presumably owing to the diffuse microscopic ossifications.

Enchondroma

Enchondromas are typically located at the costochondral junctions and occur most often in patients in the second and third decades of life. They are usually painless masses on the anterior chest wall.

On x-rays films, they appear as intramedullary radiolucencies that may thin the overlying cortex, often in an eccentric manner, but do not disrupt it. Slight or prominent stippled or matted calcifications in the tumor are frequently seen (Fig. 12–2).

On gross section, the characteristic enchondroma is composed of confluent masses of bluish semitranslucent hyaline cartilage with a distinctly lobular arrangement. The chondrocytes that make up the cellular component of a chondroma are small cells that lie in lacunar spaces and have a round regular nucleus. Because the degree of cellularity varies remarkably in chondromas, cellularity affords little help in differentiating chondroma from chondrosarcoma. If untreated, these tumors can grow to a large size, sometimes exceeding the 4-cm limit that some pathologists believe is now the upper limit of benignity.[14] Excision of the involved costal cartilage, along with a short segment of the accompanying rib, is curative.

Osteochondroma

Osteochondromas generally are identified in the first and second decades of life, and there is no sex predilection. Interestingly, the majority of rib osteochondromas are located in the first four ribs.

Many of the bone lesions heal spontaneously, but symptomatic lesions may be treated and healed by resection, curettage,

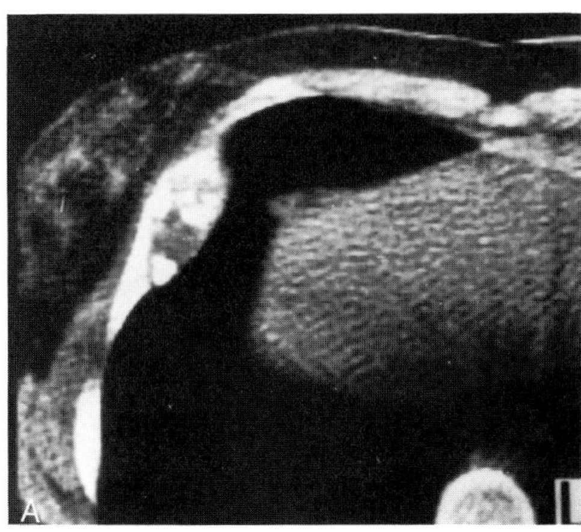
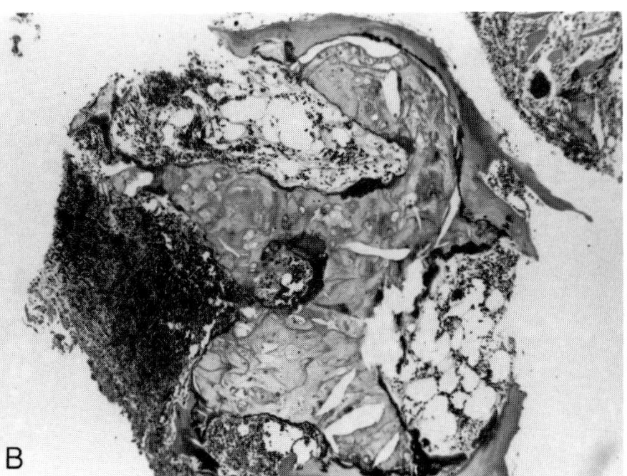

FIGURE 12–2. Chondroma. *A,* CT scan of a 3-cm chondroma of the rib. *B,* Microscopic appearance of a typical chondroma.

steroid injection, or radiation therapy in low doses.

A palpable mass is ordinarily the only finding. The characteristic appearance on roentgenogram is that of a bony projection composed of a cortex continuous with that of surrounding bone and medullary spongiosa. The cap is initially cartilaginous but irregular calcifications may be present.

The gross pathologic features confirm the roentgenologic pattern. The tumor cortex and its periosteal covering are continuous with those of the underlying bone. Microscopic studies confirm the gross appearance of regular cortical and underlying cancellous bone with its fatty or hematopoietic components differentiating from a cartilage cap by endochondral ossification (Fig. 12–3).

The presence of an osteochondroma in itself is insufficient reason for surgical extirpation because malignant transformation occurs in less than 1% of clinically recognized lesions.[19] Removal is indicated if the tumor is producing pain, has roentgenologic features suggestive of malignancy, or increases in size. Removal of the tumor at the level of the bone of origin is the treatment. The entire cartilage cap must be removed to avoid recurrence. For osteochondroma in locations such as the rib, *en bloc* excision is often necessary.

Eosinophilic Granuloma

Eosinophilic granuloma of bone accounts for 60 to 80% of all cases of histiocytosis X[19] and can be solitary or multifocal. Most patients are in the first three decades of life, the peak incidence is between 5 and 10 years, the male/female ratio is 3:2.

They are geographic lytic lesions and can be associated with a reactive sclerotic rim or have sharp punched-out areas with no sclerosis. Computed tomography often shows the extent of bone destruction much more clearly than do plain radiographs.

Grossly, the lesions contain soft gray-yellow or brownish tissue, often with necrotic areas, cysts, and hemorrhage. Microscopically, they are characterized by Langerhans-type histiocytes, which are large and ovoid and have focal collections of eosinophils.

Many of the bone lesions heal spontaneously, but symptomatic lesions may be treated by resection, curettage, steroid injection, or radiation therapy in low doses.

MALIGNANT RIB LESIONS

Chondrosarcoma

Chondrosarcoma is the most common of the primary malignant tumors of the chest wall. As for its benign counterpart (chondroma), the costochondral junction is its most frequent location. However, the tumor may occur anywhere along the course of the ribs.

Pathologic grading of the tumor is the most important curative operation. Signs of malig-

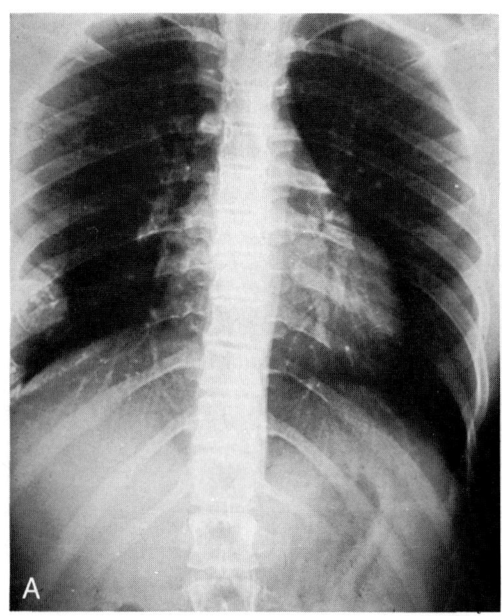

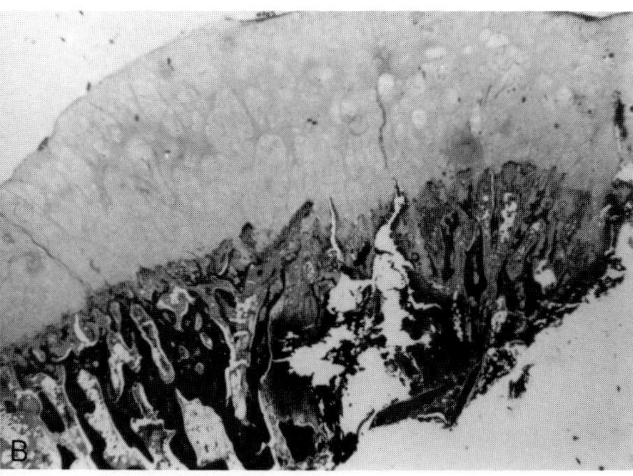

FIGURE 12–3. Osteochondroma. *A,* Radiographic appearance of an osteochondroma of the sixth rib. *B,* Microscopic appearance of regular cortical and underlying medullary bone.

nancy may be subtle and are found in only limited areas of a tumor.

The classic histologic features include the presence of many cells with plump nuclei, cells with two plump nuclei, and giant cartilage cells with large single and multiple nuclei or clumps of chromatin (Fig. 12–4). Grading of chondrosarcomas emphasizing mitotic rate and cellularity was performed by Evans and associates,[9] and a similar grading system was used by Huvos[20], and Gitelis and colleagues[10] in correlating grade with distant metastasis and survival in several large series, the following were observed: grade I chondrosarcoma—5% metastasis, 70% 5-year survival, and 50% 10-year survival; grade III chondrosarcoma—55% metastasis, 44% 5-year survival, and 28% 10-year survival.[10] As the majority of ribs lesions are grades I and II, definitive surgical resection is the treatment of choice, and the extent of resection should not be compromised because of an inability to close the chest wall defect.

Opinions differ about what constitutes a wide resection. King, reporting on the Mayo Clinic experience, advocated a minimal 2-cm margin of resection, with wider margins of resection indicated for higher-grade lesions (4 cm).[16] For rib cage resection, this includes removal of the involved ribs *in toto* and several partial ribs above and below the neoplasm.

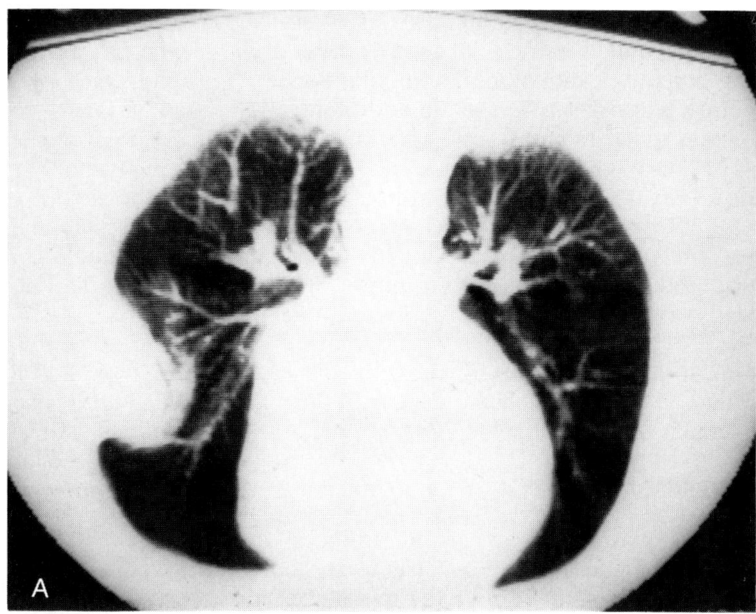

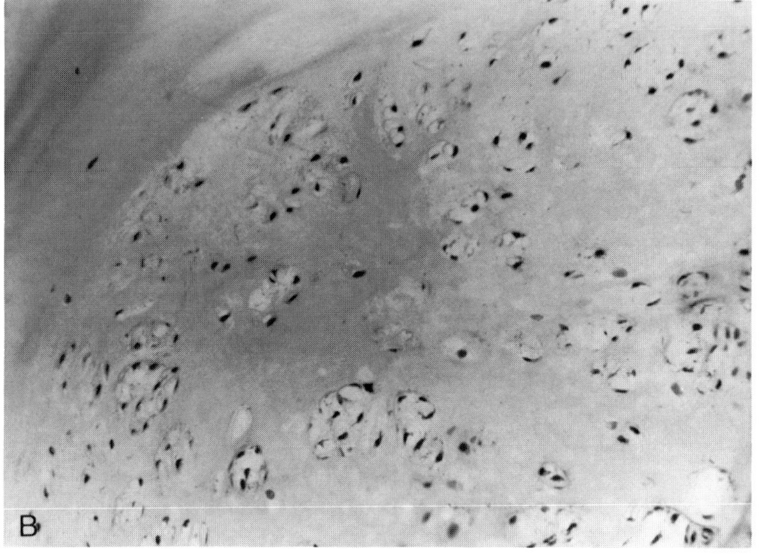

FIGURE 12–4. Chondrosarcoma. *A,* CT scan of a chondrosarcoma of the seventh rib with lung windows to rule out pulmonary metastasis. *B,* Typical microscopic appearance of a well-differentiated chondrosarcoma.

Reconstruction of these defects necessitates stabilization of the bony thorax and, in rare situations, coverage of any soft tissue defect. For anterior thoracic defects less than 5 cm in greatest diameter or posterior defects less than 10 cm in diameter, no reconstruction is usually necessary. Stabilization of the thorax has been accomplished with olefin (Marlex) mesh,[12] Marlex mesh in a methyl methacrylate sandwich,[23] polypropylene (Prolene) mesh, or most recently, using a Gore-Tex soft tissue patch.

When necessary, soft tissue reconstruction has been accomplished using pectoralis,[1] serratus anterior,[2] latissimus dorsi, and rectus abdominis muscles. All of these muscles have an axial blood supply, which permits elevation of the muscles and their rotation for a substantial distance. In selected situations, such as a previous failed muscle transfer or previous surgery and/or radiation, an omental flap[3, 15, 38] before grafting can be used in addition to free muscle transfers with vascularization.

Because chondrosarcomas are generally slow-growing malignancies with a high cure rate after adequate surgical resection, high survival rates follow resection. Five-year survival rates of 85 to 90% are common, with 10-year survival figures in most series approaching 70%.[20, 22]

At present, there is no proven efficacy of radiation therapy or chemotherapy in the management of these tumors.

Plasmacytoma

Solitary plasmacytomas arising in bone are uncommon tumors, which occur as the initial presentation in 3 to 7% of patients with plasma cell myeloma.[6, 18] Patients with the disease often have multiple myeloma, but the time to dissemination is variable and may be longer than 20 years.

Approximately 25 to 30% of all primary malignant tumors in the chest wall are plasmacytomas. Myeloma, which is familiar as multiple, punched-out lytic lesions in the skull, is not as readily recognized when it takes the form of a solitary lesion in the ribs or the sternum.[7]

The average age of patients with solitary plasmacytomas is 57 years, and men predominate in a 3:1 ratio. The ribs are the third commonest site after the spine and the pelvis. Approximately 25% of all patients have serum or urine paraprotein level elevations. The presence of paraproteins is not predictive of subsequent progression of disease.

If a skeletal radiographic series and a bone scan fail to reveal any additional lesions, a marrow specimen should be obtained by needle biopsy of the primary lesion; if the location of tumor precludes a safe approach for needle biopsy, open surgical biopsy can be accomplished.

Myeloma tissue grossly is soft, reddish gray, and friable. Microscopically, it is composed of sheets of clearly packed plasma cells, varying in maturity. Each cell contains abundant basophilic cytoplasm with a round or oval eccentric nucleus, often with two or three nucleoli.

Local control of the solitary plasmacytoma can be achieved with a high success rate by radiation therapy.[25] More radical surgical resections should be reserved for patients in whom radiation therapy has failed and those who have symptomatic localized disease.

Overall, patients with plasmacytomas have an indolent course of disease. In reviewing several reported series,[4, 5, 24, 37, 39] disease in 55% of patients progressed to systemic forms in the first 5 years after diagnosis. An additional 23% manifested systemic myeloma at a later time. At 15 years, however, 23% of all patients had no evidence of disease.

If progression of the lesions occurs, patients die of disseminated disease. There is a median survival of 47 months and a 5-year survival of 32% after progression. Overall survival for patients with solitary plasmacytomas is 75% at 5 years, 52% at 10 years, and 37% at 20 years.

Systemic chemotherapy should probably be reserved for patients with disease progression.

Ewing's Sarcoma

Ewing's sarcoma is one of the more prevalent primary bone malignancies; it has a predilection for young patients. It accounts for 6 to 7% of all primary bone malignancies and approximately 13% of all malignant tumors of the ribs. The peak incidence is at 10 to 20 years of age, and most patients are between 5 and 30 years old. Male patients are affected more commonly than female patients in a ratio of 2:1.[17]

Patients usually have pain that gradually increases in severity over several months. Other common signs and symptoms include a mass, tenderness, and local erythema. Some patients have systemic manifestations, including malaise, low-grade fever, anemia, leukocytosis, and an elevated erthrocyte sedimentation rate.

The typical plain radiographic appearance is

that of permeative bone destruction and laminated periosteal reaction (Fig. 12–5). There is frequently an associated extraosseous soft tissue mass. Incisional biopsy to establish the diagnosis is the initial step in the management of these patients. Ewing's sarcomas are grossly soft or fibrous and sometimes gelatinous. There are often areas of hemorrhagic necrosis and cyst formation.

Traditional survival rates for Ewing's sarcomas were approximately 10%. Significant improvement occurred with the advent of the combined modality approach, with 2- and 5-year survival rates of 80 and 60%, respectively.[30, 36]

Osteogenic Sarcoma

Osteosarcomas of the rib were responsible for only 10% of the malignant rib tumors reported in collected series.[7, 11, 34, 35] In the Mayo Clinic osteosarcoma series, rib tumors accounted for 1% of all lesions.[14]

There is a predilection for these tumors to occur in men, and the peak incidence is in the second decade.

Clinically, the tumor may be a painful, rapidly expanding mass. The duration of symptoms before definitive therapy may vary from a few weeks to several months.

About one half of osteosarcomas exhibit a

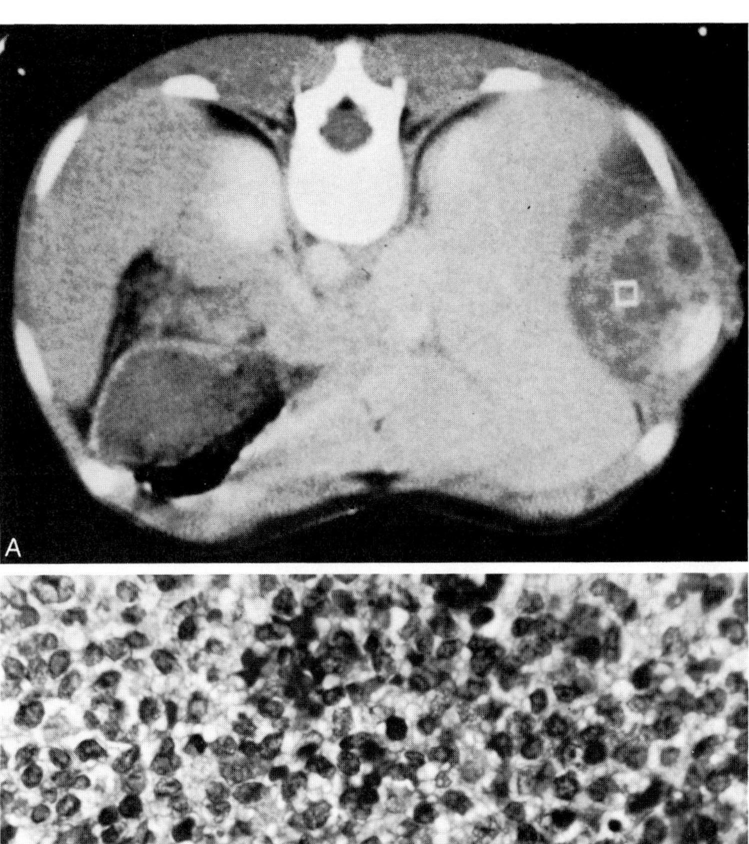

FIGURE 12–5. Ewing's sarcoma. *A*, CT scan of an extensive lesion of the ninth rib with external compression of the underlying right hepatic lobe. *B*, Microscopic appearance of multiple small round cells characteristic of Ewing's sarcoma.

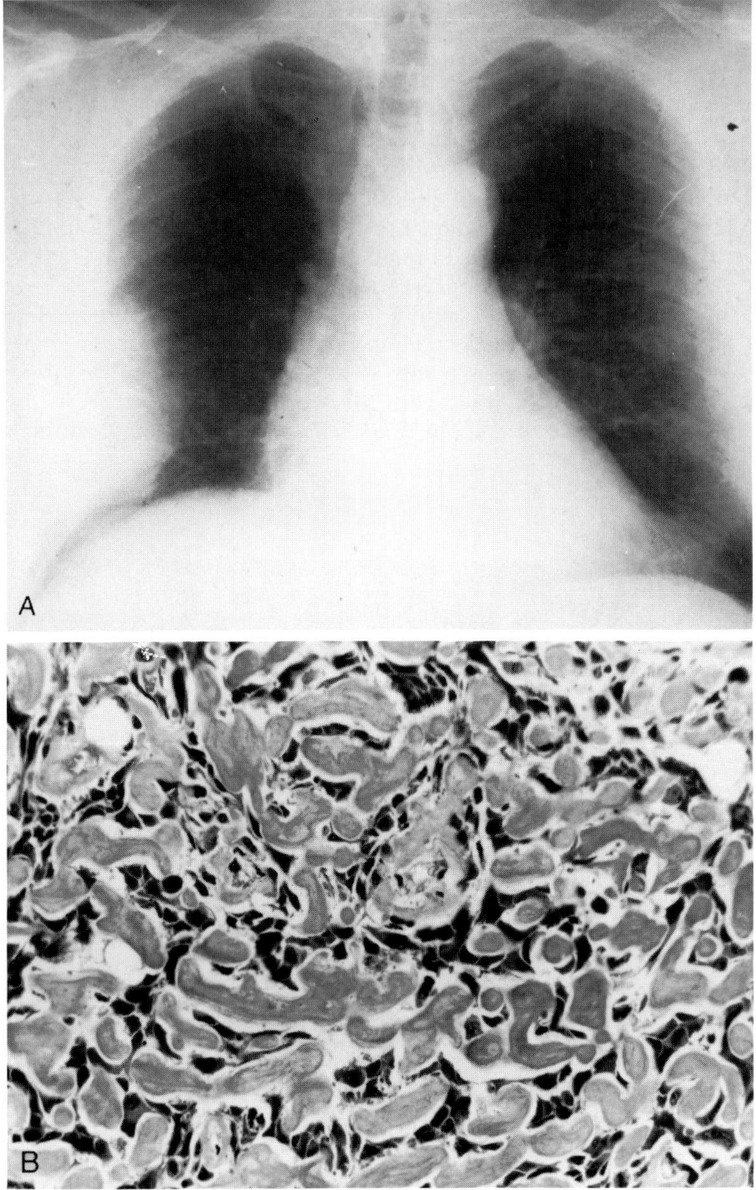

FIGURE 12–6. Osteogenic sarcoma. *A,* An extensive osteogenic sarcoma of the ribs. *B,* Photomicrograph depicting the classic microscopic appearance.

radiographic appearance typical enough to permit confident diagnosis (Fig. 12–6). The classic sunburst pattern secondary to reactive periosteal new bone is often present.

Similar to the current treatment of Ewing's sarcomas, preoperative and postoperative multidrug chemotherapy with *en bloc* resection has become the standard therapy.[31, 32]

Tumors of the Sternum

Tumors of the sternum are uncommon and the vast majority of cases are malignant. They are most likely to be metastatic and to originate from the breast, the kidney, or the thyroid.[8] Testicular, lung, gastric, and colon cancers may also metastasize to the sternum.

Primary tumors of the sternum are almost always malignant. The most common lesion is the chondrosarcoma.[21, 26, 28] Slow growth and a tendency to local recurrence after limited excision are characteristic of this tumor.

Adequate roentgenologic investigation is necessary to assess the true extent of the lesion correctly. The presenting mass is often part of a much larger tumor invading the sternum. The tumors are radioresistant and surgery is the mainstay of therapy.

The second most common group of tumors

are those of reticuloendothelial origin. This group includes Ewing's sarcomas, myelomas, and lymphomas. In the majority of these cases, the tumors are systemic, but occasionally they may be localized to the sternum. In such cases, the role of surgery is to establish the diagnosis.

Plasmacytomas may be treated with chemotherapy following radiation therapy for the localized lesion.[5, 25] *En bloc* resection of Ewing's sarcoma may be indicated in some instances, but the tumor is so radiosensitive that a course of radiation therapy between treatments with vincristine and actinomycin D (dactinomycin) is most effective.[33]

Occasionally, lesions such as angiosarcomas, neurosarcomas, and liposarcomas have been reported.[13, 29]

Benign lesions arising in the sternum include chondromas and giant cell tumors as well as inflammatory masses.

For those tumors in which resection of the sternum is indicated, the incision is carried down to the rigid chest wall, leaving any involved skin, subcutaneous tissue, or muscle adherent to the tumor. The deep aspect of the tumor is evaluated by entering a normal intercostal space. Adherent pleura or pericardium is resected with the tumor mass. If the manubrium is resected, the medial portion of the clavicles should be resected, along with the tumor mass. The tumor should be excised with a 4-cm margin of normal sternum and costal cartilage. If a portion of the sternum is preserved the sternal defect can usually be repaired with olefin (Marlex) mesh under moderate tension. When a total sternectomy is performed a Marlex and methyl methacrylate sandwich gives secure fixation and rigidity to the anterior chest wall. Secure skin closure over the area of repair can be accomplished primarily or if necessary with bipedal advancement flaps or myocutaneous flaps.

References

1. Arnold PG, Pairolero PC: Use of pectoralis major muscle flaps to repair defects of the anterior chest wall. Plast Reconstr Surg 63:205, 1974.
2. Arnold PG, Pairlero PC, Waldorf JC: The serratus anterior muscle: Intrathoracic and extrathoracic utilization. Plast Reconstr Surg 73:240, 1984.
3. Arnold PG, Witzke DJ, Frong B, Woods JE: Use of omental transposition flaps for soft tissue reconstruction. Ann Plast Surg 11:508, 1983.
4. Batkle R, Sany J: Solitary myeloma: Clinical and prognostic features of a review of 114 cases. Cancer 48:845, 1981.
5. Berysagel DE, Baily AS, Lusegly GR: The chemotherapy of plasma cell myeloma and the incidence of acute leukemia. N Engl J Med 301:743, 1979.
6. Chak L, Cox RS, Bostwick DG, Hoppe RT: Solitary plasmacytoma of bone: Treatment, progression, and survival. J Clin Oncol 5:1811–1815, 1987.
7. Corwin J, Lindberg RD: Solitary plasmacytoma of bone vs. extramedullary plasmacytoma and their relationship to multiple myeloma. Cancer 43:1007, 1979.
8. Crile G: Pulsating tumors of the sternum. Ann Surg 199:103, 1936.
9. Evans HL, Ayala AG, Romsdahl MM: Prognostic factors in chondrosarcoma of bone cancer. Cancer 40:818, 1971.
10. Gitelis S, Bertoni F, Picci P, et al: Chondrosarcoma of bone. J Bone Joint Surg 63A:1248, 1981.
11. Graeber GM: Initial and long term results in the management of primary chest wall neoplasms. Ann Thorac Surg 34:664, 1982.
12. Graham J, Usher FC, Perry SL: Marlex mesh as a prosthesis in the repair of thoracic wall defects. Ann Surg 151:469, 1960.
13. Hoop RM: Surgical Disease of the Pleura and Chest Wall. Philadelphia, WB Saunders Co, 1986.
14. Jaffe HL: Tumor and Tumorous Conditions of the Bones and Joints. Philadelphia, Lea & Febiger, 1958.
15. Jurkiewicz MJ, Arnold PG: The Omentum: An account of its use in the reconstruction of the chest wall. Ann Surg 185:548, 1977.
16. King RM: Primary chest wall tumors: Factors affecting survival. Ann Thorac Surg 41:597, 1986.
17. Kissane JM, Askin FB, Foulkes M, Stratton LB, Shirley SF: Ewing's sarcoma of bone: Clinicopathologic aspects of 303 cases from the Intergroup Ewing's Sarcoma Study. Hum Pathol 14:773, 1983.
18. Knowling MA, Harwood AR, Bergsagel DE: Comparison of extramedullary plasmacytomas with solitary and multiple plasma cell tumors at bone. J Clin Oncol 1:255–262, 1983.
19. Lichtenstein L: Bone Tumors. St Louis, CV Mosby, 1977.
20. Marcove R, Huvos A: Cartilaginous tumors of the ribs. Cancer 27:749, 1971.
21. Martini N, Huvos A, Smith J, Beattie E: Primary malignant tumors of the sternum. Surg Gynecol Obstet 138:391, 1974.
22. McAfee MK: Chondrosarcoma of the chest wall. Factors affecting survival. Ann Thorac Surg 40:535, 1985.
23. McCormack P, Bains MS, Beatle EJ, Martini N: New trends in skeletal reconstruction after resection of chest wall tumors. Ann Thorac Surg 31:45, 1981.
24. Meyer JE, Schultz MD: "Solitary" myeloma of bone. A review of 12 cases. Cancer 34:438, 1974.
25. Mill WB, Griffith R: The role of radiation therapy in the management of plasma cell tumors. Cancer 45:647, 1980.
26. O'Neal LW, Ackerman L: Cartilaginous tumors of ribs and sternum. J Thorac Surg 21:71, 1951.
27. Pasquizini CA, Dahlin DC, Clagett OT: Primary tumors of the ribs and sternum. Surg Gynecol Obstet 104:390, 1957.
28. Peabody CN: Chondrosarcoma of the sternum, report of a six year survival. J Thorac Cardiovasc Surg 61:636, 1971.
29. Pollack A: Angiosarcoma of the sternum. Am J Surg 72:522, 1949.
30. Rosen G, Caparros B, Mosende C, et al: Curability of Ewing's sarcoma and considerations for future therapeutic trials. Cancer 41:888, 1978.
31. Rosen G, Marcove R, Capanos B, et al: Primary

osteogenic sarcoma. The rationale for preoperative chemotherapy and delayed surgery. Cancer 43:2163, 1979.
32. Rosen G, Murphy ML, Huvos AG: Chemotherapy, *en bloc* resection, prosthetic bone replacement in the treatment of osteogenic sarcoma. Cancer 37:1, 1976.
33. Rosen G, Wollnen H, Tan C, et al: Disease free survival in children with Ewing's sarcoma treated with radiation therapy and adjuvant four drug sequential chemotherapy. Cancer 33:384, 1974.
34. Teitlebaum S: Twenty years experience with intrinsic tumors of the bony thorax at a large institution. Thorac Cardiovasc Surg 63:776, 1972.
35. Theikel JB, Adkins S: Primary chest wall tumors. Ann Thorac Surg 11:450, 1971.
36. Thomas PRM, Perez CA, Neff JR, Nesbit ME, Evans RG: The management of Ewing's sarcoma: Role of radiotherapy in local tumor control. Cancer Treat Rep 68:703–710, 1984.
37. Tong D, Griffin TW, Laramore GE, et al: Solitary plasmacytoma of bone and soft tissues. Radiology 135:195, 1980.
38. Vetto M, Rubin S, Bernards W: Closure of large thoracic wall defects using an omental pedicle. Am Surg 43:724, 1977.
39. Woodruff RK, Malpas JS, White FE: Solitary plasmacytoma: Solitary plasmacytoma of bone. Cancer 43:2344, 1979.

CHAPTER 13

Pelvic Tumors

MARY I. O'CONNOR
FRANKLIN H. SIM

Bone tumors involving the pelvis present a difficult diagnostic and therapeutic problem. The pelvis may be involved by many different benign or malignant osseous lesions. After the tumor has been identified, an organized and systematic approach to preoperative evaluation is mandatory.

Preoperative Assessment

The diagnosis and treatment of bone tumors involving the pelvis is very difficult. Although bone tumors involving the pelvis are relatively rare, these lesions vary greatly and have different biologic capabilities. In addition, the clinical presentation is often insidious, which makes early recognition difficult. At initial presentation, many patients have symptoms that can be attributed to various degenerative or inflammatory conditions. At times, the lesions are missed initially because of poor-quality roentgenograms. Chondrosarcoma, for instance, commonly occurs along the inner wall of the acetabulum in elderly patients—a site where symptoms may be attributed to degenerative hip disease unless the possibility of neoplasm is considered and good-quality roentgenograms are obtained (Fig. 13–1).

The evaluation of a patient with a pelvic bone tumor is divided into four phases: (1) discovery, (2) diagnosis, (3) preoperative staging, and (4) biopsy. Clinical evaluation begins with a careful history and physical examination. Plain radiographs are the key in formulating the working diagnosis. A differential diagnosis is generated by the clinical and radiographic correlation, which guides subsequent staging studies necessary to complete the preoperative phase. Careful preoperative evaluation is essential to determine evidence of occult systemic metastasis as well as the precise extent of local tumor involvement. Computed tomography (CT) is extremely sensitive in examining the lung fields for occult metastasis when a malignant lesion is suspected.

In addition to plain radiographs or tomograms of the lesion, an isotope bone scan is useful in ruling out other unsuspected bone lesions and is also helpful in assessing the degree of intraosseous extension in the pelvis. Moreover, angiography may be useful in ascertaining the relationship of the neighboring vascular structures, particularly when resection or adjunctive angiographic embolization is considered in managing a vascular primary or metastatic bone tumor. In addition, recent

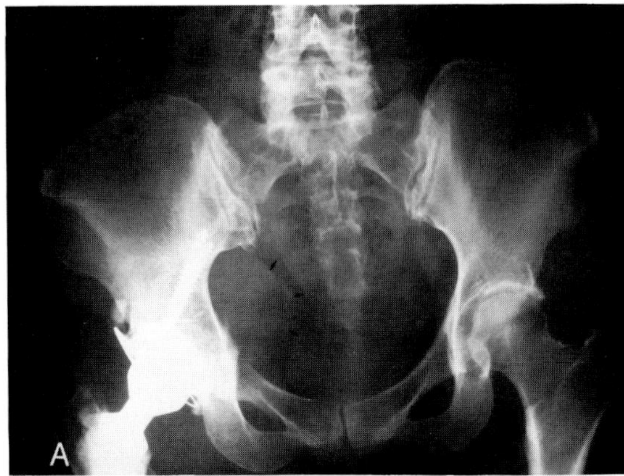

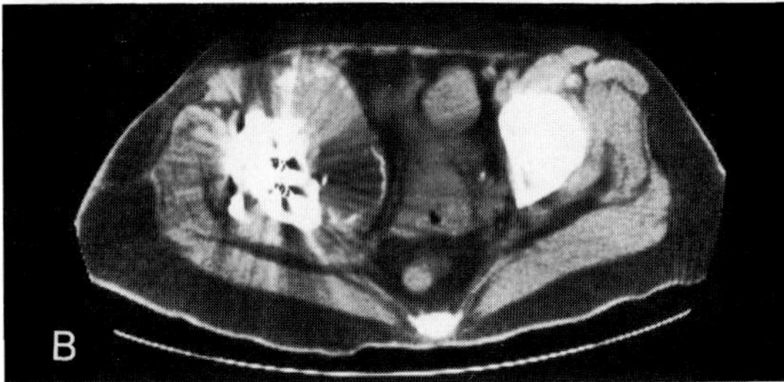

FIGURE 13–1. Chondrosarcoma. *A,* Anteroposterior (AP) view of the right hip shows total hip arthroplasty (done elsewhere) and destruction of the acetabulum by chondrosarcoma. *B,* Computed tomography (CT) scan shows large chondrosarcoma of the right acetabulum.

advances in preoperative investigative measures, particularly CT and magnetic resonance imaging (MRI), have enhanced the ability to define more accurately the anatomic confines of the lesion. These procedures help in the preoperative planning and provide information that is critical in deciding whether hemipelvectomy is necessary or limb-saving resection for a primary malignant bone tumor is possible. Excretory urography and barium enema study also provide valuable information regarding the relationship of a pelvic tumor to the visceral structures. When a lesion involves the posterior portion of the pelvis and extends into the sacrum or along the spinal column, myelography is necessary to assess the relationship to the neural contents. In addition, a liver and spleen scan, an abdominal CT scan, and a bone marrow study may be helpful when there is a disseminated sarcoma or when the pattern of spread of lymphoma or Ewing's sarcoma is assessed.

Primary Bone Tumors

BENIGN BONE TUMORS

Benign bone tumors represented 22% of the 8542 primary bone tumors in a study at the Mayo Clinic.[3] Of these, 110 (1.3%) involved the pelvis (Table 13–1). Evaluation of an osseous lesion of the pelvis necessitates that conditions simulating bone tumors be considered to eliminate confusion in diagnosis and treatment.

The goals of treatment of benign bone tumors involving the pelvis are to control the osseous lesion and to preserve and restore function. Two factors have a bearing on the surgical philosophy used in the treatment of these lesions: (1) the anatomic site and extent of pelvic involvement (based on the clinical and radiographic assessment) and (2) the natural history of the lesion (including its potential for aggressive local behavior).

A benign pelvic lesion can be managed by less radical surgery than can a malignant lesion. Most benign tumors can be managed with a relatively conservative procedure, such as curettage or marginal excision. If curettage is to be successful, adequate technique must be used, because recurrence is likely if residual tumor remains. An important factor in successful treatment is adequate exposure, which involves making a large cortical window and completely exteriorizing the tumor cavity. Failure to completely exteriorize and visualize all aspects of the tumor cavity leads almost inevitably to recurrence. After exteriorization, the tumor tissue must be thoroughly excised using a sharp curette, with care being taken to avoid contamination of the surrounding soft tissues or retroperitoneal structures. After adequate curettage, a motorized bur is used to extend the margins into the cortical bone. The cavity is cleaned with a pulsatile water lavage. In addition, the tumor cavity may be cauterized

TABLE 13–1

Distribution of Benign Pelvic Bone Tumors*

Type	Number
Osteochondroma	52
Chondroma	5
Chondroblastoma	12
Chondromyxoid fibroma	5
Osteoid osteoma	6
Osteoblastoma	4
Giant cell tumor	21
Fibrous histiocytoma	3
Hemangioma	2
TOTAL	110

*From a series of 8542 primary bone tumors in the Mayo Clinic files. Data from Dahlin DC, Unni KK: Bone Tumors: General Aspects and Data on 8,542 Cases, 4th ed. Springfield, IL, Charles C Thomas, 1986.

by chemical or thermal agents. Generally, the authors prefer local adjuvant treatment with phenol to extend the margin. After tumor excision, the integrity of the bone must be restored with bone grafts and the cavity must be filled completely with abundant bone. Autogenous or allograft bone grafts are generally used, although methyl methacrylate has recently proved useful after extensive curettage of some aggressive tumors.

Aggressive or recurrent benign lesions, particularly giant cell tumors that erode through the cortex and into the soft tissues, may necessitate *en bloc* resection with a wide margin to achieve local control. Resection of a lesion involving the acetabulum, however, necessitates major reconstruction and results in functional loss. In such cases, a more conservative approach with curettage and bone grafting or cementation is often worthwhile, with the more extensive resection procedures being used if recurrence develops.

MALIGNANT BONE TUMORS

Many different primary malignant bone tumors involve the pelvis (Table 13–2). The most frequent lesions are chondrosarcoma, osteosarcoma, and Ewing's sarcoma. Overall, primary malignant bone tumors of the pelvis are infrequent and constitute less than 10% of all malignant bone tumors. The prognosis is worse for patients with malignant lesions of the pelvis than for patients with more distal malignant tumors.

TABLE 13–2

Distribution of Malignant Pelvic Bone Tumors*

Type	Number
Primary chondrosarcoma	112
Secondary chondrosarcoma	35
Dedifferentiated chondrosarcoma	23
Mesenchymal chondrosarcoma	4
Osteosarcoma	109
Ewing's sarcoma	71
Malignant giant cell tumor	2
Malignant fibrous histiocytoma	6
Desmoplastic fibroma	2
Fibrosarcoma	31
Hemangioendothelioma	9
Hemangiopericytoma	3
TOTAL	407

*From a series of 8542 primary bone tumors in the Mayo Clinic files. Data from Dahlin DC, Unni KK: Bone Tumors: General Aspects and Data on 8,542 Cases, 4th ed. Springfield, IL, Charles C Thomas, 1986.

Hemipelvectomy

The classic treatment of primary radioresistant lesions of the pelvis has been hemipelvectomy, a debilitating and disfiguring procedure that is associated with a high incidence of postoperative morbidity. Functional results after this type of amputation are almost uniformly poor.

Limb Salvage

Previous attempts at limb salvage for malignant tumors of the pelvis resulted in a high rate of local recurrence and poor functional restoration, necessitating amputation in most patients. However, in recent years, there has been renewed interest in limb-saving resection for malignant pelvic tumors, particularly chondrosarcomas. In addition, advances in neoadjuvant chemotherapy have extended the indications for limb-sparing resections to include pelvic osteosarcomas. Moreover, recent studies suggest that Ewing's tumors in the pelvis have a better prognosis after local resection than with radiation therapy to control the primary lesion.[14] This approach extends the indications for pelvic resection further. Currently, the Intergroup Ewing's Sarcoma Study protocol recommends that patients with large pelvic tumors be given a preliminary course of multiple-drug chemotherapy in an attempt to reduce the size and extent of the lesion, after which a decision is made regarding the resectability of the lesion and postoperative radiation.[14]

For these extensive limb-sparing procedures to be a viable alternative to hemipelvectomy, they must meet two criteria. First and most important is local control of the tumor, requiring that the recurrence rate be comparable to that after hemipelvectomy. The second criterion is that the functional result be better than that after hemipelvectomy and prosthetic fitting.

Current enthusiasm for these massive resections is possible because of the recent advances in musculoskeletal oncology and the improved clinical staging made possible by CT and MRI—techniques that show the precise local extent of involvement of the tumor. Amputation surgery (hemipelvectomy) must be considered when preoperative imaging studies show involvement of the iliac vessels or the lumbosacral plexus, indicating that an adequate surgical margin cannot be achieved by limb-sparing resection. However, in many instances, the surgical margin along the bladder and the viscera is similar whether resection or amputation is performed. Moreover, in lesions of the posterior portion of the pelvis that are near the spinal column, amputation may not achieve a wider margin. In addition to the improved imaging techniques that facilitate the proper selection of patients, improved techniques of oncologic reconstruction have helped foster increased interest in limb-sparing resection for malignant pelvic tumors.

TECHNIQUE OF RESECTION

Local resection of bone tumors involving the pelvis is a demanding surgical procedure and must follow well-established principles of oncologic surgery. The surgical approach demands careful planning. An important consideration is the placement of the biopsy wound—where it can be completely circumvented at the time of definitive resection. Needle biopsy under CT guidance is particularly helpful. For a lesion in the pelvis, the biopsy site should be extrapelvic. An intrapelvic approach contaminates the retroperitoneal structures and risks local recurrence, particularly when the lesion is a chondrosarcoma, which is notorious for wound implantation. A poorly placed biopsy incision, a biopsy with extensive soft tissue dissection, or a subsequent hematoma increases tissue contamination with tumor cells and precludes successful limb-saving resection.

Resection of an osseous lesion of the pelvis is performed with the patient positioned as for hemipelvectomy. An extensive exposure provides access to both intrapelvic and extrapelvic structures. The incision is placed along the top of the pelvis, extending from the posterosuperior iliac spine along the curve of the iliac crest to the anterosuperior iliac spine. The incision is then extended distally into the thigh, coursing anterior to the greater trochanter, to below the gluteal crease. If the resection also involves the anterior pelvic arch, the incision is extended anteriorly along the inguinal ligament to expose the obturator foramen. The fascia is divided in line with the skin incision, and large flaps are developed. Posteriorly, the gluteus maximus muscle is reflected with the posterior flap to expose the sciatic nerve and the gluteal vessels. The short external rotators of the hip are divided. If the tumor does not extend externally, the gluteus medius muscle can be preserved by reflecting it from the lateral wall of the pelvis, extraperiosteally, after osteotomy of the greater trochanter.

The posterior dissection is completed after the sacrotuberous and sacrospinous ligaments, as well as the pudendal neurovascular structures, have been divided. The pelvis is exposed retroperitoneally by detaching the abdominal muscles. The femoral nerve is isolated and protected, and if the anterior arch of the pelvis is included in the resection, the iliac and femoral vessels are mobilized proximally from the bifurcation into the proximal thigh distally. When the tumor extends into the notch, the internal iliac artery and vein may be divided and ligated for exposure. When the lesion extends into the posterior portion of the pelvis or involves the sacrum, the lumbosacral plexus is mobilized from the anterior portion of the sacrum and protected during the posterior osteotomy. After the muscles around the obturator foramen have been divided, an osteotomy through the anterior portion of the pelvis may be performed with a Gigli saw, or a disarticulation may be done through the symphysis. When there is an extensive lesion involving the anterior portion of the pelvis, the osteotomy may be performed through the opposite anterior pelvic arch. The pelvic insertions of the sartorius and rectus femoris muscles are divided. The psoas muscle is divided along the brim of the pelvis, as well as at the insertion of the lesser trochanter.

The location, size, and nature of the lesion dictate the extent of the resection. If the acetabulum is involved, the preoperative assessment should determine whether an extraarticular or an intraarticular resection is necessary. In an extraarticular resection, the femoral shaft is exposed and osteotomy of the proximal femur is performed without opening the hip joint. However, if there is no joint involvement, the capsule is divided, the hip is dislocated, and the bone stock in the proximal femur is preserved to facilitate the reconstruction. When the preoperative imaging studies show a large lesion involving the iliosacral region, a hemilaminectomy of the lower lumbar spinal column and sacrum may be necessary to allow adequate resection.

Classification of resection is helpful in planning the appropriate reconstruction.[6] Type I resection involves the iliosacral or posterior region. When the surrounding gluteal musculature is resected, this becomes a type IA resection. Resection of the acetabulum is classified as type II. Preoperative staging must determine whether extraarticular resection is necessary. When this is performed, the resection is classified as type IIA. Resection involving the ischiopubic region is classified as type III. Some large lesions occupy more than one region.

METHODS OF RECONSTRUCTION

The method of reconstruction varies according to the anatomic location of the pelvic lesion and the extent of the defect. After a type I resection involving the iliosacral region, patients often do satisfactorily with no reconstruction; however, generally, the defect is closed and the remaining portion of the pelvis is approximated to the sacrum by hinging the symphysis pubis (Fig. 13–2). Fixation can be achieved with wires or screws and can be augmented with autogenous bone grafts. After a type IA resection, this type of reconstruction is necessary to restore function. Care must be taken to allow adequate room for the sciatic nerve to exit from the pelvis; this usually necessitates enlarging the inferior portion of the pelvis at this site.

Reconstruction when the lesion involves the acetabular region is problematic. If only a portion of the acetabulum is removed, the acetabulum may be reconstructed with autogenous bone grafts. However, when lesions involve the entire acetabulum and a total acetabular resection is necessary (type II), a number of reconstructive options are available.

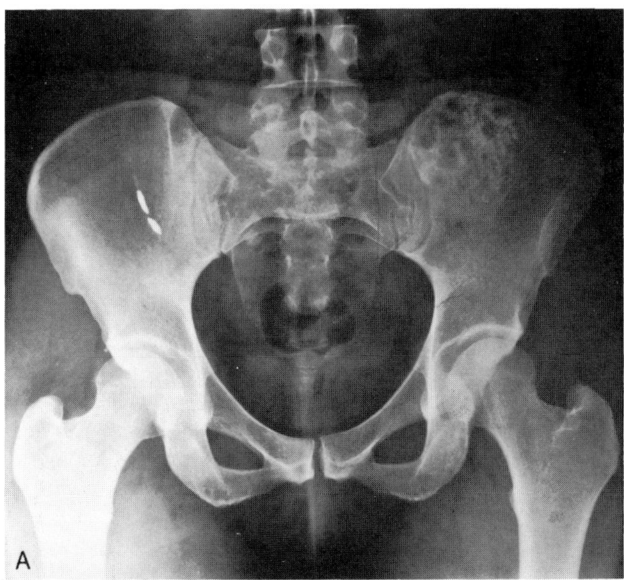

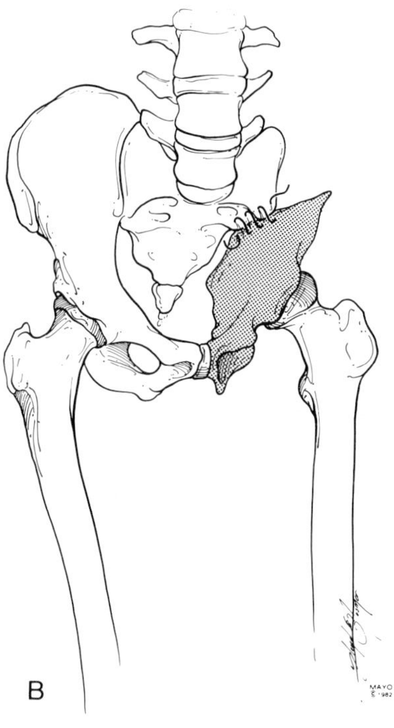

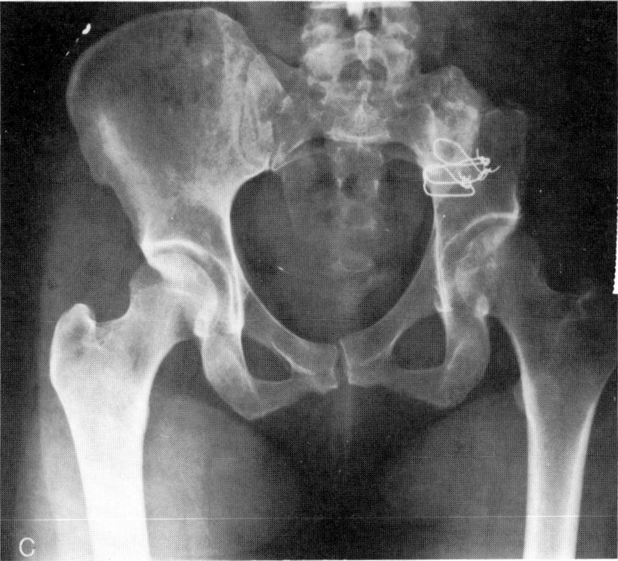

FIGURE 13–2. Iliosacral arthrodesis. *A,* AP view of the pelvis shows a large chondrosarcoma in the iliosacral region. *B,* Primary closure and wiring. (From O'Connor MI, Sim FH: Salvage of the limb in the treatment of malignant pelvic tumors. J Bone Joint Surg 71A:481–494, 1989.) *C,* AP view of the pelvis 36 months after surgery, showing solid iliosacral arthrodesis.

Enneking and colleagues popularized reconstruction by iliofemoral (Fig. 13–3) or ischiofemoral arthrodesis (Fig. 13–4).[6,7] The advantages of a durable, pain-free arthrodesis in a young active patient must be weighed against the relative disadvantages of impaired gait, limb shortening, and difficulty in obtaining fusion. An intercalary autograft or allograft may be utilized to restore the leg length discrepancy.

Capanna and colleagues, however, advocated attempted iliofemoral pseudarthrosis rather than fusion.[2] They found that the functional results are equivalent, whereas the surgical procedure is faster and less technically demanding and has potentially less risk of complications. When the remaining ilium is insufficient for an iliofemoral arthrodesis, the proximal femur may be fused to the ischium to create an ischiofemoral arthrodesis (Fig. 13–4).

Tomeno and associates advocated ischiofemoral fusion, where possible, to minimize limb shortening and to gain motion via the symphysis pubis.[16] They noted, however, that a painful symphysis developed in two of their three patients. For a lesion that requires removal of the major portion of the innominate

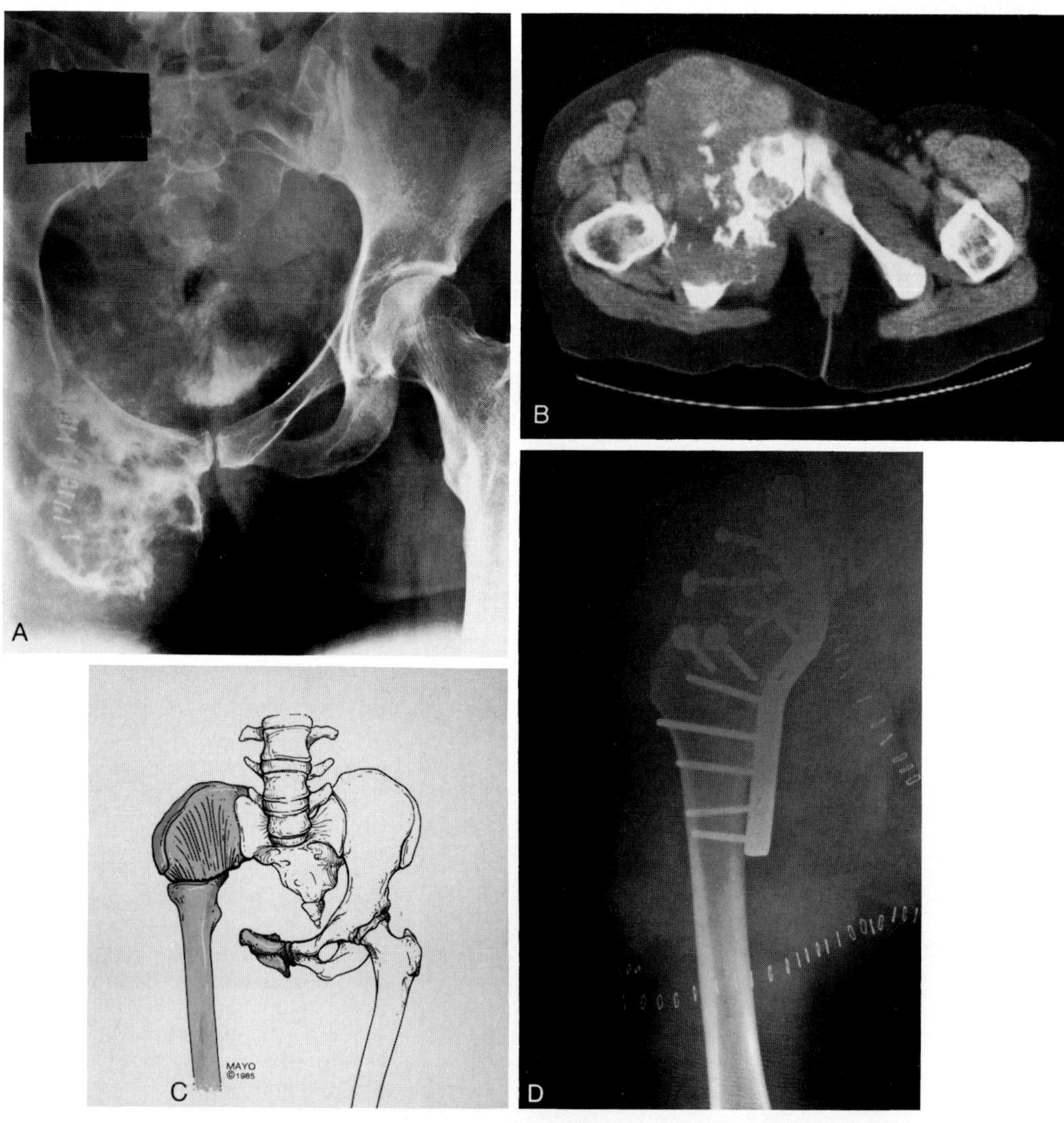

FIGURE 13–3. Iliofemoral arthrodesis. *A,* AP view of the pelvis shows a large chondrosarcoma involving the anterior pelvis and extending into the acetabulum. *B,* CT scan shows the extent of the tumor. *C,* Iliofemoral fusion. (By permission of Mayo Foundation.) *D,* AP view of the right femur after arthrodesis.

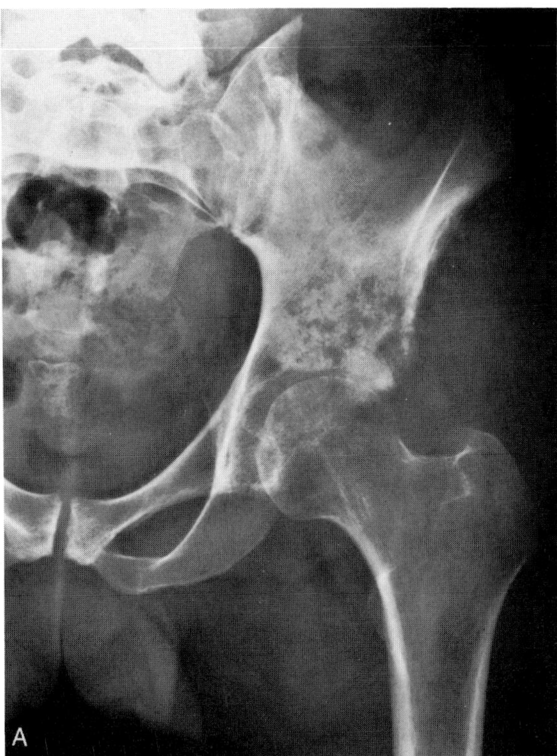

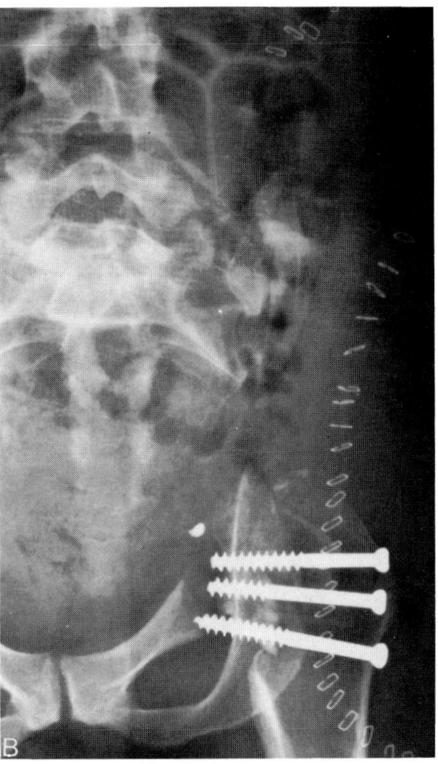

FIGURE 13–4. Ischiofemoral arthrodesis. *A,* AP view of the left hip shows chondrosarcoma involving the left acetabulum and the left ilium. *B,* AP view of the left pelvis after ischiofemoral arthrodesis with screw fixation.

bone, the limb may be left flail or reconstructed with a prosthesis or an allograft.

Reconstruction using a pelvic osteochondral allograft with or without hip prosthesis, as described by Rosenberg and Mankin,[15] may give an excellent functional result by restoring hip motion and preserving limb length, although the procedure has been complicated by high rates of infection and failure. Use of a prosthetic device, such as a modular polyacetal hemipelvis[13] or a custom-made hemipelvis,[4] is hindered by infection, prosthetic loosening, and difficulty in obtaining fixation of the prosthesis to the remaining bone. A saddle prosthesis (Fig. 13–5) may prove useful, but this design risks dislocation and loosening may be noted at long-term follow-up. Implantation of a saddle device does not significantly increase operative time and may permit the immediate use of postoperative adjuvant therapy because bone healing is not a factor. Ongoing developments in implant design and biologic methods of fixation may improve results in the future.

After resection of a lesion in the anterior portion of the pelvis (type III), reconstruction is usually not necessary.

CLINICAL SERIES

Clinical experience with malignant pelvic tumors treated by limb salvage procedures is limited to several small series. Data on 127 type II periacetabular resections from various orthopedic oncology centers were collected at the 1985 International Symposium on Limb Salvage.[1, 2, 4, 7, 13, 16] Results of type I and III resections are available from individual institutional experiences.[6] Recently, the authors reviewed experience with 60 limb-saving resections of malignant lesions of the pelvis (the findings are presented below).[13a]

Oncologic Results. The overall frequency of local recurrence after *en bloc* resection of malignant tumors of the pelvis was 17% in the authors' series and 28% in the series reported by Enneking and Dunham.[6] Most of the recurrences were found in patients who had marginal or contaminated wide margins. The influence of surgical margins was most apparent in patients with iliosacral lesions—patients in whom it is often difficult to obtain a wide margin because the tumor involves the sacrum and extends to the spinal column. For malignant iliosacral lesions, the local recurrence rate after type I or IA resections ranged from

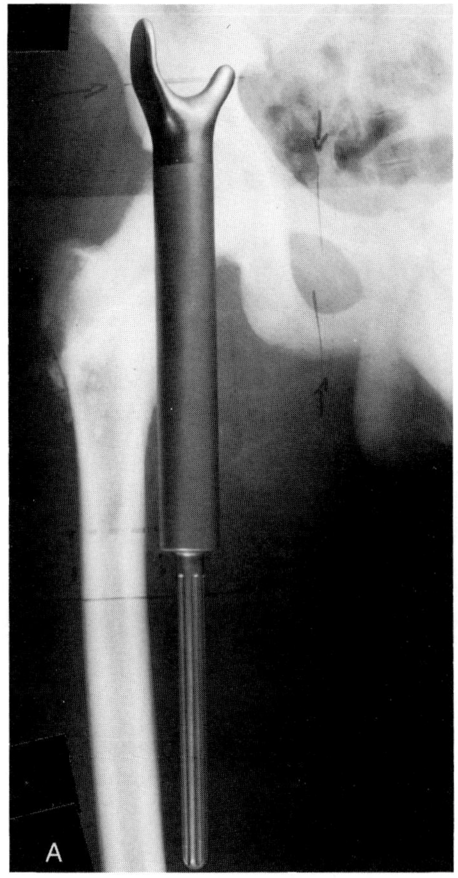

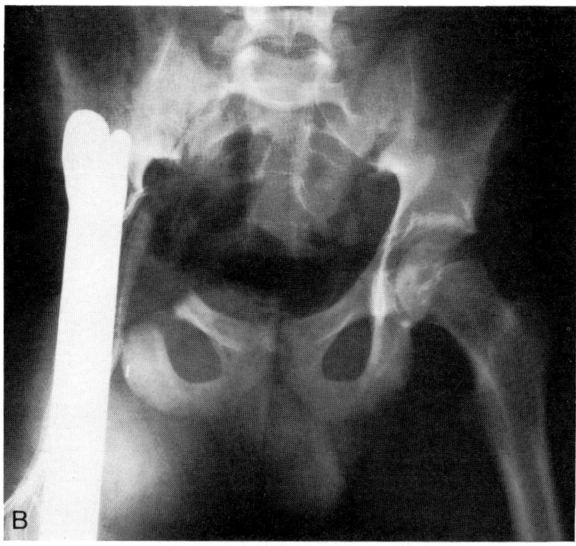

FIGURE 13–5. Saddle prosthesis. *A,* AP view of the right hip shows osteosarcoma of the proximal femur and a saddle prosthesis. *B,* AP view of the right pelvis after resection and placement of a saddle prosthesis.

27%[13a] to 50%.[6] Amputation does not improve the ability to obtain a wide margin in these patients. Adequate margins in both type II and III resections are more easily obtained. Recurrence rates after periacetabular resections have been from 8%[13a] to 24%.[1] Recurrences after *en bloc* resection of ischiopubic lesions were noted in two of ten patients in the authors' series; both patients had resection of chondrosarcoma with inadequate margins.

Functional Results. To facilitate functional analysis of various limb salvage procedures, the Musculoskeletal Tumor Society developed a standard functional evaluation system.[5a] The current modified system was used in the authors' series, as well as in those series presented at the 1985 International Symposium on Limb Salvage. Seven variables are evaluated: motion, pain, stability, deformity, strength, functional activity, and emotional acceptance. The patient receives an overall rating of excellent, good, fair, or poor.

Functional results after limb salvage of pelvic tumors vary with the type of resection and reconstruction performed. In the iliac region, results are uniformly excellent when pelvic continuity is preserved by resection above the sciatic notch. When resection includes the notch and pelvic stability is restored by iliosacral fusion, results are usually good to excellent.

At the 1985 International Symposium on Limb Salvage, analysis of reconstruction after 97 type II periacetabular resections with follow-up of longer than 20 months suggested that the best functional results were obtained after ischiofemoral arthrodesis or bone grafting with femoral prosthesis in patients with partial acetabular resection.[1] However, the numbers of patients in these two categories (seven and six, respectively) were small. The larger numbers of patients with iliofemoral arthrodesis and iliofemoral pseudarthrosis had similar functional ratings (40%, excellent to good; 60%, fair to poor). Pelvic prosthesis or allograft usually resulted in fair to poor results. When there was a flail hip or ischiofemoral pseudarthrosis, the results were worse, with poor ratings in 81 and 86% of patients, respectively. In Enneking and Menendez's analysis of their 1985 series,[7] their order of preference regarding reconstruction after periacetabular resections was as follows: ischiofemoral arthrodesis, iliofemoral arthrodesis, iliofemoral pseudarthrosis, ischiofemoral pseudarthrosis, and flail hip. The authors agree with Enneking and Menendez and prefer to stabilize the extremity by fusing the proximal femur to the remaining portion of the ischium or the ilium, depending on the type of resection performed. Unfortunately, the rate of successful arthrodesis is only 50%, which reflects the difficulty in obtaining rigid internal fixation of often narrow bone-to-bone contact areas, as well as failures resulting from infection.

Finally, after type III ischiopubic resections, functional results are uniformly excellent or good. There may be some loss of adduction power, depending on the extent of resection required.

Morbidity and Complications. Significant morbidity and a high incidence of complications may be associated with such extensive limb-sparing procedures, varying with the location of the lesion and the extent of resection. In patients who undergo extensive type I iliosacral resections, it is often necessary to sacrifice a nerve root, resulting in neurologic dysfunction. At the 1985 International Symposium on Limb Salvage, the overall complication rate for 127 periacetabular resections was 42%, graded as major in 36%.[1] These complications resulted in failure of limb salvage in less than 4% of cases, with the most frequent complications being infection, mechanical failure necessitating subsequent surgery, and flap necrosis. The incidence of these complications varied with the reconstruction method. The number of complications was significantly higher with fixation and arthrodesis than with resection without fixation. Moreover, the incidence of complications was significantly higher when an allograft or prosthesis was used. The high incidence of infection, in particular, may support a delayed reconstruction after an extensive resection.

DISCUSSION

Limb salvage in patients with malignant tumors of the pelvis continues to remain a challenge. Control of local recurrence is still a significant problem, with the location of the tumor and the surgical margin achieved being the most important factors. The local recurrence rate is particularly high with iliosacral lesions when only a lesional or marginal resection is possible, regardless of whether amputation or limb salvage is performed. This experience suggests the need for continued research into effective adjuvant treatment of these lesions. Justification for limb salvage depends on the ability to restore functional status better than that accomplished after hemipelvectomy, and to achieve local control. Reconstruction of the pelvis after resection of the tumor is a complex surgical problem that can be managed by various techniques. A major question is whether to reconstruct or not and what type of reconstruction to use.

Many factors must be considered in choosing the reconstructive method. Socioeconomic factors such as the patient's occupation may be important. If the patient has a sedentary job, a flail hip or an arthroplasty may be preferred. However, an arthrodesis of the femur to the remaining portion of the pelvis provides more stability and endurance for a patient who plans to return to vigorous activities.

Metastatic Lesions of the Pelvis

Lesions metastatic to the skeletal system are far more common than either benign or malignant primary lesions. It has been estimated that 70% of all carcinomas metastasize.[5] In addition to the vertebral bodies and skull, the pelvis is a common site of metastatic involvement. In the pelvis, metastasis may involve any of three major anatomic regions: the ischiopubic, the periacetabular, or the iliosacral. Moreover, symptoms may be influenced by the anatomic location. Metastatic foci involving the anterior ischiopubic region more commonly undergo pathologic fracture than do those located in the posterior portion of the pelvis, whereas metastatic lesions of the iliosacral region with soft tissue extension may involve the lumbosacral plexus and produce significant radicular symptoms. Metastatic deposits in the periacetabular region produce pain, which is aggravated by weight bearing and motion of the hip. Treatment of these metastatic lesions depends on a number of factors, including the anatomic location, the extent of bone destruction, and the general condition, functional level, and expected longevity of the patient.

METASTASIS WITHOUT ACETABULAR INVOLVEMENT

Metastatic lesions of the pelvis that do not involve the acetabular region are generally treated symptomatically. The pain experienced by these patients is generally caused by the metastatic lesion itself and/or a pathologic fracture. Radiation therapy is employed to control and often to alleviate the pain. Restricted weight bearing minimizes the risk of pathologic fracture or decreases the fracture-related discomfort and promotes fracture healing if a pathologic fracture is already present.

METASTASIS WITH ACETABULAR INVOLVEMENT

Treatment of metastatic disease in the acetabular region of the pelvis is primarily based on the extent of acetabular involvement and the patient's potential for prolonged survival. Reconstruction is not recommended for patients with a short life expectancy, even if acetabular involvement is present. For these patients, treatment generally consists of symptomatic measures, such as radiation therapy and protected weight bearing. In patients with massive acetabular involvement, such symptomatic measures may not provide sufficient pain relief, and a Girdlestone resection may be appropriate. Caution must be exercised, however, because the Girdlestone procedure usually does not achieve adequate pain relief and sacrifices independent ambulation in most patients.

In patients with a potential for prolonged survival, reconstruction of the acetabulum for relief of pain and improvement in function is appropriate. Both Harrington and colleagues[9–11] and Levy and associates[12] have extensive experience with management of these difficult cases, and their reconstructive approaches are discussed below.

Metastatic lesions involving only a small portion of the acetabulum have been defined by Harrington as class I (mild involvement).[9] In these cases, the superior and medial region of the acetabular globe and the lateral cortices are intact. With sufficient acetabular bone stock, conventional total hip arthroplasty is the reconstructive procedure of choice. Acetabular mesh is often used to reinforce the medial wall and to prevent cement from extruding into the pelvis. Significantly increased risk of loosening of the acetabular component has not been noted. Both Harrington[9] and Levy and coworkers[12] achieved satisfactory pain relief and adequate functional restoration in these patients after arthroplasty.

In patients with more moderate acetabular bone destruction resulting from metastatic lesions, reconstruction is more challenging. Harrington[9] categorizes these patients as class II (moderate involvement), indicating loss of the medial wall but an intact acetabular roof and rim. Both Levy and coworkers[12] and Harrington[9] advocate the use of a protrusio ring to transmit stress from the deficient medial wall to the intact peripheral cortical rim. Levy and colleagues[12] noted the need for adequate neck length of the femoral component to avoid impingement against the protrusio ring and the resultant increased risk of dislocation. Again, satisfactory pain relief and adequate functional results were reported by both Harrington and Levy and coworkers.

Consideration of reconstruction in patients with extensive metastatic involvement of the acetabulum is appropriate only in those with a prolonged life expectancy. Harrington defines this class III category as destruction of the medial wall, the superior region, and the lateral rim of the acetabulum.[9] Harrington developed specialized techniques of acetabular reconstruction and total hip arthroplasty in these patients, including placement of flexible Steinmann pins into the remaining intact superior ilium and across the sacroiliac joint.[9] These pins permit transmission of stress away from the deficient acetabular region and toward the ilium and the sacrum. Harrington noted no component loosening after eight such procedures.

The overall results in Harrington's series of 58 patients with acetabular reconstruction and hip arthroplasty for pathologic fracture or fracture-dislocation are promising.[9] Loosening of the acetabular component, caused by progression of local metastatic disease with loss of implant fixation, occurred in only 5 of the 58 patients. Good to excellent pain relief was obtained in 67% of the patients for at least 6 months and in 43% of the patients at 2 years. In terms of functional level, 80% of the patients were ambulatory at 6 months and 45% remained so at 2 years. Mean survival of the patients in the series was 19 months.

Finally, occult metastasis to the periacetabulum merits review. Metastatic lesions of the proximal femur have a high incidence of acetabular involvement.[8, 10] Habermann and associates reported that 80% of patients with metastatic disease of the proximal femur had biopsy-proven acetabular involvement, despite normal plain roentgenograms for many patients.[8] Because acetabular involvement is often not appreciated on the plain films, it may be necessary to perform tomography, isotope bone scanning, CT, or MRI to determine the amount of acetabular bone destruction. If acetabular disease is present, total hip arthroplasty is preferred to hemiarthroplasty. Although hemiarthroplasty (femoral endoprosthesis) and postoperative radiation therapy may give a good result initially, the hyperemic radiation-induced bone softening, coupled with progression of the acetabular metastasis, may cause a delayed intrapelvic protrusion of the endoprosthesis and resulting disability and pain. In the authors' experience with 35 total hip arthroplasties after pathologic fracture of the proximal femur, excellent results were achieved.

Summary

Management of bone tumors involving the pelvis begins with a complete assessment. In most patients, biopsy is mandatory to confirm the diagnosis. Treatment of most benign lesions consists of thorough curettage or marginal excision, followed by bone grafting. Aggressive or recurrent benign tumors may require *en bloc* resection with a wide margin to achieve local control. If the preoperative evaluation of a primary malignant lesion indicates that a satisfactory margin may be achieved by *en bloc* resection, limb salvage should be strongly considered. However, if an appropriate margin cannot be achieved by resection, amputation is preferred. Amputation, however, may not provide a better margin than limb salvage when lesions involve the iliosacral region, and this fact highlights the need for continued research into effective adjuvant treatment of these lesions.

Reconstruction after limb salvage varies according to the location of the lesion and the extent of the defect. In general, the authors favor reconstruction of femoropelvic continuity via arthrodesis. Definitive reconstructive procedures may be delayed until there is no evidence of wound infection or wound-healing problems.

Patients who have metastatic lesions of the pelvis but no acetabular involvement are generally treated symptomatically. In selected patients with prolonged life expectancy who have metatasis involving the acetabulum, satisfactory results may be achieved by one of many reconstructive procedures.

References

1. Campanacci M, Capanna R: Closing remarks. *In* Enneking WF (ed): Limb Salvage in Musculoskeletal Oncology. New York, Churchill Livingstone, 1987, p 190.
2. Capanna R, Guernelli N, Ruggiere P, Biagini R, Toni A, Picci P, Campanacci M: Periacetabular pelvic resections. *In* Enneking WF (ed): Limb Salvage in Musculoskeletal Oncology. New York, Churchill Livingstone, 1987, pp 141–146.
3. Dahlin DC, Unni KK: Bone Tumors: General Aspects and Data on 8,542 Cases, 4th ed. Springfield, IL, Charles C Thomas, 1986.
4. Dunham WK Jr: Acetabular resections for sarcoma. *In* Enneking WF (ed): Limb Salvage in Musculoskeletal Oncology. New York, Churchill Livingstone, 1987, pp 170–184.
5. Enneking WF: Clinical Musculoskeletal Pathology. Gainesville, FL, Shorter Printing Company, 1986, p 358.
5a. Enneking WF: Modification of the system for functional evaluation of surgical management of musculoskeletal tumors. *In* Enneking WF (ed): Limb Salvage in Musculoskeletal Oncology. New York, Churchill Livingstone, 1987, pp 626–639.
6. Enneking WF, Dunham WK: Resection and reconstruction for primary neoplasms involving the innominate bone. J Bone Joint Surg 60A:731–746, 1978.
7. Enneking WF, Menendez LR: Functional evaluation of various reconstructions after periacetabular resection of iliac lesions. *In* Enneking WF (ed): Limb Salvage in Musculoskeletal Oncology. New York, Churchill Livingstone, 1987, pp 117–135.
8. Habermann ET, Sachs R, Stern RE, Hirsh DM, Anderson WJ Jr: The pathology and treatment of metastatic disease of the femur. Clin Orthop 169:70–82, 1982.
9. Harrington KD: The management of acetabular insufficiency secondary to metastatic malignant disease. J Bone Joint Surg 63A:653–664, 1981.
10. Harrington KD, Johnston JO, Turner RH, Green DL: The use of methylmethacrylate as an adjunct in the internal fixation of malignant neoplastic fractures. J Bone Joint Surg 54A:1665–1676, 1972.
11. Harrington KD, Sim FH, Enis JE, Johnston JO, Dick HM, Gristina AG: Methylmethacrylate as an adjunct in internal fixation of pathological fractures: Experience with three hundred and seventy-five cases. J Bone Joint Surg 58A:1047–1055, 1976.
12. Levy RN, Sherry HS, Siffert RS: Surgical management of metastatic disease of bone at the hip. Clin Orthop 169:62–69, 1982.
13. Mutschler W, Burri C, Kiefer H: Functional results after pelvic resection with endoprosthetic replacement. *In* Enneking WF (ed): Limb Salvage in Musculoskeletal Oncology. New York, Churchill Livingstone, 1987, pp 156–166.
13a. O'Connor MI, Sim FH: Salvage of the limb in the treatment of malignant pelvic tumors. J Bone Joint Surg 71A(4):481–494, 1989.
14. Nesbit ME, Perez CA, Tefft M, Burgert ED, Vietti

TJ, Kissane J, Pritchard DJ, Gehan EA: Multimodal therapy for the management of primary nonmetastatic Ewing's sarcoma of bone. An Intergroup study. NCI Monogr 56:259, 1986.

15. Rosenberg AG, Mankin HJ: Complications of allograft surgery. *In* Epps CH Jr (ed): Complications in Orthopedic Surgery, 2nd ed, Vol 2. Philadelphia, JB Lippincott, 1986, pp 1385–1417.

16. Tomeno B, Languepin A, Gerber C: Local resection with limb salvage for the treatment of periacetabular bone tumors: Functional results in nine cases. *In* Enneking WF (ed): Limb Salvage in Musculoskeletal Oncology. New York, Churchill Livingstone, 1987, pp 147–156.

CHAPTER **14**

Hand Tumors

JACK CHOUEKA
MICHAEL R. HAUSMAN

The presence of a mass or swelling in the hand is one of the most common complaints seen by the hand specialist. Confronted with such a patient, the surgeon must make two fundamental, though not necessarily simple, decisions. First, while the exact diagnosis may not be immediately apparent, one must decide if the lesion is obviously benign or if a biopsy is required. Second, one must decide upon the appropriate treatment. Here again, the problem is somewhat simpler than may appear. Most benign hand tumors are adequately treated by intralesional or marginal resection, while malignant lesions require wide or radical extirpation, the parameters of which are discussed later. While the variety of tumors is great, in most cases a reasoned analysis of demographic, physiologic, and radiologic data, in conjunction with the physical examination, can usually yield an accurate diagnosis and determination of the necessity for a biopsy.

Important information should be gleaned from the history including the age of the patient, duration of the mass, the presence of pain (and pain at night), exacerbating factors such as cold, associated neurologic or vascular abnormalities, and any associated systemic medical conditions. The possibility of myeloma or metastatic disease from the breast, lung, or kidney should also be kept in mind.[69]

The physical examination is facilitated by comparison with the opposite side. Usually, the swelling of the tumor is not subtle. In equivocal cases, Littler's method of measuring the circumference with ½-inch paper tape is useful and reproducible. In addition to the size, location, color, texture, mobility, and tenderness, any motion observed in conjunction with adjacent tendons or joints is important. Joint range of motion should be recorded, along with sensibility changes reflected in the two-point or moving two-point discrimination test. The Allen test is helpful when vascular involvement is suspected.

Radiography is suggested in all but the most obvious cases. Even apparently simple problems, such as a wrist ganglion or mucous cyst, may be manifestations of underlying conditions such as arthritis, carpal instability, or intraosseous ganglion.[132] Such knowledge would help refine the treatment to deal with the underlying pathology as well as the manifestation. Xeroradiography has not been particularly useful in our experience, but computed tomography (CT) and magnetic resonance imaging (MRI) are excellent for bone and soft tissue lesions, respectively. MRI may be particularly helpful for palmar or wrist lesions, where it is important to know the extent of the lesion and whether or not it has violated the carpal canal.

Angiography may also be useful in planning the resection and is mandatory if some type of flap or microvascular reconstruction is anticipated.

In pragmatic terms, one may consider hand tumors in three broad categories: skin lesions, bone lesions, and those affecting the intervening connective tissue. Speaking in broad terms, it is not entirely absurd to generalize that malignant skin lesions are ugly or dark, malignant bone lesions are painful, and those of the intervening tissues are large, firm, and/or painful. These simple rules, melded with a bit of common sense, will serve surprisingly well. One should bear in mind that statistically, the overwhelming majority of tumors (94 to 95%) are benign.[11, 18, 104] Furthermore, in the hand, the distinction between benign and malignant tumors is usually obvious. The appearance and presentation of a ganglion or synovial cyst should allow for immediate diagnosis and reassurance. Widely accepted distinctions between benign and malignant processes generally apply to the hand as well. Thus, well-circumscribed, slow-growing lesions are generally benign. Pain associated with benign processes in the hand is usually due to adjacent structures or underlying pathology and is subtly different from that associated with malignancy. A truly "waxing and waning" lesion that grows and diminishes in size is almost certainly a benign ganglion or cystic process communicating with a joint.

Skin Lesions

The relative mobility of the skin in relation to the underlying structures in the hand usually permits easy determination of whether or not the lesion originates in the skin or underlying tissue. A history of chemical or radiation exposure (including solar) should alert one to the possibility of malignancy. The family history may also be pertinent because certain types of melanoma are thought to be inherited.[72]

BENIGN LESIONS

Common benign conditions include common warts, epidermoid inclusion cysts (nearly always with a history of trauma), actinic keratosis, knuckle pads, and keratoacanthoma.

Warts are caused by a papovirus and usually resolve spontaneously with time.[89] Other treatments include freezing with liquid nitrogen, electrocautery, and surgical excision.[2, 111] Cauterization of periungual warts should be done with care to avoid scarring and contracture of the eponychial fold or even damage to the geminal matrix. These are vexing complications of treatment. Our personal preference is for repeated application of liquid nitrogen, which seems to afford better control over the degree of destruction and is less uncomfortable for the patient.

Actinic keratoses occur on the dorsum of hands in an older population[128] exposed to the elements or arsenical compounds. While considered benign, these lesions should be observed for any signs of malignant degeneration, heralded by bleeding, deeper ulceration, or centrifugal growth. If there is any doubt, biopsy is appropriate.

Inclusion cysts are usually associated with a history of penetrating trauma, which is thought to "plant" or "seed" epithelial cells in deeper layers. They are more common in areas of glabrous skin. The collection of cells produces the characteristic "cheesy" keratin, and treatment is by simple surgical excision.

Keratoacanthoma is another lesion found on the dorsum of the hand, as well as the face (Fig. 14–1). Differentiation from squamous cell carcinoma is difficult, even on histologic section.[76] Typically, keratoacanthoma has a more rapid onset and a keratin plug that may be removed from the center of the lesion. This is not characteristic of squamous cell carcinoma. In situations of doubt, wide excision is the safest course.

MALIGNANT LESIONS

The most common malignant skin tumors are Bowen's disease, squamous cell carcinoma,

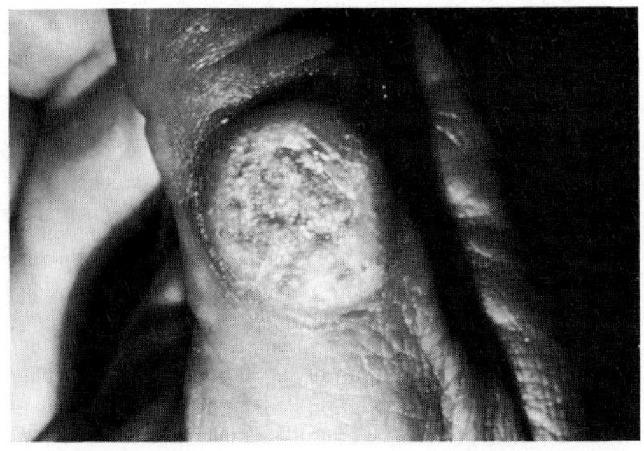

FIGURE 14–1. Typical "heaped-up" appearance of keratoacanthoma.

basal cell carcinoma, malignant melanoma, and sweat gland carcinoma. Metastatic soft tissue lesions of the hand are extremely rare. *Squamous cell carcinoma* accounts for 90% of malignant skin lesions.[18, 58] Sunlight, ionizing radiation, and arsenical chemicals are risk factors. Prior to our appreciation of the dangers of ionizing radiation, squamous cell carcinoma was frequently seen in dentists and shoe salesmen using fluoroscopy in fitting shoes. Squamous cell carcinoma begins as a superficial, scaly lesion that is slightly indurated and is resistant to local therapy. As it grows, it becomes increasingly indurated and develops a center ulceration or crater (Fig. 14–2).[2]

Bowen's disease, or intraepidermal squamous cell carcinoma, may be thought of as a forme fruste of squamous cell carcinoma. It is frequently associated with carcinoma of the viscera.[100] Surgical excision is the recommended treatment.

Another variant is the *subungual squamous cell carcinoma,* which is frequently confused with fungal disease.[59] Refractory "chronic paronychia" may ultimately require biopsy. In general, squamous cell carcinoma affects the dorsum of the hand, and treatment is wide excision and primary closure or skin grafting.

The incidence of lymph node metastases with squamous cell carcinoma and the role of lymphadenectomy are disputed.[53, 58] Spread to the regional nodes probably occurs in 5 to 15% of cases.[9, 53, 58] Lymph node dissection is not routinely necessary, but is reserved for those with demonstrable lymphadenopathy.[53, 58, 68] Enlarged axillary nodes may be seen with CT and may help in evaluating the need for lymph node biopsy or lymphadenectomy.

Basal cell carcinoma is, as elsewhere in the body, much less aggressive than squamous cell carcinoma. Clinically, it appears as a well-marginated, firm, "pearly" lesion. Excision with a margin of normal tissue is adequate treatment for this less aggressive lesion.

Malignant melanoma is becoming increasingly prevalent, and roughly 16% of melanomas are found in the hand and arm.[6, 122] Various types are described, including superficial spreading melanoma, nodular melanoma (which tends to grow deeper at an early stage and thus has a poorer prognosis), lentigo maligna melanoma (which develops within a Hutchinson freckle), and acral lentiginous melanoma (which occurs on the glabrous skin of the hands and feet and has an extremely poor prognosis) (Fig. 14–3).[28, 50, 127]

Two staging systems are widely used. The Clark system refers to the depth of invasion as follows: level I—epidermis; level II—papillary dermis; level III—interface of papillary and reticular dermis; level IV—reticular dermis but no fat; level V—invading subcutaneous tissue.[27] The Breslow system refers simply to the depth of the lesion as measured with a special optical micrometer.[15, 16] The stages are highly significant prognostically.[6]

Treatment is by wide excision. Lesions less than 0.76 mm thick may be excised with margins of 1 to 2 cm of normal tissue. Deeper lesions should have wider margins.[26, 39, 110] The

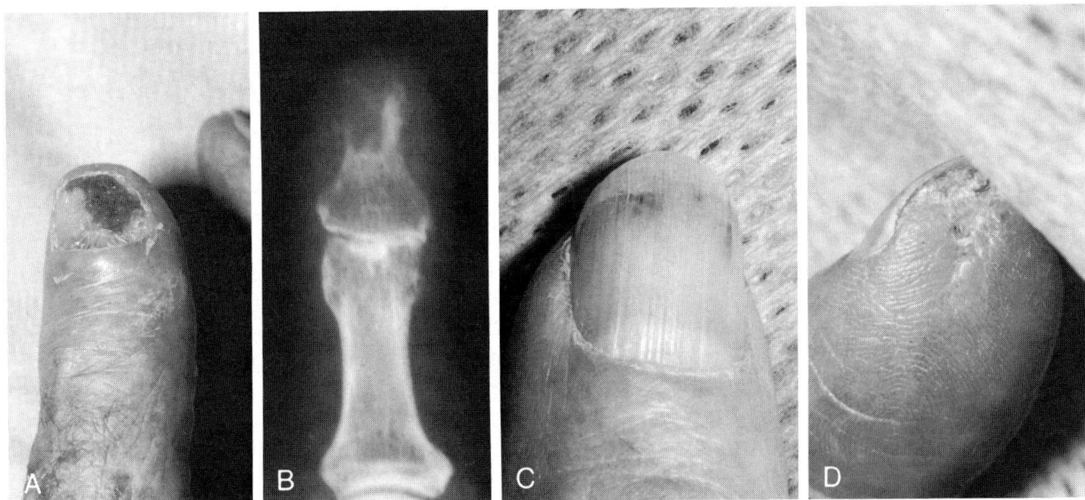

FIGURE 14–2. *A*, Squamous cell carcinoma of the nail bed. *B*, Radiograph shows degree of bony destruction. *C* and *D*, A more subtle appearance is also possible.

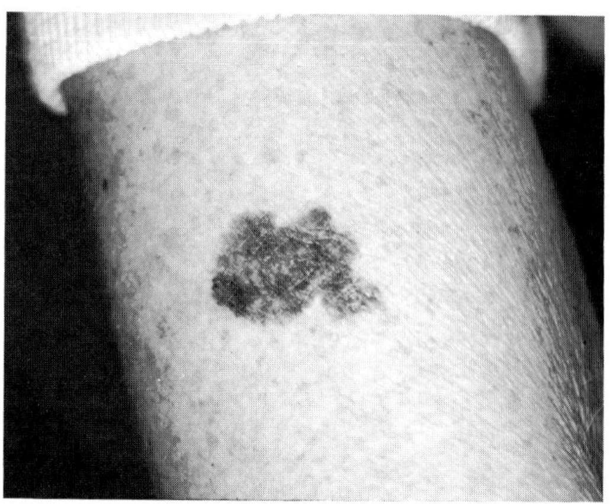

FIGURE 14–3. Melanoma *in situ*. The appearance of melanoma varies widely, and suspicious or changing lesions should be biopsied.

role of axillary lymphadenectomy is also debatable but is probably of value in deeper lesions, 60% of which may be associated with metastases. However, this has not been conclusively demonstrated and must be individualized on a case-by-case basis.[6, 107, 131]

A final category of malignant skin tumors is the *sweat gland carcinoma*. An extremely rare occurrence in the hand, only 26 cases have been reported.[136] The natural history is early metastasis to the regional lymph nodes, bone, and lung; the prognosis is poor.[29, 76] A disease of later decades, the sweat gland carcinoma appears as a nodular ulceration. Treatment requires early detection and wide excision.[29]

Bone Tumors

BENIGN TUMORS

Benign tumors of bone include enchondroma, osteochondroma, unicameral bone cyst, osteoid osteoma, osteoblastoma, aneurysmal bone cyst, intraosseous ganglia, and giant cell tumor of bony origin (which should be distinguished from those of tendon sheath). The tumors may be indolent and present serendipitously or as pathologic fractures. The radiograph and history are usually sufficient to distinguish benign from malignant processes.

Enchondroma is the most common bony tumor of the hand and usually affects 20- to 50-year-old persons. The hand, especially the proximal phalanx, is the site of 62% of all enchondromas (Fig. 14–4).[113] The lesions are well marginated, and the classic "ground glass" appearance on radiography is distinctive. Numerous treatments have been advocated, but most authors recommend curettage and bone grafting. Malignant degeneration of a solitary enchondroma is exceedingly rare.[30, 32] However, those with multiple enchondromas, as occurs in Maffucci's syndrome (multiple enchondromata and hemangiomata), have a higher risk of malignant degeneration and must be closely followed for clinical or radiographic changes. Malignant transformation occurs in approximately 18.6% of patients with Maffucci's syndrome.[46, 78] Such patients should be closely monitored for signs of further growth of the tumor, pain, or increased activity on bone scan.

The next most common benign bony tumor of the hand is the *osteochondroma*. They are found almost exclusively in patients with multiple osteochondromatosis and occur in the metaphyseal area of long bones.[71, 84] Such tumors usually present with mechanical symptoms or swelling and may cause angular deformities of the long bones or limitation of range of motion.[66] Malignant degeneration in the hand is exceedingly rare and is heralded by growth after skeletal maturity and new onset of pain.[51] Surgical treatment is most predictable after skeletal maturity, but earlier intervention is advocated in cases of progressive angular deformity. A variant of the tumors is the subungual osteochondroma, which can occur in the hand as well as the great toe. Again, treatment is by local excision.[41]

Unicameral bone cysts appear during the first and second decades of life and have a male predilection of 3:1.[113] They have a characteristic eccentric, metaphyseal radiolucent appearance that is frequently septated.[86] Although the lesions may be large, they should not exceed the diameter of the epiphyseal plate. Several authors report success with methylprednisolone injection.[112] The likelihood of success increases as the patient approaches skeletal maturity. Failures can be treated successfully with curettage and bone grafting.

In general, benign lesions such as enchondromata and unicameral bone cysts presenting as pathologic fractures should be managed conservatively and allowed to heal prior to treatment of the tumor. This makes the surgery technically easier and permits earlier rehabilitation to minimize postoperative adhesions and stiffness.

Aneurysmal bone cysts, while rare in the hand,[33, 64] constitute a considerable therapeutic challenge. These usually occur in the second

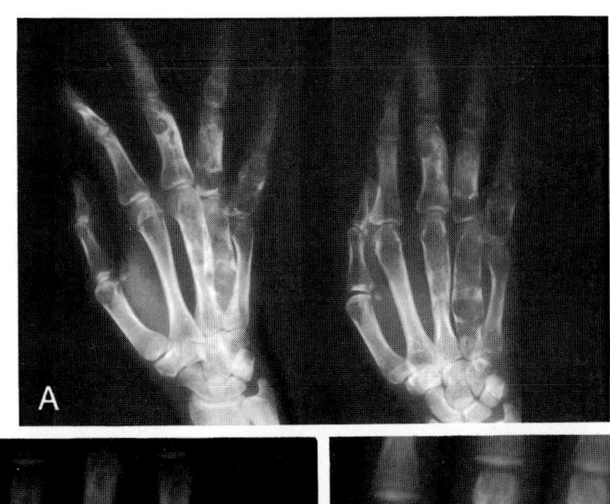

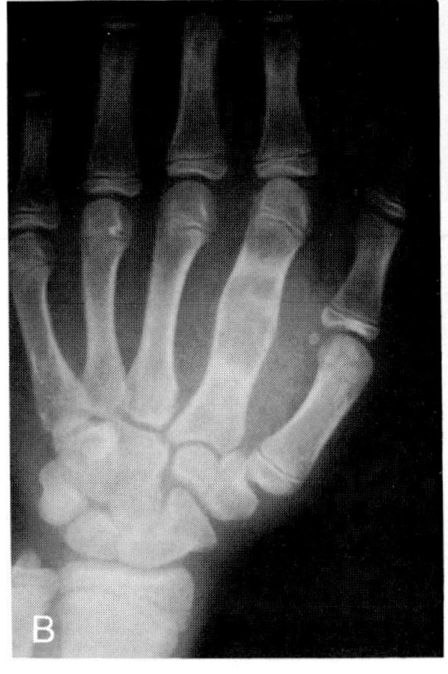

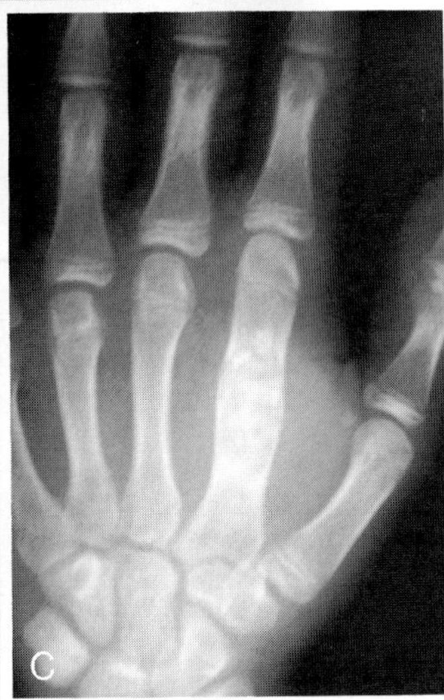

FIGURE 14–4. *A,* Radiograph shows the multiple enchondromata associated with Ollier's disease. There is a broad spectrum of lesions represented in this patient, ranging from a small, well-circumscribed benign lesion, to much larger, more aggressive tumors. *B* and *C,* Treatment is curettage, or curettage and grafting. In the case of pathologic fractures, surgery is best deferred until after healing has occurred. Suspicious lesions should be biopsied and the entire specimen carefully reviewed for foci of malignancy.

or third decades and affect males and females in equal numbers. Aneurysmal bone cysts can occur in the distal phalanx and destroy the bone sufficiently so as to appear malignant. The radiographic appearance of a "ballooned-out," large metaphyseal lesion is well described.[33, 64] The lesion may appear quite aggressive and may show an associated Codman's triangle. The epiphysis will only be affected after skeletal maturity.[33] Tumors of the phalanges may be difficult to extirpate while preserving the digit. Some advocate preoperative arterial embolization.[42] Because the lesion is benign, marginal or even intralesional resection and grafting are worthwhile, despite the high incidence of recurrence.[7] The aggressive appearance of this lesion requires that a specimen be examined microscopically. In cases of *en-bloc* resections, reconstruction with allograft or nonvascularized autograft is disappointing. Vascularized bone graft may lead to better results in the future if the articular surfaces can be spared.

Osteoid osteoma may be found in the long bones or carpal bones during the first two decades. The classic history of pain relieved by aspirin should raise a high index of suspicion. Bone scan is uniformly "hot" and complex motion tomography is useful.[55, 73] CT scan, while helpful in larger bones, has not been as useful in the hand. Treatment is complete excision.[21, 126] The technique of intraoperative quantitative measurement with radionuclide scanning and scintigraphy is useful in confirming the complete extirpation of the tumor if there is doubt.[56, 96, 129]

Osteoblastoma, while related to osteoid osteoma, is histologically distinct. It has not been reported in the carpus. Treatment is curettage and grafting.[41]

Other, more unusual tumors include the nonossifying fibroma, Brown tumor of hyperparathyroidism, and the inclusion cyst. *Nonossifying fibroma* is seen in the hand in the first two decades as an eccentrically located radiolucent, metaphyseal lesion. It may regress spontaneously, and recidivist cases can be treated with curettage and grafting.[115] *Brown tumors* are multiple osteolytic, cortex-expanding lesions associated with hyperparathyroid-

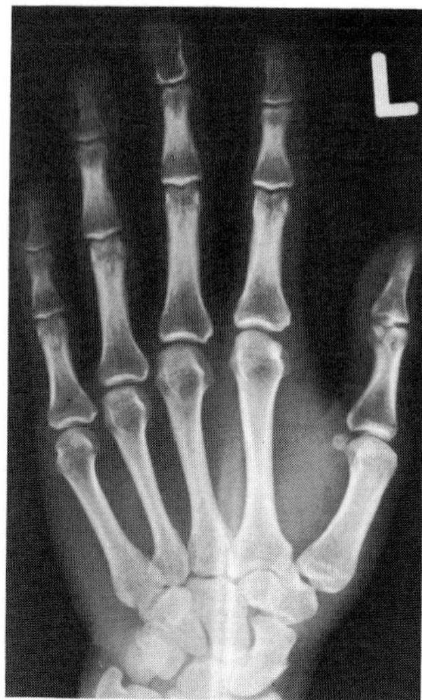

FIGURE 14–5. Radiographic appearance of the epidermoid inclusion cyst. The lesion may grow quite large and involve the cortex, but the remaining cortical borders appear benign. Local excision and curettage with grafting suffice for treatment.

ism. The characteristic radiographic appearance and associated elevated PTH, calcium, alkaline phosphatase, and decreased phosphate levels are diagnostic.[106] *Inclusion cysts* may be intraosseous and are seen in the distal phalanx. They are usually associated with some history of penetrating trauma, which is thought to drive epidermal elements into the bone. The spherical, well-marginated appearance on radiography is usually diagnostic (Fig. 14–5).[75]

Giant cell tumor (GCT) of bone (Fig. 14–6) must be distinguished from the giant cell tumor of tendon sheath, which, while histologically similar, has a different prognosis. At times GCT has a paradoxically aggressive behavior, and malignant degeneration has been reported.[4] According to Schajowicz, a progressive, potentially malignant process can recur in about 50%, sarcomatous transformation in about 10%, and metastases can be produced without apparent previous malignant changes.[113] GCT tends to appear in the third and fourth decades and seems to have a slight female predominance. GCT of the hand may also be associated with other sites.[99] Its radiographic appearance as an expansile, eccentric metaphyseal lesion is distinctive but can be confused with a simple bone cyst, aneurysmal bone cyst, or even an enchondroma that has been previously fractured.[34, 80, 116] The cortex is thinned or breached, and little periosteal reaction is provoked. Giant cell tumors have been graded by Jaffe,[63] but the prognostic utility of this distinction is disputed.[91, 99, 123]

Treatment may be begun with curettage and either autogenous or allograft grafting if the lesion is not extensive. Cryosurgery has a high complication rate.[87, 88] Others have advocated

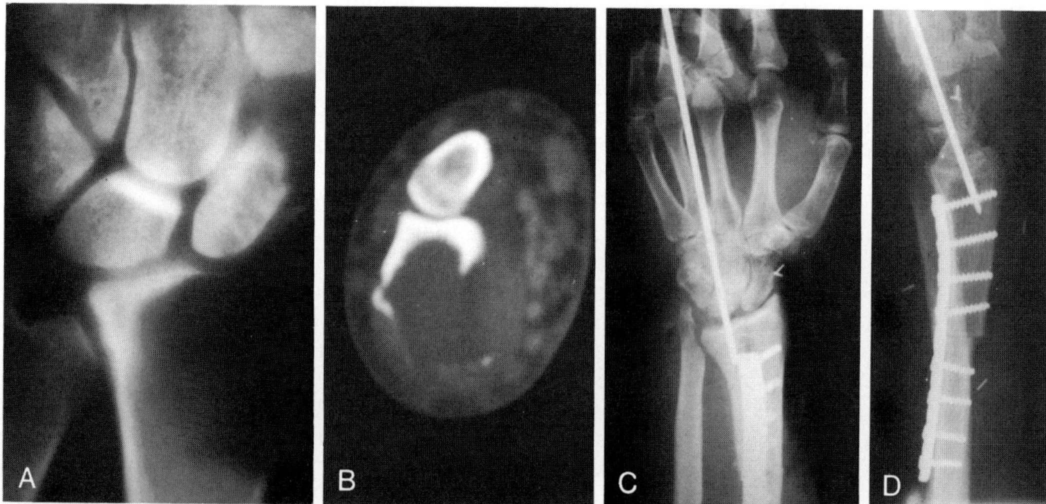

FIGURE 14–6. *A,* This radiograph is typical of the expansile, metaphyseal giant cell tumor, causing cortical expansion, thinning and, at times, infraction. The lesion can be treated by curettage and grafting or cementing. *B,* Recurrent giant cell tumor of the distal radius. Pathologic examination suggested an aggressive, though not frankly malignant lesion. *C, En-bloc* resection and allograft reconstruction were performed. The contralateral radius is used in the reversed position to provide additional volar buttressing against subluxation. *D,* Follow-up at 1 year shows good incorporation of the graft and excellent function.

curettage and cementing with methylmethacrylate. Multiple recurrences or a change to more aggressive behavior is an indication for *en-bloc* resection. Reconstruction with allograft or vascularized autogenous graft can offer excellent results.[94, 120, 133]

MALIGNANT TUMORS

Pain, rapid growth, and aggressive radiographic features are hallmarks of malignancy. Worrisome lesions should be staged and biopsied. Staging includes a blood count, chemistries, alkaline phosphatase, erythrocyte sedimentation rate, serum protein electrophoresis for myeloma, bone scan, and chest CT. The surgeon ultimately responsible for definitive treatment should take specimens for histologic examination by using longitudinally oriented incisions that will not compromise subsequent definitive care.

Enneking has devised a grading system with prognostic significance.[47] Based on the surgical stage, incorporating the degree of malignancy and whether the tumor is intra- or extracompartmental, a surgical procedure may be devised. One must consider that the anatomy of the hand and digits tends to defy the standard definition of tissue compartments, making strict application of staging and margin definitions difficult.

Surgical excision may be intralesional (as in curettage), marginal, wide (an *en-bloc* resection with normal tissue), or radical, usually involving substantial ablation in the hand. In dealing with malignant tumors, intralesional and marginal resections are most always inadequate and one should aim to achieve a wide excision. Preoperative chemotherapy may be of use in certain large lesions to shrink the tumor and thus facilitate limb-sparing surgery.[62, 108]

The most common malignant primary bone tumors in the hand are chondrosarcoma, osteosarcoma, and Ewing's sarcoma. Other lesions such as fibrosarcoma, hemangiosarcoma, and metastatic disease, including myeloma, are rare but must be included in the differential diagnosis.

Chondrosarcoma is a tumor of the later decades. It may appear similar to an enchondroma or appear very large and aggressive with considerable calcification (Fig. 14–7). Soft tissue chondrosarcoma also occurs in the hand (Fig. 14–8).[36, 98, 130] The issue of malignant degeneration of preexisting enchondromas is not entirely resolved, but this is probably rare. This does occur, however, in Maffucci's syndrome of multiple enchondromata and hemangiomata,[30, 46, 78] and the treatment of choice is *en-bloc* resection with adequate margins and not intralesional curettage.

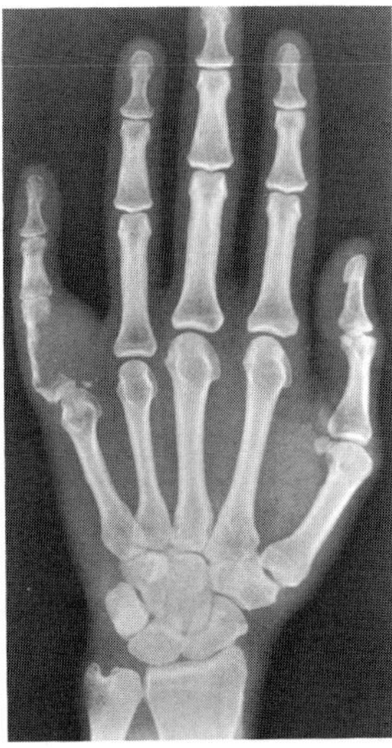

FIGURE 14–7. Radiograph shows the aggressive nature of malignant cartilage tumors. The soft tissue extension can be quite large and may require resection of neurovascular structures or tendons from adjacent fingers.

Osteogenic sarcoma is uncommon in the hand but may occur in the distal radius. Like chondrosarcoma, it shows a predilection for the proximal phalanges and metacarpals. However, it usually occurs in the first two decades of life.[24, 52] Radiographically the lesions appear as a blastic or mixed blastic/lytic, aggressive, expansile lesion. Adequate biopsy is always required, as extirpation usually requires ray amputation, at least, in a young person. The role of adjuvant chemotherapy has been explored.[62, 108]

Ewing's sarcoma also occurs during the first decade of life. It is a soft tissue swelling, usually warm; frequently there is an elevation of the sedimentation rate and a radiographic appearance as a permeative, lytic lesion with periosteal reaction that resembles osteomyelitis. Sickle cell dactylitis is another condition that may resemble Ewing's sarcoma.[43, 67] Definitive diagnosis is by open biopsy, and treatment is wide resection or amputation. Adjuvant chemotherapy is routine. The prognosis for peripheral lesions is better than for those that are centrally located.[85]

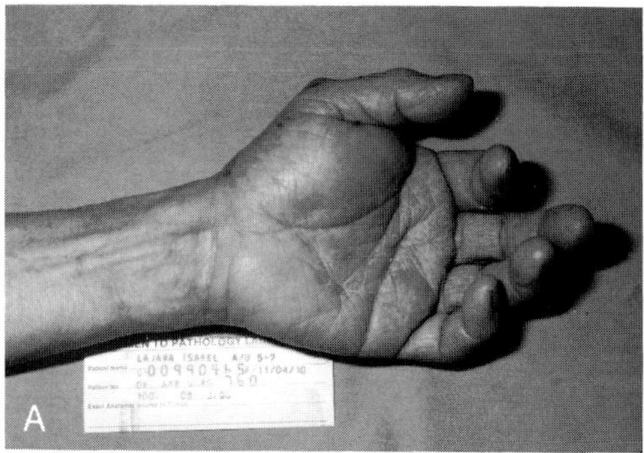

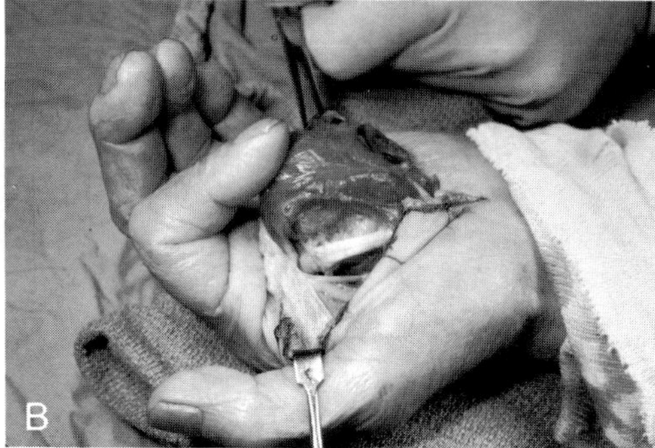

FIGURE 14–8. *A,* Large mass in the first web-space is an extraskeletal chondrosarcoma. This older patient was blind and refused amputation. *B, En-bloc* resection was performed, and there was no recurrence at 8 months.

While uncommon, the presence of a malignant-appearing lesion in the hand should also raise the question of metastatic disease, especially if the lesion is in the distal phalanx.[69, 121, 138] Lesions of the breast, lung, and kidney are most commonly metastatic to the hand bones.[14, 31, 69] Obviously, investigation of the primary tumor is imperative, and open biopsy may offer useful information. Treatment is by wide excision or amputation.

Treatment of Malignant Bone Tumors

Generally, while intralesional or marginal resection suffices for benign tumors, the treatment of malignant lesions is much more involved and is dictated by distinct considerations and principles. With the realization that these are life-threatening disorders, the primary goal of treatment is eradication of the tumor. While peripheral variants of certain tumors, such as Ewing's sarcoma, seem to have a better survival rate, the malignant potential of these lesions should not be underestimated. In addition, the ability of the hand to resume excellent function after deletion of one or even two rays must be borne in mind when the lesions are present in the digits. Carpal, metacarpal, or thumb lesions are more challenging reconstructive problems and may require considerable ingenuity, including the use of microvascular free tissue transfer, to preserve or restore function.

The treatment of malignant lesions of the hand was discussed by Smith in 1977,[119] and the use of open biopsy to insure representative material was encouraged. Design of the biopsy incision should permit subsequent *en-bloc* resection, and all bleeding must be controlled to prevent contamination by subcutaneous hematoma. The use of a tourniquet is controversial, but no study has ever demonstrated an increased incidence of metastasis with a tourniquet.[118] In general, we would recommend use of the tourniquet for more precise surgery with less trauma. We do not use a tourniquet for the biopsy and do not recommend using an Esmarch bandage to exsanguinate the hand and arm.

In defining an adequate wide or radical excision, the tumor should not be visualized during the resection. Ray amputation is an adequate resection for digital and some less aggressive metacarpal lesions (Figs. 14–9 and 14–10). One must, however, recall the fascial planes and spaces in the hand. Thus, cortical breakthrough of a metacarpal lesion may produce contamination of the carpal canal, necessitating complete amputation.

Lesions about the dorsum of the hand, carpus, or distal forearm require special consideration. One must consider the three aspects of reconstruction: skin coverage, skeletal support, and functional restoration. Adjacent skin flaps are not desirable in tumor reconstruction because of the possibility of contamination of adjacent areas. We prefer skin grafting, when feasible, or remote microvascular free tissue transfer if more extensive or durable coverage is required. In such cases, care should be taken to use separate instruments and avoid contamination of other areas.

Loss of bony support may be reconstructed by a variety of techniques, including fusion to adjacent structures, autograft or allograft replacement, or composite free tissue transfer including bone and muscle or skin. For example, the radius with GCT can be reconstructed with creation of a one-bone forearm, allograft replacement, fibular vascularized, or nonvascularized autograft. Replacement of a single digit or even two digits is generally not indicated, except in the case of the thumb, where secondary reconstruction with a toe-to-thumb transfer may be considered after final pathology is reviewed and the prognosis appears favorable. With all methods of reconstruction, the foremost objective must be obliteration of the disease. Furthermore, one should bear in mind that a hand with four or even three good digits is more useful than a stiff, scarred, insensate hand with a full complement of fingers. Thus, while cosmetic considerations may argue for or against a particular reconstruction, a reasonable balance should be sought.

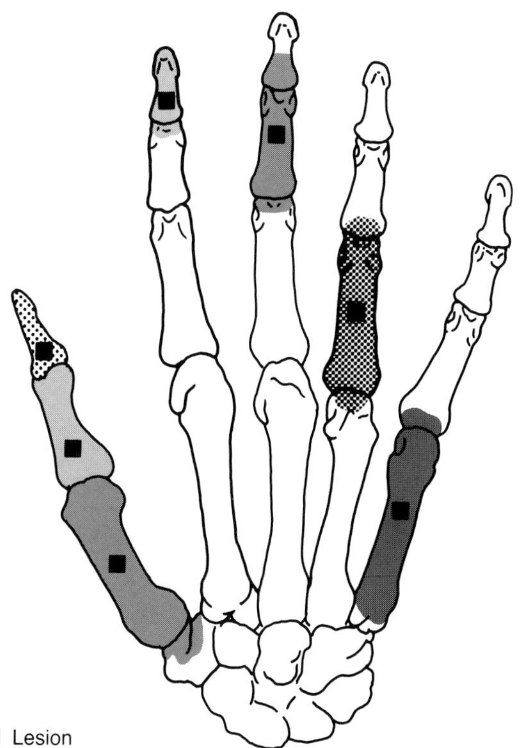

FIGURE 14–9. Intracompartmental bony lesions may be treated by the margins indicated in the shaded areas. Practically, resection frequently includes structures distal to the involved bone, although reconstruction is feasible in some cases, particularly metacarpal lesions. Treatment must be individualized. For instance, a low-grade metaphyseal lesion may permit sparing of the articular surfaces, facilitating reconstruction. If, however, the lesion is extracompartmental and high-grade, the treatment scheme for soft tissue malignancy outlined in Figure 14–10 applies.

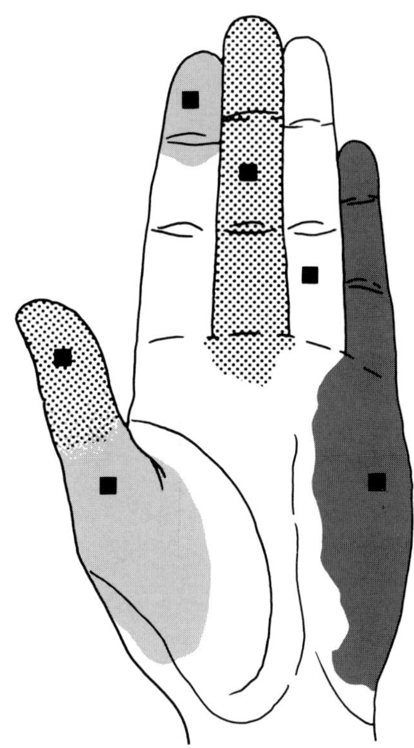

FIGURE 14–10. Guidelines for resection of malignant soft tissue tumors of the hand. Although lesions at the middle phalangeal level are usually treated adequately by disarticulation at the metacarpophalangeal level, cosmesis and function may be better if ray amputation is performed, particularly in the central digits. A lesion in the metacarpal area usually required ablation of at least part of the adjacent ray and may necessitate removal of the hand if it extends into the carpal canal. Lesions in the thumb metacarpal area are treated with resection of the thenar musculature. Thumb lesions may often be reconstructed with microvascular toe transfer.

Soft Tissue Tumors

Of the three categories, soft tissue tumors are the least obvious to diagnose. Soft tissue tumors are not grossly evident and because they often have the same radiodensity as the surrounding structures, they are not often evident on radiography.

BENIGN TUMORS

Most soft tissue tumors in the hand are benign. In general, if the tumor is smaller than 2 cm, is not ulcerated or painful, and is not fixed to the surrounding structures, it is probably benign. If one is concerned about malignancy, a biopsy will be necessary in addition to routine laboratory and staging studies discussed in the section on malignant bone tumors. MRI scan is excellent for defining the extent of soft tissue tumors of the hand. Imaging with special coil will permit identification of fascial planes and spaces of the hand, as well as adjacent tendons, vessels, and nerves. Such information is critical in planning the extent of a resection.

However, if malignancy is not suspected, then the differential diagnosis is narrowed considerably. Treatment is also simplified, as management of benign soft tissue tumors in the hand is almost always excisional biopsy or "marginal" excision.

Ganglia represent 50 to 70% of all soft tissue tumors of the hand[90] and usually afflict women between the ages of 20 and 50.[8, 139] A ganglion most often originates in the dorsum of the wrist, in particular the scapholunate ligament and joint complex.[3] Dorsal wrist ganglia constitute 60 to 70% of all ganglions.[139] Volar wrist ganglia make up 20% of the ganglia and usually arise from the tendon sheaths or capsule adjacent to the radial flexor tendon.[139] Other, less common sites, include the flexor tendon sheaths of the fingers and the distal interphalangeal joints. The latter are often referred to as mucous cysts. These later cysts are associated with osteoarthritis of the distal interphalangeal joint and osteophytes (Figs. 14–11 and 14–12).

Ganglia may be associated with weakness and, if present in the volar side of the wrist, can mimic carpal tunnel syndrome.[61] The onset, duration, and any associated symptoms, especially any history of inciting trauma that may suggest underlying carpal instability, should be recorded. The physical examination should concentrate on definitive identification of the lesion and evaluation of the neurovascular status of the extremity. Transillumination with a penlight will positively distinguish cystic from solid lesions. Treatment should be individualized for each patient. An asymptomatic patient can be left untreated and reassured that the ganglion is not malignant. Some studies show spontaneous regression.[12, 104] Numerous nonsurgical therapies involving rupture of the cyst have been tried over the centuries. Today the most effective nonsurgical treatment is aspiration followed by steroid injection. When nonsurgical therapy is ineffective, complete ganglionectomy is recommended. This procedure should include resection of 1 to 2 mm of the weakened capsule or ligament and repair using nonabsorbable suture.

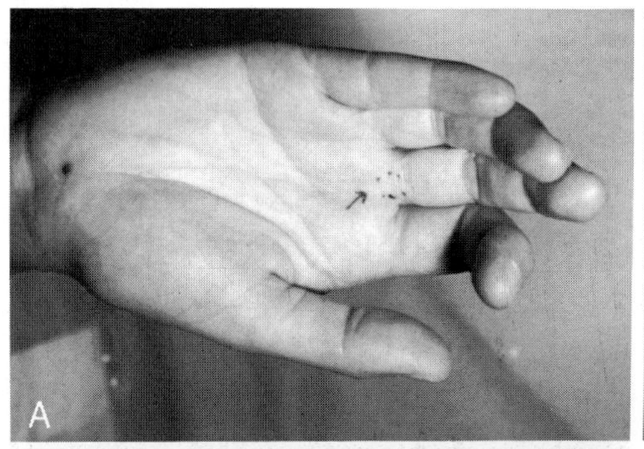

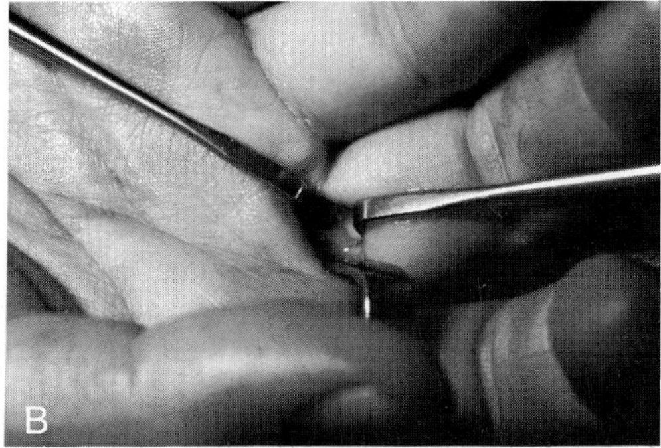

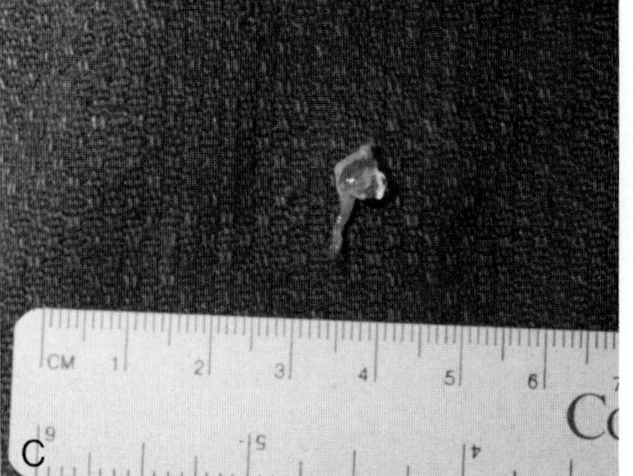

FIGURE 14–11. *A* to *C*, The firm, tender, centrally located nodule at the palmodigital crease is classic for a synovial cyst.

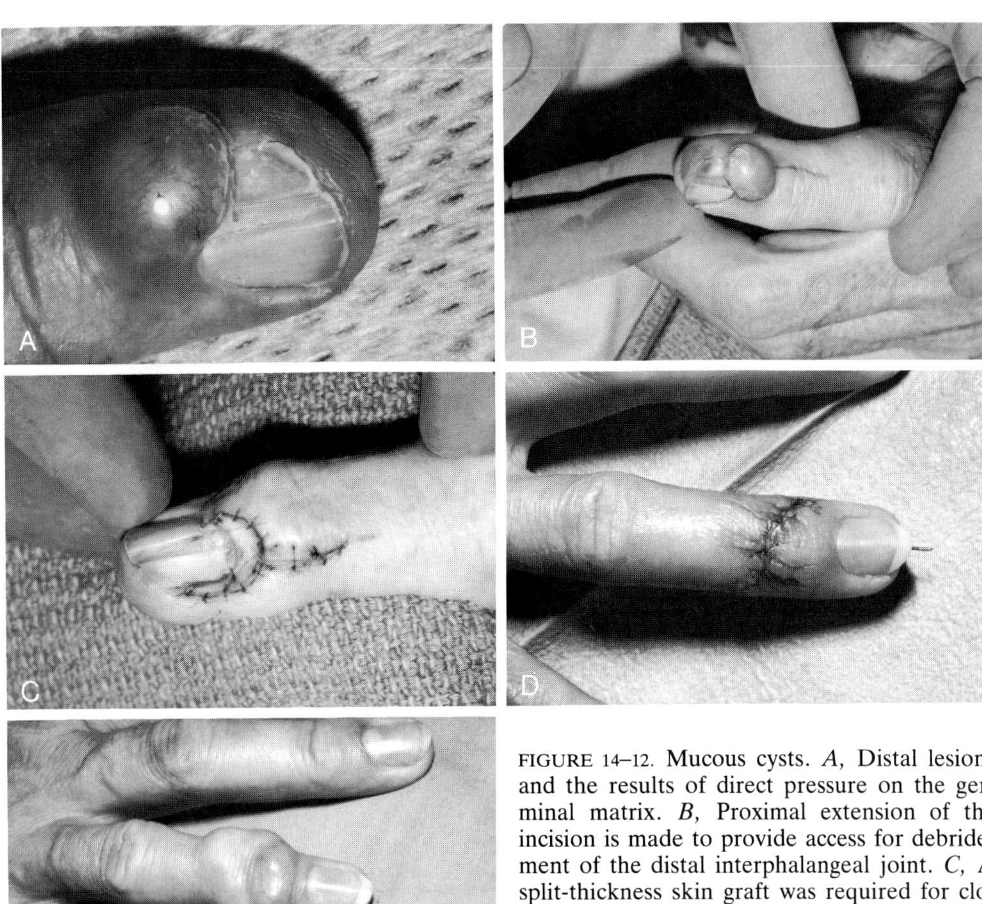

FIGURE 14–12. Mucous cysts. *A,* Distal lesions and the results of direct pressure on the germinal matrix. *B,* Proximal extension of the incision is made to provide access for debridement of the distal interphalangeal joint. *C,* A split-thickness skin graft was required for closure. *D,* Direct closure was possible, and the finger was temporarily pinned to protect the terminal slip of the extensor mechanism. *E,* Multiple mucous cysts.

Giant cell tumor of tendon sheath, the second most common soft tissue tumor found in the hand (Fig. 14–13),[104] is characteristically benign because of its tendency toward indolent, painless growth. It occurs most frequently in the fourth and fifth decades, and the physical examination is often all that is necessary to establish the diagnosis. Although the etiology is unclear, it is generally accepted that it is a reactive inflammatory-type lesion.[90] These lesions are encapsulated; therefore, proper treatment requires excision of the entire tumor within its capsule. Recurrence is seen in 10 to 17% of cases and is managed by repeat excision.[65] Careful pathologic examination is required, as malignancy has been reported, although this is disputed by Schajowicz.[113]

Lipomata are easily diagnosed by their characteristic soft texture. Difficulty may arise in diagnosis if they are deep-seated, in which case they will appear firm. They can appear on both dorsal and volar aspects of the hand. Patients with lipomata will remain asymptomatic unless the mass grows in such a way as to compress adjacent nerves or vessels.[74, 102] Radiographic analysis reveals a characteristic lucency referred to as "water clear."[54] Caution should be taken when attempting to excise these lesions, for they often encompass neighboring vessels and nerves. Malignant degeneration has never been reported, and recurrences are not an issue. Lipomata may occur in the carpal canal and present as carpal tunnel syndrome.

Soft tissue chondromata affect the hand in 64% of cases.[37] They tend to appear during the third or fourth decade as small, round soft tissue radiodensities that may be present within the tendon sheath. Treatment is by excisional biopsy.

Vascular tumors should come to mind if a

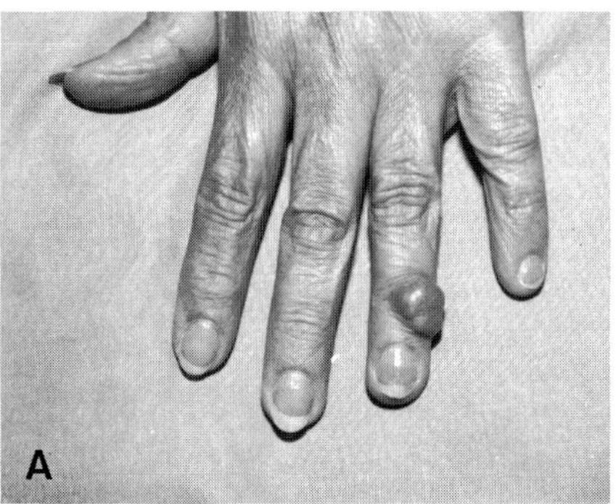

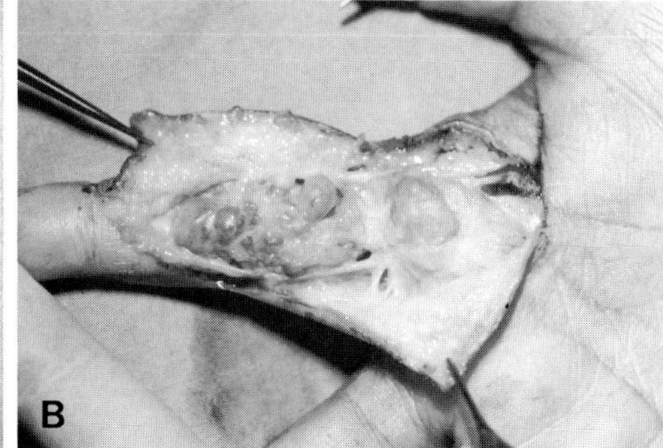

FIGURE 14–13. *A*, The preoperative diagnosis of this firm, nodular swelling of the finger was giant cell tumor of the tendon sheath. *B*, The lesions may be dorsal or volar, and must be carefully and thoroughly excised from the adjacent structures. This xanthoma is characteristically yellow-brown.

mass is pulsatile or changes shape when placed in a dependent position. An intensive study of the vascular supply may include Doppler, isotope studies, and angiography. Hemangiomas are by far the most common type of vascular tumors, comprising 63% of all vascular tumors of the hand and forearm (Fig. 14–14).[97] They present as an enlarging mass associated with throbbing pain and often appear dark blue or red. Treatment of choice is surgical excision, requiring the ligation of vessels that enter and exit the mass. Hemangiomas that appear in childhood should be observed and not surgically treated because they tend to regress spontaneously.[97] Malignant vascular tumors are rare but do exist and should be suspected in a recurrent lesion after surgical treatment. Kaposi sarcoma, a malignant vascular tumor, appears in the immunocompromised patient and has had a renewed interest recently owing to its high incidence among patients with acquired immune deficiency syndrome (AIDS). The other common malignant tumors include hemangioendothelioma and hemangiosarcoma.

Glomus tumors may also be considered with vascular tumors because of their probable origin from the neuromyoarterial glomus.[103] A history of intense pain produced by the cold is common. They are usually located beneath the sterile matrix of the nail but can occur in the bone.[25] Careful comparison of high-quality lateral radiographs of the involved and contralateral digits may reveal a slightly increased distance between the nail plate and dorsal cortex of the distal phalanx. MRI and bone scan have also been used. Occasionally, the lesion can be seen as a discoloration beneath the nail plate. Treatment is by local excision either by removing the nail plate or by Littler's midlateral approach beneath the sterile matrix (Fig. 14–15).[81]

Nerve tumors of the hand are extremely uncommon,[83] their incidence being about 1% of all tumors originating in the hand.[125] Malignant degeneration is rare unless the tumor is

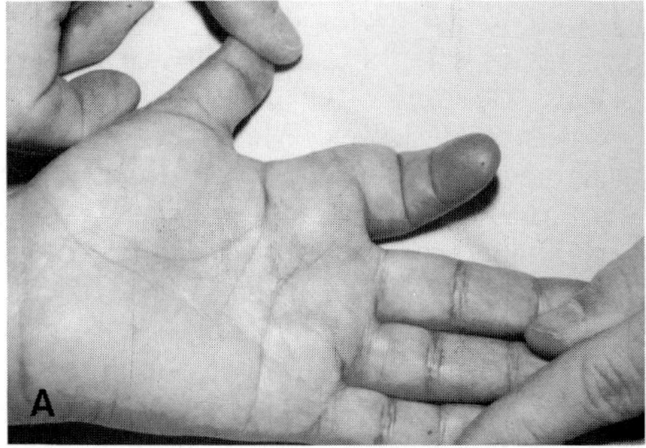

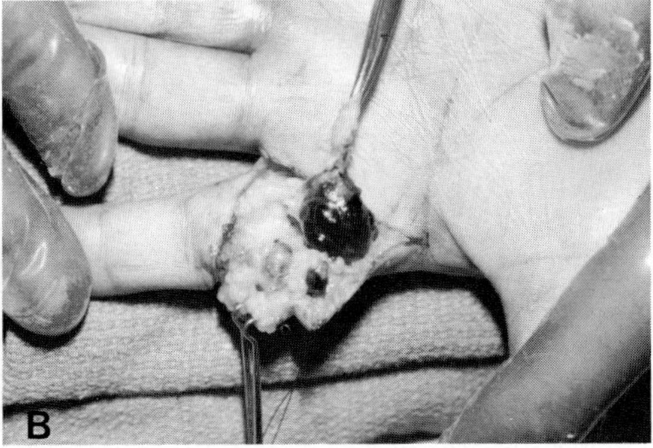

FIGURE 14–14. *A* and *B*, Benign hemangioma treated by surgical excision. Intimate involvement with the neurovascular structures may be present.

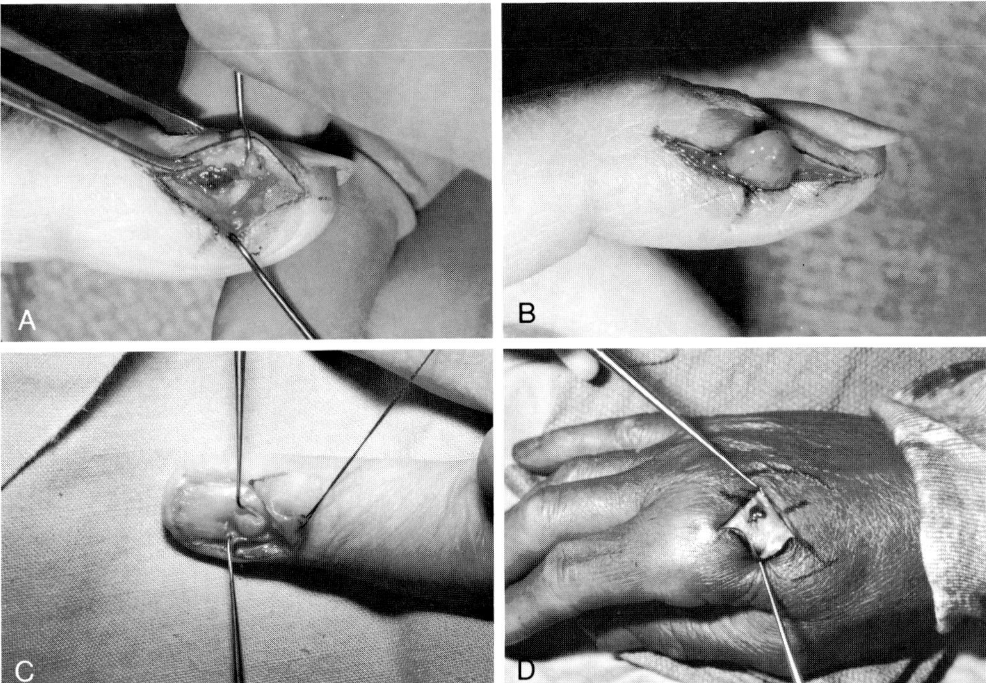

FIGURE 14–15. *A*, Glomus tumor with subungual location and brownish color. Resection can be performed by a midlateral approach, with sparing of the nail *(B)* or by the more direct dorsal approach with removal of the nail plate *(C)*. *D*, The tumor may also occur in other locations.

associated with von Recklinghausen's disease.[83] In general, these tumors should be observed for malignant changes and then removed. The onset of symptoms also mandates treatment.

Amputation neuromas are benign tumors, which, as the name suggests, are secondary to nerve trauma. The neuroma is formed at the proximal cut end of nerve. Axons attempting to regenerate become involved in adjacent, hypertrophic scar tissue. They can become extremely painful if sensory fibers are present and if the tumor is located in a position where it is repeatedly traumatized. Treatment should be aimed at removal of the painful neuroma. The development of a new neuroma in the same location can be avoided by destroying the axons around the neuroma by lightly crushing them and then removing the lesion.[93] Other methods proposed include placing a silicone cap on the cut end of the nerve or injecting the nerve with alcohol.[117] Recently, Dellon and colleagues[40] have studied the growth of neuromas in various environments and suggest that implantation into bone or muscle is superior. Also, Lluch and Beasley[82] have written on the role of overlapping cutaneous nerve territories in dysesthesias associated with lesions of the superficial radial nerve. They suggest that the lateral antebrachial cutaneous nerve be sectioned in addition to transposing the neuroma.

Neurilemomas are the most common nerve tumors.[19] They are benign and encapsulated and grow within the sheath of a peripheral nerve without involving the nerve fibers.[19, 83] They more commonly affect flexor surfaces of the upper extremity.[124] Neurilemomas usually occur as solitary lesions but in rare instances can be multiple;[101] they may also be intraosseous.[77] Benign schwannomas may grow quite large. The important consideration in treating them is to realize the nature of the tumor, which takes its origin from the Schwann cells, and usually grows eccentrically, thus displacing the axonal elements (Fig. 14–16). Recognition of this fact generally permits microdissection of the nerve, removal of the tumor, and preservation of at least some neural function.

Neurofibromas may appear single or multiple as part of von Recklinghausen's disease.[83] Presentation is dependent on whether or not nerve compression has occurred. Malignant transformation can occur with inadequate excision of this lesion.[19] Also malignant degeneration is more likely when associated with

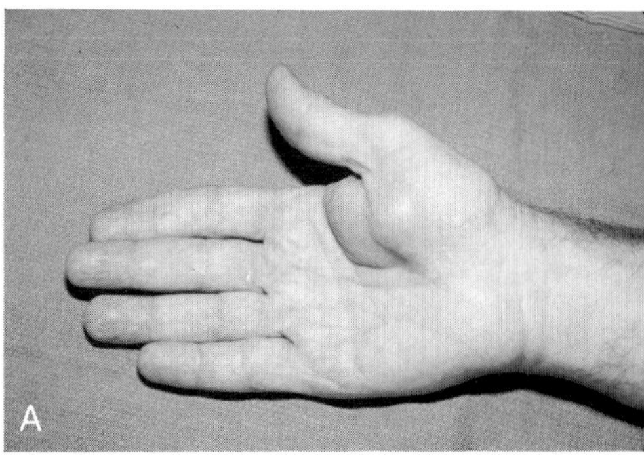

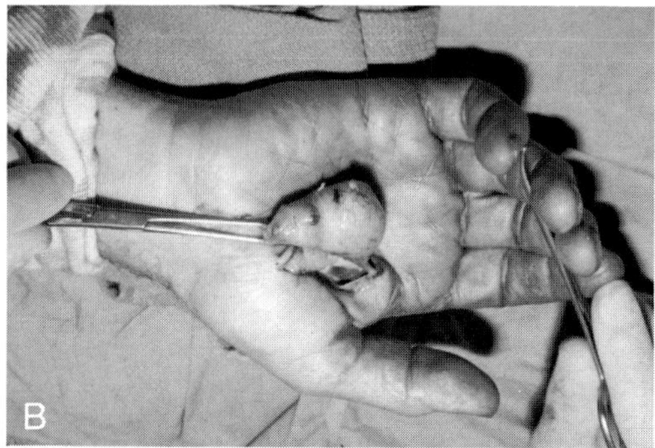

FIGURE 14–16. Clinical appearance *(A)* and intraoperative photograph *(B)* of a large schwannoma. Correct diagnosis and careful dissection with the microscope, if necessary, will generally permit resection and preservation of nerve function.

von Recklinghausen's disease.[13, 38] Unlike the neurilemoma, neurofibromas involve the nerve fascicles. Thus, nerve function cannot be preserved and reconstruction, often involving nerve grafting, is required.

Neurofibrosarcoma is a malignant nerve tumor that may arise *de novo* or from a previously benign nerve tumor. A more radical excision is warranted.

MALIGNANT TUMORS

Although uncommon, malignant soft tissue tumors are troublesome in diagnosis, behavior, and treatment. They comprise under 5% of all upper extremity tumors.[90] The more common malignant tumors include epithelioid sarcoma, synovial sarcoma, rhabdomyosarcoma, and malignant fibrous histiocytoma.

There is some controversy over the benign or malignant nature of *desmoid*. Extra-abdominal desmoid of the hand and forearm represents only 4.6% of extra-abdominal desmoid.[49] There have been no reported cases of metastasis from these lesions; however, their locally aggressive behavior and their tendency toward local recurrence make the treatment of desmoid a challenge. The patient usually presents with a firm, painless, poorly circumscribed mass that has grown insidiously over several weeks; pain may be a late finding. Because of its aggressive nature, desmoid should be treated as any other malignant soft tissue tumor.

Rhabdomyosarcomas are malignant tumors that arise from striated muscle, with 7.4% of them arising in the upper extremity.[49] Although they grow rapidly, they are consistently nonpainful unless nerve compression results. They are classified into four types: embryonal, pleomorphic, alveolar, and botryoid; the botryoid cell type is regarded as a variant of the embryonal type.[105] Of the four types, the alveolar rhabdomyosarcoma is the most common in the hand.[49] It is a common soft tissue malignancy that affects adolescents and young adults. Widespread metastases have been reported in rhabdomyosarcoma of the hand.[105]

Epithelioid sarcoma in the hand more often involves the tendon sheaths or fascia on the volar surface of the fingers and palms.[104] It is the third most common malignant soft tissue tumor,[17] and 57% of cases occur in the hand and forearm.[48, 49] It begins as a raised painless nodule, originating from the deep dermis or subcutaneous layer which, if left untreated, may ulcerate. Incisional biopsy should be performed to establish the diagnosis. In treating this tumor, the importance of taking wide margins must be emphasized. According to Enzinger, the recurrence rate is 85%.[48] This is an extremely malignant tumor, and radical amputation is not unreasonable because of the dismal results with recurrent or metastatic disease.

Synovioma, despite its name, does not arise from synovium but may arise from any structure, including joint capsules, bursae, and tendon sheaths.[104] The extremities account for 83% of synovial sarcoma, but the most common site is around the knee.[45] The tumor is most common in the third, fourth, and fifth decades and may be slow-growing. MRI is the study of choice. In late stages this is an aggressive tumor; however, early on it may follow an indolent course. Metastasis by hematogenous route to the lungs is usual. Schajowicz cites a local recurrence rate greater than 50% but states that the results of amputation are no better because of the high incidence of metastasis.[113] Cutaneous metastasis to the surrounding area is less common.[20]

Malignant fibrous histiocytoma in the past has been misdiagnosed as liposarcoma, fibrosarcoma, or rhabdomyosarcoma, but now it is accepted as a discrete entity[95, 134] and is considered to be the most common soft tissue sarcoma of late adult life.[134] The size of the tumor and its histologic grade are significant to the incidence of recurrence and metastases.[38] Treatment of choice is wide local excision.

References

1. Adeyemi-Doro HO, Durosimi-Etti FA, Olude O: Primary malignant tumors of the hand. J Hand Surg 10A:815, 1985.
2. Allen AC: The Skin: A Clinicopathological Treatise, 2nd ed. New York, Grune and Stratton, 1967.
3. Angelides A, Wallace PF: The dorsal ganglion of the wrist: Its pathogenesis, gross and microscopic anatomy and surgical treatment. J Hand Surg 1:228, 1976.
4. Averill RM, Smith RJ, Campbell CJ: Giant-cell tumors of the bones of the hand. J Hand Surg 5:39, 1980.
5. Balch CM: Surgical management of regional lymph nodes in cutaneous melanoma. J Am Acad Dermatol 3:511, 1980.
6. Balch CM, Murad TM, Soong SJ, et al: A multifactorial analysis of melanoma: Prognostic histopathological features comparing Clark's and Breslow's staging methods. Ann Surg 188:732, 1978.
7. Barbieri CH: Aneurysmal bone cyst of the hand: An unusual situation. J Hand Surg 9B:89, 1984.
8. Barnes WE, Larson RD, Posch JL: Review of ganglia of the hand and wrist with analysis of surgical treatment. Plast Reconstr Surg 34:570, 1964.
9. Bean DJ, Rees RS, O'Leary O, Lynch JB: Carcinoma of the hand: A 20 year experience. South Med J 77:998, 1984.
10. Beasley RW, Ristow BVB: Malignant tumors of the hand. *In* Andrade R, Gumport SL, Popkin GL, Rees TD (eds): Cancer of the Skin. Philadelphia, WB Saunders, 1976.
11. Bogumill GP, Sullivan DJ, Baker GI: Tumors of the hand. Clin Orthop 108:214, 1975.
12. Boyes JH: Bunnell's Surgery of the Hand, 5th ed. Philadelphia, JB Lippincott, 1970, p 669.
13. Brasfield RO, Das Gupta TK: Von Recklinghausen's disease: A clinico-pathological study. Ann Surg 175:86, 1972.
14. Brason FW, Eschner EG, Sanes S, Milkey G: Secondary carcinoma of the phalanges. Radiology 57:864, 1951.
15. Breslow A: Tumor thickness, level of invasion and node dissection in stage I cutaneous melanoma. Ann Surg 182:572, 1975.
16. Breslow A: Thickness cross-sectional areas and depth of invasion in the prognosis of cutaneous melanoma. Ann Surg 172:902, 1970.
17. Bryan RS, Soule EH, Dobyns JH, et al: Primary epithelioid sarcoma of the hand and forearm: A review of thirteen cases. J Bone Joint Surg 56A:458, 1974.
18. Butler ED, Hammill JP, Seipel RS, De Lorimier AA: Tumors of the hand: A ten-year survey and report of 437 cases. Am J Surg 100:293, 1960.
19. Byrne JJ: Nerve tumors. *In* Flynn JE (ed): Hand Surgery, 3rd ed. Baltimore, Williams & Wilkins, 1982.
20. Cameron HU, Kostuik JP: A long term follow-up of synovial sarcoma. J Bone Joint Surg 56B:613, 1974.
21. Carroll RE: Osteoid osteoma in the hand. J Bone Joint Surg 35A:888, 1953.
22. Carroll RE: Squamous cell carcinoma of the nailbed. J Hand Surg 1:92, 1976.
23. Carroll RE: Tumors of the hand skeleton. *In* Flynn JE (ed): Hand Surgery, 3rd ed. Baltimore, Williams & Wilkins, 1982.
24. Carroll RE: Osteogenic sarcoma in the hand. J Bone Joint Surg 35A:325, 1957.
25. Carroll RE, Berman AT: Glomus tumors of the hand. J Hand Surg 54:691, 1972.
26. Cascinelli N, Van der Esch EP, Breslow A, et al: Stage I melanoma of the skin: The problem of resection margin. Eur J Cancer 16:1079, 1980.
27. Clark WH, From L, Bernardino EA, Milne MC: The histogenesis and biologic behavior of primary human malignant melanomas of the skin. Cancer Res 29:705, 1969.
28. Coleman W, Loria PR, Reed RJ, Krementz ET: Acral lentiginous melanoma. Arch Dermatol 116:773, 1980.
29. Cooper PH: Carcinoma of sweat glands. Pathol Annu 22:83, 1987.
30. Culver JE Jr, Sweet DE McCue FC: Chondrosarcoma of the hand arising from a pre-existent benign solitary enchondroma. Clin Orthop 113:128, 1975.
31. Dahlin DC: Bone Tumors. Springfield, IL Charles C Thomas, 1957.
32. Dahlin DC: Bone Tumors, 2nd ed. Springfield, IL, Charles C Thomas, 1973.
33. Dahlin DC, Bess E, Pugh DG, Ghormley RK: Aneurysmal bone cysts. Radiology 64:56, 1955.
34. Dahlin DC, Cupps RE, Johnson EW: Giant cell tumor: A study of 195 cases. Cancer 25:1061, 1970.
35. Dahlin DC, Henderson ED: Chondrosarcoma: A surgical and pathological problem. J Bone Joint Surg 38A:1025, 1956.
36. Dahlin DC, Salvador AH: Chondrosarcoma of bones of the hands and feet: A study of thirty cases. Cancer 34:755, 1974.
37. Dahlin DC, Salvador AH: Cartilaginous tumors of the soft tissues of the hands and feet. Mayo Clin Proc 49:721, 1974.
38. Das Gupta TK: Tumors of Soft Tissue. Norwalk, CT, Appleton-Century-Crofts, 1983.
39. Day CL, Mihm MC, Sobert AJ, et al: Narrower margins for clinical stage I malignant melanoma. N Engl J Med 306:479, 1982.
40. Dellon AL, Mackinnon S, Pestronk A: Implantation of sensory nerve into muscle: Preliminary clinical and experimental observations on neuroma formation. Ann Plast Surg 12:30, 1984.
41. Dick HM: Bone Tumors. *In* Green DP (ed): Operative Hand Surgery. New York, Churchill Livingstone, 1988.
42. Dick HM, Bigliani LU, Michelsen Y, Stinchfield FE: Adjuvant arterial embolization in the treatment of benign primary bone tumors in children. Orthop Trans 1:249, 1977.

43. Dick HM, Francis KC, Johnston AJ: Ewing's sarcoma of the hand. J Bone Joint Surg 53A:345, 1971.
44. Dick HM, Malinin TI, Mnaymneh WA: Massive allograft implantation following radical resection high grade tumors requiring adjuvant chemotherapy treatment. Clin Orthop 197:88, 1989.
45. Eilber FR, Morton DL, Sondak VK, Economou JS: The Soft Tissue Sarcomas. Orlando, FL, Grune and Stratton, 1987.
46. Elmore SM, Cantrell WC: Maffucci's syndrome. Case report with a normal karyotype. J Bone Joint Surg 48A:1607, 1966.
47. Enneking WF, Spanier SS, Goodman MA: The surgical staging of musculoskeletal sarcoma. Clin Orthop 153:106, 1980.
48. Enzinger FM: Recent developments in the classification of soft tissue sarcoma. *In* Management of Primary Bone and Soft Tissue Tumors. Year Book, Chicago, 1977.
49. Enzinger FM, Weiss SW: Soft Tissue Tumors, 2nd ed. St. Louis, CV Mosby, 1988.
50. Feibleman CE, Stoll H, Maize JC: Melanomas of the palm, sole and nailbed: A clinicopathologic study. Cancer 46:2492, 1980.
51. Feldman F: Primary bone tumors of the hand and carpus. Hand Clin 3:269, 1987.
52. Fleegler EJ, Marks KE, Sebek BA, et al: Osteosarcoma of the hand. Hand 12:316, 1980.
53. Forsythe RL, Bajaj P, Engeron O, Shadid EA: The treatment of squamous cell carcinoma of the hand. Hand 10:104, 1978.
54. Froimsen Al: Benign solid tumors. Hand Clin 3:213, 1987.
55. Ghiam GF, Bora FW: Osteoid osteoma of the carpal bones. J Hand Surg 3:280, 1978.
56. Gille P, Nachin P, Aubert D, et al: Intraoperative radioactive localization of osteoid osteomas: Four case reports. J Pediatr Orthop 6:596, 1986.
57. Gunther SF: The occult scapholunate ganglion. Orthop Trans 4:94, 1980.
58. Haber MH, Alter AH, Wheelock MC: Tumors of the hand. Surg Gynecol Obstet 121:1073, 1965.
59. Hazelrigg DE, Renne JW: Squamous cell carcinoma of the nailbed. J Dermatol Surg Oncol 8:200, 1982.
60. Holdsworth BJ: Nerve tumors in the upper limb: A clinical review. J Hand Surg 10B:236, 1985.
61. Hvid-Hansen O: On the treatment of ganglia. Acta Chir Scand 136:471, 1970.
62. Jaffe HL, Frei E, Trageis D, Bishop Y: Adjuvant methotrexate and citrovorum factor treatment of osteogenic sarcoma. N Engl J Med 291:994, 1974.
63. Jaffe HL, Lichtenstein L, Portis R: Giant cell tumor of bone. Arch Pathol 30:993, 1940.
64. Johnston AD: Aneurysmal bone cyst of the hand. Hand Clin 3:299, 1987.
65. Jones FE, Soule EH, Coventry MB: Fibrous xanthoma of synovium (giant cell tumors of tendon sheath, pigmented nodular synovitis). J Bone Joint Surg 51:76, 1969.
66. Karr MA, Aulicino PL, Dupuy TE, Gwathmey FW: Osteochondromas of the hand in hereditary multiple exostosis: Report of a case presenting as a blocked proximal interphalangeal joint. J Hand Surg 9A:264, 1984.
67. Kedar A, Bialik V, Fishman J: Ewing sarcoma of the hand. Literature review and a case report of nonsurgical management. J Surg Oncol 25:25, 1984.
68. Kendall TE, Robinson DW, Masters FW: Primary malignant tumors of the hand. Plast Reconst Surg 44:37, 1969.
69. Kerin R: The hand in metastatic disease. J Hand Surg 12A:77, 1987.
70. Kerin R: Metastatic tumors of the hand. J Bone Joint Surg 40A:263, 1958.
71. Kettlekamp DB, Mills WJ: Tumors and tumor-like conditions of the hand. NY State J Med 66:363, 1966.
72. Kopf AW, Hellman LJ, Rogers GS: Familial malignant melanoma. JAMA 256:1915, 1986.
73. Lamb DW, DelCastillo F: Phalangeal osteoid osteoma in the hand. Hand 13:291, 1981.
74. Leffert RD: Lipomas of the upper extremity. J Bone Joint Surg 54A:1262, 1972.
75. Lerner M, Southwick WO: Keratin cyst in phalangeal bones. J Bone Joint Surg 50:365, 1968.
76. Lever WF: Histopathology of the Skin, 4th ed. Philadelphia, JB Lippincott, 1967.
77. Lewis HH, Korbin HT: Neurilemoma of the first metacarpal: A case report. Clin Orthop 82:67, 1972.
78. Lewis RJ, Ketcham AS: Maffucci's syndrome: Functional and neoplastic significance—case report and review of the literature. J Bone Joint Surg 55:1465, 1973.
79. Lichtenstein L: Bone Tumors. St Louis, CV Mosby, 1972.
80. Lichtenstein L: Aneurysmal bone cyst, a pathological entity commonly mistaken for giant cell tumor and occasionally for hemangioma and ostegenic sarcoma. Cancer 3:279, 1950.
81. Littler, JW: Unpublished data, 1985.
82. Lluch AL, Beasley RW: Treatment of dysesthesia of the sensory branch of the radial nerve by distal posterior interosseous neurectomy. J Hand Surg 14A:121, 1989.
83. Louis DS: Peripheral nerve tumors in the upper extremity. Hand Clin 3:311, 1987.
84. Lucas GL: Hand tumors: A quick guide to types and treatment. Res Staff Phys 25:76, 1979.
85. MacIntosh DJ, Price CHG, Jeffree GM: Ewing's tumor: A study of behavior and treatment in forty-seven cases. J Bone Joint Surg 57B:331, 1975.
86. Mangini U: Tumors of the hand. Surg Gynecol Obstet 64:129, 1937.
87. Marcove RC, Abou Zahr K, Huvos AG, Ogihara W: Cryosurgery in osteogenic sarcoma: Report of three cases. Compr Ther 10:52, 1984.
88. Marcove RC, Weiss LD, Vaghaiwalla MR, et al: Cryosurgery in the treatment of giant cell tumors of bone: A report of 52 consecutive cases. Cancer 41:957, 1978.
89. Matthews RS, Shirodaria PV: Study of regressing warts by immunofluorescence. Lancet 1:689, 1973.
90. McFarland GB Jr.: Soft tissue tumors. *In* Green DP (ed): Operative Hand Surgery. New York, Churchill Livingstone, 1988.
91. McGrath PM: Giant cell tumours of bone: An analysis of fifty-two cases. J Bone Joint Surg 52B:216, 1972.
92. Mosher JF, Peckhan AC: Osteoblastoma of the metacarpal: A case report. J Hand Surg 3:358, 1978.
93. Munro D, Mallory GK: Elimination of so-called amputation neuromas of divided peripheral nerves. N Engl J Med 260:358, 1959.
94. Noellert RC, Louis DS: Long term follow-up of nonvascularized fibular autografts for distal radial reconstriction. J Hand Surg 10A:335, 1985.
95. O'Brien JE, Stout AP: Malignant fibrous xanthomas. Cancer 17:1445, 1964.
96. O'Brien TM, Murray TE, Malone LA, et al: Osteoid

osteoma: Excision with scintimetric guidance. Radiology 153:543, 1984.

97. Palmieri TJ: Vascular tumors of the hand and forearm. Hand Clin 3:225, 1987.
98. Palmieri TJ: Chondrosarcoma of the hand. J Hand Surg 9A:332, 1984.
99. Peimer CA, Schiller AL, Mankin HJ, Smith RJ: Multicentric giant-cell tumor of bone. J Bone Joint Surg 62A:652, 1980.
100. Peterka ES, Lynch FW, Goltz RW: An association between Bowen's disease and internal cancer. Arch Dermatol 84:623, 1953.
101. Phalen GS: Neurilemomas of the forearm and hand. Clin Orthop 114:219, 1976.
102. Phalen G, Kendrick J, Rodriguez J: Lipomas of the upper extremity: A series of fifteen tumors in the hand and wrist and six tumors causing nerve compression. Am J Surg 121:298, 1971.
103. Popoff NW: The digital vascular system with reference to the state of the glomus in inflammation, arteriosclerotic gangrene, thromboangiitis obliterans and supernumerary digits in man. Arch Pathol 18:294, 1934.
104. Posch JI: Soft tissue tumors of the hand. *In* Flynn JE (ed): Hand Surgery, 3rd ed. Baltimore, Williams & Wilkins, 1982.
105. Potenza AD, Winslow DJ: Rhabdomyosarcoma of the hand. J Bone Joint Surg 43A:700, 1961.
106. Pugh DG: The roentgenographic diagnosis of hyperparathyroidism. Surg Clin North Am 32:1017, 1958.
107. Raderman O, Giles S, et al: Late metastases (beyond ten years) of cutaneous malignant melanoma. J Am Acad Dermatol 15:374, 1986.
108. Rosen G, Murphy ML, Huvos AG, et al: Chemotherapy, en bloc resection and prosthetic bone replacement in the treatment of osteogenic sarcoma. Cancer 37:1, 1976.
109. Roses DF, Harris MN, Hidalgo D, et al: Primary melanoma thickness correlated with regional lymph node metastases. Arch Surg 117:921, 1982.
110. Roses DF, Harris MN, Rigel D, et al: Local and in-transit metastases following definitive excision for primary cutaneous malignant melanoma. Ann Surg 198:65, 1983.
111. Sanders BB, Stretcher GS: Warts: Diagnosis and treatment. JAMA 235:2859, 1976.
112. Scaglietti O, Marchetti PG, Bartolozzi P: The effects of methylprednisolone acetate in the treatment of bone cysts: Results of three years follow up. J Bone Joint Surg 61B:200, 1979.
113. Schajowicz F: Tumors and Tumorlike Lesions of the Bone and Joints. New York, Springer-Verlag, 1981.
114. Schajowicz F, Rebecchini AC, Bosch-Mayol G: Intracortical hemangioma simulating osteoid osteoma. J Bone Joint Surg 61B:94, 1979.
115. Selby S: Metaphyseal cortical defects in the tubular bones of growing children. J Bone Joint Surg 43:395, 1961.
116. Shaw JA, Mosher JF: A giant-cell tumor in the hand presenting as an expansile diaphyseal lesion: Case report. J Bone Joint Surg 65A:692, 1983.
117. Smith JW, Guthrie RH: Tumors of the hand. *In* Grabb WC, Smith JW (ed): Plastic Surgery, 3rd ed. Boston, Little, Brown Company, 1979.
118. Smith RJ: Benign and malignant bone tumors of the hand. *In* McCarthy JG (ed): Plastic Surgery, vol 8. Philadelphia, JB Lippincott, 1990.
119. Smith RJ: Tumors of the hand: Who is best qualified to treat tumors of the hand? J Hand Surg 2:251, 1977.
120. Smith RJ, Mankin HJ: Allograft replacement of the distal radius for giant cell tumor. J Hand Surg 2:299, 1977.
121. Smithers DW, Woodhouse Price LR; Isolated secondary deposit in a terminal phalanx in a case of squamous cell carcinoma of the lung. Br J Radiol 18:299, 1945.
122. Sober AJ, Fitzpatrick TB: Melanoma fact sheet. Cancer 29(5):276, 1979.
123. Spjut HJ, Dorfman HD, Fechner RE, Ackerman LV: Tumors of bone and cartilage. *In* Atlas of Tumor Pathology, 2nd series, fascicle 5. Washington, DC, Armed Forces Institute of Pathology, 1971.
124. Stout AP: The peripheral manifestations of specific nerve sheath tumor (neurilemoma). Am J Cancer 24:251, 1935.
125. Strickland JW, Steichen JB: Nerve tumors of the hand and forearm. J Hand Surg 2:285, 1977.
126. Sullivan M: Osteoid osteoma of the fingers. Hand 3:175, 1971.
127. Taylor DR, South DA: Acral lentiginous melanoma. Cutis 26:35, 1980.
128. Tindall JP, Smith JG Jr: Skin lesions of the aged and their association with internal changes. JAMA 186:1039, 1963.
129. Todd BD, Godfrey LW, Bodley RN: Intraoperative radioactive localization of an osteoid osteoma: A useful variation in technique. Br J Radiol 62:187, 1989.
130. Trias A, Basora J, Sanchez G, Madarnas P: Chondrosarcomas of the hand. Clin Orthop 134:297, 1978.
131. Veronesi U, Adamus J, Bandiera DC, et al: Inefficacy of immediate node dissection in stage I melanoma of the limbs. N Engl J Med 297:627, 1977.
132. Watson HK, Rogers WD, Ashmead D 4th: Reevaluation of the cause of the wrist ganglion. J Hand Surg 14:812, 1990.
133. Weiland AJ, Kleinert HE, Kutz JE, Daniel RK: Free vascularized bone grafts in surgery of the upper extremity. J Hand Surg 4:129, 1979.
134. Weiss SW, Enzinger FM: Malignant fibrous histiocytoma: An analysis of 200 cases. Cancer 41:2250, 1978.
135. Wilner D: Radiology of Bone Tumors and Allied Disorders. Philadelphia, WB Saunders, 1982.
136. Wilson KM, Jubert AV, Joseph JI: Sweat gland carcinoma of the hand (malignant acrospiroma). J Hand Surg 14:531, 1989.
137. Wu KK, Frost HM, Guise EE: A chondrosarcoma of the hand arising from an asymptomatic benign solitary enchondroma of 40 years duration. J Hand Surg 8:317, 1984.
138. Wu KK, Guise ER: Metastatic tumors of the hand: A report of six cases. J Hand Surg 3:271, 1978.
139. Young L, Bartell T, Logan SE: Ganglions of the hand and wrist (review article). South Med J 81:751, 1988.

CHAPTER 15

Tumors and Tumor-like Conditions of the Shoulder Girdle

SAMUEL KENAN
FREDRIC A. KLEINBART
MICHAEL LEWIS

Tumors and tumor-like conditions are commonly found around the shoulder girdle. These disorders may initially produce disabling pain, which can interfere with normal activities. Occasionally, there may be just a vague discomfort or even an incidental finding of the lesion. In most situations, a presumptive differential diagnosis can be based on the clinical and radiologic work-up. Other situations, however, can represent challenging diagnostic problems. This chapter provides an overview of the diagnostic work-up, the more significant tumor and tumor-like disorders of the shoulder girdle, and the different surgical procedures available.

DIAGNOSIS

Anatomic Considerations

The shoulder girdle includes the proximal humerus, the scapula, the clavicle, and the surrounding muscles and axillary contents. The shoulder girdle also includes three synovial joints: the glenohumeral, the sternoclavicular, and the acromioclavicular. There is one articulation: the gliding scapulothoracic. The stability of the glenohumeral joint depends essentially on its muscular arrangement (i.e., the rotator cuff). The bony architecture plays a lesser role in stability, because unlike the situation in other joints, in the shoulder, only a limited portion of the humeral head articulates with the glenoid cavity throughout the range of motion.[63]

Certain anatomic facts about the shoulder girdle are important with respect to tumor management. The proximal humerus is intimately related to the axillary neurovascular structures, anatomically creating poor compartmentalization between the humerus and the axillary fossa. Any malignant or aggressive bone tumor in the proximal humerus therefore has an increased likelihood of extending into the surrounding soft tissue and encroaching on the neurovascular structures. If this occurs, it creates complex surgical problems and may make local tumor eradication by limb-sparing techniques difficult. Conversely, the deltoid muscle protects the lateral aspect of the glenohumeral joint by producing one closed compartment.[63] This becomes important when one is planning biopsy sites.

The scapula lies on the posterior chest wall, with which it forms a gliding articulation. It is suspended by a group of muscles that permit stable movement in all directions; these muscles form a well-compartmentalized structure.

Malignant tumors of the scapula, even those with soft tissue extension, usually remain confined to the compartment.[24]

The clavicle articulates medially with the sternum and laterally with the acromion. It provides sites for muscular attachments, protects the underlying neurovascular structures, and adds stability to the shoulder girdle. The sternoclavicular joint is the only joint connecting the shoulder to the axial skeleton. The clavicle is poorly compartmentalized, therefore early invasion of the deep structures is not uncommon. This implies that even a radical resection may not obtain an adequate surgical margin.[63]

Patient Evaluation

Patient evaluation should include a complete medical history and physical examination. Pain is the initial symptom in most cases. Degenerative and inflammatory symptoms are often difficult to distinguish from those of neoplasm. Therefore, it is essential to determine the nature of the pain and its location, distribution, onset, and relationship to joint motion. Pain associated with degenerative or inflammatory disorders is usually activity related, is aggravated by joint motion, and is relieved by rest and nonsteroidal antiinflammatory drugs (NSAIDs). For example, patients with rotator cuff injuries complain of pain with throwing or overhead activities and joint tenderness over the supraspinatus insertion, both of which are relieved by rest and NSAIDs. It is also important to rule out cervical radiculopathy when evaluating shoulder pain. The differential diagnosis is usually based on the character of the pain and its relationship to cervical motion. The cause of pain in most nontumorous disorders is inflammation of synovial membranes and bursae.

Tumor pain often is (1) progressive, (2) constant (day and night), (3) usually not associated with activity or joint motion, (4) insidious in nature, and (5) characterized by a lack of a history of trauma, although minor trauma may be the reason the patient seeks medical attention. Certain tumors have characteristic histories, such as osteoid osteomas. Typically, the patient complains of both day and night pain, which is usually relieved by aspirin.[22, 63]

The patient's age is important in the differential diagnosis because most tumors have an age predilection. In general, osteosarcoma, Ewing's sarcoma, and benign lesions are seen in patients younger than 30 years of age, whereas fibrosarcoma, chondrosarcoma, and metastatic disease are prevalent in patients older than 40 years of age. An exception is round cell tumors other than Ewing's sarcoma, which can be seen in both young and adult patients. In all age groups, tumor-like disorders are much more common than neoplasia and must be included in the differential diagnosis of a painful shoulder. In young children, osteomyelitis, congenital malformations, and pathologic fractures through bone cysts should be considered. In active adolescents, trauma and sports injuries are part of the differential diagnosis. In adults, degenerative joint disease and metastasis far outnumber primary bone tumors and must be ruled out.[36, 61, 62]

Diagnostic Studies

Because the scapula and the clavicle are often difficult to see fully on regular roentgenograms, special views should be obtained. Additionally, the clavicle is best visualized by plain tomography and computed tomography (CT). For the scapula, an oblique tangential roentgenogram and CT scan provide additional information. For the proximal humerus, an anterolateral and two oblique roentgenograms are sufficient. Magnetic resonance imaging (MRI) is the best modality for differentiating soft tissue structures. It provides important information about the extent and the anatomic relationship of the different structures. A technetium bone scan should be included as part of the work-up, especially if a round cell tumor is suspected, as this lesion is poorly visualized through alternative radiographic modalities. The bone scan also can aid in determining the activity of the lesion and detect possible other pathologic foci. Arteriography is useful in evaluating the vascularity of the lesion and its relationship to the nearby neurovascular bundle. This is essential in preoperative surgical planning, especially if limb salvage is being contemplated.

Biopsy

A biopsy is performed most often after a thorough and nonsurgical work-up and after formulation of the definitive surgical treatment plan. The biopsy site should be planned carefully. The skin incision should be small, longitudinal, and resectable. The surgery must be performed with minimal soft tissue dissection and meticulous hemostasis. The tissue obtained should be representative of the tumor. Frozen section examinations may be performed to confirm that representative tissue has been biopsied. The choice of open biopsy versus needle biopsy is based on the individual situation, the preference of the surgeon, and the confidence of the pathologist. Needle biopsies can usually be done on an outpatient basis, as they are well tolerated by the patient and carry a low risk of contamination. In the proximal humerus, the biopsy site can be over the anteromedial margin of the deltoid muscle, not in the deltopectoral groove overlying the neurovascular structures. In growing children, special precautions should be taken to avoid growth plate injury. A biopsy from the clavicle should be in the direction of its long axis.[54, 76]

Classification

DISORDERS AFFECTING THE PROXIMAL HUMERUS

The proximal humerus is a common site of benign and malignant neoplasms as well as tumor-like conditions.

Tumor-like Conditions

Hematologic Disorders. Sickle cell anemia[12, 31] and Gaucher's disease[10] may be manifested in bone by foci of osteosclerosis and osteonecrosis. Osteonecrosis, early in the disease process, is diagnosed roentgenographically as subchondral sclerosis, and later in its course as a crescentic subchondral fissure line with irregular patchy calcifications. Some patients with Gaucher's disease have symptoms resembling those of osteomyelitis. Hemophilic joints may be associated with intraarticular pseudotumor masses.[3, 64] Recurrent hemarthrosis may produce joint space narrowing with intraosseous cyst formation.

METABOLIC DISORDERS: PERIARTICULAR TUMOROUS CRYSTALLINE DEPOSITS

Several metabolic alterations may produce periarticular deposits resembling neoplasm, including tophaceous gout, calcium pyrophosphate dihydrate [CPPD] deposition disease (pseudogout), and tumoral calcinosis.

Tophaceous Gout. Tophaceous gout is produced by the deposition of sodium urate crystals in the joint synovium and cartilage. The crystals are phagocytized by polymorphonuclear leukocytes, which initiate a local inflammatory process by releasing proteolytic enzymes and chemotactic factors. The tophi are foreign body granulomas containing urate crystals.[22, 50, 51, 70]

Pseudogout. CPPD deposition is a crystalline disorder that presents as an acute attack of synovitis. The mechanism of its inflammatory process is similar to that of gout. Rarely in CPPD, a tophus or calcific mass forms, but when this occurs, it is difficult to differentiate it from a tumor. A biopsy must be performed before any definitive surgical procedure.[17, 22, 51]

Tumoral Calcinosis. Tumoral calcinosis is a rare condition, seen most commonly in black patients during the first and second decades of life. Most likely, it results from a defect in phosphate reabsorption in the proximal renal tubule. Affected patients have hyperphosphatemia, normal serum calcium levels, and normal parathyroid hormone levels. They report a progressively enlarging and painful calcified mass near the large joints. Marginal excision alone has been reported to result in a high rate of recurrence, but in combination with dietary restriction of phosphate and the use of phosphate-binding antacids, it has been effective.[22, 35, 42, 59]

PAGET'S DISEASE

Paget's disease is a disorder of unknown cause and is characterized by a disturbance in bony architecture resulting from an imbalance in the rate of bone tissue breakdown and formation. Virtually any bone in the body may be affected, including the shoulder girdle (Fig. 15–1). It may involve either a single bone or multiple bones. Roentgenographically, Paget's disease is characterized by thickening of the cortex, with focal areas of sclerosis intermingled with radiolucent areas. Approximately 1% of diagnosed cases of Paget's disease undergo malignant transformation into a nontypical osteosarcoma (i.e., one with a mixed mesenchymal pattern). Clinically, malignant transformation should be suspected if a patient with pagetoid disease experiences new pain. The prognosis for Paget's sarcoma is poor.[68]

BROWN TUMOR OF HYPERPARATHYROIDISM

Brown tumor of hyperparathyroidism is seen roentgenographically as a generalized or unifocal area of radiolucency; it can involve any part of the shoulder girdle. An early sign

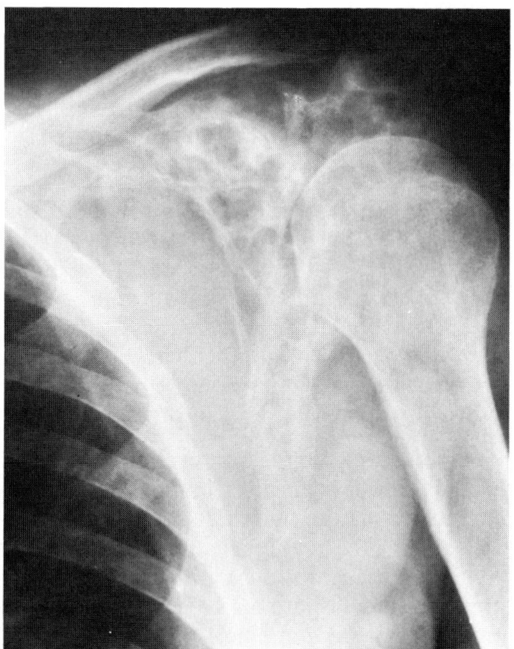

FIGURE 15–1. A 75-year-old man with Paget's sarcoma involving the scapula.

of hyperparathyroidism roentgenographically, which aids in the diagnosis, is subperiosteal resorption along the radial border of the index finger.[35, 67]

INFECTIOUS CONDITIONS

Osteomyelitis. Osteomyelitis may resemble an aggressive neoplasm such as osteosarcoma or Ewing's sarcoma. The clinical presentation and anatomic location vary according to the patient's age. This is due to age-related blood supply patterns and the varying predilection of different organisms for various age groups.[5, 40, 74]

Brodie's Abscess. Brodie's abscess is the self-limited end result of suppurative osteomyelitis. It is most frequently located in the metaphyseal portion of a long tubular bone. In the disease's early phase, it appears roentgenographically as a radiolucent area without periosteal reaction, resembling an eosinophilic granuloma. In later stages, these radiolucent areas are surrounded by reactive sclerotic bone. Roentgenographically, a Brodie's abscess in its later stage may resemble an osteoid osteoma. Culture of biopsy specimens is usually negative.[5, 22]

Tuberculosis. Tuberculosis is most frequently seen in the third decade of life. It has a predilection for the major joints, including the hip, the knee, and the shoulder. The joint space is invaded either by the hematogenous route or indirectly from lesions in the epiphysis that erode into the joint space. The metaphyseal and epiphyseal ends of the bone, as well as the joint surfaces, show varying degrees of erosion, initially without significant marginal reaction.[21]

NEUROPATHIC JOINT DISEASE

Certain conditions, such as trauma, infection, and tumor, can produce syringomyelia, which at a later stage produces neuropathic joint disease. Clinically, neuropathic joint disease of the shoulder is characterized by progressive joint destruction, instability, and effusion. This clinical picture of an enlarging mass may resemble that of a neoplasm. The minimal or absent pain associated with a neuropathic joint is much less than that expected for such extensive destruction. The neurologic changes may be variable, and usually symptoms are minimal for several years after the onset of the disease. Plain roentgenograms of the shoulder yield the most information (Fig. 15–2 *A, B*). The roentgenographic features include disorganization of the joint space and fragmentation with multiple bone fragments in the soft tissue. MRI of the cervical spine may reveal a syringomyelia (Fig. 15–2*C*). The differential diagnosis includes traumatic arthritis, pyogenic arthritis, and soft tissue sarcoma.[72]

Tumorous Conditions

SIMPLE BONE CYST

Simple bone cyst is also referred to as a unicameral bone cyst (UBC). Simple bone cysts most commonly occur in the first or second decade of life, with more than 50% of these lesions occurring in the proximal humerus (Fig. 15–3*A*). Occasionally, simple bone cysts may be asymptomatic and are seen as an incidental roentgenographic finding, but usually, they are symptomatic and they even result in pathologic fractures. On roentgenograms, they appear as a central fusiform cystic lesion located in the metaphyseal region. Simple bone cysts are classified as either active or not active, depending on their relationship to the growth plate. An active lesion is located next to the growth plate, whereas an inactive lesion is not abutting the physis. Active simple bone cysts are most frequently seen in children younger than 10 years of age. Curettage and bone grafting have been reported to yield good results (Fig.

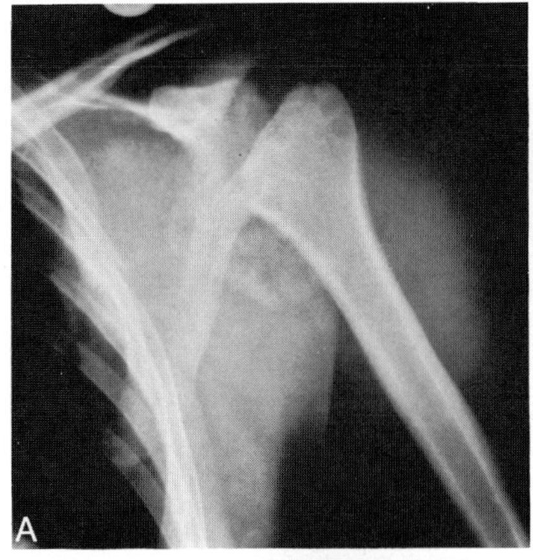

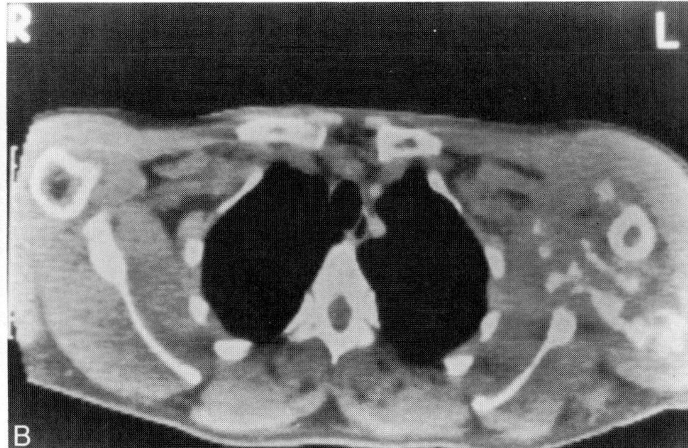

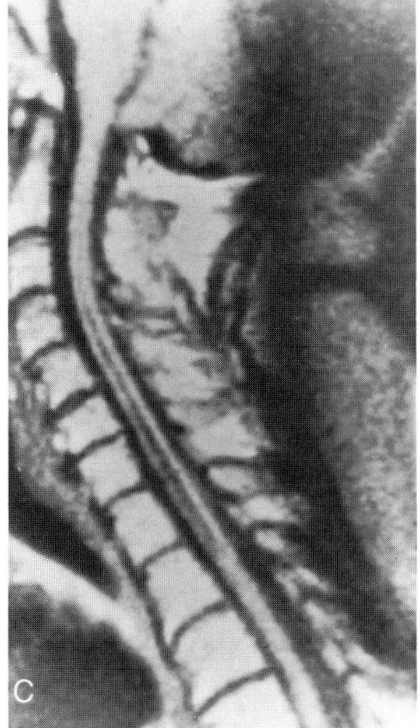

FIGURE 15–2. A 40-year-old man with neuropathic joint disease involving the glenohumeral joint. *A*, Plain x-ray film shows flattening of the humeral head. *B*, Computed tomography (CT) scan shows calcification and debris in the surrounding soft tissue. *C*, Magnetic resonance imaging (MRI) scan reveals cervical syringomyelia.

15–3*B*, *C*). Scaglietti and associates reported similar results with intralesional steroid injections.[73a] If an active lesion is treated, it is recommended that it be approached through a small cortical window to protect the growth plate. Occasionally, some of the cysts that produce pathologic fractures may heal without surgical intervention.[8, 11, 26, 29]

ANEURYSMAL BONE CYST

Aneurysmal bone cyst (ABC) is seen most frequently in the first and second decades of life. It usually involves the metaphyseal area of long tubular bones and flat bones. The proximal humerus is a common site (Fig. 15–4*A*). Roentgenographically, ABCs have an eccentric, expansile, lytic appearance. The most common patient complaints are pain or pathologic fracture through the cyst. The initial treatment of choice is curettage and bone grafting (Fig. 15–4*B*, *C*). The younger the patient, the higher the rate of recurrence is.

GIANT CELL TUMOR

Giant cell tumor (GCT) usually occurs during the third and fourth decades of life, and approximately 10% of all GCTs are located in the proximal humerus. They are locally aggressive neoplasms. Roentgenographically, GCTs appear as active, large, and expansile lesions close to the subchondral plate (Fig. 15–5*A*). In some cases, they extend through the cortex into the soft tissue or joint cavities; they may result in a pathologic fracture. Treatment with curettage alone has been reported to have a high recurrence rate, but this can be reduced

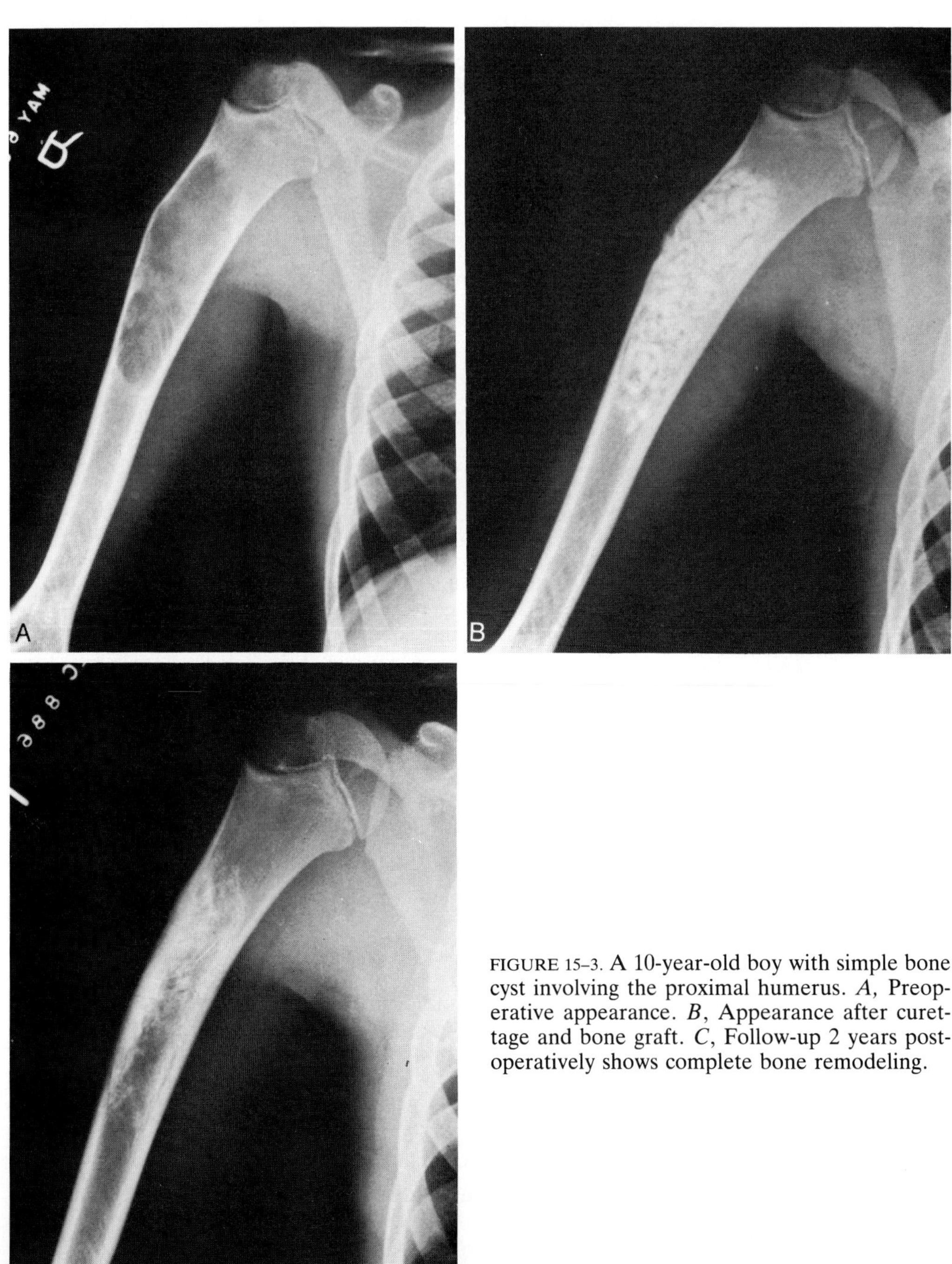

FIGURE 15–3. A 10-year-old boy with simple bone cyst involving the proximal humerus. *A*, Preoperative appearance. *B*, Appearance after curettage and bone graft. *C*, Follow-up 2 years postoperatively shows complete bone remodeling.

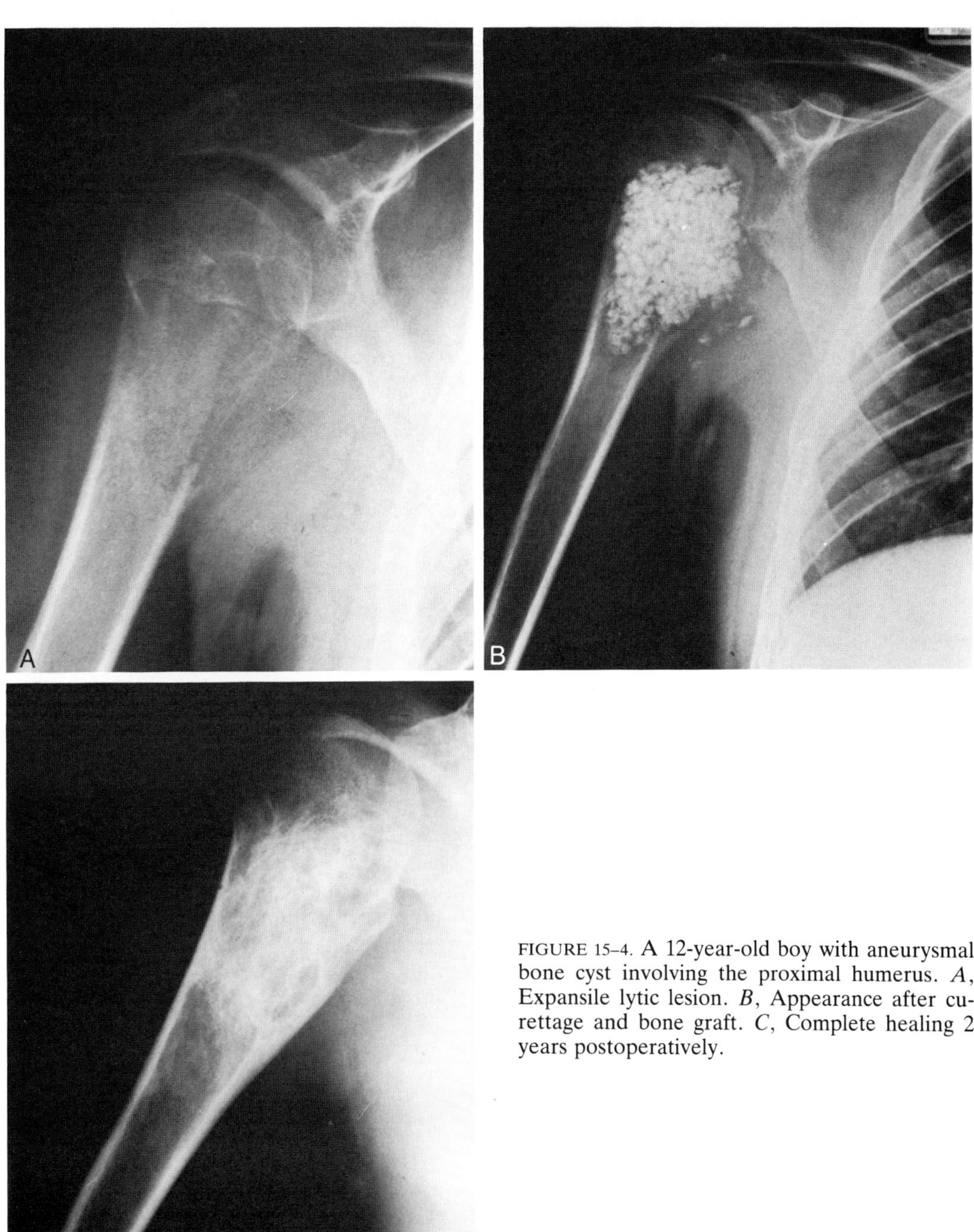

FIGURE 15–4. A 12-year-old boy with aneurysmal bone cyst involving the proximal humerus. *A*, Expansile lytic lesion. *B*, Appearance after curettage and bone graft. *C*, Complete healing 2 years postoperatively.

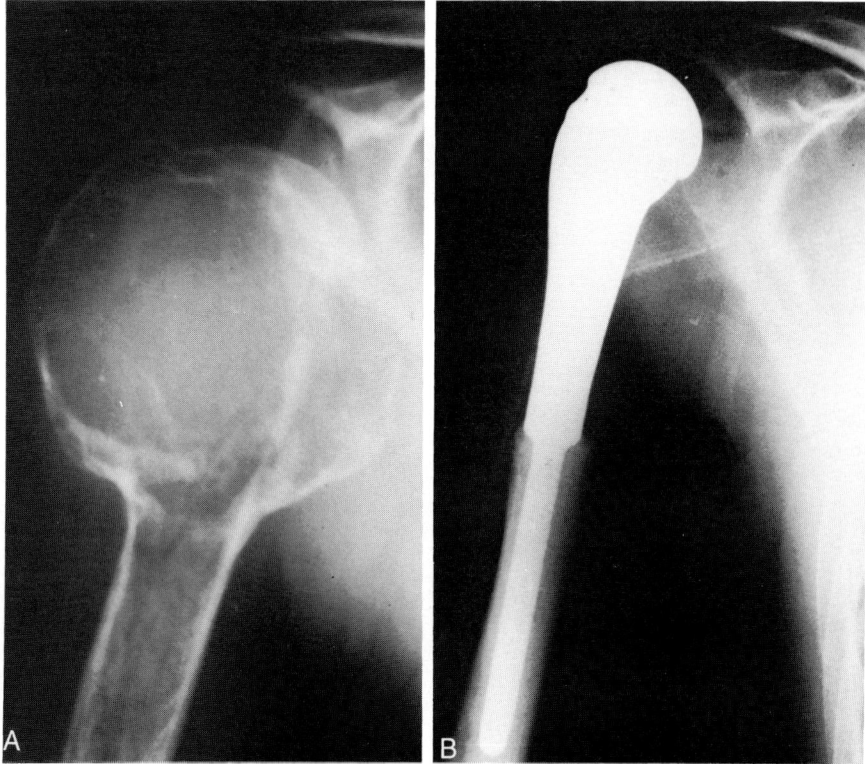

FIGURE 15–5. A 45-year-old man with giant cell tumor. *A*, Expansile radiolucent lesion. *B*, Appearance after *en bloc* resection of the proximal humerus.

with the addition of bone grafting and/or the use of polymethyl methacrylate (PMMA). For aggressive GCTs and in cases of local recurrences, wide resection may be necessary[21, 52] (Fig. 15–5*B*).

BENIGN OSSEOUS TUMORS

Benign osseous tumors around the shoulder girdle are uncommon, representing less than 5% of skeletal lesions occurring in the shoulder. These include osteoid osteoma and osteoblastoma.

OSTEOSARCOMA

Osteosarcoma is most frequently seen in the first or second decades of life. It is the most common malignant bone tumor in the proximal humerus, with approximately 10 to 15% of all osteosarcomas occurring in this region. Osteosarcomas in the proximal humerus are usually high-grade, stage IIB lesions. Roentgenographically, they appear as sclerotic (35%), lytic (25%), or mixed lesions in the metaphysis with an aggressive periosteal reaction and Codman's triangle (Fig. 15–6). Osteosarcomas are classified by their clinical behavior and histologic features. The authors' current treatment protocol is perioperative adjuvant chemotherapy, combined with wide resection, which is often limb sparing. In unusual instances, radical resection is done. During the past decade, there has been dramatic improvement in the surgical management and survival rate of osteosarcomas. At present, the 5-year survival rate using a combination of chemotherapy and surgery is approximately 75%.[18, 19, 71]

CARTILAGINOUS TUMORS

Cartilaginous neoplasms of all kinds are often seen in the shoulder girdle.[15, 23, 33, 34, 58, 73]

Osteochondroma. Osteochondroma is usually seen during the second and third decades of life. It is the most common benign growth involving the shoulder girdle. The patient usually complains of a mass without pain. The majority of osteochondromas located in the proximal humerus are broad based and may attain large sizes (Fig. 15–7). Growth of an osteochondroma is rarely seen after the physes close. The treatment of choice is marginal excision.[15] Malignant degeneration occurs in

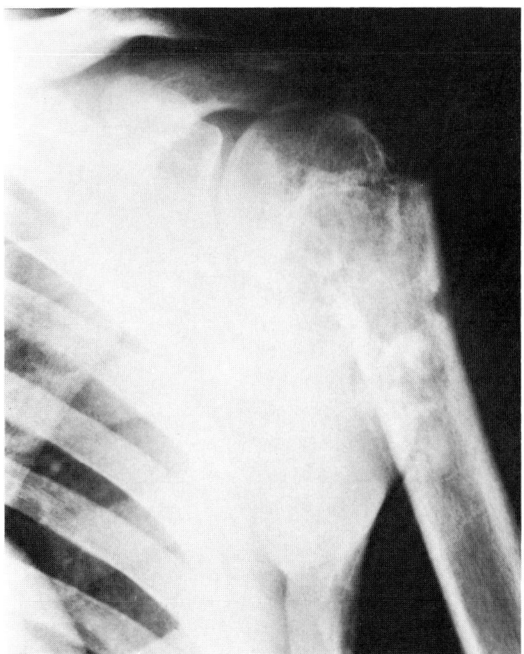

FIGURE 15–6. A 15-year-old male adolescent with osteosarcoma involving the proximal humerus. Aggressive periosteal reaction with pathologic separation of the growth plate is evident.

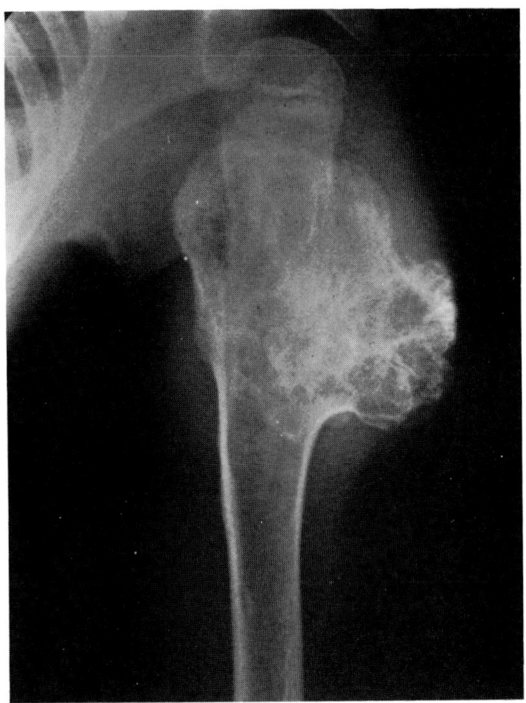

FIGURE 15–7. A 16-year-old male adolescent with broad-based osteochondroma.

less than 1% of all osteochondromas. Roentgenographically, malignant change should be suspected whenever an osteochondroma enlarges after the closure of the patient's growth plate and its cartilage cap widens with peripheral stippling-like calcifications.

Periosteal Chondroma. Periosteal chondroma is most commonly found in the proximal humerus. It appears roentgenographically as a shallow, cup-shaped depression (2 to 3 cm) in the metaphyseal region, surrounded by a buttress of periosteal reaction (Fig. 15–8). The treatment of choice is marginal or intralesional excision. Local recurrence after surgical treatment is uncommon.[23]

Chondroblastoma. Chondroblastoma is seen most frequently in the second and third decades of life. The lesion has a predilection for the upper end of the humerus. Roentgenographically, chondroblastoma presents as a radiolucent eccentric lesion of variable size, located in the epiphysis (Fig. 15–9*A*). Intralesional curettage and bone grafting is the treatment of choice (Fig. 15–9*B*), but recurrence can occur.[33]

Enchondroma. Enchondroma is a lesion most frequently seen in adults, with the proximal humerus being one of the most common sites. Enchondromas are usually asymptomatic and are found incidentally on roentgenograms. They are seen roentgenographically as patchy ringlike calcifications in the metaphyseal region (Fig. 15–10). Bone scan shows a moderate increase in uptake. In some cases, it is difficult to differentiate between an enchondroma and

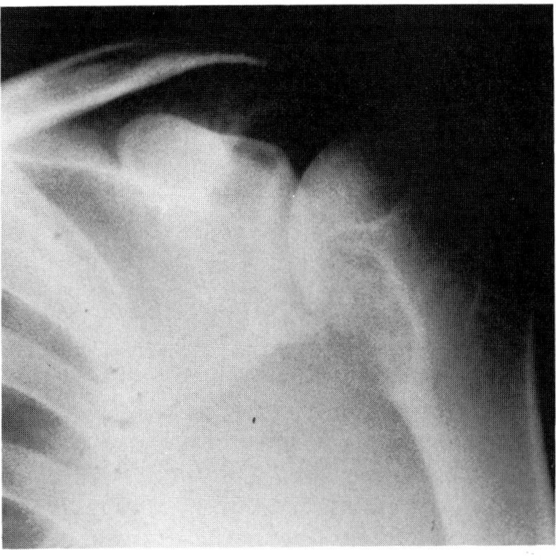

FIGURE 15–8. A 35-year-old man with periosteal chondroma. Cupped-out cortical erosion is noted.

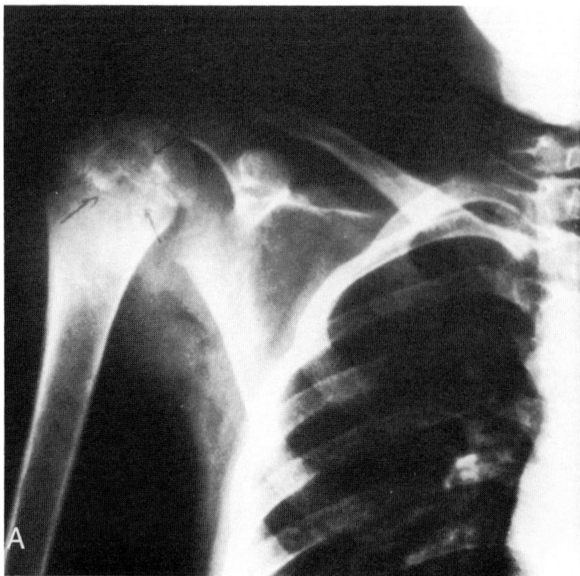

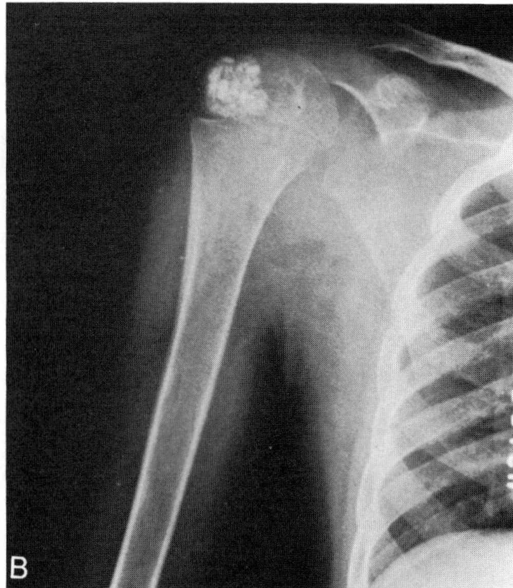

FIGURE 15–9. A 10-year-old boy with chondroblastoma. *A*, Radiolucent eccentric lesion in the physis. *B*, Appearance after curettage and bone graft.

a low-grade chondrosarcoma. In that circumstance, the open biopsy establishes the nature of the lesion.

Chondrosarcoma. Chondrosarcoma is a malignant tumor that produces cartilage. It is seen most frequently in adults older than the age of 30 years. Chondrosarcoma occurs frequently in the proximal femur and the proximal humerus. Patients usually complain of a pain and swelling. Roentgenographically, it characteristically appears as a permeative, radiolucent lesion with cortical thickening, inner cortical scalloping, popcorn-like calcifications, and a soft tissue mass (Fig. 15–11*A*). Bone scans show a marked increase in uptake. Chondrosarcomas constitute a large group of entities with variable presentation and prognosis. Generally, they do not respond to chemotherapy and irradiation, and the treatment of choice is a wide surgical resection[73] (Fig. 15–11*B*).

FIBROUS LESIONS

Benign and malignant fibrous lesions are not common in the shoulder girdle.

Fibrous Dysplasia. Fibrous dysplasia is seen most frequently in the first two decades of life. It may occur in monostotic or polyostotic forms or as part of Albright's syndrome. Patients are usually asymptomatic, but occasionally they have a pathologic fracture. Roentgenographically, fibrous dysplasia classically appears as a radiolucent fusiform enlargement with a ground-glass appearance (Fig. 15–12). Bony deformity, on roentgenogram, is a hallmark finding. Malignant degeneration is rare.

Fibrosarcoma and Malignant Fibrous Histiocytoma. Fibrosarcoma and malignant fibrous

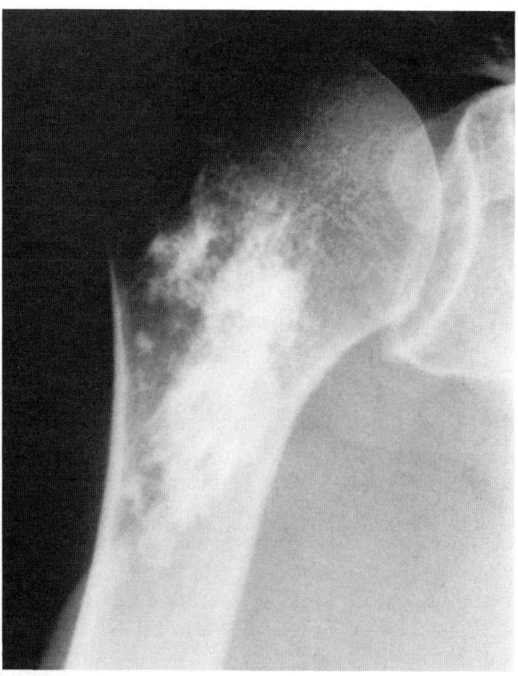

FIGURE 15–10. A 45-year-old woman with enchondroma. Patchy, ringlike calcifications are noted.

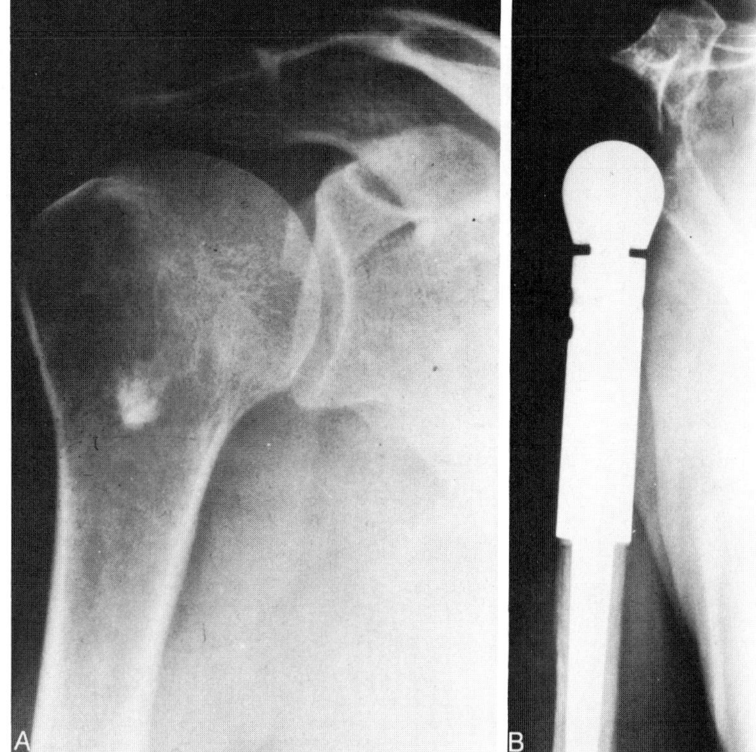

FIGURE 15–11. A 65-year-old man with chondrosarcoma involving the proximal humerus. *A*, Radiolucent lesion with patchy calcification is noted. *B*, Appearance after wide *en bloc* resection.

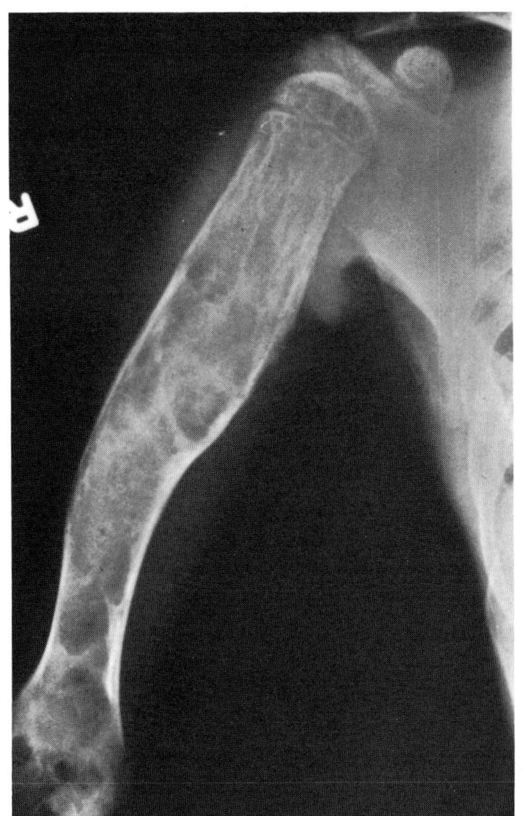

FIGURE 15–12. A 15-year-old male adolescent with fibrous dysplasia. Ground-glass radiolucent lesion with bone deformity is noted.

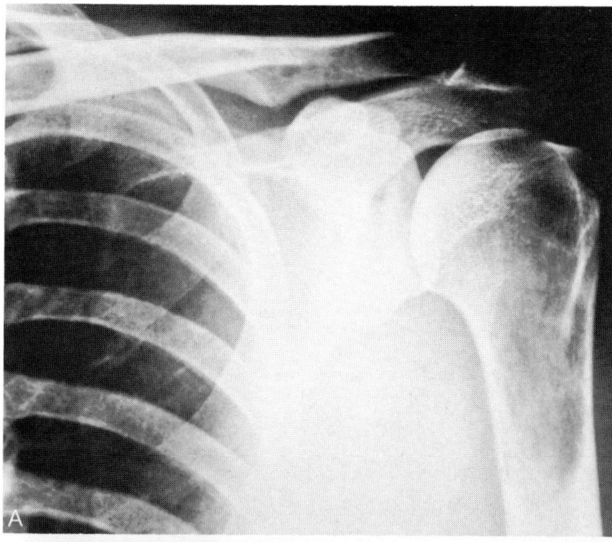

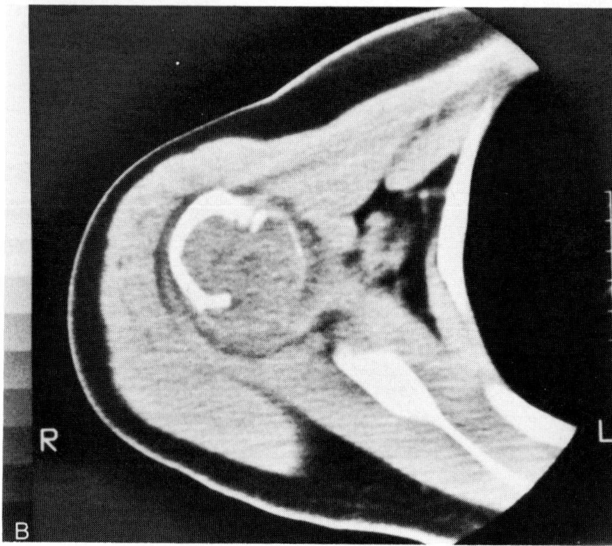

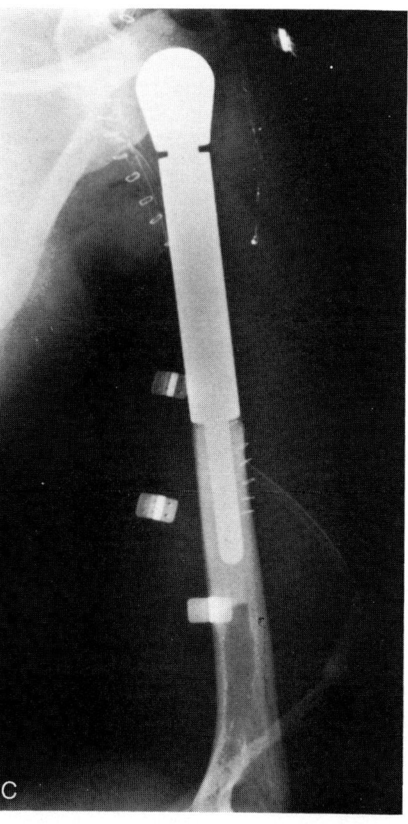

FIGURE 15–13. A 45-year-old man with malignant fibrous histiocytoma. *A*, Lytic radiolucent lesion. *B*, CT reveals cortical destruction and extent of soft tissue involvement. *C*, Appearance after wide *en bloc* resection.

histiocytoma (MFH) are rare tumors seen most frequently in adults. Patients complain of pain and swelling and, not uncommonly, have a pathologic fracture. Roentgenographically, fibrosarcoma and MFH are typically radiolucent lesions with cortical destruction located in the metaphyseal region of long bones (Fig. 15–13*A*, *B*). The treatment of choice is wide excision[37] (Fig. 15–13*C*).

ROUND CELL LESIONS

Round cell lesions are common in the shoulder girdle.

Ewing's Sarcoma. Ewing's sarcoma is essentially a tumor of childhood. Approximately 10 to 15% of all cases of Ewing's sarcoma occur in the proximal humerus. Patients may have fever, anemia, leukocytosis, elevated erythrocyte sedimentation rate, and occasionally a pathologic fracture. This presentation is often difficult to differentiate clinically and roentgenographically from that of osteomyelitis. On roentgenograms, Ewing's sarcoma appears as a lytic, moth-eaten lesion, classically with a laminated "onionskin" periosteal reaction (Fig. 15–14). There is a high incidence of early metastasis. The treatment of choice is a combination of chemotherapy, radiotherapy, and wide surgical resection.[38]

Primary Lymphoma of Bone. Primary bone lymphoma occurs in both young and adult patients, usually involving the metaphyseal region of long and flat bones (Fig. 15–15). Patients without systemic involvement have a

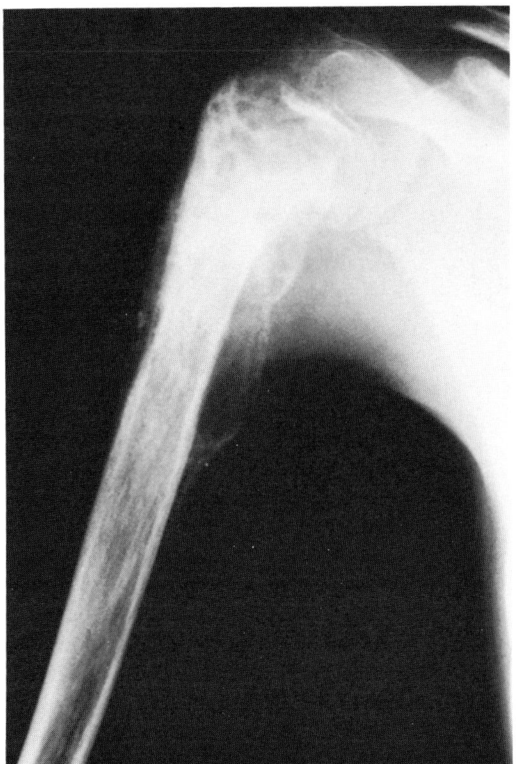

FIGURE 15–14. A 14-year-old female adolescent with Ewing's sarcoma of the proximal humerus.

better prognosis. The treatment of choice is local irradiation and chemotherapy. If there is a large lytic lesion and impending or actual fracture, internal fixation or wide resection with appropriate reconstruction may be necessary. Wide excision is indicated for a large lytic lesion with an impending fracture.[60]

Multiple Myeloma. Multiple myeloma is seen most frequently in patients older than 40 years of age. Multiple myeloma is found in bones that contain active hematopoietic marrow, such as the spine, the pelvis, and the shoulder girdle. Roentgenographically, it is characterized by multiple punched-out lesions. Radiation therapy and chemotherapy protocols have been effective in prolonging survival; the surgical approach is similar to that for primary lymphoma.[57]

CONDITIONS AFFECTING THE CLAVICLE

The clavicle is an uncommon location for tumors and tumor-like conditions. The lateral third of the clavicle is the most common site of involvement. The frequently reported lesions include Ewing's sarcoma (Fig. 15–16), lymphoma (Fig. 15–17), myeloma, metastatic disease, osteomyelitis, and eosinophilic granuloma. Malignant tumors occur more frequently than benign lesions. Among the benign conditions, aneurysmal bone cyst (Fig. 15–18) and eosinophilic granuloma (Fig. 15–19) are the most common. Both of these are visualized on roentgenograms as expansile lytic lesions in the lateral one third of the clavicle.[77] Monostotic fibrous dysplasia is extremely rare in the clavicle but has a unique roentgenographic appearance, consisting of fusiform enlargement of the entire clavicular shaft.[30]

In the clavicle, several uncommon tumor-like conditions have been described.[1, 2, 6, 9, 65, 77–79]

STERNOCLAVICULAR HYPEROSTOSIS

Sternoclavicular hyperostosis is characterized by a marked bilateral hyperostosis of the clavicles. The sternum and the upper ribs may also be involved. This disorder is seen most frequently in patients of Japanese ancestry older than 40 years of age. The condition may represent a type of nonsuppurative inflammation.

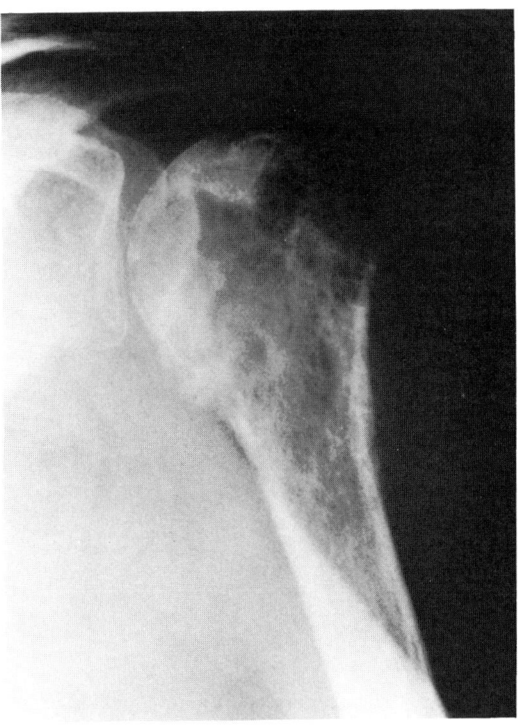

FIGURE 15–15. A 60-year-old female patient with malignant lymphoma. Multiple moth-eaten radiolucencies are noted.

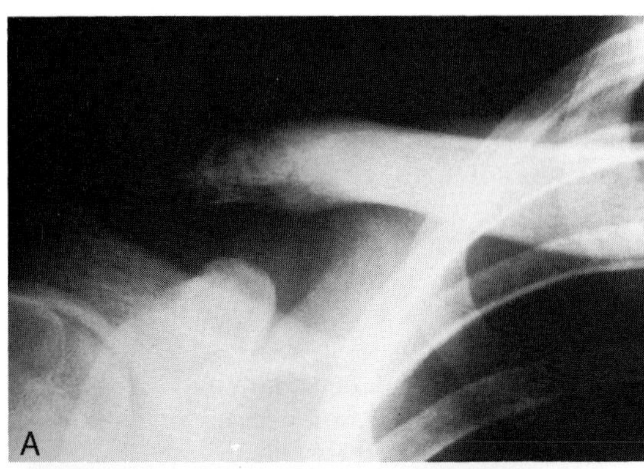

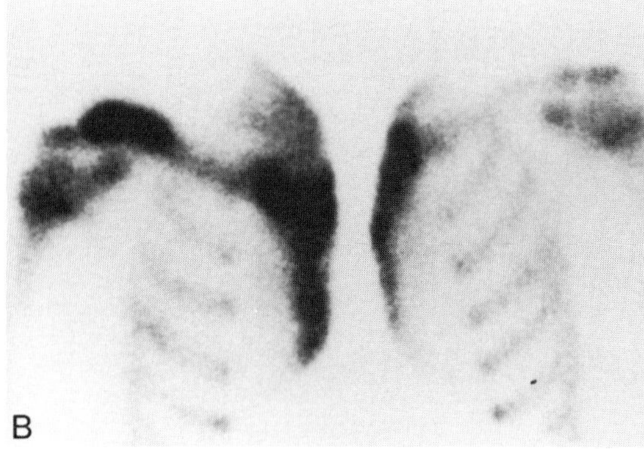

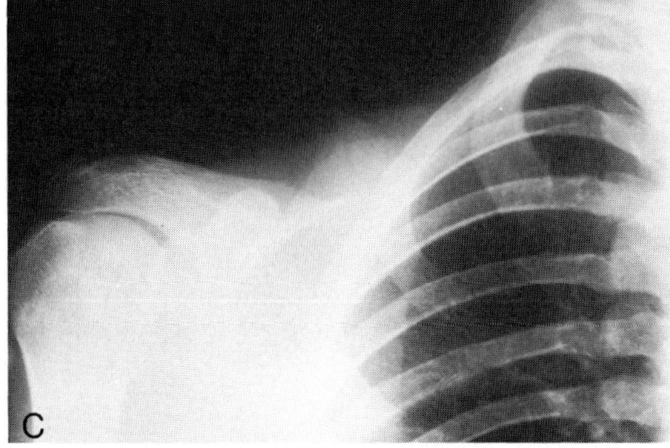

FIGURE 15–16. An 8-year-old girl with Ewing's sarcoma of the clavicle. *A*, Thickening of the lateral third of the clavicle is noted. *B*, Bone scan shows pathologic increased uptake. *C*, Appearance after wide *en bloc* resection of the clavicle.

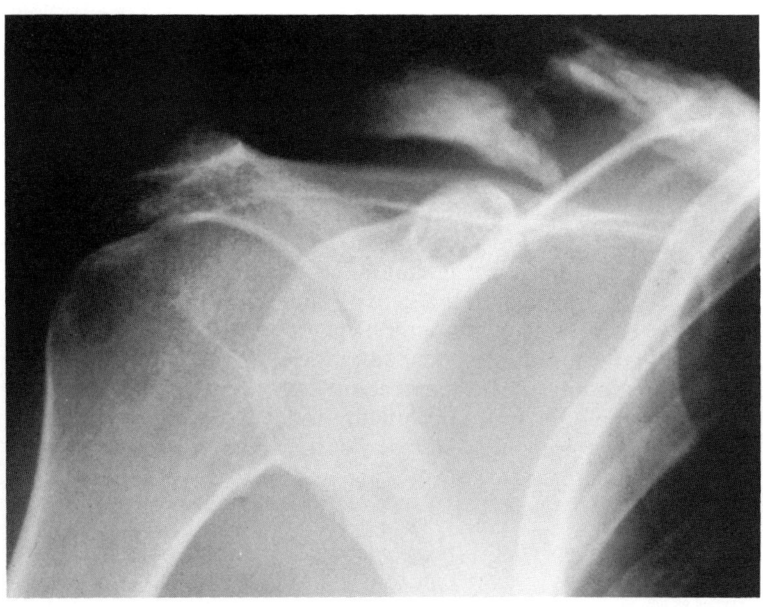

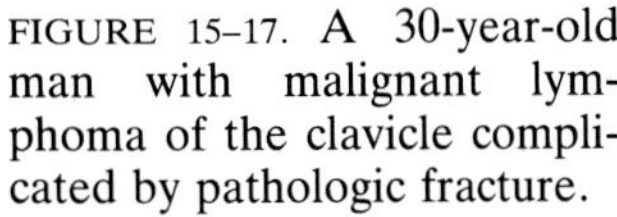
FIGURE 15–17. A 30-year-old man with malignant lymphoma of the clavicle complicated by pathologic fracture.

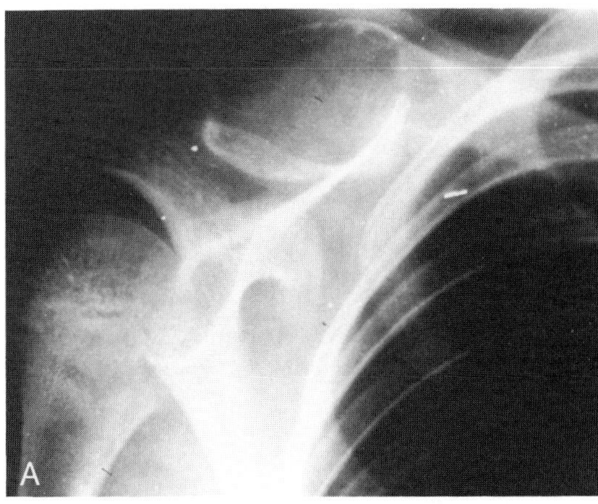

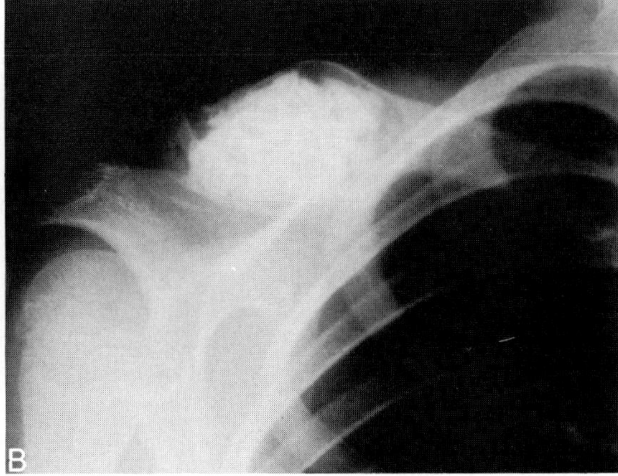

FIGURE 15–18. A 9-year-old girl with aneurysmal bone cyst of the lateral clavicle. *A*, Expansile lytic lesion. *B*, Appearance after curettage and bone graft.

In these patients, an elevated erythrocyte sedimentation rate, elevated alkaline phosphatase levels, and positive HLA-B27 finding may be seen. Cultures of biopsy specimens are usually negative.[32, 39, 69, 80]

CONDENSING OSTEITIS

Condensing osteitis of the clavicle is most frequently found in female patients older than 40 years of age. The patients usually complain of swelling and tenderness over the sternoclavicular joint. Roentgenographically, there is a hyperdense sclerotic lesion with osteophytes along the medial portion of the clavicle, without involvement at the sternum. Bone scan shows focal increased uptake. The differential diagnosis includes degenerative arthritis, Paget's disease, metastatic osteoblastic tumors, and Friedrich's disease. Biopsy reveals thickened cancellous bone without evidence of tumor.[4, 13]

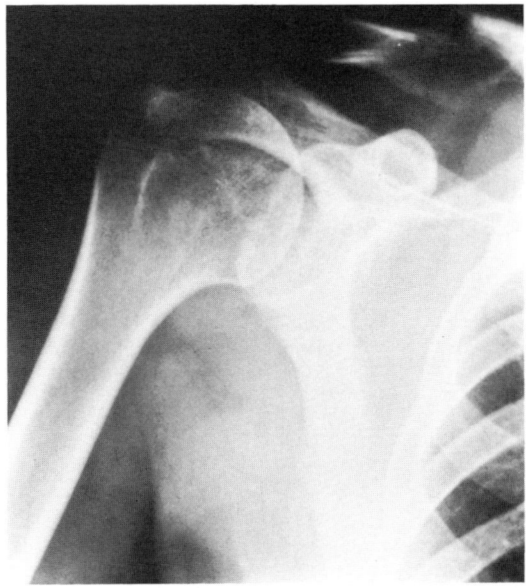

FIGURE 15–19. A 20-year-old man with eosinophilic granuloma of the clavicle complicated by fractures.

CHRONIC RECURRENT MULTIFOCAL OSTEOMYELITIS

Chronic recurrent multifocal osteomyelitis is a rare condition of unknown cause seen most frequently in childhood. Patients complain of tenderness over the affected clavicle. Roentgenograms show widening of the clavicle with periosteal reaction, more commonly seen along the medial segment of the clavicle (Fig. 15–20). Ewing's sarcoma, eosinophilic granuloma, and osteosarcoma should be considered in the differential diagnosis. Cultures of biopsy and blood specimens are usually negative.[66]

FRIEDRICH'S DISEASE

Friedrich's disease is defined as aseptic necrosis of the medial segment of the clavicle. The patient most often has a history of tenderness and swelling over one side of the sternoclavicular joint. Roentgenographically, it appears as focal radiodense areas with patchy calcifications. Biopsy reveals necrotic bone fragments.[27]

DISAPPEARING CLAVICLE SYNDROME

Disappearing clavicle syndrome, or posttraumatic osteolysis of the distal clavicle, is a self-

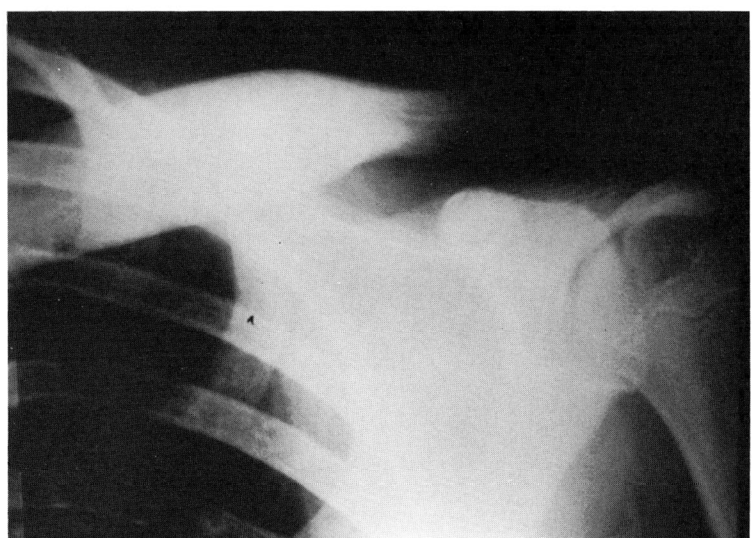

FIGURE 15–20. A 12-year-old girl with chronic osteomyelitis of the clavicle. Radiodense widening of the clavicle is noted.

limited disorder; it is defined roentgenographically by marked bone loss of the distal third of the clavicle. Biopsy reveals a chronic inflammatory process and cultures are negative. Other disorders of the distal clavicle known to produce a radiolucent lesion should be considered in the differential diagnosis, including Brown's tumor, eosinophilic granuloma, myeloma, and metastatic hypernephroma.[7, 43]

BROWN'S TUMOR

Brown's tumor is most commonly seen over the lateral segment of the clavicle. Roentgenographically, it appears as a radiolucent lesion (Fig. 15–21). Roentgenograms of the hand may show the typical subperiosteal resorption of Brown's tumor along the radial margin of the middle phalanges of the index finger.[35, 75]

DISORDERS AFFECTING THE SCAPULA

The most common malignant tumors involving the scapula are round cell tumors, metastatic carcinoma, and chondrosarcoma, and the most common benign lesion is an osteochondroma. Osteochondromas of the scapula are usually broad-based lesions located along the thoracic

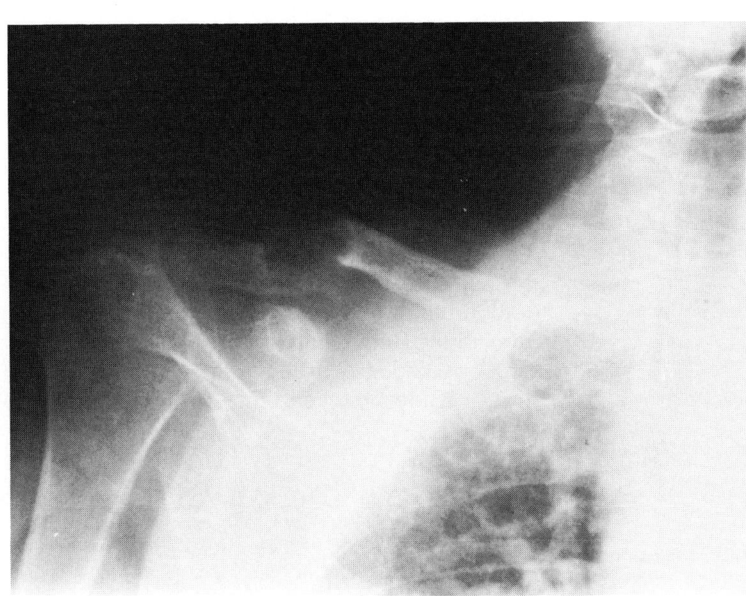

FIGURE 15–21. A 50-year-old man with Brown's tumor of the clavicle complicated by fracture.

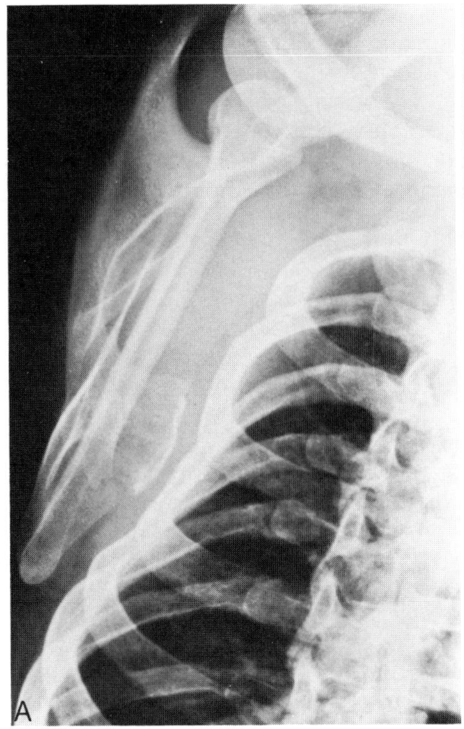

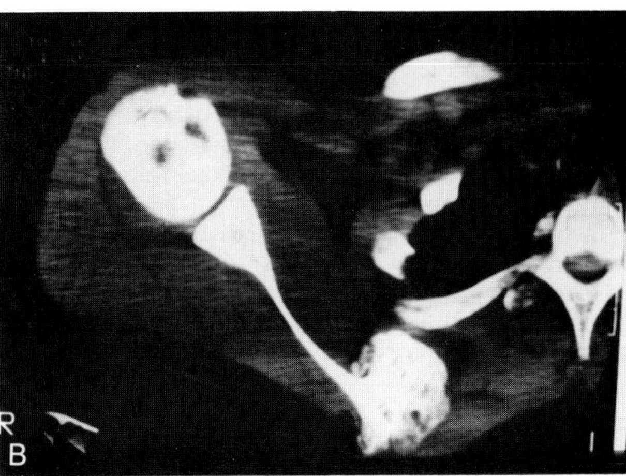

FIGURE 15–22. *A*, X-ray, and *B*, CT scan of an 18-year-old male adolescent with osteochondroma of the medial margin of the scapula.

surface of the distal portion of the scapula (Fig. 15–22). The rate of malignant transformation of an osteochondroma occurring in the scapula is higher than for an osteochondroma in the extremities. Other benign lesions found in the scapula are aneurysmal bone cyst, which is seen in the scapular spine and the acromion (Fig. 15–23); osteoid osteoma; osteoblastoma; and intraosseous ganglion, which is usually located in the neck of the scapula just behind the glenoid.[24]

Surgical Management

SHOULDER GIRDLE LESIONS

The goal of any surgical procedure is to eradicate local disease and to restore as much as

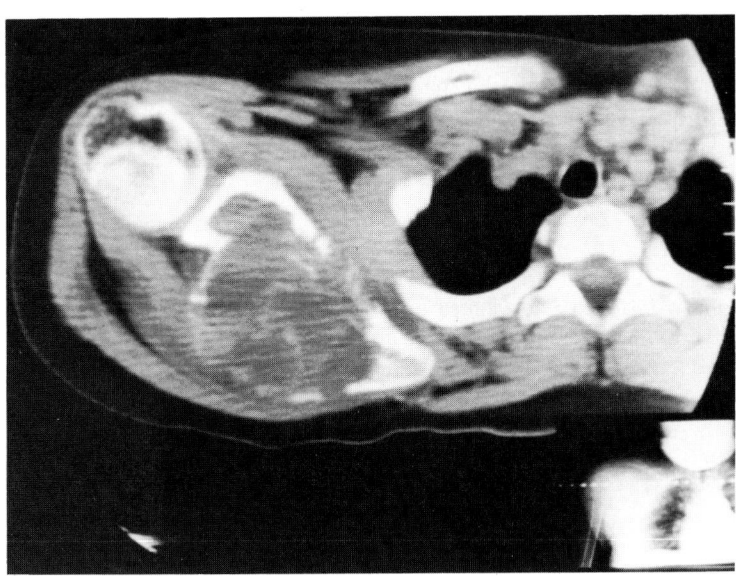

FIGURE 15–23. A 12-year-old girl with aneurysmal bone cyst involving the scapula. An aggressive expansile radiolucent lesion is noted.

possible a painless and functional upper extremity. The main objective of the limb-sparing procedure is preservation of arm and hand function. The treatment protocol depends on the nature of the disease, the age and occupation of the patient, and the anticipated functional demands on the shoulder.[28]

Recent advances in reconstructive surgery and surgical oncology have encouraged limb-sparing procedures as an alternative to forequarter amputation.[41, 44–46] All surgical procedures should follow strict oncologic surgical technique.

Staging

An effective staging system for musculoskeletal neoplasms was introduced by Enneking and associates in 1980.[25]

Benign lesions are classified as follows:

Stage 1: latent
Stage 2: active
Stage 3: aggressive

Malignant lesions are categorized as follows:

Stage IA: Low grade intracompartmental
Stage IB: Low grade extracompartmental
Stage IIA: High grade intracompartmental
Stage IIB: High grade extracompartmental
Stage III: With metastasis

Benign Latent Lesion. An example of a stage 1 lesion is a simple bone cyst. Benign latent lesions can be treated conservatively by intralesional curettage and bone grafting (see Fig. 15–3). The rate of local recurrence after such treatment is low.

Benign Active Lesions. Stage 2 lesions include disorders such as eosinophilic granuloma, chondroblastoma, and certain giant cell tumors of bone. Benign active lesions can be treated by aggressive curettage and bone grafting and/or the use of PMMA, especially for GCT (see Fig. 15–4).

Benign Aggressive Lesions. Examples of stage 3 lesions are aggressive forms of GCT and osteoblastoma. These lesions show extensive bone destruction, cortical erosions with soft tissue masses, and joint space invasion. Aggressive benign lesions are commonly associated with pathologic fractures. The treatment of choice is marginal or wide excision (see Fig. 15–5).

Low-Grade Malignant Tumor. Low-grade chondrosarcoma, paraosteal osteosarcoma, and low-grade fibrosarcoma are included in stages IA and IB. Low-grade malignant tumors are treated by wide *en bloc* excision (see Fig. 15–11). The extent of the normal soft tissue collar resected with the specimen is variable and depends on the extent of soft tissue involvement and anatomic boundaries.

High-Grade Malignant Tumors. Representative lesions of stages IIA and IIB include conventional osteosarcoma, Ewing's sarcoma, chondrosarcoma, and MFH. High-grade tumors are treated by extended wide *en bloc* excision or radical resection (see Fig. 15–13). Surgery consists of either limb-sparing procedure or amputation. When indicated, adjuvant chemotherapy is part of the treatment protocol. Whenever the lesion is suspected to involve the articular surface in the proximal humerus, the glenohumeral joint is resected *en bloc* to ensure against any intraarticular microscopic dissemination.

Metastatic Tumor. Treatment of all metastatic lesions should be individualized according to the tumor's origin, anatomic location, and clinical course as well as the patient's age. The goal of treatment is to relieve pain and to return the patient to his or her previous functional status as much as possible, especially because these patients have an increased morbidity and mortality with prolonged bed rest.

A single metastatic lesion, such as hypernephroma, can be treated surgically by wide excision for local cure. Patients with multifocal bone metastases should be treated palliatively by a combination of local irradiation when appropriate, internal fixation (often with PMMA) (Fig. 15–24), and occasionally, selective resection with appropriate reconstruction. Intramedullary nailing augmented with methyl methacrylate is usually the preferred method of internal fixation, because, with some plate fixation, there is a tendency for the bone to fracture above or below the fixation device.[36, 61]

Surgical Classification of Resections

During the past decade, there have been dramatic improvements in the surgical management of shoulder girdle tumors.[41, 44, 55] Malawer and associates introduced an effective classification system of the different surgical procedures employed around the shoulder girdle.[53] This system permits a more precise description of the type of resection performed and allows

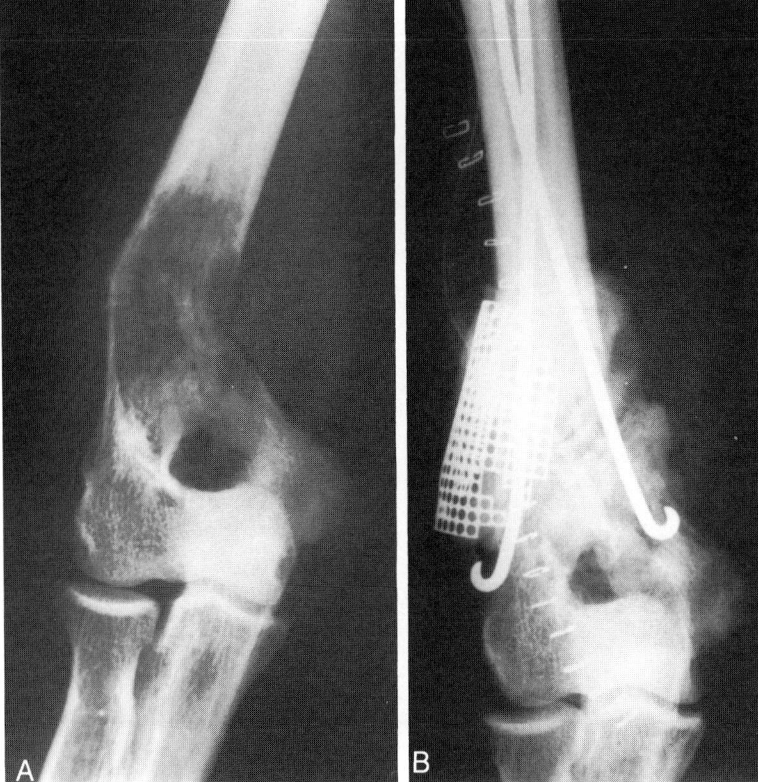

FIGURE 15–24. A 60-year-old male patient with metastatic renal cell carcinoma of the right distal humerus. *A*, Pathologic fracture is noted. *B*, Appearance after internal fixation augmented with methyl methacrylate.

a more accurate comparison of functional results for each type of resection.

Type I Resection. Type I resection includes the proximal humerus without the glenoid (see Fig. 15–13). It is indicated in aggressive benign, low-grade malignant, or high-grade malignant tumors without extraosseous involvement. When only a small segment of the proximal humerus needs to be resected and the rotator cuff can be preserved, surgical reconstruction can be achieved by arthroplasty and/or placement of an allograft. In cases involving resection of large segments of the proximal humerus and when the rotator cuff can not be preserved, arthroplasty is contraindicated because it has a high incidence of failure. The increased failure rate is thought to be due to loss of muscular integrity and secondary glenohumeral joint instability. The surgical goal in patients with large resections is pain relief and restoration of motion. In these cases, the proximal humerus can be reconstructed with a metallic spacer or an allograft. These patients have full function of the hand and the elbow and may regain limited active and passive shoulder motion (Fig. 15–25).

Type II Resection. Type II resection involves the lower half of the scapula. The glenoid cavity and the coracoid process remain intact. Such patients do not require reconstruction and usually regain full range of shoulder motion.

Type III Resection. Total scapulectomy is indicated for aggressive lesions when an adequate soft tissue cuff can be obtained, resulting in a free surgical margin.

Type IV Resection. Type IV resection involves total scapulectomy and resection of a short segment of the proximal humerus and the deltoid muscle. Reconstructive surgery can be done by medial displacement of the humerus against the chest wall and reattachment of the biceps longus tendon through a humeral tunnel to the lower margin of the clavicle.[63] The lateral segment of the clavicle can be resected for improved cosmesis. After type IV shoulder girdle resections, patients can expect to regain some passive motion of the shoulder with good function of the hand and the elbow.

Type V Resection. Modified Tikhoff-Linberg resection includes resection of a long

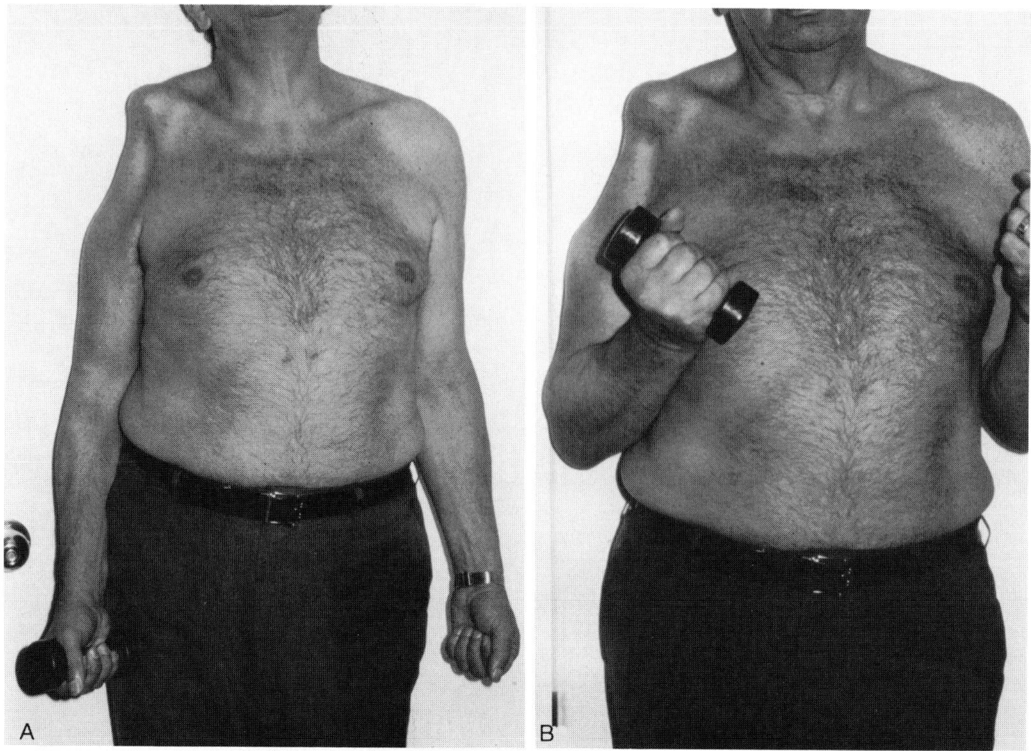

FIGURE 15–25. Same patient as in Figure 15–11. The functional result after type I resection.

segment of the proximal humerus and glenoid, including the deltoid muscle and the rotator cuff (Fig. 15–26). This resection is indicated in a high-grade lesion close to the glenohumeral joint. Reconstructive options include arthrodesis, placement of a passive spacer, or flail shoulder,[48] each of which preserves hand and elbow function.[56]

SHOULDER ARTHRODESIS. Arthrodesis can give good functional results in properly selected cases. The patient may regain abduction through the scapulothoracic articulation. Functionally, the patient can usually raise the hand to the mouth and the head, grasp objects, and push and pull forcefully. Reconstruction is achieved by allograft or dowel fibular graft. The recommended position for arthrodesis is 15 to 20 degrees of abduction, 25 to 30 degrees of forward flexion, and 45 degrees of internal rotation.[14, 24]

PASSIVE SPACER. The insertion of a passive spacer, such as an allograft or a metallic spacer, produces better upper extremity cosmesis and stabilizes the elbow to permit passive range of shoulder motion and better function of the hand. Adult patients who are not involved in strenuous work achieve passive motion, which allows them to perform activities of daily living (see Fig. 15–25). In cases in which the glenoid is also resected, there is the risk of chronic subluxation or dislocation of the spacer, which may cause a painful shoulder.[24]

FLAIL SHOULDER. Patients with flail shoulder have a functionally normal elbow and hand, but as they have no active motion of the shoulder, they have poor control of proximal limb motion (Fig. 15–26). Patients with flail shoulders usually do not complain of significant pain, and certainly there is no comparison with forequarter amputation.[24]

Type VI Resection. Type VI resection is a feasible alternative to forequarter amputation. The extended Tikhoff-Linberg resection involves removal of the entire scapula and wide resection of a long segment of the proximal humerus and the deltoid muscle (Fig. 15–27).

This procedure is indicated for high-grade malignant tumors involving the proximal humerus and the scapula, which are extracompartmental. In elderly patients whose functional demands are minimal, reconstructive surgery may not be indicated after an extended Tikhoff-Linberg resection. If no reconstruction is performed, the result is a flail shoulder.

Other Surgical Considerations. Several additional procedures are important in shoulder tumor management, including intercalary resection of the humerus and forequarter amputation. *Intercalary resection* of the humerus is indicated for aggressive and malignant neoplasms involving the humerus when the proximal humeral metaphysis is disease free. Reconstructive surgery consists of placement of an intercalary allograft, an autograft, or a vascularized fibula graft.

Forequarter amputation is indicated for (1) tumor involvement of both the scapulohumeral articulation with a large soft tissue extension and the neurovascular structures, thus precluding limb sparing; and (2) most cases of local recurrence. The procedure consists of removal of the entire upper extremity with the axillary contents, the scapula, and most of the clavicle. Two major surgical approaches have been described, the indication for each depending on the size and location of the tumor. Both the anterior and the posterior approach were first described in 1882, the anterior by Berger and

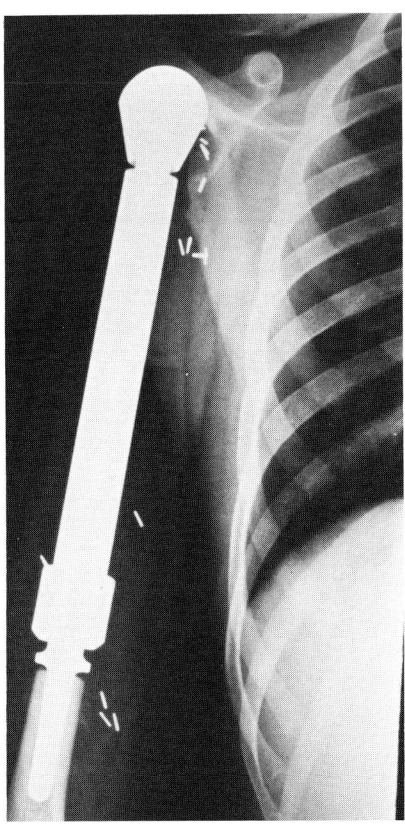

FIGURE 15–26. A 16-year-old male adolescent after type V resection for osteosarcoma.

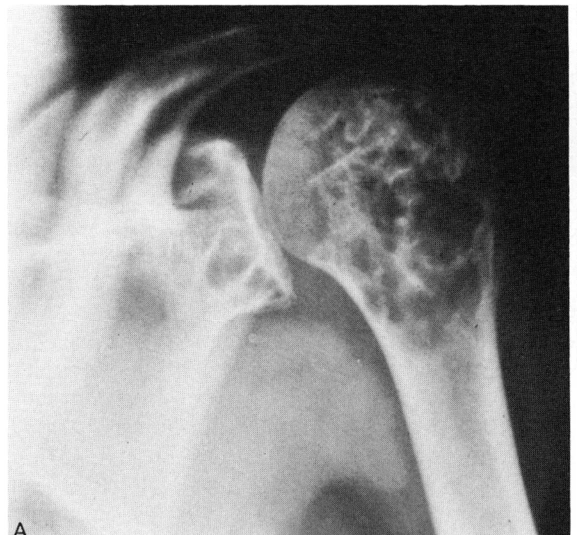

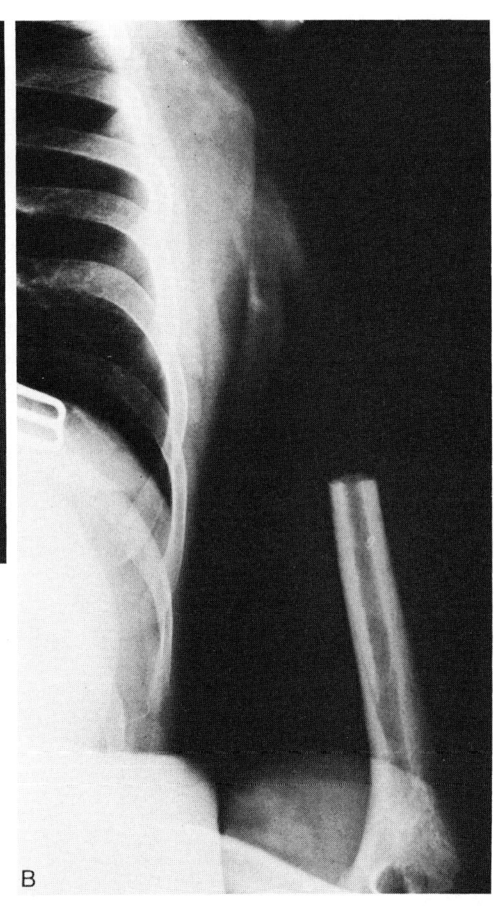

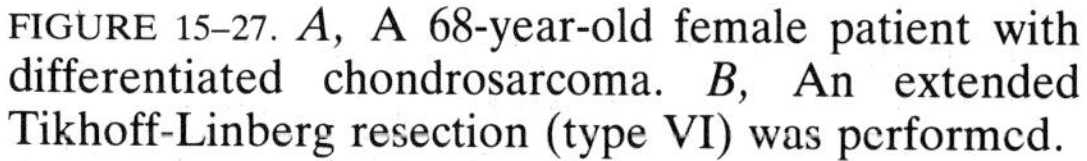
FIGURE 15–27. *A,* A 68-year-old female patient with differentiated chondrosarcoma. *B,* An extended Tikhoff-Linberg resection (type VI) was performed.

the posterior by Littlewood. The anterior technique is more direct, with the major vessels being identified and ligated first. The posterior approach is said to be easier and less time consuming, but the neurovascular bundle is not identified and ligated until the last part of the procedure.[49]

ISOLATED CLAVICULAR LESIONS

Most benign conditions involving the clavicle can be treated by intralesional curettage and bone grafting. Chronic osteomyelitis is best approached by partial clavicular resection or subperiosteal excision.[81] One advantage of leaving a periosteal tube is that it may allow clavicular regrowth and its muscle attachments may compensate for the structural loss of the clavicle. In malignant neoplasms, radical *en bloc* excision is effective in properly selected patients. Patients who undergo radical clavicular resection have some weakness of shoulder abduction and flexion, but the functional deficits usually are clinically insignificant. They commonly have a full range of motion of the shoulder joint and an acceptable cosmetic result.[16, 47, 81]

References

1. Aprin H, Calandra J, Mir R, Lee JY: Radiation-induced chondrosarcoma of the clavicle complicating Hodgkin's disease. A case report. Clin Orthop 209:189, 1986.
2. Bernard TN, Haddad R: Enchondroma of the proximal clavicle, an unusual cause of pathologic fracture-dislocation of the sternoclavicular joint. Clin Orthop 167:239, 1982.
3. Boldero JL, King HS: The early bone and joint changes in haemophilic and similar blood dysplasia. Br J Radiol 39:172, 1960.
4. Brower AC, Sweet DE, Keats TE: Condensing osteitis of the clavicle. A new entity. Am J Roentgenol Radium Ther Nucl Med 121:17–21, 1979.
5. Butt WP: The radiology of infection. Clin Orthop 96:20–30, 1973.
6. Byrd T, Gleis GE, Johnson JR: Primary osteogenic sarcoma of the clavicle. A case report. Orthopedics 9:1717, 1986.
7. Cahill BR: Osteolysis of the distal part of the clavicle in male athletes. J Bone Joint Surg 64A:1053–1058, 1982.

8. Capana R, Monte AD, Gitelis S, Campanacci M: The natural history of unicameal bone cyst after steroid injection. Clin Orthop 166:204–211, 1982.
9. Cervenansky J, Pavlis S: Clavicular neoplasms. Acta Chir Orthop Traumatal Cech 37:170, 1970.
10. Chang-Lo M, Yam LT, Rubenstone AI: Gaucher's disease. Review of the literature and report of twelve new cases. Am J Med Sci 254:303–315, 1967.
11. Chigira M, Maehara S, Arita S, Udagawa E: The aetiology and treatment of simple bone cysts. J Bone Joint Surg 65B:633–637, 1983.
12. Chung SMK, Ralston EL: Necrosis of the humeral head in sickle cell anemia and its genetic variant. Clin Orthop 80:105–107, 1971.
13. Cone RO, Resnick D, Goergen TG, et al: Condensing osteitis of the clavicle. Am J Radiol 141:387–388, 1983.
14. Conrad EU, Enneking WF: Shoulder arthrodesis following tumor resection. Presented to American Academy of Orthopaedic Surgeons, February 1986.
15. Cooley LH, Torg JS: Pseudowinging of the scapula secondary to subscapular osteochondroma. Clin Orthop 162:119–124, 1982.
16. Copland SM: Total resection of the clavicle. Am J Surg 72:280, 1946.
17. Currey HLF: Pyrophosphate arthropathy and calcific periarthritis. Clin Orthop 71:70–80, 1970.
18. Dahlin DC, Conventry MB: Osteosarcoma: A study of 600 cases. J Bone Joint Surg 49A:101–110, 1967.
19. Dahlin DC, Unni KK: Osteosarcoma of bone and its important recognizable varieties. Am J Surg Pathol 1:61–72, 1977.
20. Dahlin DC, Cupps RE, Johnson EW: Giant cell tumor: A study of 195 cases. Cancer 25:1061, 1970.
21. Davidson PT, Horowitz I: Skeletal tuberculosis, a review with patient presentations and discussion. Am J Med 48:77–84, 1970.
22. DePalma AF: Surgery of the Shoulder, 3rd ed. Philadelphia, JB Lippincott, 1983.
23. DeSantos LA, Spjut HJ: Periosteal chondroma: A radiographic spectrum. Skeletal Radiol 6:15, 1981.
24. Enneking WF: Musculoskeletal tumor surgery. New York, Churchill Livingstone, 1983.
25. Enneking WF, Spainier SS, Goodman MA: A system for the surgical staging of musculoskeletal sarcomas. Clin Orthop 153:106, 1980.
26. Fahey JJ, O'Brien ET: Subtotal resection and grafting in selected cases of solitary unicameral bone cyst. J Bone Joint Surg 55A:59–68, 1973.
27. Fischel RE, Bernstein D: Friedrich's disease. Br J Radiol 48:318–319, 1975.
28. Francis EC, Worcester JN: Radical resection for tumors of the shoulder with preservation of a functional extremity. J Bone Joint Surg 44A:1423–1430, 1962.
29. Gartland JJ, Cole FL: Modern concepts in the treatment of unicameral bone cysts of the proximal humerus. Orthop Clin North Am 6:487–498, 1975.
30. Gibson MY, Middlemass JH: Fibrous dysplasia of bone. Br J Radiol 44:1, 1971.
31. Golding JS, MacIver JE, Went LN: The bone changes in sickle cell anemia and its genetic variants. J Bone Joint Surg 41B:711–718, 1959.
32. Goossens M, Vanderstraeten C, Claessens H: Sternoclavicular hyperostosis. Clin Orthop 194:164–168, 1985.
33. Green P, Whittaker RP: Benign chondroblastoma. J Bone Joint Surg 57A:418, 1975.
34. Gudmundrsen TE, Siewers PB: Synovial chondromatosis of the shoulder. A case report. Acta Orthop Scand 58:419–420, 1987.
35. Harkess JW, Peters HJ: Tumoral calcinosis. A report of six cases. J Bone Joint Surg 49A:721–731, 1967.
36. Harrington KD, Sim FH, Enis JE, et al: Methylmethacrylate as adjunct in internal fixation of pathological fractures. J Bone Joint Surg 58A:1047, 1976.
37. Huvos AG, Higinbotham NL: Primary fibrosarcoma of bone. Cancer 35:837, 1975.
38. Jurgens H, Exner U, Gadner H, et al: Multidisciplinary treatment of primary Ewing's sarcoma of bone. Cancer 61:23–32, 1988.
39. Jurik AG, Moller BN: Inflammatory hyperostosis and sclerosis of the clavicle. Skeletal Radiol 15:284, 1986.
40. Kelly PJ: Osteomyelitis in the adult. Orthop Clin North Am 6:983, 1975.
41. Kenan S, Jones C, Lewis MM: Limb sparing reconstructive surgery in malignant and aggressive benign bone tumors of the extremities. J Surg Round for Orthop, August 1987.
42. Kirk TS, Simon MA: Tumoral calcinosis. J Bone Joint Surg 63A:1167–1169, 1981.
43. Levine AH, Pais MJ, Schwartz EE: Post traumatic osteolysis of the distal clavicle with emphasis on early radiologic changes. Am J Roentgenol 127:781–784, 1976.
44. Lewis MM: An approach to the treatment of malignant bone tumors. Orthopedics 8:655–656, 1985.
45. Lewis MM: The use of an expandable and adjustable prosthesis in the treatment of childhood malignant bone tumors of the extremity. Cancer 57:499–502, 1986.
46. Lewis MM: Bone Tumor Surgery: Limb Sparing Techniques. Philadelphia, JB Lippincott, 1988.
47. Lewis MM, Ballet FL, Kroll PG, Bloom N: *En bloc* clavicular resection: Operative procedure and postoperative testing of function. Clin Orthop 193:214–220, 1985.
48. Linberg BE: Interscapulo-thoracic resection for malignant tumors of the shoulder joint region. J Bone Joint Surg 10:344–349, 1928.
49. Littlewood H: Amputations at the shoulder and the hip. Br Med J 1:381, 1922.
50. McCarthy DJ: Phagocytosis of urates in gouty synovial fluid. Am J Med Sci 243:285–288, 1962.
51. McCarthy DJ: Pseudogout syndrome. Bull Rheum Dis 14:331–334, 1964.
52. McCarthy EF: Giant cell tumor of bone. An historical perspective. Clin Orthop 153:14, 1980.
53. Malawer MM, Sugarbaker PH, Lampert M, et al: The Tikhoff-Linberg procedure. Report of the patients and presentation of a modified technique for tumors of the proximal humerus. Surgery 97:518–528, 1985.
54. Mankin HJ, Lange TA, Spanier SS: The hazards of biopsy in patients with malignant primary bone and soft tissue tumors. J Bone Joint Surg 64:1121–1127, 1982.
55. Marcove RC: Neoplasms of the shoulder girdle. Orthop Clin North Am 6:541–555, 1975.
56. Marcove RC, Lewis MM, Huvos AG: *En bloc* humeral interscapulo-thoracic resection. Clin Orthop 124:219–228, 1977.
57. Meis JM, Butler JJ, Osborne BM, et al: Solitary plasmacytoma of bone and extramedullary plasmacytoma. Cancer 59:1475–1485, 1987.
58. Milgran JW: Synovial osteochondromatosis. J Bone Joint Surg 59A:792–901, 1977.
59. Mitnick PD, Goldfarb S, Slatopolsky L, et al: Calcium and phosphate metabolism in tumoral calcinosis. Ann Intern Med 92:482–487, 1980.
60. Ostrowski ML, Unni KK, Banks PM, et al: Malignant lymphoma of bone. Cancer 58:2646–2655, 1986.

61. Parrish FF, Murray JA: Surgical treatment for secondary neoplastic fractures. J Bone Joint Surg 53A:605, 1979.
62. Pearson C, Dick WC (eds): Current management of rheumatoid arthritis. Clin Rheum Dis 1:367–400, 1975.
63. Post M (ed): The Shoulder: Surgical and Nonsurgical Management, 2nd ed. Philadelphia, Lea & Febiger, 1988.
64. Post M, Telfer MC: Surgery in hemophilic patients. J Bone Joint Surg 57A:1136–1145, 1975.
65. Pratt GF, Dahlin DC, Ghormley RJ: Tumors of scapula and clavicle. Surg Gynecol Obstet 106:536, 1958.
66. Probst FP, Bjorksten B, Gustavson KH: Radiological aspects of chronic recurrent multifocal osteomyelitis. Ann Radiol (Paris) 21:115–125, 1978.
67. Pugh DG: Subperiosteal resorption of bone: Roentgenologic manifestation of primary hyperparathyroidism and renal osteodystrophy. Am J Roentgenol Radium Ther 66:577–586, 1951.
68. Rebel A, Basle M, Pouplard A, et al: Bone tissue in Paget's disease of bone. Arthritis Rheum 23:1104, 1980.
69. Resnick D: Sternoclavicular hyperostosis. AJR 135:1278, 1980.
70. Riddle JM, Bluhm GB, Barnhart MD: Ultrastructural study of leukocytes and urates in gouty arthritis. Ann Rheum Dis 26:3897, 1967.
71. Rosen G, Marcove RJ, Huvos AG, et al: Primary osteogenic sarcoma: Eight years experience of adjuvant chemotherapy. J Cancer Res Clin Oncol 106:55–67, 1983.
72. Sackellares JC, Swift TR: Shoulder enlargement as the presenting sign of syringomyelia. Report of two cases and review of the literature. JAMA 236:2878, 1976.
73. Sanerkin NG, Gallagher P: A review of the behavior of chondrosarcoma of bone. J Bone Joint Surg 61B:395, 1979.
73a. Scaglietti O, Marchetti PG, Bartolozzi P: Final results in the treatment of bone cysts with methylprednisolone acetate. Clin Orthop 165:33–42, 1982.
74. Schmitt D, Mubarak S, Gelberman R: Septic shoulders in children. J Pediatr Orthop 1:67–72, 1981.
75. Schwartz EE, Lantieri R, Teplick JG: Erosion of the inferior aspect of the clavicle in secondary hyperparathyroidism. AJR 129:291–295, 1977.
76. Simon MA: Biopsy of muscoloskeletal tumors. J Bone Joint Surg 64A:1253–1257, 1982.
77. Smith J: Aneurysmal bone cyst of clavicle. Br J Radiol 50:706–709, 1977.
78. Smith J, Yuppa F, Watson RC: Primary tumors and tumor-like lesions of the clavicle. Skeletal Radiol 17:235–246, 1988.
79. Smith J, McLachlau D, Huvos AG, Higinbotham NL: Primary bone tumors of the clavicle and scapula. AJR 124:113, 1975.
80. Sonozaki H, Mitsui H, Miyanaga Y: Clinical features of 53 cases with pustolotic arthroosteitis. Ann Rheum Dis 50:547, 1981.
81. Spar J: Total claviculectomy for pathological fractures. Clin Orthop 129:236, 1977.

CHAPTER 16

Malignant and Benign Primary Tumors of the Proximal Femur

STEVEN G. ROBBINS
DALE B. GLASSER
JOSEPH M. LANE
FRANK P. CAMMISA, Jr.

The diagnosis and the treatment of tumors of the proximal femur are based on well-established oncologic principles. Great strides have recently been achieved in the care of both benign and malignant conditions, with improved survival and function resulting. This chapter discusses the current general concepts of diagnosis, tumor staging, and treatment options, including limb preservation, as well as the most common malignant and benign bone tumors of the proximal femur.

The relevant history, physical examination, and basic radiologic assessment are always used initially. With information obtained with these basic tools, the physician must decide if further investigation or treatment is warranted. Treatment possibilities with these tumors or tumor-like lesions range from reassurance and observation to wide ablative surgery with reconstruction, depending on the diagnosis.

SPECIAL CONSIDERATIONS IN THE PROXIMAL FEMUR

The bone marrow begins serving the function of hematopoiesis *in utero*. With aging, there is a conversion of red hematopoietic marrow to fatty yellow marrow. In adults, hematopoietic, or red, marrow predominates in the axial skeleton (spine, pelvis, ribs, sternum, and skull) and the proximal portions of the femur and humerus.[42] Certain types of tumors, either related to their derivation from cells of the red marrow or to their transport to these locations by the marrow vasculature, predominate in these locations.[24] Ewing's sarcoma, metastatic disease, plasma cell myeloma, and histiocytic lymphoma are examples of tumors that have an affinity for localizing in regions of hematopoietic marrow. The proximal femur lies deeply contained in a well-muscled envelope. This may allow extracompartmental soft tissue extension of an osseous neoplasm to escape detection for an extended period as compared with the more superficial location of the distal femur or the proximal tibia, where soft tissue extension is readily palpable or even visible to the patient or the examining physician. Multiple vascular perforations along the femoral neck allow early extraosseous extension of tumor from this location.[8] The hip joint may become involved when tumor spreads from the femoral head along the ligamentum teres. The groin-femoral triangle is, by Enneking's definition,[10] an extracompartmental location, and because of the important neurovascular struc-

Supported by the Greenwall Foundation.

tures that pass through the region surrounding the proximal femur, special considerations are required when planning surgical procedures (see below).

Biomechanically, the medial aspect of the femoral neck is exposed to high compressive loads with muscular contraction and weight-bearing activities (2½ times body weight standing; 10 times body weight stepping off a curb). This predisposes to a high incidence of pathologic fractures through benign or malignant neoplasms in this location, often with minimal antecedent trauma.[18, 28, 41] Prophylactic use of orthoses or internal fixation may be required after biopsy or definitive surgery (e.g., curettage and bone grafting).

Clinical Features

The most common symptoms in patients with bone tumors are progressive pain and an enlarging mass.[25, 27] Classically, the pain is unrelieved by changes in position and may occur at night. Dull, aching pain may mimic that of degenerative arthritis of the hip in the elderly. Classically, the pain may be referred to the medial thigh or the knee. Occasionally, lesions may not be active enough to cause symptoms and are diagnosed incidentally on a radiograph for an unrelated problem. Pathologic fracture presents with typical pain and deformity.[28, 41] The medical history is usually not helpful in patients with primary disease, although it may reveal the location of a primary malignancy in those with metastatic lesions. There is a history of trauma in approximately 30% of cases, but evidence suggesting it as an etiologic factor is scant. Physical examination is usually nonspecific; a mass, if present, may not be tender. Lymphadenopathy is rare with primary bone tumors, except for embryonal rhabdomyosarcoma and certain soft tissue sarcomas.[11, 17] Some limitation in range of motion may occur with tumors that mechanically encroach on the hip joint or with osteoid osteoma, in which synovitis of the hip may occur. Changes in neurovascular function of the extremity due to extrinsic compression of vital structures by extracompartmental tumor spread may be detectable.

Diagnostic Studies

The single most useful test in the diagnosis of bone lesions is the conventional biplane roentgenogram.[21] It usually suggests whether the process is benign or malignant and indicates a differential diagnosis. The location of a lesion (epiphyseal, metaphyseal, or diaphyseal) is of diagnostic importance. Epiphyseal and trochanteric apophyseal locations suggest chondroblastoma in the pediatric population. The round cell tumors (Ewing's sarcoma, lymphoma, and metastatic neuroblastoma) tend to originate at a diaphyseal location, whereas osteogenic sarcoma and chondrosarcoma are found in the metaphysis.

The radiographic appearance of the solitary lesion can reveal much as to its eventual growth or activity.[25, 27] Benign lesions are suggested by small size and elongated shape with well-defined margins. A sclerotic edge at the lesion's periphery indicates a slow process to which the normal bone outside the lesion has successfully created a reactive margin. Malignant pathologic change is suggested by large size, a wide zone of transition with cortical breakthrough, and soft tissue involvement, which may elevate the periosteum (Codman's triangle). The presence or absence of calcification, reactive bone, sarcomatous bone formation, and pure lysis may help in differentiating the specific type of tumor. There are enough exceptions to the rules to force the surgeon to perform bone biopsy to establish a definitive diagnosis. However, some lesions, such as osteochondroma and fibrous cortical defects, can be diagnosed radiographically with extremely high certainty. Some tumors are commonly associated with benign bone diseases, such as the association of malignant fibrous histiocytoma with aseptic necrosis or the malignant degeneration of Paget's disease.

Serologic, biochemical, and immunologic studies have limited value in the diagnosis.[21] The erythrocyte sedimentation rate is nonspecific, although it may be elevated in round cell tumors such as Ewing's sarcoma and non-Hodgkin's lymphoma of bone. The alkaline phosphatase level is commonly elevated in patients with osteoblastic osteogenic sarcoma. Bone marrow biopsies may assist in diagnosing metabolic bone disease or leukemia and in staging the extent of disease during work-up for Ewing's sarcoma. Patients with chondrosarcoma may have a normal blood glucose level in the face of an abnormal glucose tolerance test.[36]

If at this stage the diagnosis can be made with confidence, and particularly if the lesion is benign, further investigations may not be required. If, however, major surgery is required to remove the lesion, further radiologic and nuclear imaging studies may be helpful in determining the extent of the tumor and its relationship to the neurovascular structures.[50] Tomography may be used to accurately localize the nidus of an osteoid osteoma. Biplane peripheral arteriography outlines the extent of the accompanying soft tissue mass and the relationship of the tumor to the major vessels and nerves (e.g., displacement of the femoral artery as it passes through the femoral triangle). The soft tissue extent can be distinctly demonstrated by computed tomography (CT) (with or without contrast material), and more importantly, the relationship of the tumor to the neurovascular structures can be assessed. In staging the tumor (see below), the CT scan is significantly superior to arteriography and has essentially little or no morbidity. In comparison with magnetic resonance imaging (MRI), CT is superior in evaluating the bony architecture (see below). Lymphangiography is generally not indicated in primary bone tumors, except in the case of lymphoma of bone, to help in staging. MRI is an important tool in investigating the intramedullary extent of tumor, the presence of skip lesions, and the relationship of the surrounding soft tissue structures. The great advantages of this modality are the following: no exposure to ionizing radiation, ease of coronal or sagittal reconstruction, and clear definition of bone marrow involvement. MRI can identify trabecular bone quite well; however, it cannot adequately visualize cortical bone, which appears as a signal void. Areas of destruction or replacement of trabecular bone with hematoma, serous fluid, or tumor may be visualized quite effectively. CT scans and MRI images together can unequivocally indicate involvement of a joint by tumor, and they therefore constitute the most important staging modalities for tumors about the hip.

The search for distant or multiple bone disease should include a technetium TC-99m polyphosphate bone scan.[50] In addition to detecting distant disease, it assists in accurately localizing the primary lesion, as well as identifying skip lesions. Gallium scans are helpful in assessing the soft tissue component of the tumor and in clarifying the contribution of disuse osteoporosis to abnormal findings on a technetium bone scan. Whole lung tomography is helpful in detecting pulmonary metastases so that appropriate staging can be accomplished. CT lung scans may be too sensitive and in certain centers yielded significant false-positive findings. Technologic advances in scanners and more experience may significantly improve accuracy.

Staging

Malignant Lesions. With data from the investigations described above, it should be possible to determine a surgical stage for malignant tumors. Enneking and associates devised a system for the staging of musculoskeletal sarcomas.[10] In this system, neoplasms are histologically graded on their biologic aggressiveness as low grade (I) or high grade (II). In general, low-grade malignant lesions have a lower risk for metastasis (less than 25%) and a higher 5-year survival rate. They can usually be managed by relatively conservative procedures. High-grade lesions (grade II) have significantly higher incidence of metastasis and, therefore, require more aggressive procedures to achieve local control and the use of neoadjuvant chemotherapy to eradicate microscopic systemic spread. In addition to grading the neoplasm, the physician assesses its anatomic extent. If it is confined to a well-defined anatomic compartment, it is designated intracompartmental (A). A lesion in two or more anatomic compartments is designated extracompartmental (B). An example of the latter is an intraosseous lesion that lifts the periosteum from cortical bone. A superficial lesion that penetrates the deep fascia is also extracompartmental. Staging of the tumor is based on two considerations, grading and anatomic extent. The stages are subdivided as follows: IA—low-grade tumor within a compartment, IB—low-grade tumor in two or more functional compartments, IIA, intracompartmental high-grade tumor, IIB—high-grade tumor in two or more compartments, and III—any grade tumor with regional or distant metastasis. Intrapelvic lesions and femoral triangle tumors are, by definition, extracompartmental and are classified as B. The unique extensive placement of the femoral head and neck within the hip joint leads to easier and earlier joint extension of malignant and benign lesions as compared with those of the knee and shoulder joints.

Benign Lesions. Benign tumors can be graded into three levels of activity. Grade 1 tumors (latent), such as fibrous cortical defects, are intracompartmental lesions with little or no chance of expansion. Grade 2 benign lesions (active), such as lipoma or simple (unicameral) bone cyst, are intracompartmental lesions with a tendency for slow continuous growth. Grade 3 benign lesions (aggressive) are lesions with a tendency to extend beyond the anatomic compartment, to recur frequently, and occasionally to transport cells to the lungs, as with chondroblastomas or giant cell tumors. The treatment, in general, of grade 1 tumors is observation or incisional curettage; grade 2 lesions, curettage or marginal excision; and grade 3 lesions, excision or curettage beyond the pseudocapsule or reactive bone margin.

Surgical Procedures. Along with this surgical staging system for musculoskeletal tumors, a system for classifying surgical procedures was devised.[10] *En bloc* excisions and amputations may be classified with the same four types of margins. A procedure with an intralesional margin enters the tumor and leaves gross or macroscopic tumor behind. An example is curettage or a debulking procedure. In a marginal procedure, there is reactive tissue or pseudocapsule at the margin. The possibility of leaving satellite lesions or microscopic tumor in the pseudocapsule is high. In a wide excisional procedure, there is a margin of normal, nonreactive tissue completely surrounding the resected lesion. A radical procedure removes the entire involved compartment. In some cases of intralesional or marginal procedure, the margin may be extended with a surgical adjuvant, such as cryosurgery. Malignant lesions require wide removal to completely ablate the local disease.

Biopsy

In many circumstances, one can confidently diagnose certain benign lesions (e.g., fibrous cortical defects and osteochondromas) from the clinical and radiologic appearances. If these lesions are found incidentally and are not the source of the patient's symptoms, further investigation and/or surgery is not indicated. If, however, a lesion does not have one of the classic benign radiographic appearances or locations or is growing or causing symptoms, a biopsy is mandatory.[32, 49] Symptomatic osteochondromas may be treated by excisional biopsy, with care being taken to completely excise the perichondrium to minimize recurrence. Excisional biopsy is also adequate for treatment of other lesions, such as osteoid osteoma, that have little potential for recurrence.

An incisional biopsy is the most commonly employed type of open biopsy.[25, 27, 32, 49] It is the procedure of choice for open biopsy of most malignant tumors. The placement of the biopsy incision is crucial, as the biopsy scar together with the biopsy track must be excised *en bloc* with the malignant tumor at the definitive surgical procedure. The biopsy incision should be longitudinal, along the lines of anticipated extensile exposure needed for potential *en bloc* resection. Poorly placed biopsy scars may jeopardize further exposure for *en bloc* resection and indeed a large transverse scar may preclude the possibility of performing a limb-sparing resection and necessitate amputation. The smallest incision that is compatible with adequate exposure is preferred. The periphery of any malignant tumor offers the best and most representative tissue. The center may be necrotic. A small segment of bone may be carefully excised, using a sharp osteotome after predrilling multiple small holes. The biopsy specimen should be round or oval to decrease local stress concentrations. In addition to specimens for permanent sections, frozen sections should be obtained to confirm accurate location and adequacy of the biopsy. Special studies such as electron microscopy and lymphona typing may be necessary and can be suggested by the frozen section examination results. Multiple cultures for aerobic, anaerobic, and acid-fast bacilli, as well as fungal cultures, should be obtained. Consequently, antibiotics should not be given before biopsy. Tumor blood can also be sent for biochemical analysis (e.g., acid and alkaline phosphatase determinations). Very high values of alkaline phosphatase may be seen in osteosarcomas. Care must be taken to minimize tumor spillage. Meticulous hemostasis during wound closure is of paramount importance, as the larger the postoperative hematoma, the greater is the contamination of soft tissues with neoplastic cells. Plugging of the biopsy hole with absorbable gelatin sponge (Gelfoam) with thrombin, microcrystalline collagen, or methyl methacrylate may be necessary. Selective use of a drain along the line of biopsy incision (and rapid removal) may be indicated. After biopsy, it is important that the limb is protected to prevent a pathologic fracture.

Percutaneous needle biopsies may be performed in some specialized centers, but again the placement of the needle should be carefully planned so that the needle tract may be excised *en bloc.*[40] The needle biopsy should be considered a "small" open biopsy. The diagnostic accuracy with percutaneous needle biopsies is approximately 80% compared with a 98% accuracy with an open biopsy. The accuracy and method of the biopsy significantly affects the ultimate outcome.

The proximal femur requires special considerations for biopsy. If the lesion is in the intertrochanteric area, a laterally placed biopsy tract through the greater trochanter causes little structural weakness and preserves most options for *en bloc* resections. The subtrochanteric area can be reached through such an approach as well. Lesions of the head and neck can be addressed either through a lateral opening with a long intramedullary approach or directly through the proximal arm of an anterolateral incision. Efforts to stay outside the hip joint are critical. A biopsy at the lateral anterior base of the neck significantly weakens the femur and requires postoperative protection. Lesions distal to the lesser trochanter are best approached laterally or anteriorly; however, the femur is structurally weakened, as in the neck, and requires postoperative protection as well.

After the pathologic grade of the tumor is determined, the tumor may be staged either as IA, IB, IIA, IIB, or III.[10] This system of surgical staging assists in the decision of whether a limb-sparing procedure is feasible or an amputation is necessary. Stage III lesions with pulmonary metastasis may be considered for limb-sparing procedure, as, in many circumstances, the pulmonary metastasis may be amenable to chemotherapy followed by surgical excision with or without chemotherapy.[27]

Treatment

BENIGN LESIONS

Benign lesions showing indisputable diagnostic radiologic characteristics (e.g., asymptomatic nonossifying fibroma or asymptomatic osteochondroma) do not require surgical treatment or even a biopsy.[21, 25, 27] If, however, any doubt about the benign nature of the lesion exists, a biopsy should be performed. Symptomatic osteochondromas may be treated by excisional biopsy (i.e., marginal excision). Most of the other grade 1 or 2 benign tumors are adequately treated by standard procedures, such as curettage and packing with bone chips or by small *en bloc* excisions. Simple curettage can be extended for aggressive benign lesions, such as aneurysmal bone cysts, by utilizing cryosurgery, phenolization, or thermal cautery with methyl methacrylate. (A more detailed discussion follows for specific tumors.) Simple (unicameral) bone cysts have been successfully treated by repetitive intralesional injection with 40 to 80 mg of crystalline methylprednisolone acetate. Currently being investigated at the authors' center is the use of bone marrow injections into these cysts.[19] In the course of curettage or resection, the resulting surgical osseous defects represent significant stress risers and may give rise to pathologic fractures about the hip. Femoral head and neck lesions can be supported with threaded Knowles pins or cannulated screws. Defects from the base of the neck to the lesser trochanter should be protected with appropriately sized hip compression screws with side plates. Lesser trochanteric and proximal diaphyseal lesions are aided by interlocking intramedullary devices such as the Zickel nail or interlocking femoral rods. If the diagnosis is in question, staged procedures are preferred to prevent inadvertent contamination of the entire femoral medullary canal with an undiagnosed malignancy at the time of initial biopsy.

Surgical Considerations

When treating lesions of the proximal femur, the primary postoperative considerations are maintenance of hip joint stability and preservation of motion. Bone grafting and internal fixation along with protected weight bearing are indicated to prevent pathologic fracture following curettage, cryosurgery, or excision. Consideration should be given to removal of internal fixation devices after healing and remodeling are complete in young people.

Benign Bone-Forming Tumors

The two lesions in this class that affect the proximal femur are osteoid osteoma and, rarely, osteoblastoma.[5, 21, 27]

OSTEOID OSTEOMA

Slightly fewer than 25% of osteoid osteomas involve the proximal femur.[5] The lesion is characterized by a nidus measuring approximately 1 cm in diameter surrounded by a sclerotic rim of differing thickness. Pain at night, relieved with aspirin, has been the classic presentation, but this combination is not found in the vast majority of cases. The lesion is found predominantly in children and young adults from 10 to 25 years.

The radiographic appearance of osteoid osteoma is quite helpful. The nidus is surrounded by a rim of reactive sclerotic cancellous bone in the spongiosa or reactively thickened periosteal new bone if it occurs in the cortex. The nidus is a clear radiolucent area, which may become radiopaque as the nidus matures. The excessive, reactive bone may obscure the nidus. Bone scanning and tomography may be helpful in such cases.[50] A "double-density sign" with an area of increased radionuclide uptake and a second area of increased uptake superimposed on the radionuclide scan has been described to differentiate osteoid osteoma from osteomyelitis and may aid in accurate preoperative localization of the nidus.[20] Angiography demonstrates an intense blush because of the hypervascularity of the nidus. Osteoid osteomas in juxtaarticular situations may be difficult to diagnose. The osteoblastic reaction may be blunted or missing and the lesion may give rise to inflammatory changes within the hip joint.

The treatment of osteoid osteomas is wide surgical excision of the nidus with a surrounding rim of perilesional sclerotic bone and curettage of the adjacent bone. Radiographic control to locate the area of the nidus is mandatory. Drill holes or needle markers are commonly used with intraoperative radiographs to ensure exact placement of the incision. Commonly, if the lesion is cortical, the periosteal reactive bone appears as a roughened raised surface over the nidus. The intact *en bloc* excision of the nidus and surrounding bone may be examined radiologically during surgery to ensure complete removal of the nidus. Recently, the use of intraoperative radionuclide localization of the tumor has been helpful in identifying the prospective site of resection and confirming that the tumor has been resected. In addition, reports suggest that tetracycline and ultraviolet light (Wood's lamp) may be helpful.[1] At Memorial Sloan-Kettering Cancer Center, the majority of osteoid osteomas about the hip occurred in the medial aspect of the femoral neck. A modified Ludloff approach, either superior or inferior to the adductor lateralis, provides excellent exposure. Resections usually necessitate bone grafting and stabilization of the hip, with either a spica cast, Knowles pins, or a hip screw with a side plate, depending on the location of the lesion and the age of the patient. Conservative management of primary or recurrent osteoid osteomas is based on nonsteroidal therapy. Osteoid osteomas produce excessive prostaglandins locally. Long-acting nonsteroidal agents may not only control the symptoms, but also diminish the hip inflammatory reaction.

OSTEOBLASTOMA

Osteoblastoma[5, 21, 27] is a benign bone-forming lesion that is related histologically to the osteoid osteoma. It rarely occurs in the hip region; less than 1% of these lesions occur in the proximal femur.[5] It is larger than the 1 cm nidus of osteoid osteoma and does not have as much perilesional reactive bone nor as much pain. This uncommon lesion is found in children and young adults, usually in the metaphysis or the diaphysis. The lesions are well circumscribed, 2 to 12 cm in diameter, expansile, and radiolucent, with differing amounts of mottled calcification. The bone scan and angiogram are often useful in delineating the extent of the lesion. The treatment of choice is resection of the lesion and stabilization of the femur, as is accomplished for osteoid osteoma. Curettage is associated with a recurrence rate of 25%.[31] A small percentage (less than 2%) may become malignant.

Benign Cartilage-Forming Tumors

The benign cartilage-forming tumors affecting the region of the proximal femur include osteochondroma, enchondroma, chondroblastoma, and chondromyxoid fibroma.[5, 21, 27]

OSTEOCHONDROMA

The osteochondroma is a bony mass, either sessile or pedunculated, whose growth is produced by enchondral ossification of a cartilage cap (Fig. 16–1). This is the most common benign bone tumor. Slightly more than 8% occur in the region of the proximal femur.[5] This benign growth is usually asymptomatic and is not seen or treated by the physician. Others may be palpable beneath the skin. A few may give rise to symptoms resulting from pressure on nearby structures, such as nerves or vessels, or cause significant limitation of hip movement. When following patients with symptomatic osteochondromas older than 30 years of age, one should carefully evaluate for malignant transformation (cartilage cap greater than 0.5 cm), particularly in proximally located lesions. Excisional biopsy should in-

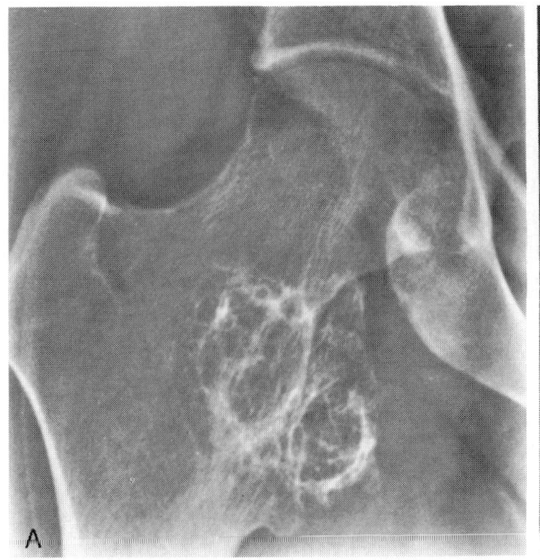

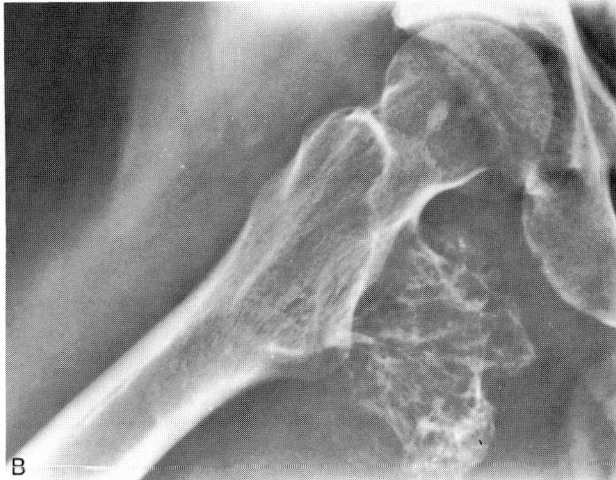

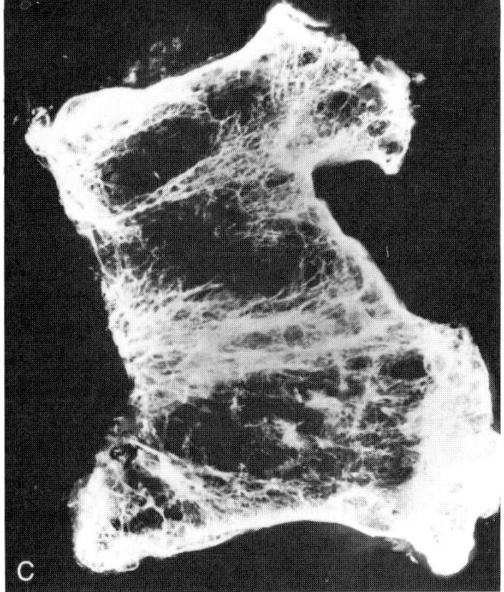

FIGURE 16–1. Osteosarcoma. *A*, *B*, Two views of a large osteochondroma arising from the posterior aspect of the lesser trochanter in a 36-year-old man with signs and symptoms of sciatic nerve irritation. *C*, The lesion was excised and the specimen radiograph is depicted. The lesion was 7.5 × 5.0 × 5.0 cm in size, with a cartilaginous cap that measured 0.2 cm over most of the lesion (and 0.5 cm at its maximal diameter). The diagnosis of benign osteochondroma was confirmed.

clude the perichondrial lining layer. MRI has been reported to show the essential anatomic features of these lesions and was especially useful in evaluating the presence and thickness of the cartilage cap. The cartilage cap can be seen as a region of high signal intensity on T2-weighted images. The intact perichondrium, a superficial zone of low-signal intensity that covered the cartilage cap, was also detected on MRI.[30] Changes in the MRI signal of the cartilage cap may suggest malignant degeneration. Indications for surgical excision include suspicion of malignant degeneration (wide excisional biopsy), pain, limitation of hip motion, and pressure on vital structures. The osteochondroma should be removed *in toto* to the base of the osseous neck. The perichondrium must be included in the resection or recurrence will occur.

ENCHONDROMA

Enchondromas are benign cartilage tumors that probably represent developmental cartilage rests.[21, 27] They are frequently found incidentally. Approximately 7% of solitary enchondromas occur in the proximal femur.[5] Enchondromas are characterized by calcified cartilage within the metaphysis. Endosteal scalloping, cortical breakthrough, lucency, and localized pain are all suggestive of malignant degeneration.

Bone scans remain abnormal well into early adulthood. Benign enchondromas require no surgical treatment, unless they are associated with impending or completed pathologic fractures. In these cases, curettage with bone grafting should be curative. Very-low-grade chondrosarcomas and aggressive (recurrent) enchondromas can be cured with extensive curettage and cryosurgery. Care should be taken to prevent pathologic fractures after cryosurgery. The bone should be protected until osseous remodeling has occurred.

CHONDROBLASTOMA

Chondroblastomas occur in the epiphysis and the apophysis (Fig. 16–2) in late adolescence and rarely occur in patients older than 25 years of age.[22] Slightly less than 10% occur about the proximal femur.[5] The lesion may be associated with an aneurysmal bone cyst component in 20 to 25% of cases. Treatment consists of thorough curettage and bone grafting. The results of adjuvants to curettage such as phenol application or cryosurgery are still uncertain. Occasionally, chondroblastoma may be transported to the lung and must be resected with thoracotomy. Rarely, the chondroblastoma can degenerate into a sarcoma.

CHONDROMYXOID FIBROMA

Chondromyxoid fibromas involve the proximal femur in fewer than 1% of cases.[5] Aggressive curettage cures the lesion, but sometimes marginal resection with reconstruction is needed.

Other Benign Lesions

FIBROUS DYSPLASIA

Fibrous dysplasia is a benign developmental condition, which may be monostotic or polyostotic. The disease begins in childhood but usually becomes clinically apparent in young adulthood during an incidental radiographic examination. Fibrous dysplasia in the proximal femur can cause the progressive varus "shepherd's crook" deformity associated with shortening of the leg, limping, and occasional chronic fatigue fractures with disabling pain. The appearance is that of a radiolucent cystic lesion with deformity and diffuse enlargement of the bone contour (Fig. 16–3). Treatment is indicated for pathologic fracture or progressive deformity. Cortical bone grafting without curettage, excision, or internal fixation in symptomatic patients with fibrous dysplasia of the femoral neck has been recommended by Enneking and Gearen[9]; however, other physicians suggest adding internal fixation to curettage and bone grafting to improve satisfactory results.[52] Curettage, bone grafting, and stabilization with either bracing or internal fixation until the osseous remodeling has been completed is the approach used at Memorial Sloan-Kettering Cancer Center. Frequently, the fibrous dysplasia recurs, even in the face of thorough curettage and bone grafting. The osteogenic cells that replace and incorporate the graft arise from the bed of fibrous dysplasia. This accounts for the frequent resorption of the graft and led to the recommendation of cortical bone by Enneking (see above). The triad of café au lait skin lesions, polyostotic fibrous dysplasia, and endocrinopathy constitute Albright's syndrome.

FIBROUS CORTICAL DEFECTS

Fibrous cortical defects (nonossifying fibromas) occur in approximately one third of all children, and spontaneous regression of this asymptomatic focus of periosteal fibrous tissue is usual. Approximately 6% of cases occur in the proximal femur.[21] Curettage is recom-

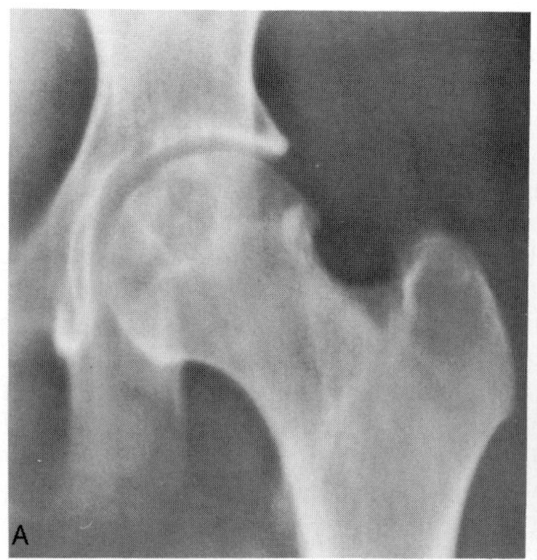

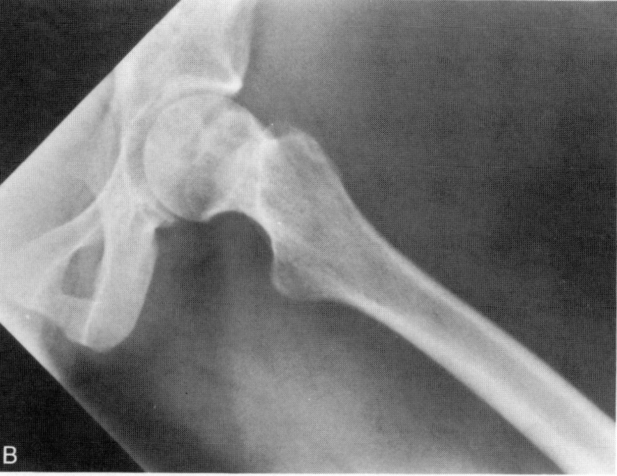

FIGURE 16–2. *A*, AP view, and *B*, Lateral view of chondroblastoma of the head of the femur in a 17-year-old male adolescent.

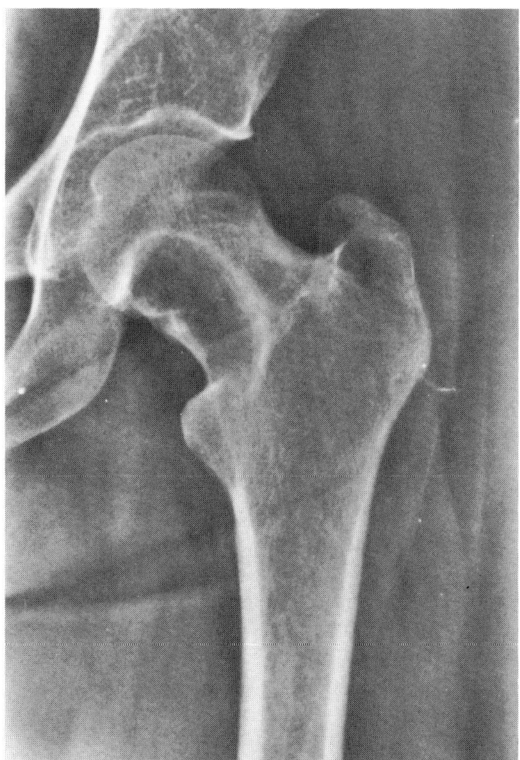

FIGURE 16–3. Fibrous dysplasia of the femoral neck in a 23-year-old woman. The radiograph shows a well-circumscribed lytic lesion of the femoral neck with a sclerotic border. The lesion was treated with curettage, bone graft, and a slide screw and plate device for fixation.

mended for large symptomatic lesions in which a pathologic fracture is imminent. Reinforcement of the femur with Knowles pins or a nail plate may be necessary in cases of impending fracture.

ANEURYSMAL BONE CYST

Aneurysmal bone cyst is one of the most rapidly growing destructive lesions of bone. Approximately one third of cases are in association with other entities, such as nonossifying fibroma, fibrous dysplasia, chondroblastoma, giant cell tumor, and solitary bone cyst. For this reason, aneurysmal bone cyst is frequently described as an arteriovenous malformation engrafted on other primary processes.[21] Approximately 3.5% occur in the region of the proximal femur[5]; 85% occur before the age of 20 years. Roentgenographic features include eccentric soap bubble appearance often associated with obvious soft tissue extension formed by periosteal new bone (Fig. 16–4*A*). Aneurysmal bone cysts may grow rapidly and be mistaken for a telangiectatic osteogenic sarcoma. Treatment consists of curettage and bone grafting (Fig. 16–4*B*). At Memorial Sloan-Kettering Cancer Center, the judicious use of cryosurgery significantly decreases the recurrence rate. Internal fixation or postoperative orthoses may be required to prevent fracture.

SIMPLE CYSTS

Simple, or unicameral, bone cysts are relatively common lesions, occurring in the first two decades of life (Fig. 16–5). After the proximal humerus, the proximal femur is the second most common location of these cysts. A disturbance of growth at the epiphyseal plate is the theorized origin of simple cysts. Males predominate by a 2:1 ratio. "Active" cysts abut a growth plate and tend to recur more frequently than do "latent" cysts, which are separated from the plate by normal bone. Curettage and grafting carries recurrence rates of approximately 25%. Scaglietti and colleagues advocated injecting the cysts with 80 to 200 mg of methylprednisolone acetate, using a two-needle technique, and reported 80 to 90% satisfactory results with multiple injections; however healing occurred in only 55% of cases.[2, 47, 48] Healey, at the authors' institution, reported the use of autologous osteogenic marrow grafting, using a similar two-needle technique, and noted more rapid healing and more frequent bone formation and patients required fewer injections.[19] A needle biopsy at the time of the first encounter is suggested to rule out the rare possibility of telangiectatic osteogenic sarcoma. Partial or complete subperiosteal diaphysectomy of the cyst walls lowers recurrence rates to approximately 5%.[14] Simple (unicameral) bone cysts of the proximal femur frequently result in pathologic fractures. The limb should be immobilized for 3 weeks to allow partial healing and skeletal continuity before initiating treatment of the primary lesion.

EOSINOPHILIC GRANULOMA

Eosinophilic granuloma occurs most commonly in the first decade of life. Lesions are relatively common in the supraacetabular area. The proximal femoral metaphysis and diaphysis are rarely involved. A combination of bone scanning and skeletal radiographic survey is necessary to determine the presence of multifocal disease because neither method alone is

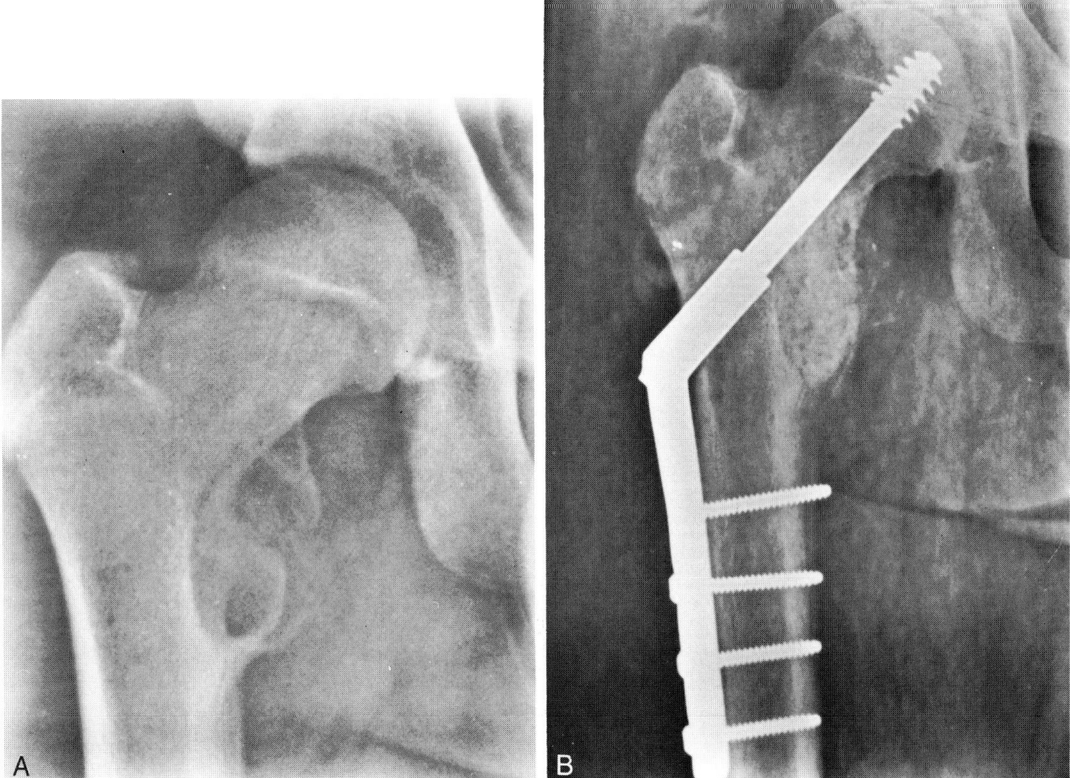

FIGURE 16–4. Aneurysmal bone cyst in the area of the lesser trochanter. *A*, A bubbly lesion with destruction of the cortex and periosteal reaction in the proximal medial femoral shaft. *B*, The lesion was treated with curettage, cryosurgery, irradiated cancellous bone graft, and internal fixation.

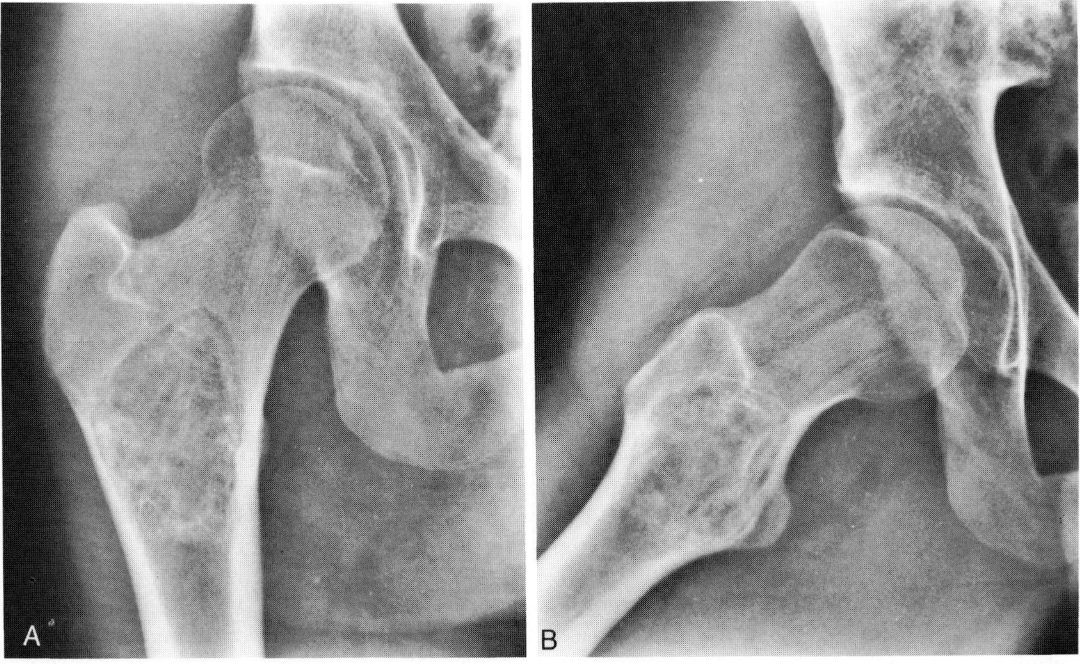

FIGURE 16–5. Incidental finding of a large cyst in the neck and proximal shaft of the femur in a 16-year-old male adolescent. There is marked thinning of the cortex. The lesion proved to be a unicameral bone cyst.

sufficiently sensitive. Treatment consists of curettage, bone grafting, and rarely, low-dose radiation. Low-dose chemotherapy is necessary for the treatment of multiple lesions. The prognosis is good. Hip lesions significantly weaken the bone; thus, protective ambulation is required until osseous reconstitution has taken place.

GIANT CELL TUMOR

Giant cell tumors of bone most frequently occur in patients older than 20 years of age and are one of only two primary bone tumors that occur more frequently in females than in males (the other is juxtacortical osteogenic sarcoma).[21] The proximal femur accounts for approximately 5% of these tumors.[5, 16, 21] Roentgenographically, they appear as radiolucent epiphyseal lesions, eccentric to the long axis of the bone, and may expand the cortex (Fig. 16–6). Occasionally, giant cell tumors may undergo sarcomatous change, especially if they have been irradiated. The local recurrence rates after curettage alone are greater than 80% within 2 years. The addition of bone grafting results in lower recurrence rates (40 to 60%), in part related to a more thorough curettage.[16] Marcove and associates, at the authors' institution, pioneered the use of cryosurgery with liquid nitrogen at temperatures of −20° C after curettage[33] and lowered the recurrence rate to 12% in 52 consecutive cases of giant cell tumor.[38] The current recommendation from the Musculoskeletal Tumor Society is to perform a thorough curettage through a wide cortical window and insert methyl methacrylate into the cavity. The cement works in an adjuvant manner by causing some degree of thermal necrosis of the surrounding bone and provides structural support around the defect.[18] Cure rates of better than 80% have been reported and recurrences are easily detectable. Although this method has a lower cure rate than with cryosurgery, the complications are fewer. In large recurrent tumors, or Campanacci stage 3 lesions (cortical break-

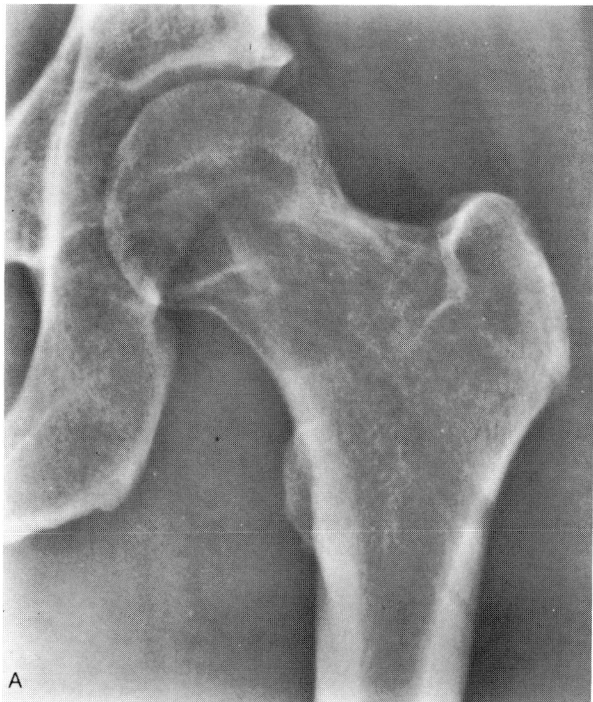

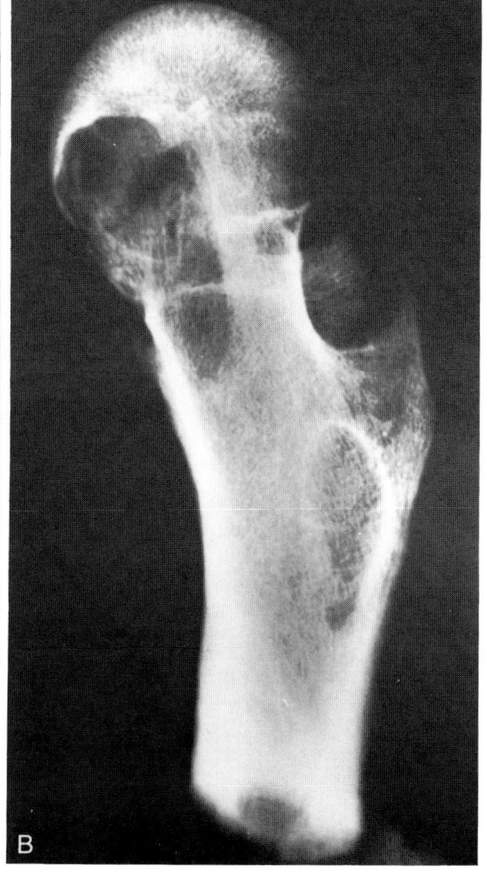

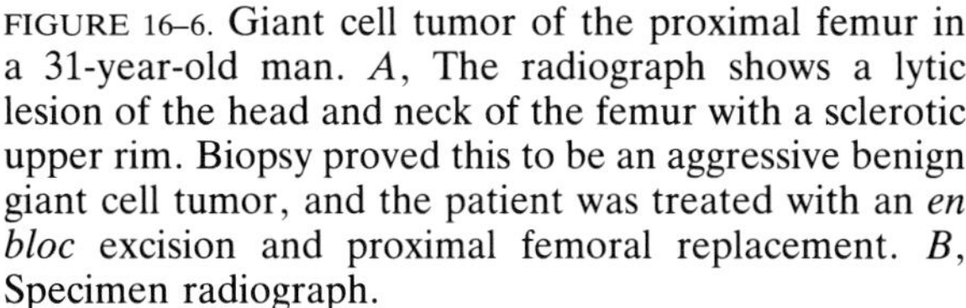
FIGURE 16–6. Giant cell tumor of the proximal femur in a 31-year-old man. *A*, The radiograph shows a lytic lesion of the head and neck of the femur with a sclerotic upper rim. Biopsy proved this to be an aggressive benign giant cell tumor, and the patient was treated with an *en bloc* excision and proximal femoral replacement. *B*, Specimen radiograph.

through), wide *en bloc* excision and proximal femoral replacement may be indicated.

MALIGNANT LESIONS

Dramatic advances in the treatment of high-grade malignant lesions have been made since the mid-1970s. They include the development of sophisticated adjuvant multiagent chemotherapeutic protocols and refinement of surgical techniques for local control of these lesions.[13]

Chemotherapy

With modern multidrug chemotherapy, increasing numbers of patients with malignant bone tumors are now expected to be disease-free survivors after amputation or *en bloc* resection. In earlier reports, the 5-year cure rate for patients with osteogenic sarcoma was between 15 and 20%, and for those with Ewing's sarcoma, it was 5 to 15%, despite amputation or high-dose radiation.[6, 21, 34] Formerly, all patients with malignant lesions of the extremities were treated by amputation. In the past decade, increasing numbers of tumors were successfully treated with limb preservation. In addition to greatly improved survival rates, an enhanced quality of life for many survivors was also achieved.[46]

It is assumed that, at the time of diagnosis of certain sarcomas, patients already have microscopic foci of disease in their lungs. Although surgery can eliminate the primary tumor, chemotherapy is used to destroy these microscopic but undetectable areas of disease. In addition to its use as an adjuvant modality for micrometastases in the treatment of primary bone tumors, chemotherapy is employed preoperatively to rapidly shrink bulky primary and metastatic tumors.[12, 43, 45, 51]

Many centers now give adjuvant chemotherapy to all patients with high-grade spindle cell sarcomas, which include osteogenic sarcomas and high-grade chondrosarcomas.[12, 43] Small cell sarcomas, including Ewing's sarcoma, non-Hodgkin's lymphoma, and rhabdomyosarcoma, are highly malignant and are very sensitive to modern multidrug chemotherapy.[11, 17, 44] In addition to surgery and chemotherapy, radiation therapy is used to help obtain local control of primary small cell sarcomas.

Osteogenic sarcoma is the most frequently occurring primary malignant tumor of bone in children and adolescents. The current approach to osteogenic sarcoma[43] is to treat all patients preoperatively with multicycle high-dose methotrexate with citrovorum factor rescue; bleomycin, cyclophosphamide, and actinomycin D (BCD); and doxorubicin (Adriamycin). This protocol is used for patients scheduled to have either amputation or a limb-sparing procedure. The effect of 4 to 8 weeks of preoperative chemotherapy is assessed by the histologic examination of the resected primary tumor. A grading system based on the extent of tumor necrosis has been devised by Huvos:[43, 45] grade I—little or no effect of chemotherapy noted (0 to 50% tumor necrosis); grade II—a partial response, with the majority of the tumor being necrotic; grade III—only microscopic foci of tumor remain (greater than 90% necrosis in each histologic section); and grade IV—no viable-appearing tumor cells noted in any of the histologic specimens (minimum of 30 sections). In osteogenic sarcoma, patients with grade III or IV response continue to receive the same chemotherapy as preoperatively. Patients with a grade I or II effect of preoperative chemotherapy on the primary tumor are placed on a regimen containing cisplatin with mannitol diuresis combined with doxorubicin (Adriamycin).

Combination chemotherapy is also used in the treatment of small cell sarcomas.[44] The patient is given early aggressive chemotherapy to eliminate micrometastases. Large bulky tumors usually reduce significantly in size. Local therapy is planned for approximately 6 to 10 weeks after the initiation of treatment, except if there is a poor response of the tumor as judged by frequent clinical examination results, radionuclide imaging, and/or roentgenograms. In these cases, immediate surgical attention to the primary tumor is preferable.

Although multidrug chemotherapy has provided major advances in the treatment of cancer in general, it is associated with considerable toxicity. High-dose methotrexate with citrovorum rescue had a mortality of approximately 6% in the early days of its use.[23] Mortality due to chemotherapy has declined with experience, and there have been no deaths associated with the use of high-dose methotrexate at the authors' center for more than 10 years; however, significant temporary morbidity often exists. High-dose methotrexate may be associated with transient, and rarely permanent, central nervous system toxicity.

Doxorubicin (Adriamycin) in high cumulative doses may produce irreversible cardiomyopathy and bleomycin may lead to pulmonary fibrosis. Cisplatin can cause permanent renal toxicity and ototoxicity. Bone healing may be delayed so that grafting procedures after resections require prolonged periods of immobilization. Skin healing is protracted; consequently, chemotherapy should not be resumed for 2 weeks after surgery. Skin sutures are usually left in place for approximately 6 weeks to prevent wound dehiscence.

Surgical Treatment

The choice of surgical procedures for malignant lesions depends on a number of factors. Accurate histologic diagnosis and surgical staging are of paramount importance.[10] The size and extent of both osseous and soft tissue involvement can be determined by biplane roentgenograms, arteriograms, bone scans, and gallium scans together with CT and MRI scans.[25, 27] Perfusion CT scanning is particularly sensitive in determining whether the major neurovascular structures are involved and assists in the decision about the resectability of the lesion versus the necessity for amputation. MRI has surpassed CT in delineating soft tissue involvement. Preoperative chemotherapy may reduce the size of a tumor, rendering it resectable.[43, 45] The age of the patient has a major role in determining the type of surgical procedures that should be employed. The projected limb length discrepancy in actively growing, very young children may make amputation the only realistic choice in proximal femoral lesions, although an expandable prosthesis has been used.

Despite the advances in chemotherapy, amputation remains a common surgical procedure for malignant tumors. The level of amputation is selected after careful study of roentgenograms, bone scans, and MRI images. The bone scans and MRI images are particularly helpful in providing a good approximation of the proximal margin of the involved bone.

Limb-sparing procedures employing *en bloc* resection are a valid alternative to amputation in carefully selected cases.[13, 26, 27, 46] Local resection of malignant lesions is still at the developmental stage and should be done only in centers experienced with these techniques. In general, limb-sparing procedures using *en bloc* excisional surgery may be considered in individuals with low-grade malignant neoplasms and carefully selected, localized high-grade malignancies. These patients must have a potentially normal cuff of tissue around the tumor, no neurovascular involvement, and adequate skin coverage. Plastic surgical techniques to cover large skin defects, especially myocutaneous "free flaps" performed using microsurgical techniques, have expanded the indications for limb salvage. The first objective in tumor surgery in patients without evidence of skip areas or metastases is to obtain local control and avoid local recurrence. The second is to preserve as much function as possible without jeopardizing survival. Local recurrence after resection of a high-grade sarcoma is associated with a poor chance of long-term survival. Limb-sparing surgery for malignant tumors should be applied with caution and only after careful evaluation of imaging studies, including biplane roentgenograms and arteriograms and bone, gallium, CT, and MRI scans.

Wide *en bloc* resection of malignant tumor entails the removal of the lesion with an intact cuff of normal tissue that completely surrounds the lesion. Careful judgment is required in deciding to proceed with such procedures. The patient and the family should understand realistic functional goals of limb-sparing surgery. The patient will have definite impairment. Consent for an alternative procedure such as amputation, if it becomes necessary, should be obtained preoperatively. *En bloc* resection of carefully selected malignant tumors employs the same principles that are applied to all tumor surgery (i.e., the tumor must never be violated and a surrounding margin of normal soft tissue and bone must be removed *en bloc* with the lesion).[10]

Neoplasms of the hip region necessitating amputation can be surgically treated by a hip disarticulation or hemipelvectomy (hindquarter amputation). Proximal femoral lesions with involvement of the joint capsule necessitate hemipelvectomy to achieve a wide margin. The classic hemipelvectomy involves removal of the leg and the pelvis through the sacroiliac joint and the symphysis pubis. The modified hemipelvectomy leaves the superior wing of the ilium and provides for increased ease of prosthetic fit. The extended hemipelvectomy includes part of the sacrum in the resection to achieve a wide margin.

If the neurovascular structures are not involved, or the vessels can be grafted, *en bloc* excision is possible. Options in this area include wide excision of the proximal femur and/or periacetabulum, depending on the extent of the lesion. For large lesions, a classic hemipelvectomy may not provide better tumor margins medially than an *en bloc* excision. Other reconstructive options for this region are resection arthroplasty (pseudarthrosis), implant arthroplasty (with biologic or nonbiologic replacements), arthrodesis, or hip rotationplasty.

A discussion of reconstructive options in this area is extremely complex. The choice of procedure must be individualized to the resection performed. The first priority is to perform an adequate ablative tumor procedure and achieve wide margins, and thoughts about reconstruction must be secondary. The authors found that the most important consideration is the achievement of stability for the extremity, although motion may have to be sacrificed. It may be technically possible to reconstruct almost any defect; however, careful consideration must be given to whether the patient's function, life style, and comfort are being compromised by any option.

Excisions of lesions in this area may be subdivided into three major categories: limited extracapsular excision of the hip joint and proximal femur, resection of the inferior hemipelvis distal to the level of the sciatic notch (including resection of the femoral head and neck), and resection of nearly the entire hemipelvis, including the femoral head and neck. At the authors' institution, several reconstructive alternatives have been employed. A Girdlestone-like pseudoarthrosis has been tried. Although patients achieved ambulation with gait aids, the lack of stability has not allowed for optimal function. A large functional leg length discrepancy is apparent. Patients complain of instability and "telescoping" of the extremity during ambulation. Alternatives have been sought that would allow more proximal stability.

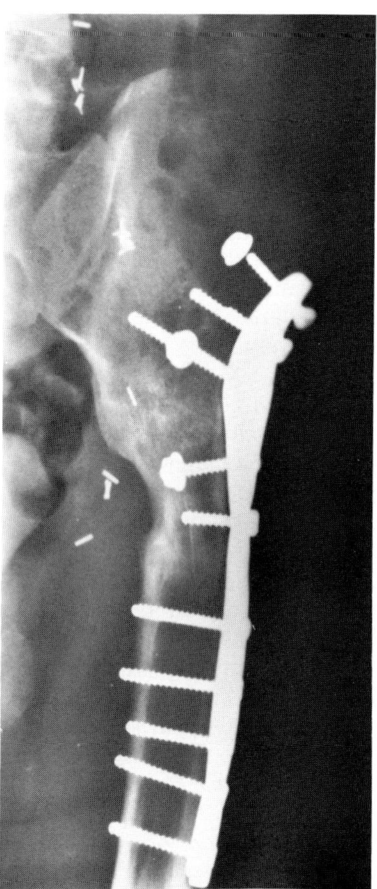

FIGURE 16–7. An internal hemipelvectomy with iliofemoral fusion using a vascularized iliac crest bone graft and Cobra plate. This procedure was performed to treat an osteogenic sarcoma of the femoral head in a 16-year-old male adolescent. He experienced a pathologic fracture of the neck of the femur while receiving preoperative chemotherapy. Pathology examination revealed involvement of the hip joint. This view depicts a healed fusion (and a fracture of a screw) just before the removal of hardware.

Iliofemoral fusion often necessitates a segmental graft to bridge the resection gap, preferably a vascularized pedicle graft (Fig. 16–7). All patients on whom the authors have used this method have received chemotherapy both before and after resection. Delays have been experienced in achieving union in these patients; however, all have experienced bone union after supplemental bone grafting and exhibited good function and excellent stability. The authors believe that arthrodesis provides an excellent pain-free and functional reconstructive choice for young patients. New methods of employing vascularized iliac crest grafts and better methods of fixation are currently being explored. Pelvic allografts have been employed to reconstruct massive defects of the pelvis combined with proximal femur allograft or, preferably, allograft pelvis and bipolar proximal femoral replacement. Resorption of allograft, fractures, dislocations, and infection have also been commonly seen with pelvic allografts. Only one of four cases was ultimately successful, but that one case required a femoral prosthetic conversion. Because of major problems with pelvic allografts, the authors prefer alternatives if possible. If a limited excision of the proximal femur is possible, a long-stem segmental proximal femoral replacement is used. The authors designed a custom modular segmental replacement system for this application and similar systems were described by others.[4, 29] A significant rate of dislocation may be seen, owing to the necessity of resecting musculature. Immobilization for 6 weeks in a single-leg spica or a hip dislocation abduction orthosis often precluded this problem. The addition of porous ingrowth, whether intramedullary or extramedullary, may enhance fixation. At this time, fewer than 5% of prostheses have failed over 5 years. Abduction is achieved by meticulous attention to attachment of the abductors to the prosthesis.

Allografts to reconstruct intercalary segments for diaphyseal resections remain an excellent option for reconstruction.[31] Intramedullary fixation with interlocking femoral and reconstruction nails is preferable. Bone grafting at the host-allograft junction increases the rate and quality of the osteosynthesis. Reports describing healing of allografts both with and without the use of adjuvant chemotherapy have been published.[7, 39] Proximal femoral allografts combined with proximal femoral prosthesis (the bioimplant) have advantages in that soft tissue may be easily reattached to the allograft and bone stock is augmented for future revision and reconstructive procedures (Fig. 16–8).

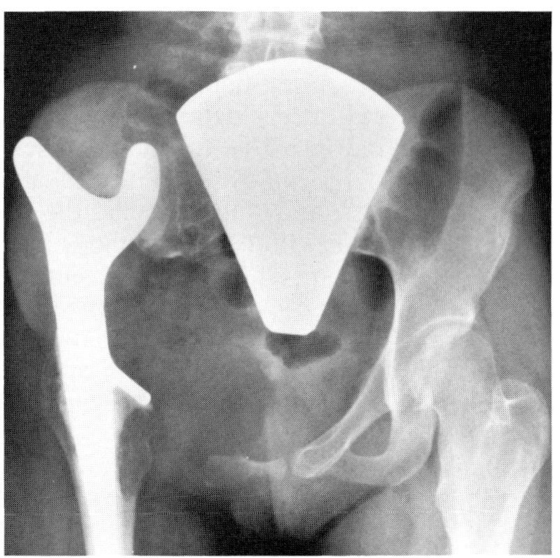

FIGURE 16–9. A saddle prosthesis was used to reconstruct a large defect involving the femoral head, the ischium, and the pubis resulting from *en bloc* excision of a chondrosarcoma.

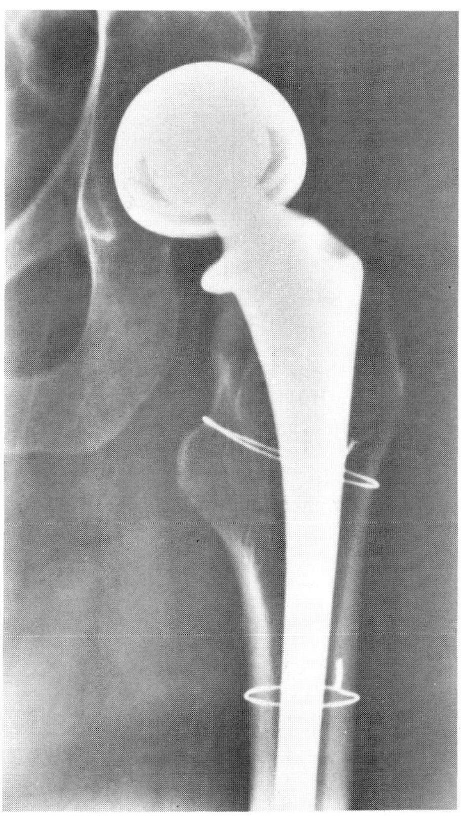

FIGURE 16–8. A composite prosthesis-allograft reconstruction in a 22-year-old woman who had a wide *en bloc* excision for a low-grade malignant fibrous histiocytoma. Originally, a proximal femoral replacement was used in conjunction with a proximal femoral allograft. A later revision included an acetabular component.

A less desirable salvage reconstruction for severe acetabular deficit is the saddle prosthesis (Fig. 16–9). The crook of the prosthesis articulates with an arc created in the ilium. This procedure does not provide true hip motion, but a gliding motion at the bone-prosthesis junction does occur. Experience with this device is limited, and follow-up is too short to draw conclusions. At Memorial Sloan-Kettering Cancer Center, three of four patients achieved assisted ambulation (single cane), but long-distance ambulation was compromised and rehabilitation requirements were extensive.

A recent development has been a report from Germany using a modification of the Van Nes rotationplasty. An *en bloc* excision is performed, and the distal femur, knee, and leg are rotated 180 degrees and fused to the ilium. In this position, the knee functions as a pseudohip, and the ankle functions as a pseudoknee. The authors have no experience with this method of reconstruction.

The authors are currently in the process of measuring performance capabilities for patients who have had amputations and various types of *en bloc* excisions and reconstructions to determine the most functionally advantageous procedure. Assessment includes clinical evaluation as well as evaluation in a pathokinesiology laboratory. The functional assessment suggested by Enneking is helpful as a gross estimate of function; however, the authors used a more objective method. Gait analysis, including measurements of symmetry and velocity, and energy expenditure measurement, using oxygen consumption data, are helpful in evaluating the efficiency of ambulation. Because of the multiplicity of reconstructive procedures employed, there are as yet too few patients in each category to make any statements with statistical significance. However, preliminary analysis suggests that, in limited resections of the proximal femur, endoprosthetic replacement provides an excellent functional result. For major resections of the periacetabular area, arthrodesis seems to provide the best result.

TYPES OF MALIGNANT LESIONS

Osteogenic Sarcoma

Osteogenic sarcoma is the most common primary malignant sarcoma of the skeletal system.[21, 23, 25, 31] Approximately 5% of primary osteogenic sarcomas occur in the proximal femur[5, 21] (Fig. 16–10). The hip area is the third most common region of involvement by tumors, after the knee region and the proximal humerus.[21] The mean age of involvement is 18 years for males and 17 years for females. Characteristically, the tumor is located in the metaphyseal area, causes trabecular destruction, breaks through the cortex, has little or no margination, elevates the periosteum (Codman's triangle), and usually has evidence of sarcomatous bone formation (except in telangiectatic osteogenic sarcomas, which are purely lytic). The majority of osteogenic sarcomas are either stage IIB or stage III lesions.

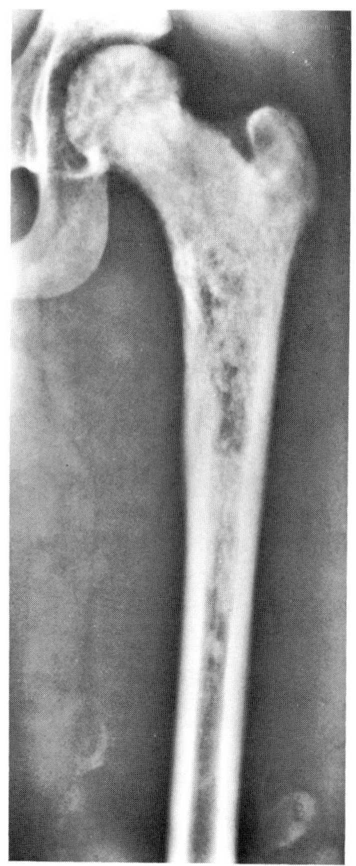

FIGURE 16–10. A chondroblastic type of osteogenic sarcoma (stage IIB) in an 18-year-old female adolescent. The radiograph depicts the extensive involvement of the proximal femur and the proximal diaphysis. An *en bloc* excision of the proximal femur (26 cm) and the acetabulum was performed and reconstructed with a custom prosthesis. Pathology examination confirmed extension of tumor into the hip joint at the femoral neck. The patient received preoperative and postoperative chemotherapy in accordance with the Memorial Sloan-Kettering Hospital T10 protocol.

Before 1973, the overall 5-year survival rate was 10 to 25%, depending on the source of data,[34] and significantly less than 6% for the femur. Currently, overall 10-year disease-free survival rates of close to 70% for stage II lesions of the proximal femur have been achieved at Memorial Sloan-Kettering Cancer Center. Unfortunately, the proximal femur has a disturbingly high local recurrence rate (21%) and a lower long-term disease-free survival rate as compared with other anatomic sites (82% disease free in tibia and humerus). In recent series, all local recurrences in the proximal femur (with the exception of one) occurred when pathologic examination indicated that wide surgical margins were achieved. It was noted clinically that local recurrence often occurred along the iliopsoas muscle and might represent soft tissue skip lesions. When performing a wide local excision, extra care should be taken to continue the resection proximally to include this area.

Chondrosarcoma

Approximately 13% of primary and secondary chrondrosarcomas occur in the proximal femur.[3, 5, 15, 35] The tumor occurs commonly in the fourth to sixth decades of life. Fewer than 10% of chondrosarcomas are seen in the pediatric age group. When occurring in the younger age group, these sarcomas are often the result of malignant degeneration of a preexisting benign cartilaginous lesion. Careful follow-up is indicated for benign cartilaginous growths, especially those occurring in the axial skeleton or the proximal appendicular skeleton, because these are associated with the highest rate of malignant transformation. Chondrosarcomas are suggested over enchondromas when there is endosteal erosion, cortical breakthrough, areas of lysis, persistent pain (especially at night), and changes on serial radiographs. Although chondrosarcomas have abnormal bone scans, benign enchondromas in adolescents and young adolescents can also have abnormal scans. Chondrosarcomas require wide surgical excision. Grade I and II tumors do not respond to chemotherapy. In high-grade chondrosarcomas, only the nonchondroid spindle cell component may be affected by adjuvant chemotherapy. Resections about the proximal femur follow the principles described above (see discussion of osteogenic sarcoma). Borderline and low-grade chondrosarcomas have been treated successfully by thorough curettage, extensive cryosurgery, and stabilization with methyl methacrylate and internal fixation. Although resections result in cure rates of 95% for grade I chondrosarcomas versus 75% cure rates with cryosurgery, the latter preserves the hip, and secondary resections are still possible in cases of local recurrence.[3, 15, 35, 37]

Ewing's Sarcoma

Ewing's sarcoma is most frequently seen in flat bones or in the diaphyses of long bones. Approximately 10% occur in the proximal femur.[5] If the proximal femoral diaphysis is included, 27% of the Memorial Sloan-Kettering Cancer Center series[21] and an additional 8% of the Mayo Clinic series[5] occurred in this location. It is most commonly seen between the ages of 5 and 20 years. The tumor arises in the marrow space and invades the cortex via the haversian system. Frequently, there is soft tissue extension. The tumor is a permeative destructive lesion (Fig. 16–11), which can give rise to serial elevations of the periosteum and reactive bone formation ("onionskinning"). The tumor can spread to the lungs and may generally invade the bone marrow (3%). The common diaphyseal location of this tumor makes it particularly amenable to wide *en bloc* excision and intercalary allograft reconstruction, using various forms of interlocking intramedullary nails for fixation or proximal femoral replacement hemiarthroplasty. Formerly, this tumor had a grim prognosis (15% 5-year survival). Recently, with the advent of combination chemotherapy and radiation (50 Gy), the 5-year survival rate is approximately 60%. However, a continual fall-off occurs even after 5 years, and a local recurrence rate of 21% after radiation therapy has given rise to preference for wide surgical excision of the tumor mass coupled with chemotherapy and the use of radiation to the resection bed (30 Gy). Particular

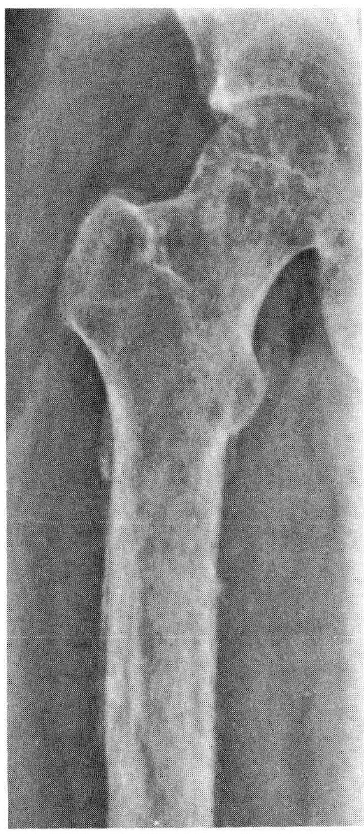

FIGURE 16–11. A permeative lesion with periosteal reaction in a 22-year-old man. Biopsy confirmed Ewing's sarcoma. The patient was treated with an *en bloc* excision of the proximal femur, reconstruction with a custom endoprosthesis, and preoperative and postoperative chemotherapy.

problems about the proximal femur are frequent pathologic fractures and significant limb shortening after radiation. Thus, in young children, surgical resection is preferred. Expandable femoral endoprostheses can compensate for growth deficiency. The potential for local recurrence in the groin or along Hunter's canal necessitates radiation of these areas.

Malignant Fibrous Histiocytoma

Malignant fibrous histiocytoma of bone, with its classic storiform pattern of fibrogenic histologic differentiation, occurs in the proximal femur in approximately 9% of cases.[5] On x-ray film, these tumors are permeative, destructive lesions without significant periosteal or endosteal bone production. They may show mottling with ill-defined hazy areas of increased radiodensity, suggesting the fibrous component. These high-grade lesions are presently treated at Memorial Sloan-Kettering Cancer Center with preoperative multiagent chemotherapy with high-dose methotrexate, wide *en bloc* surgical excision or amputation, and postoperative adjuvant chemotherapy.

Summary

This chapter describes the staging and classification of benign and malignant tumors of the proximal femur. The principles of diagnostic work-up, including the critical biopsy, and the current strategies of treatment are outlined. Survival has recently improved for the high-grade malignant tumors coupled with the preservation of limb. These advances have resulted from the combined use of definitive surgery, adjuvant chemotherapy, and radiotherapy. Some guarded optimism is currently warranted.

References

1. Ayala AF, Murray JA, Erling MA, Raymond AK: Osteoid-osteoma: Intraoperative tetracycline-fluorescence demonstration of the nidus. J Bone Joint Surg 68A:747–751, 1986.
2. Campanacci M, Di Sessa L, Trentani C: Scaglietti's method for conservative treatment of simple bone cysts with local injections of methylprednisolone acetate. Ital J Orthop Traumatol 3:27–36, 1977.
3. Campanacci M, Guernelli N, Leonessa D: Chondrosarcoma: A study of 133 cases, 80 with long-term follow-up. Ital J Orthop Traumatol 1:387–414, 1975.
4. Chao EYS, Sim FH: Modular prosthetic system for segmental bone and joint replacement after tumor resection. Orthopedics 8:641–651, 1985.
5. Dahlin DC: Bone Tumors, General Aspects and Data on 8,542 Cases, 4th ed. Springfield, IL, Charles C Thomas, 1986.
6. Dahlin DC, Coventry MB: Osteosarcoma: A study of 600 cases. J Bone Joint Surg 49A:101–110, 1967.
7. Dick HM, Malinin TI, Mnaymneh WA: Massive allograft implantation following radical resection of high-grade tumors requiring adjuvant chemotherapy treatment. Clin Orthop 197:88–95, 1985.
8. Enneking WF: Musculoskeletal Tumor Surgery. New York, Churchill Livingstone, 1983, p 531.
9. Enneking WF, Gearen PF: Fibrous dysplasia of the femoral neck: Treatment by cortical bone-grafting. J Bone Joint Surg 68A:1415–1422, 1986.
10. Enneking WF, Spanier SS, Goodman M: Current concepts review: Surgical staging of musculoskeletal sarcoma. J Bone Joint Surg 62A:1027–1030, 1980.
11. Enzinger FM: Soft Tissue Tumors. St Louis, CV Mosby, 1983.
12. Eilber FR: Adjuvant treatment of osteosarcoma. Surg Clin North Am 61:1371–1378, 1982.
13. Eilber FR, Grant T, Eckhardt J: The evolution of limb salvage at UCLA. Presented at 2nd International Workshop on Design and Application of Tumor Prostheses for Bone and Joint Reconstruction, Vienna, September 5, 1983.
14. Fahey JJ, O'Brien ET: Subtotal resection and grafting in selected cases of solitary unicameral bone cyst. J Bone Joint Surg 55A:59, 1973.
15. Gitelis S: Chondrosarcoma of bone. The experience at the Instituto Orthopedico Rizzoli. J Bone Joint Surg 63A:1248–1257, 1981.
16. Goldenberg RR, Campbell CJ, Bonfiglio M: Giant cell tumor of bone. An analysis of 218 cases. J Bone Joint Surg 52A:619–664, 1970.
17. Hajdu SI: Pathology of Soft Tissue Tumors. Philadelphia, Lea & Febiger, 1979.
18. Harrington KD, Sim FH, Enis JE, Johnston JO, Dick HM, Gristina AG: Methylmethacrylate as an adjunct in internal fixation of pathological fractures. J Bone Joint Surg 58A:1047–1054, 1976.
19. Healey JH, Bowen MK, Lane JM, Boland P: Osteogenic marrow grafting to heal refractory unicameral bone cysts. Orthop Trans 12:402, 1988.
20. Helms CA, Hattner RS, Vogler JB III: Osteoid osteoma: Radionuclide diagnosis. Radiology 151:779–784, 1984.
21. Huvos AC: Bone Tumors. Diagnosis, Treatment and Prognosis. Philadelphia, WB Saunders Co, 1979.
22. Huvos AC, Marcove RC: Chondroblastoma of bone. A critical review. Clin Orthop 95:300–312, 1973.
23. Jaffee N, Frei E, Traggis D, Bishop Y: Adjuvant methotrexate and citrovorum-factor treatment of osteogenic sarcoma. N Engl J Med 29A:994–997, 1974.
24. Kricun ME: Red-yellow marrow conversion: Its effect on the location of some solitary bone lesions. Skeletal Radiol 14:10, 1985.
25. Lane JM: Malignant bone tumors. *In* Alfonson AE, Gardner E (eds): The Practice of Cancer Surgery. New York, Appleton-Century-Crofts, 1982, pp 307–324.
26. Lane JM: Custom prosthetic segmental bone and joint replacement in malignant bone tumor patients. *In* Chao EYS, Ivins J (eds): Tumor Prosthesis—The Design and Application. New York, Thieme-Stratton, 1983.
27. Lane JM, Boland PJ: Tumors of bone and cartilage.

In Goldsmith HS (ed): Practice of Surgery. Philadelphia, Harper & Row, 1983.
28. Lane JM, McCormack RR, Sundaresan N, Hurson B, Boland PJ: Treatment of pathological fractures. *In* Whitkoff H (ed): Current Concepts of Diagnosis and Treatment of Soft Tissue and Bone Tumors. New York, Springer-Verlag, 1984.
29. Langlais F, Aubriot JH, Postel M, Tomeno B, Vielpeau C: Prosthetic reconstruction of the proximal femur after tumor resection: A review of 20 cases. Rev Chir Orthop 72:415–425, 1986.
30. Lee JK, Yao L, Wirth C: MR imaging of solitary osteochondromas: Report of eight cases. AJR 149:557–560, 1987.
31. Mankin HJ, Doppelt SH, Sullivan TR, Tomford WW: Osteoarticular and intercalary allograft transplantation in the management of malignant tumors of bone. Cancer 50:613–630, 1982.
32. Mankin HJ, Lange L, Spanier SS: The hazards of biopsy in patients with malignant primary bone and soft tissue tumors. J Bone Joint Surg 64A:1121–1127, 1982.
33. Marcove RC, Lyden JP, Huvos AG, Bullough PB: Giant cell tumors treated by cryosurgery: A report of twenty-five cases. J Bone Joint Surg 55A:1633, 1973.
34. Marcove RC, Mike V, Hajek JV, et al: Osteogenic sarcoma under the age of 21. A review of 145 preoperative cases. J Bone Joint Surg 52A:411–423, 1970.
35. Marcove RC, Mike V, Hutter RVP: Chondrosarcoma of the pelvis and upper end of the femur. An analysis of factors influencing survival time in 113 cases. J Bone Joint Surg 54A:53–54, 1974.
36. Marcove RC, Shaji H, Arlen M: Altered carbohydrate metabolism in cartilaginous tumors. Contemp Surg 5:53–54, 1974.
37. Marcove RC, Stoveli PB, Huvos AG: The use of cryosurgery in the treatment of low and medium grade chondrosarcoma. Clin Orthop 122:147–156, 1977.
38. Marcove RC, Weis LD, Vaghaiwalla MR, et al: Cryosurgery in the treatment of giant cell tumors of bone. A report of 52 consecutive cases. Cancer 41:957–969, 1978.
39. Mnaymneh W, Malinin TI, Makley JT, Dick HM: Massive osteoarticular allografts in the reconstruction of extremities following resection of tumors not requiring chemotherapy and radiation. Clin Orthop 1978:76–87, 1985.
40. Moore TM, Myers MH, Patzakis MJ, Terry RT, Starvey JP Jr: Closed biopsy of musculoskeletal lesions. J Bone Joint Surg 61A:375–380, 1979.
41. Parrish FF, Murray JA: Surgical treatment for secondary neoplastic fractures. J Bone Joint Surg 52A:665–686, 1970.
42. Piney A: The anatomy of the bone marrow. Br Med J 2:792, 1922.
43. Rosen G, Caparros B, Huvos AG, et al: Preoperative chemotherapy for osteogenic sarcoma. Selection of postoperative adjuvant chemotherapy, based upon the response of the primary tumor to preoperative chemotherapy. Cancer 49:1221–1230, 1982.
44. Rosen G, Caparros B, Nirenberg N, et al: Ewing's sarcoma: Ten-year experience with adjuvant chemotherapy. Cancer 47:2204–2213, 1981.
45. Rosen G, Marcove RC, Caparros B, et al: Primary osteogenic sarcoma. The rationale for preoperative chemotherapy and delayed surgery. Cancer 43:2163–2177, 1979.
46. Rosen G, Murphy ML, Huvos AG, et al: Chemotherapy, *en bloc* resection, and prosthetic bone replacement in the treatment of osteogenic sarcoma. Cancer 37:1–11, 1976.
47. Scaglietti O, Marchetti PG, Bartolozzi P: The effects of methylprednisolone acetate in the treatment of bone cysts: Results of three years follow-up. J Bone Joint Surg 61B:200, 1979.
48. Scaglietti O, Marchetti PG, Bartolozzi P: Final results obtained in the treatment of bone cysts with methylprednisolone acetate (depo-medrol) and a discussion of results achieved in other bone lesions. Clin Orthop 165:33, 1982.
49. Simon MA: Current concepts review. Biopsy of musculoskeletal tumors. J Bone Joint Surg 64A:1253–1257, 1982.
50. Simon MA, Kirchner PT: Scintigraphic evaluation of primary bone tumors. J Bone Joint Surg 62A:758–764, 1980.
51. Souhami RL: What has adjuvant chemotherapy of osteosarcoma achieved? (Discussion paper.) J R Soc Med 76:943–946, 1983.
52. Stephenson RB, London MD, Hankin FM, Kaufer H: Fibrous dysplasia: An analysis of options for treatment. J Bone Joint Surg 69A:400–409, 1987.
53. Sweetnam R: Amputation in osteosarcoma. J Bone Joint Surg 55B:189–192, 1973.

CHAPTER 17

Surgical Considerations in Tumors About the Knee

CARL BARBERA
MICHAEL M. LEWIS

The human knee enables mobility and provides strength and stability. The bony structures are able to tolerate the forces produced across the various articular surfaces both by the stresses of weight bearing and by the muscular actions on the joint throughout a wide range of motion.

Abnormalities in the structures of the knee—even if such abnormalities are comparatively small in anatomic terms—can produce significant symptomatic and functional disability. Conversely, patients are able to compensate for remarkable alterations in structure or function and tolerate them well. Thus it is understandable why some musculoskeletal conditions will require attention early in their course while others go unnoticed until they reach an advanced stage.

Presentation

Most primary tumors and tumorlike conditions of bone, and many of soft tissue, have an affinity for the various structures that compose the knee.[5] Of all areas in the musculoskeletal system, therefore, the knee is one of the most commonly affected by tumors and tumorlike conditions.

For the purpose of tumor diagnosis and treatment, the knee region has several distinct components. Bony portions include the distal femur, proximal tibia, patella, and proximal end of the fibula. Lesions may also occur within the joint cavity itself, arising from the soft tissue deep to the fibrous capsule. Superficial to the capsule, neoplastic disease can originate in any of the supporting structures, muscular components, skin, subcutaneous tissue surrounding the knee, or neurologic or vascular structures that traverse the popliteal fossa (Fig. 17–1).

Pain, a common finding, may vary in intensity from mild to severe, in character from dull to aching to sharp, in duration from days to months and from constant to occasional, and in location from ill-defined and generalized to precise. Some pain patterns, such as that associated with osteoid osteoma, are characteristic (Fig. 17–2); others are less predictable. Though some patients do not initially complain of pain, they may recognize retrospectively that they experienced discomfort in the knee for a variable time. In addition, the onset of a new pain in an area that is mechanically weakened by a lesion may herald an impending pathologic fracture or indicate that a subclinical one has already occurred. Occasionally a

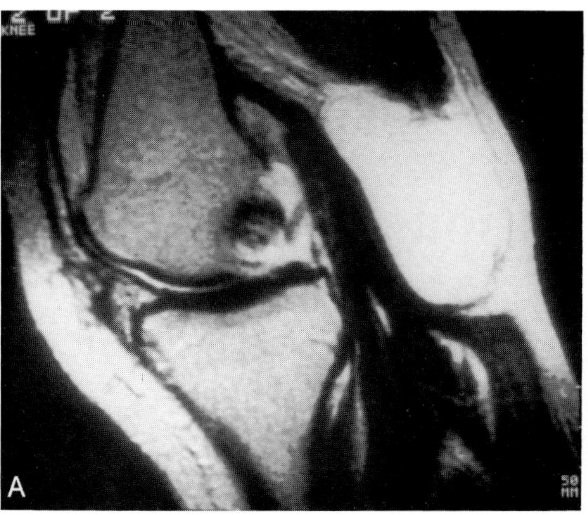

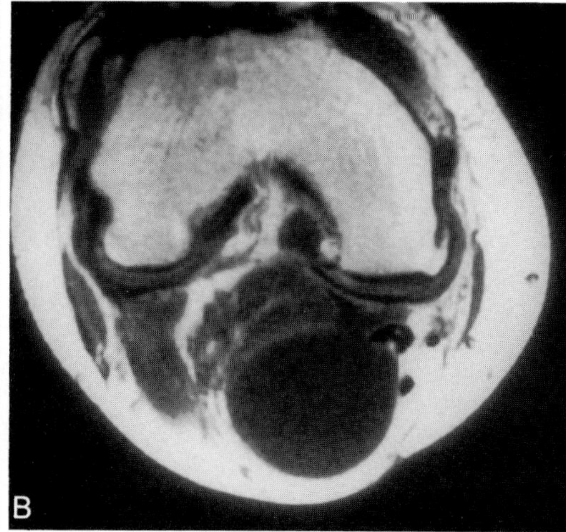

FIGURE 17–1. Baker's cyst. *A,* 50-year-old female patient with pain and swelling at the popliteal fossa. *A, B,* MRI scans reveal a round, well-defined, homogeneous, low-signal mass in T1 and a high-signal mass in T2 image.

fracture may occur without warning and reveal the presence of a bony lesion.

The first sign of abnormality may be the presence of a mass, the size of which is not necessarily an indicator of diagnosis or prognosis. Small malignant lesions may be discovered early when in an accessible, superficial location, whereas benign masses deep in the popliteal space have grown to considerable size before being discovered.

A more reliable impression can be formulated from careful physical examination combined with a history of the behavior and rate of growth of the mass. It may be an unfortunate oversight, for instance, to assign the diagnosis of Baker's cyst to any mass that arises

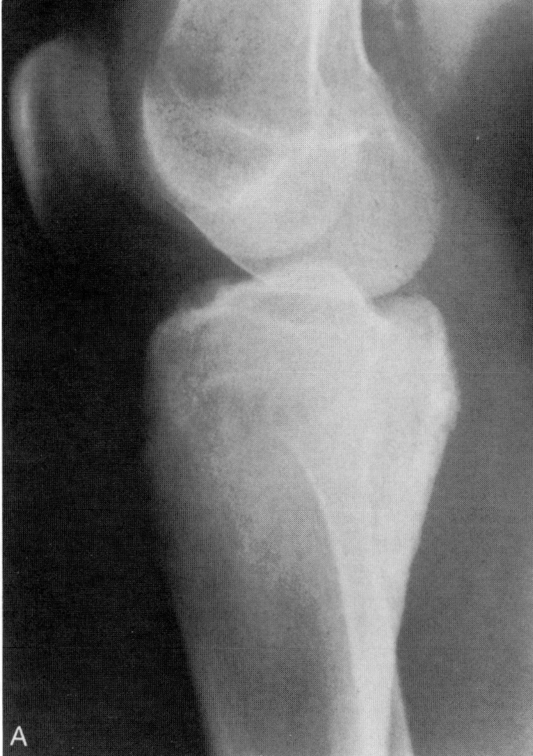

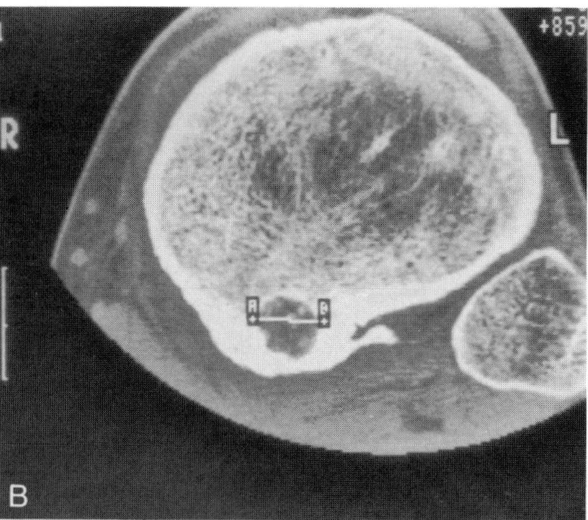

FIGURE 17–2. Osteoid osteoma. A 24-year-old male patient with day and night knee pain, which responds to aspirin. Plain roentgenogram (*A*) and CT scan (*B*) reveal a small radiolucent nidus surrounded by sclerotic margin.

behind the knee (Fig. 17–3), as fewer than half of all posterior knee masses are actually Baker's cysts.

Because of the anatomy peculiar to the knee and a lesion's effect on joint function, mechanical impairment is a common symptom at presentation. Depending upon their location, neoplastic lesions in the knee can produce a variety of neurovascular, physiologic, or purely mechanical disturbances.

Osteochondroma, for instance, may be seen as a mass but commonly presents with pain attributable to an inflamed overlying bursa. Osteochondromata may interfere with the motion of normal structures, occasionally cause motor or sensory disturbances from pressure effects on adjacent nerves, and rarely cause vascular interruption (Fig. 17–4).

Painless popliteal lesions are often discovered because they interfere with full flexion, even before they are easily palpable. Intra-articular lesions can mimic internal derangements such as torn cartilage of the joint. Motion can be inhibited, pain present, or effusions produced. These effects can be a recognized part of the disease, such as the boggy joint fullness and blood-tinged effusion associated with pigmented villonodular synovitis (Fig. 17–5). On the other hand, extra-articular tumors may produce a "sympathetic" effusion as part of the synovial reaction to their presence.

An effusion, especially if it contains gross blood or marrow fat, can indicate that a bony lesion has involved the joint, through either direct invasion or fracture.

Finally, lesions can be discovered incidentally during routine physical examination or on screening radiographs or bone scans obtained for other reasons.

Staging and Diagnostic Studies

Proper treatment of tumors or tumorlike conditions requires an accurate assessment of diagnosis and extent of disease. Although the ultimate diagnosis usually relies upon histologic examination of lesional tissue, the approach and method for obtaining such tissue, as well as timing in relation to additional treatment, surgical or otherwise, should be based upon an accurate preoperative impression of probable diagnosis. An educated evaluation of the various investigative studies available is the cornerstone of such an impression.[10]

In addition, these studies provide the only

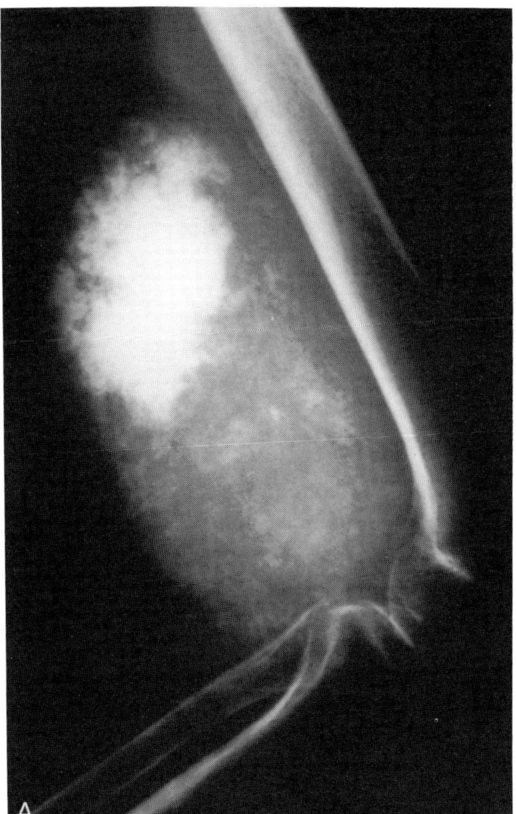

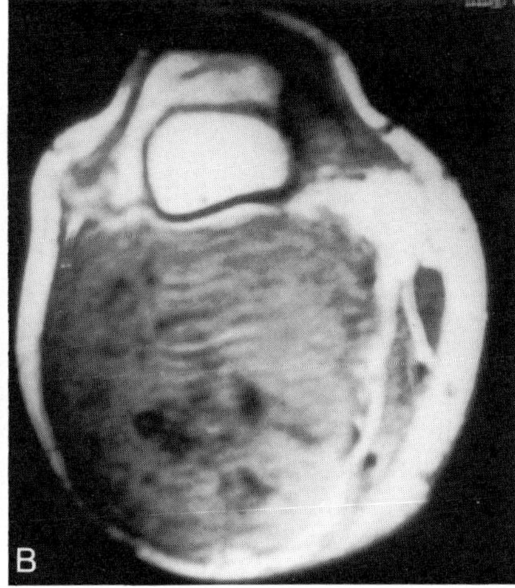

FIGURE 17–3. Soft tissue chondrosarcoma. A 60-year-old male patient with a long history of swelling along the posterior thigh. *A,* Plain roentgenogram reveals a soft tissue mass containing diffuse calcification. *B,* MRI reveals the mass to be solid, with matrix calcification, and separate from the adjacent femur.

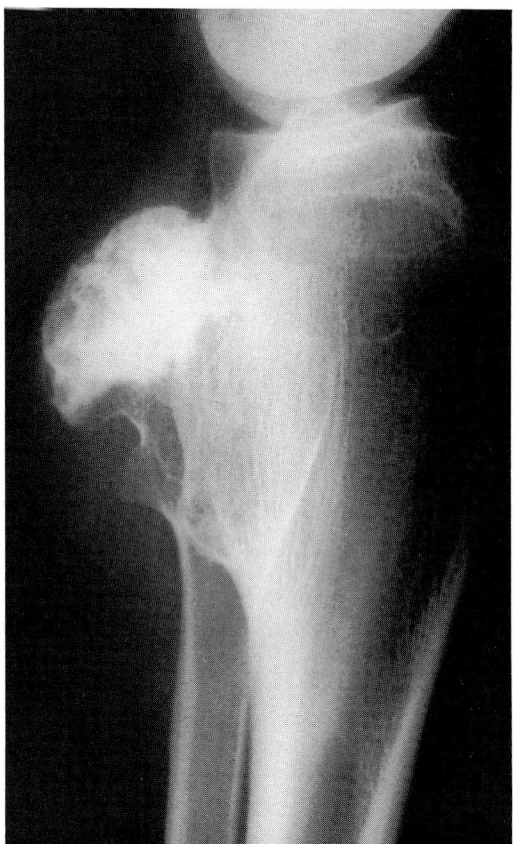

FIGURE 17–4. Familial multiple osteochondromatosis. A 22-year-old with osteochondroma arising from the proximal fibula, causing compression of the common peroneal nerve.

accurate method of measuring the extent of disease, both locally and systemically. Often such decisions as the need for surgical treatment, the feasibility of obtaining adequate surgical margins through limb-sparing surgery, or the need for amputation to provide local tumor control will be based upon findings of these staging studies.[26, 30, 31]

Different imaging techniques have relative strengths and weaknesses regarding the accuracy and sensitivity with which they provide information about the various tumors that appear about the knee. They are best when used in concert to provide answers to specific questions raised by the physician.

STANDARD RADIOGRAPHS

Plain radiographs are widely available, safely and easily obtained, and indispensable in the evaluation of neoplastic lesions of the extremities. They should not be overlooked in favor of more sophisticated studies, as they remain the single most useful study for evaluation of lesions of bone. In most cases, a likely diagnosis can be established on the basis of the x-ray alone or the differential diagnosis narrowed to a few conditions.[22]

In addition, the clinical course of several diseases can be easily and reliably monitored through radiographic changes alone. At times, such as with stress fractures or occult osteomyelitis, the diagnosis may not be clear at first but revealed only through sequential radiographic examination.[1]

Plain films are quite sensitive in detecting the subtle periosteal reaction that often is the first indication of bony disease or the reaction of bone to an adjacent soft tissue mass. An exception to this is behind the knee, where the posterior portion of the distal femur is poorly invested with periosteum. Radiographic evidence of periosteal response may, therefore, be obviously less than otherwise expected.

ISOTOPE STUDIES

Bone-seeking isotopes have proved useful in the assessment of musculoskeletal tumors and are well suited for studies of the knee region. Although nonspecific, they are sensitive in detecting an otherwise undemonstrable bony process or early involvement of bone by soft tissue disease. Some assessment of intraosseous tumor extent can be made through isotope scanning, though it is less useful in detecting soft tissue disease. Inflammatory responses and areas of hypervascularity will also be well identified, especially when they are differentially active on the early phase of bone scanning.

The bone scan is less useful, however, in detecting the precise demarcation between tumor, reactive changes, or even disuse osteoporosis, which will commonly exhibit moderately increased isotope uptake.[32] For this purpose, computed tomography or magnetic resonance imaging may be more helpful.

The bone scan can also be of help in determining the metabolic activity of bone lesions. An example would be an incidentally discovered abnormality of the distal femoral metaphysis, which radiographically could be consistent with either a bone infarct or chondrosarcoma. Although both lesions can exhibit increased isotopic activity, lack of uptake would suggest a less aggressive approach to the lesion.

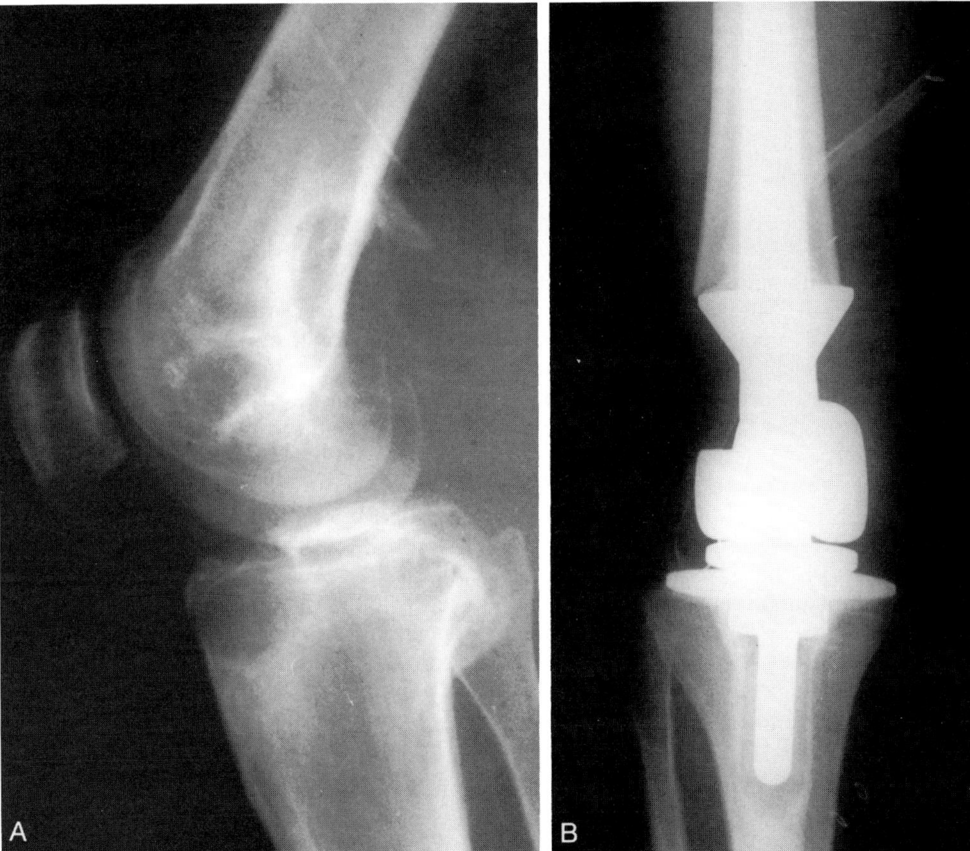

FIGURE 17–5. *A,* Aggressive villonodular synovitis presenting as a large popliteal mass eroding into the distal femur and the proximal tibia. *B,* Wide resection of the knee joint was performed, reconstructed by a rotating hinge prosthesis.

A drawback of this study is encountered when it is used to investigate extremely lytic tumors as well as tumors in the immature skeleton. Growing physes exhibit intense activity and could obscure the lesion itself or its true extent toward the joint. Alternative studies will generally be needed to obtain this information.

COMPUTED TOMOGRAPHY

Computed tomography (CT) is extremely useful in studying lesions that occur in areas about the knee that are otherwise difficult to image. The ability of CT to display anatomic information in three dimensions is a distinct advantage in the multiplanar architecture of the knee joint.[28] CT also usually provides a good demonstration of the soft tissue component that accompanies a bony lesion and may be able to localize the neurovascular structures in relation to the mass.

The main advantage of CT, however, is the bony detail it can provide: for example, the presence or absence of a reactive shell of bone about a lesion; unsuspected cortical breaches or matrix calcifications; or a small lesion's true location in relation to the endosteum, cortex, and periosteum. In addition, an estimate of the volumetric extent of a mass can be formulated and an inference made regarding the mechanical strength of the involved bone.

CT is also useful in presurgical planning. The intramedullary extent of tumor can be assessed, and the bony level of resection for local procedures, limb sparing, or amputations can be determined.

A disadvantage of this study is that it scans the knee in the horizontal plane, which is coincident with the tibiofemoral articulation. Coronal and sagittal CT reconstructions are decidedly inferior to the axial images, and the result is that it is difficult to conceptualize the longitudinal extent of the disease. Lesions that are epiphyseal are not ideally demonstrated, and their relation to the subchondral bone, physeal plate, or the joint itself may not be truly represented.

MAGNETIC RESONANCE IMAGING

Although the magnetic resonance imaging (MRI) does not provide the bony detail available with CT, it can complement some of the CT's weaknesses. It can study the knee in sagittal and coronal planes as well as in the axial, and it can also demonstrate marrow infiltration by tumor, thereby delineating intramedullary extent of disease (Fig. 17–6).

Discrete soft tissue lesions are well visualized, and comparison of the differing signal characteristics of the mass on T1, T2, and proton density techniques may help identify the lesion's composition. The homogeneity of the matrix can be studied as well.[33–35]

At present, neither MRI nor CT is an ideal study or generally applicable for all needs. Although one may be preferred over the other in any particular situation, they provide more information when used in concert.

ANGIOGRAPHY

An important determinant of the feasibility of local excision of tumors about the knee is the existence of a plane of surgical dissection between the lesion and the major vascular structures of the leg.

The popliteal artery and vein are relatively tethered within the popliteal space, proximally by the adductor canal and distally by the anterior tibial artery and soleus tunnel. Because malignant tumors of the distal femur and proximal tibia commonly extend in the posterior direction and many benign and malignant lesions occur there primarily, the question of vascular involvement by disease often arises.

An accurate method of determining this is through angiography. In addition, soft tissue extent is reflected by this study, as is the inherent vascularity of the lesion, which may be of diagnostic value (Fig. 17–7). Careful examination of the neovascularity demonstrated by the angiogram may be able to identify or rule out bone involvement by an adjacent soft tissue lesion.

It may be difficult, however, to identify

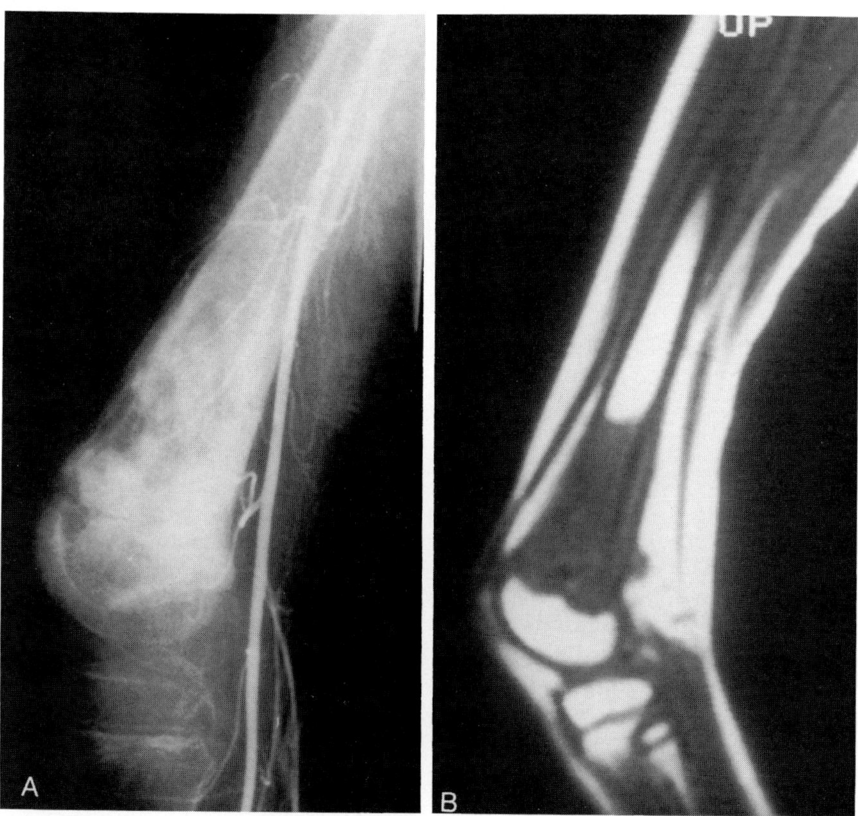

FIGURE 17–6. Osteosarcoma. *A,* An 11-year-old female patient with a blastic lesion of the distal femur. *B,* MRI demonstrates the medullary extent of the tumor.

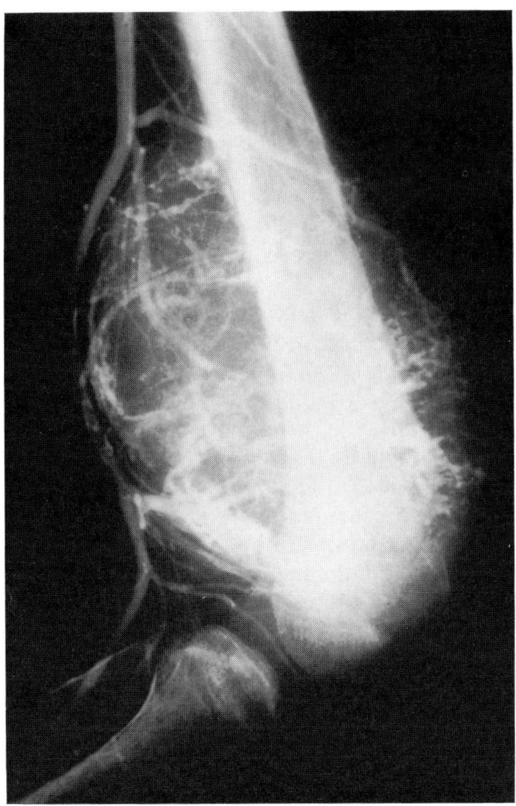

FIGURE 17–7. Osteosarcoma. A 16-year-old male patient with large associated soft tissue mass. Arteriogram demonstrates the relationship of the main popliteal artery and the vascularity of the tumor.

intraarticular extension as reliably as intraosseous extension, as the vascularity inherent in the synovial lining of a large joint could easily mimic neoplastic vasculature. This is especially true if there is an element of inflammatory reaction or redundancy of the synovial lining.

Furthermore, if a lesion is eccentric in location or wraps around one or both of the femoral or tibial condyles, it may be inadequately represented in the standard biplanar angiographic projections. Three-dimensional studies would generally provide more information in these situations.

ARTHROGRAPHY

Injection of contrast material into the knee joint entails little risk of tumor contamination, even if there is joint invasion by a malignant lesion, and may provide the necessary documentation of such invasion where other studies would not.

Finer detail of the intraarticular architecture may be obtainable with contrast material than with other studies and can be accomplished either with standard radiography after injection or CT. In addition, sometimes a communication between the joint cavity and lesion can be demonstrated, such as with synovial cyst.

COMMON TUMOR IMPERSONATORS

Radiographic abnormalities are often detected in the area of the knee either incidentally or coincidentally with or related to a patient's specific complaints. Often these findings are suggestive of or compatible with a diagnosis of neoplasia. Stress fracture in the proximal tibia may present with periosteal reaction without history of trauma, therefore resembling neoplasm.[6, 7]

HISTOLOGIC EXAMINATION

In the area of the knee, as in other regions of the musculoskeletal system, the general principles of obtaining safe and adequate specimens for histologic examination pertain. The choice of open or needle biopsy must be individualized. Small longitudinal incisions should be used with open biopsy and placed in locations which, if subsequent wide local excision is planned, can be excised *en bloc* with the specimen. Also, if subsequent wide amputation should be necessary, the biopsy tract should be placed so that its excision does not compromise the amputation flaps.[25]

If a large area of tissue, especially skin and subcutaneous tissue, must be removed with the biopsy tract at the time of excision, difficulties in wound closure may be encountered. A particular surgical defect in an area of the body where soft tissue is plentiful or mobile may be closed primarily, whereas the same defect about the knee will require local or free vascularized tissue transfer to obtain coverage. For this reason, care must be taken at the time of biopsy to minimize both the size of biopsy tract and contamination of the surrounding tissues.

A soft tissue lesion is best approached directly, usually overlying its greatest prominence. If malignancy is suspected, incisional-type biopsy should be performed. An excisional biopsy, or "shelling out," does not add to diagnosis, is inadequate for local tumor control, and may compromise subsequent wide excision.

Surgical Management

SOFT TISSUE

When soft tissue neoplasms are located in the tissues about the knee, their surgical excision poses several unique difficulties. Ideally, the surgeon would prefer to be able to obtain adequate surgical margins than to compromise them in the interest of preserving maximum function. This is complicated by the fact that the periarticular soft tissues of the knee often do not present as clear a definition between individual structures, either normal or pathologic, compared with other areas of the musculoskeletal system (Fig. 17–8).

When lesions are located in the popliteal fossa, the possibility of obtaining true wide margins is less predictable than for lesions in other areas of the knee (Fig. 17–9). The floor of the fossa, composed of the posterior knee capsule and the muscular medial and lateral heads of the gastrocnemius muscle, provide some barriers to tumor extension. The capsule and muscular fascia may be used as a margin, carrying the surgical dissection deep to these structures. More proximally, the biceps femoris laterally and the hamstrings medially provide less reliable and identifiable barriers. In the longitudinal dimension, the tissues provide less barrier for tumor containment. Furthermore, the difference between a neoplasm, the reactive zone, and normal tissue can easily be obscured in the areolar tissue of the popliteal fossa.

The neural and vascular structures traversing this area are also enveloped by soft areolar and fatty tissue. Though not a particularly good barrier to tumor extension, this tissue often permits the development of an adequate surgical plane of dissection. If such dissection is not possible, the popliteal artery, vein, or both can be segmentally excised with the resection specimen, although this is an uncommon situation. Loss of the popliteal vein can be tolerated, though chronic edema and venous insufficiency can ensue if collateral drainage is inadequate.

The artery can be reconstructed with satisfactory results.[11] Predictably, the reconstruction is more reliable if the distal level of arterial

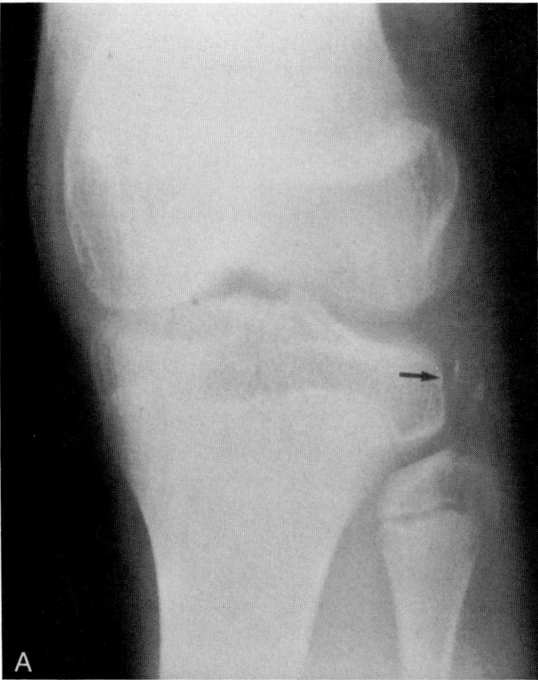

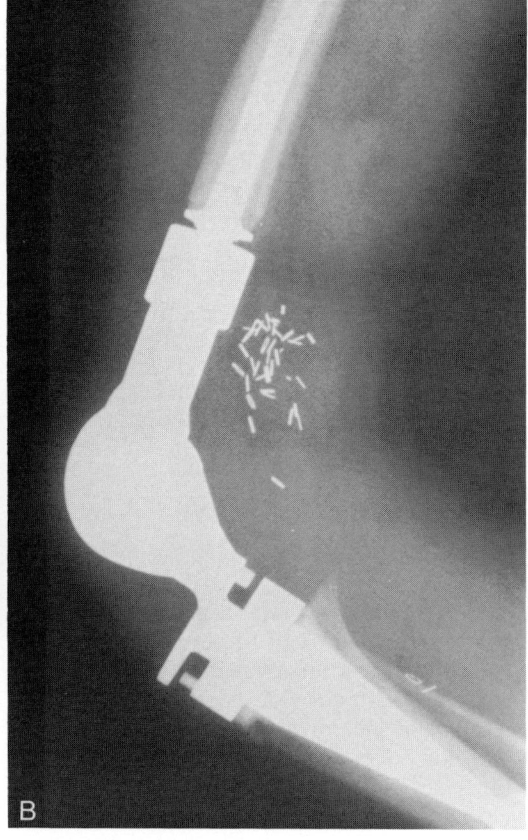

FIGURE 17–8. Synovial sarcoma. A 16-year-old male patient with a history of knee pain. *A,* Plain roentgenogram reveals a calcified soft tissue mass at the lateral aspect of the knee joint (*arrow*). *B,* Wide *en bloc* resection of the knee joint and reconstruction by expandable prosthesis.

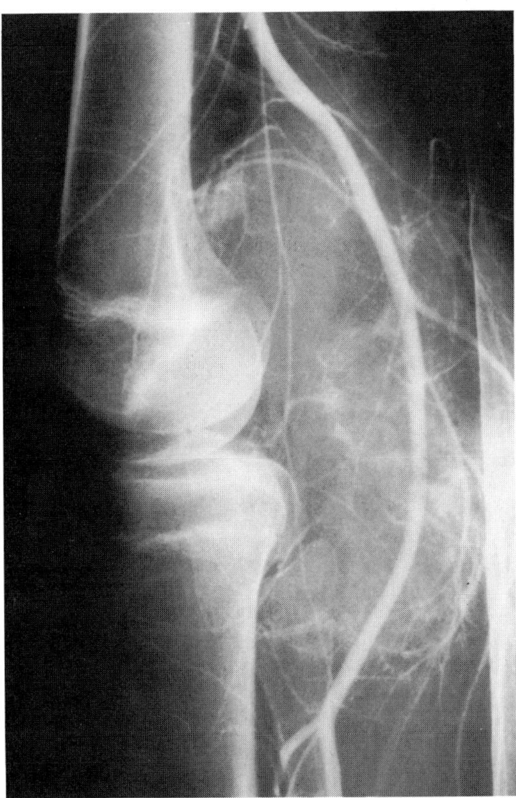

FIGURE 17–9. Synovial sarcoma. A 15-year-old female patient with large popliteal mass. Arteriogram reveals encasement of the popliteal artery.

resection remains proximal to the origin of the anterior tibial artery. Factors of age and the presence of coincident peripheral vascular disease must be taken into account when considering the feasibility of such a reconstruction.

The sciatic nerve can often be freed from the neoplasm, though this sometimes requires intraneural dissection. When necessary, sacrifice of the peroneal nerve can be reasonably well tolerated by the patient, with the resultant foot drop compensated for, as needed, with external supports.

Loss of tibial nerve function is less well tolerated, however, and results in plantar foot anesthesia and muscular deficiency that is difficult to compensate for. Sacrifice of the sciatic nerve in its entirety produces an anesthetic extremity with poor muscular control and often chronic edema. Better functional results can be expected in such an instance with above-the-knee amputation.

The desire to preserve the lower limb if at all possible is a strong one, but for reasons already mentioned, one must weigh cautiously the decision to rely upon adjuvant treatments for local tumor control if satisfactory surgical excision is impossible.

DISTAL FEMUR

Benign intraosseous lesions are usually suited to intralesional curettage either with manual instruments, such as curettes, or with power instruments, such as burs (Fig. 17–10). Meticulous care should be taken to perform a thorough mechanical excision of the lesion while scrupulously avoiding penetration either through the articular surface into the knee joint or transcortically into soft tissue. This danger is especially true posteriorly, where soft tissue recurrence in the popliteal fossa may be difficult to control without extensive surgery. Care should also be taken to control seeding of the lesion locally in the surgical field.

Supplemental bone grafting can be desirable for many of these lesions, and both autogenous and allogenic grafts (especially for the larger defects) have been used with success. Postoperative protection of the limb is often required until graft incorporation occurs. Special considerations pertain in the immature skeleton, especially where curettage would risk damage to the physeal plate.

When feasible, more indolent lesions that do not immediately threaten pathologic fracture can be observed until skeletal growth distances them from the physis. If prior treatment is necessary, care should be taken to avoid mechanical damage to the growth plate. If the physis is violated either by the lesion or surgically, central defects seem to produce fewer complications and less angular deformity than do peripheral ones. Fat grafts can be employed in the region of the growth plate disruption to help avoid formation of transphyseal bars and resultant growth arrest. Bone grafting across the physis should be avoided.

In most instances, however, it is possible to proceed with a careful intralesional excision and also consider the use of local mechanical adjuvants. Polymethylmethacrylate has been used with success to provide both immediate structural support and thermal necrosis of suspected microresiduals of tumor (Fig. 17–11). Cryosurgical techniques are reported to provide local tumor control but are associated with a high incidence of complications, which often themselves can produce significant disability.

If there is evidence of compromise of the integrity of the subchondral plate or cortical

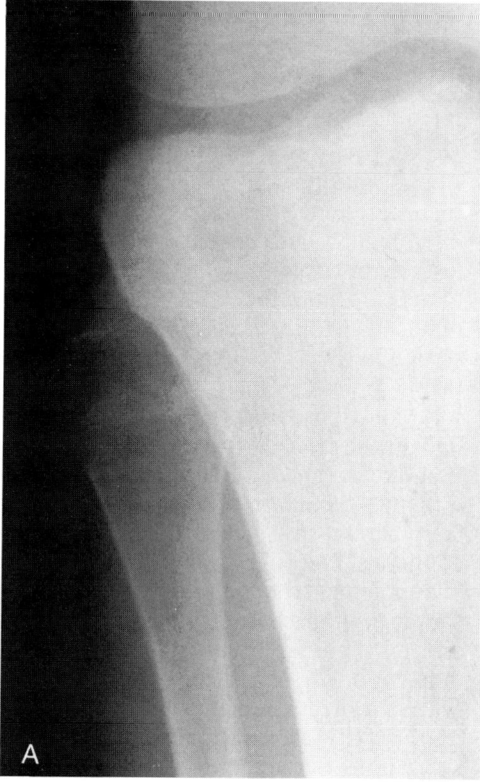

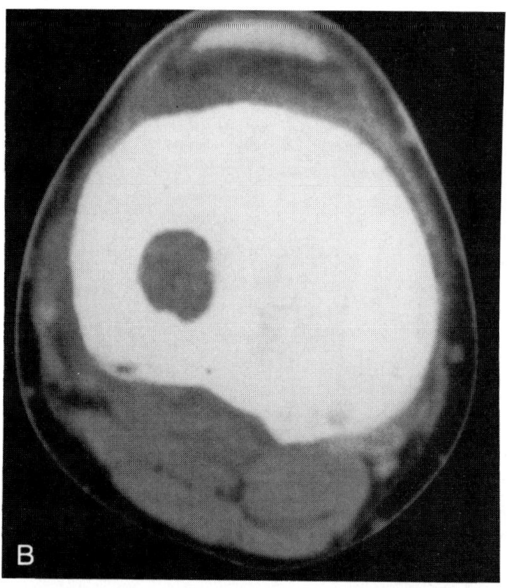

FIGURE 17–10. Chondroblastoma. A 16-year-old male patient with subchondral radiolucent lesion over the lateral tibial condyle (*A*). *B*, CT scan demonstrates the anatomic location and configuration of the lesion.

erosion (with intact periosteum), the surgeon must weigh the risk of pathologic fracture, late condylar collapse, or extraosseous dissemination of tumor by curettage. It may be prudent in these instances to perform a more extensive marginal or wide excision with a more reliable reconstruction (Fig. 17–12).

When a wide margin is required, it can be obtained by amputation, unicondylar resection, or complete distal femoral resection.[4, 13] This latter procedure has been performed through several surgical exposures.[19, 21] A straight longitudinal anterior midline incision permits the elevation of medial and lateral myocutaneous flaps, except when the tumor has a significant anterior soft tissue component. These flaps can be sufficiently retracted posteriorly to permit visualization of the popliteal neurovascular structures.

Alternatively, the popliteal fossa can be approached through a medial-posterior approach. The medial head of the gastrocnemius is detached from the femur and retracted distally, and the popliteal fossa entered. This permits immediate control of the vascular structures, which can then be dissected free from the tumor and retracted posteriorly, with ligation of geniculate and neovascular vessels as needed. In addition, adequate vascular control in this manner permits performance of the procedure without use of a tourniquet.

When lesions of the distal femur are found to be unresectable, it is almost invariably the result of involvement of the neurovascular structures. Early exploration of these structures permits application of limb-sparing techniques to any locally resectable lesion.

After vascular control is obtained, the anterior myocutaneous flap is raised, sparing as much of the extensor mechanism of the knee as possible. Adequate lateral exposure can be obtained through this approach, and dissection about the tumor is continued. The peroneal nerve is identified and protected if it can be spared.

The knee is then disarticulated by division of the capsule and the collateral and cruciate ligaments. The posterior capsule and lateral gastrocnemius are generally left until the end, so that the tibia can be subluxated anteriorly to help protect the peroneal nerve and posterior structures.

If extraarticular resection is required because of contamination of the knee joint by the tumor, a transverse osteotomy through the proximal tibia is made just distal to the insertion of the joint capsule.[15]

The femur is then retracted anteriorly and

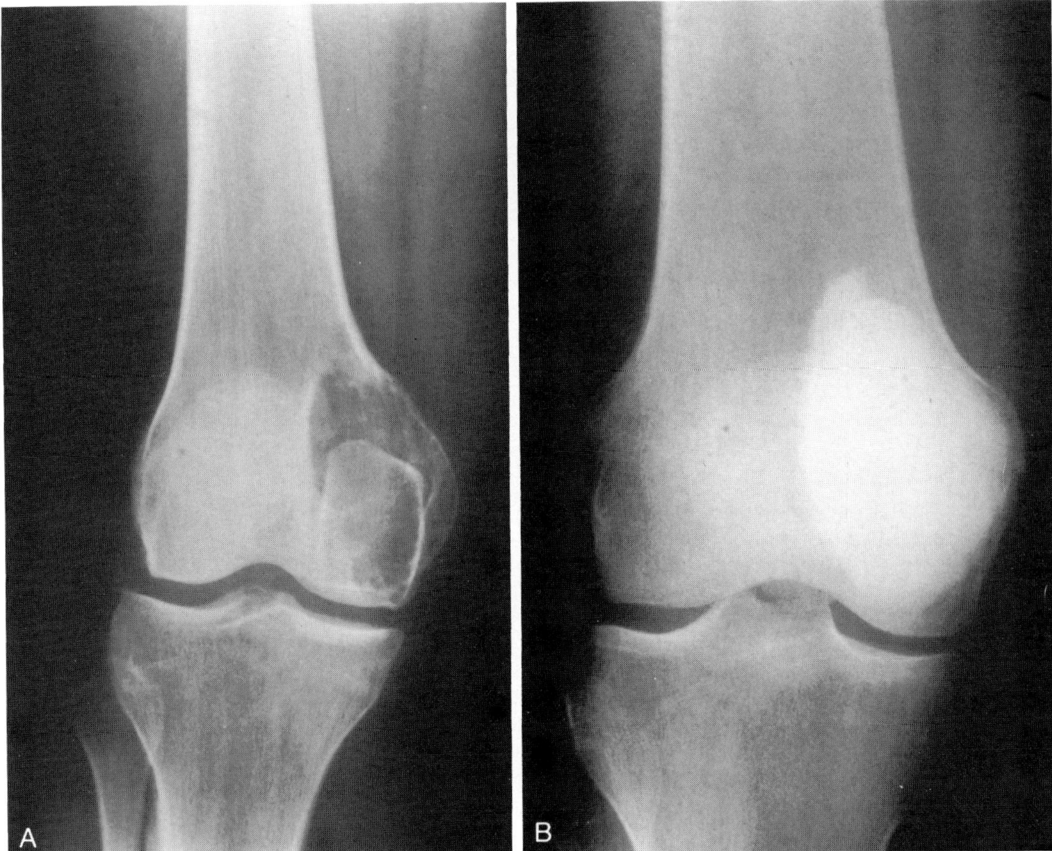

FIGURE 17–11. Giant cell tumor. A 35-year-old female patient with radiolucent lesion occupying the medial femoral condyle (*A*). *B,* Following curettage and filling of the cavity by cement.

medially, and dissection is continued proximally to the predetermined level of bony resection. Osteotomy can then be performed, and the specimen delivered and examined (Fig. 17–13).

PROXIMAL TIBIA

Benign tumors of the proximal tibia may be treated in an analogous fashion to those in the femur. In fact, the surgical approach to intraosseous lesions of the tibia is generally more straightforward than those of the femur. In the growing child, for instance, most epiphyseal defects may be approached directly, without the need to violate either the joint or the growth plate, which is not true in the femur.

When wide margins are necessary or desirable, unicondylar or total proximal tibial resection can be performed (Fig. 17–14). As in the distal femur, extraosseous extension of proximal tibial lesions tends to be more prominent posteriorly. This may be due to the fact that because the anterior tibia is relatively superficial, masses in this location are identified earlier and at a smaller size than those that originate posteriorly.[23, 29]

Tibial lesions differ from femoral ones in that the anatomic structures about the tibia are more confined. The tibial nerve and the posterior tibial artery are relatively tethered by their entry into the soleus tunnel. The anterior tibial artery is held in place by its entry into the anterior compartment; in turn this limits posterior surgical retraction of the popliteal artery. These anatomic situations can make resection of tibial neoplasms a more difficult undertaking than resection of their femoral counterparts.

Wide excision of the proximal tibia can be performed through incisions like those used for the distal femur. The incision is shortened proximally and then extended distally along the anterior midline. Again, use of a tourniquet is possible but can usually be avoided.

The popliteal artery is dissected free distally to the origin of the anterior tibial artery. The sciatic nerve and the peroneal nerve, which is

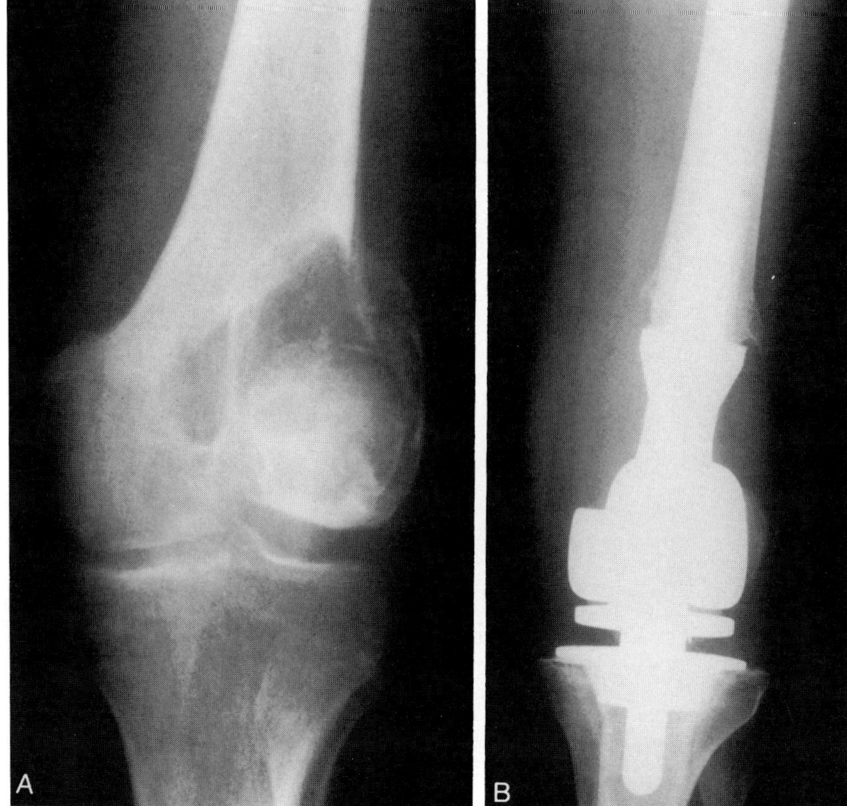

FIGURE 17–12. Giant cell tumor. *A,* Plain roentgenogram reveals an ill-defined radiolucent lytic lesion with fracture of the lateral femoral condyle. *B,* A marginal resection of the distal femur reconstructed by a custom rotating hinge prosthesis was performed.

usually salvageable, are dissected free and protected. The soleus tunnel is opened, and the posterior tibial artery vein and nerve are dissected distally to the level of bony resection. If a large segment of tibia must be resected, it may also be necessary to dissect and protect the peroneal vessels.

The knee is then disarticulated, and the distal tibial osteotomy performed. If there is minimal or no lateral tumor extension, it is desirable to preserve the fibula and the anterior tibial artery. The artery is identified in the anterior compartment and dissected proximally to where it penetrates the interosseous membrane. The proximal tibiofibular joint is then disarticulated.

If the anterior tibial artery is involved by tumor, it can be ligated proximally and posteriorly, where it branches from the popliteal artery, and also can be ligated in the anterior compartment, distal to the tumor, then segmentally excised with the specimen. If the fibula is not salvageable, it can be osteotomized distally and disarticulated at the level of the knee.

In either case, the specimen is then unconstrained and careful dissection through the remaining soft tissues can be performed by alternately rotating the specimen medially and laterally for exposure.

A difficulty more often encountered after tibial than after femoral resection is the inability to achieve primary wound closure. Often local or distant myocutaneous flaps are needed to achieve coverage, and this possibility must be taken into account when planning surgery.[12]

Reconstruction

Several techniques are available for restoring function to the lower extremity after local tumor excisions in the knee area.[26] The various reconstructions differ in their relative abilities to provide motion and stability and in the rate and nature of complications commonly encountered.

The choice of reconstruction in any particular patient must be based upon life style and functional needs, life expectancy, expected fur-

FIGURE 17-13. Osteosarcoma. An 18-year-old male patient with a mixed sclerotic and lytic lesion of the distal femur (*A*). *B,* Following wide resection and reconstruction by distal femur prosthesis.

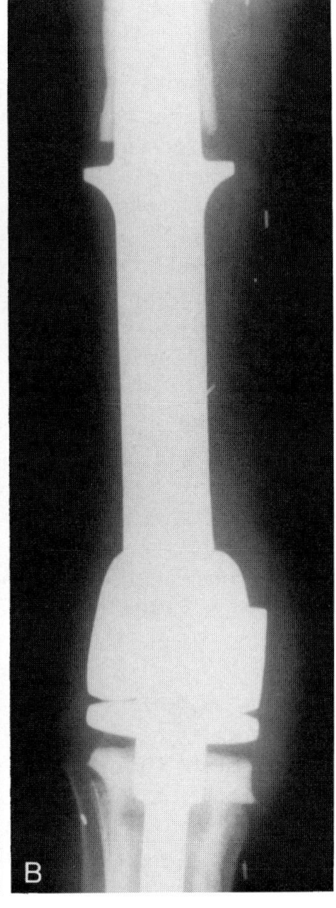

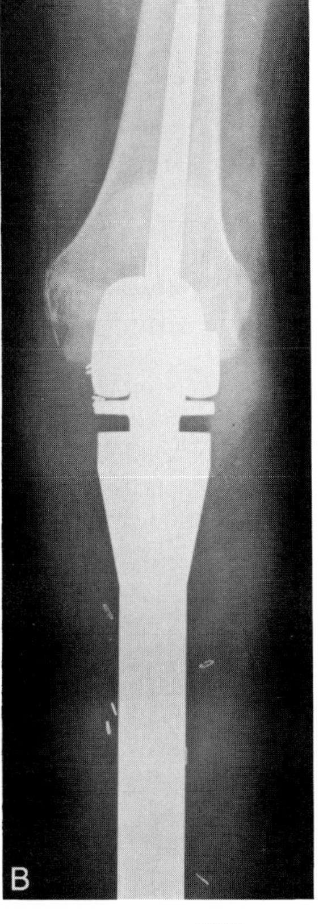

FIGURE 17-14. Chondrosarcoma. A 40-year-old male patient with large radiolucent lesion over the proximal tibia (*A*). *B,* Following proximal tibia replacement.

ther treatment (both surgical and adjunctive), and reasonable expectations of the success of the reconstruction.[3, 9, 13, 17]

The functional deficiencies to be expected from loss of soft tissue structures about the knee can be predicted rather well from an understanding of the functional anatomy involved. Whether specific treatment is required for these deficiencies is a clinical judgment.

Ligamentous stabilizing structures can, in many instances, be sacrificed with surprisingly little adverse effect if a constrained prosthesis, an appropriate allograft, or both are utilized. Uncommonly, secondary reconstruction can be performed as a delayed procedure according to established techniques.

If reconstruction of supporting ligaments is considered at the time of excision, the value of the expected added stability must be weighed against the risk of occult tumor dissemination due to the added dissection. Reconstruction should neither compromise wound closure nor sacrifice structures that may be needed for wound coverage. If a choice must be made between wound healing and ligament reconstruction, the former should take priority.

Patients tolerate loss of hamstring function quite well and generally do not require treatment. Likewise, even large segments of the lateral musculature can be sacrificed with little functional consequence. With loss of vastus medialis, however, resulting in abnormal patella tracking or frank subluxation, external bracing may be required if the patient is symptomatic. Rarely, surgical realignment or internal splinting of the quadriceps mechanism may be undertaken as a delayed procedure.

Sacrifice of part or all of the extensor mechanism of the knee carries with it a more pronounced disability, resulting in absent or significantly lessened active knee extension. The life style and demands of the patient will determine whether external bracing is required and, if so, whether it is sufficient. If stability is a greater priority than motion, knee fusion is a reliable means of treatment.

Multiple options are available for the reconstruction of bony defects. Available materials include autogenous bone, allograft bone, and synthetic prosthetics, used alone or in combination. The use of allografting for large defects can be a successful option. Appropriate patient selection seems to be essential to obtaining satisfactory results with this technique. The incidence of complications—including infection, failure of union of the osteosynthesis, and allograft fracture—are all significant. This is especially true with concurrent administration of systemic chemotherapy and/or local irradiation of the graft and its surrounding bed.[2, 4, 24, 27]

Implant technology has enjoyed remarkable advances recently, and prosthetic reconstruction of massive bony defects is an available option. This technique affords greater and more rapid achievement of joint motion, a shorter period of immobilization after surgery, and a more rapid return to function. As with any implant, deep infection is a concern, as is the problem of prosthetic loosening. Long-term good results can and have been obtained; experience with prosthetic replacement, both cemented and uncemented, for such large defects, in what frequently is a younger age group, is still being analyzed.

Their use in a selected patient population can be viewed as a temporary measure (though their "temporary lifespan" may, in fact, be quite long) until advances in technique or technology, particularly intramedullary or extramedullary direct bone fixation, make it more feasible to expect reliable satisfactory long-term results.

What implant technology can provide is an alternative to amputation in the pediatric population. Neither arthrodesis nor allograft reconstruction provides for continued longitudinal growth of the affected extremity with the patient's skeletal growth if the epiphyseal plate has been resected. Use of an expandable, adjustable prosthesis has been a realistic alternative to amputation in this patient population.[20]

Specific Considerations

Nonarticular defects are quite amenable to grafting, with appropriate internal fixation as needed. The most common sources of autogenous graft are cancellous or corticocancellous iliac bone and fibula. Allogeneic bone is also well suited to this application in the appropriate clinical setting.

Articular reconstruction is more challenging, and the results are less reliable. Unicondylar femoral defects lend themselves well to allograft reconstruction. Adequate fixation of the graft is more easily obtained in this area, and achieving bone union is generally less of a problem. A significant incidence of ultimate articular degeneration and joint stiffness does exist with mode of treatment, however.

Similar difficulties are encountered when replacing the entire distal femur with an osteoarticular allograft. Articular degeneration seems to be minimized when there is a close correlation between the dimensions of the femoral allograft and the host tibia, but the mechanical problems of stiffness, joint instability, and nonunion of the allograft-host osteosynthesis persist.

Allograft reconstruction of unicondylar tibial defects has met with less satisfying results than those in the femur. Fixation and union are achievable, but loss of articular cartilage and subsequent joint degeneration are greater than in the corresponding femoral condylar allograft. These complications are also encountered when attempting allograft replacement of the entire proximal tibia.

Alternatives are replacement of a single tibial plateau with the articular surface of the patella, the use of autograft or allograft to support the patella in position, or prosthetic replacement of the entire proximal tibia. This prosthetic technique can also be used after total proximal tibial resection. A drawback of this technique is the lack of a fully reliable method for permanent attachment of the extensor mechanism to the prosthesis where the quadriceps mechanism has not been resected.

Custom prosthetic distal femoral replacements are hinged at the knee joint, and some permit an element of tibial rotation. The axis of the extremity permits passive locking of the device in the extended position during the stance phase. Thus the ability to ambulate without aids is generally attainable. The use of an external brace is always possible if the stability of the extremity is insufficient for ambulation, but it is not needed in the majority of patients.

If priorities lie with obtaining an extremity that can provide long-term stability and load-bearing capacity at the expense of motion, an arthrodesis can be performed. Whether bone loss is subsequent to femoral resection, tibial resection, or both (due to extraarticular resection), the techniques for achieving arthrodesis are multiple and varied. Most rely upon the maintenance of length and alignment with an intramedullary device spanning the defect from femur to tibia. The bony defect is reconstituted either with autogenous graft material or allograft.[3, 9]

Autograft material may be local, utilizing hemicortical portions of the remaining normal tibia or femur as intercalary or "sliding" grafts. Otherwise, one or both fibulae, either vascularized or not, can be used to span the defect. Appropriate internal fixation is used to fix the graft, which is then usually supplemented with iliac bone.

The extremity is then immobilized or protected as needed until sufficient incorporation of the graft is present to permit graduated weight bearing and eventual return to full function.

Summary

Surgical extirpation of neoplasms about the knee and subsequent reconstruction of the extremity require a special understanding of the anatomy and function of the joint and its components.[14, 16, 18] If patients are treated with a mind to the considerations elaborated in this chapter, the goal of achieving adequate local disease control combined with optimal functional status can be realized.[8]

References

1. Barbera C, Lewis MM: Office evaluation of bone tumors. Orthop Clin North Am 19:821–838, 1988.
2. Benjamin RS: Chemotherapy for osteosarcoma. *In* Unni KK (ed): Tumors. New York, Churchill Livingstone, 1988, pp 149–156.
3. Campanacci M, Cerellati C, Guerra A, et al: Knee resection-arthrodesis. *In* Enneking WF (ed): Limb Salvage in Musculoskeletal Oncology. New York, Churchill Livingstone, 1987, pp 364–378.
4. Campanacci M, Laus M: Local recurrence after amputation for osteosarcoma. J Bone Joint Surg 62B:201–207, 1980.
5. Dahlin DC, Unni KK: Bone Tumors: General Aspects and Data on 8542 Cases, 4th ed. Springfield, IL, Charles C Thomas, 1986.
6. Devas MB: Stress fractures in children. J Bone Joint Surg 45B:528, 1963.
7. Engh CA, Robinson RA, Milgram J: Stress fractures in children. J Trauma 10:532, 1970.
8. Enneking WF: Modification of the system for functional evaluation of surgical management of musculoskeletal tumors. *In* Enneking WF (ed): Limb Salvage in Musculoskeletal Oncology. New York, Churchill Livingstone, 1987, p 626.
9. Enneking WF, Shirley PO: Resection arthrodesis for malignant and potentially malignant lesions about the knee using an intramedullary rod and local bone grafts. J Bone Joint Surg 59A:223–236, 1977.
10. Enneking WF, Spanier SS, Goodman MA: Current concepts review: The surgical staging of musculoskeletal sarcoma. J Bone Joint Surg 62A:1027–1030, 1980.
11. Imperato AM, Roses DF, Francis KC, Lewis MM: Major vascular reconstruction for limb salvage in patients with soft tissue and skeletal sarcomas of the extremities. Surg Gynecol Obstet 147:891, 1978.
12. Frykman GK, Leung VCL: Free vascularized flaps for

lower extremity reconstruction. Orthopaedics 9:841–848, 1986.

13. Gebhardt MC, Goorin AM, Triana J, et al: Long-term results of limb salvage and amputation in extremity osteosarcoma. *In* Yamamuro T (ed): New Development for Limb Salvage in Musculoskeletal Tumors. Tokyo, Springer-Verlag, 1989, pp 99–109.
14. Ivins JC, Taylor WF, Golenzer H: A multi-institutional cooperative study of osteosarcoma. *In* Yamamuro T (ed): New Development for Limb Salvage in Musculoskeletal Tumors. Tokyo, Springer-Verlag, 1989, pp 61–69.
15. Kenan S, Jones C, Lewis MM: Limb sparing reconstructive surgery in malignant and aggressive benign bone tumors of the extremities. Surg Rounds Orthop. pp. 25–33, August 1987.
16. Klein JK, Kenan S, Lewis MM: Osteosarcoma: Clinical and pathological considerations. Orthop Clin North Am 20:327–345, 1989.
17. Kotz R, Salzer M: Rotationaplasty for childhood osteosarcoma of the distal part of the femur. J Bone Joint Surg 64A:959, 1982.
18. Lane JM, Hurson B, Boland PJ, Glasser DB: Osteogenic sarcoma. Clin Orthop 204:93, 1986.
19. Lewis MM: An approach to the treatment of malignant bone tumors. Orthopaedics 8:655–656, 1985.
20. Lewis MM: The use of an expandable and adjustable prosthesis in the treatment of childhood malignant bone tumors of the extremities. Cancer 57:499–502, 1986.
21. Lewis MM: Bone Tumor Surgery: Limb Sparing Techniques. Philadelphia, JB Lippincott, 1988.
22. Lodwick GS: A systematic approach to the roentgen diagnosis of bone tumors. *In* MD Anderson Hospital: Tumors of Bone and Soft Tissue. Chicago, Year Book Medical Publishers, 1965, p 49.
23. Malawer MM, McHale KA: Limb sparing surgery for high grade malignant tumors of the proximal tibia: Surgical technique and method of extension mechanism reconstruction. Clin Orthop 237:68–85, 1988.
24. Mankin H, Fogelson F, Thrasher A: Massive allograft transplanation for bone tumors. J Bone Joint Surg 57A:1171, 1975.
25. Mankin HJ, Lange TA, Spanier SS: The hazards of biopsy in patients with malignant primary bone and soft tissue tumors. J Bone Joint Surg 64A:1121–1127, 1982.
26. Marcove RC, Lewis MM, Rosen G, et al: Total femur and total knee replacement. Clin Orthop 126:147–152, 1977.
27. Neff JR: Experience in the use of a custom modular titanium intramedullary rod in resection/arthrodesis of the knee. *In* Yamamuro T (ed): New Development for Limb Salvage in Musculoskeletal Tumors. Tokyo, Springer-Verlag, 1989, p 264.
28. Schreiman JS, Crass JR, Wick MR, et al: Osteosarcoma: Role of CT in limb sparing treatment. Radiology 161:485–488, 1986.
29. Sim FH, Chao EYS: Prosthetic replacement of the knee and a large segment of the femur or tibia. J Bone Joint Surg 61A:887–892, 1979.
30. Simon MA: Limb salvage for osteosarcoma. *In* Yamamuro T (ed): New Development for Limb Salvage in Musculoskeletal Tumors. Tokyo, Springer-Verlag, 1989, pp 71–72.
31. Simon MA, Aschliman MA, Thomas N: Limb salvage treatment vs amputation for osteosarcoma of the distal end of the femur. J Bone Joint Surg 68A:1331–1337, 1986.
32. Simon MA, Kirchner PT: Scintigraphic evaluation of primary bone tumors. J Bone Joint Surg 68A:1458, 1986.
33. Sundaram M, McGuire MH, Harold DR, et al: Magnetic resonance imaging in planning limb salvage surgery for primary malignant tumors of bone. J Bone Joint Surg 68A:809–819, 1986.
34. Taminiav AHM, Bloem JL: The impact of MRI on staging malignant musculoskeletal tumors. *In* Yamamuro T (ed): New Development for Limb Salvage in Musculoskeletal Tumors. Tokyo, Springer-Verlag, 1989, pp 111–114.
35. Zimmer WD, Berquist TH, McLeod RA, et al: Magnetic resonance imaging of osteosarcoma: Comparison with computed tomography. Clin Orthop 208:289–299, 1986.

CHAPTER 18

Tumors of the Foot and Ankle

JOHN F. WALLER
MICHAEL CLAIN

Foot Deformities and Pseudotumors

Hallux Valgus. Hallux valgus, a common disorder that causes the so-called bunion of the forefoot, is the complex deformity that results from the appearance of the first metatarsophalangeal joint with medial prominence of the metatarsal head. This condition may be on a neuromuscular basis, such as in cerebral palsy, may appear "as an adolescent bunion," or more commonly may be a congenital condition that progresses with age.

Spasm of the Extensor Digitorum Brevis. The extensor digitorum brevis muscle arises from the superior and lateral surfaces of the calcaneus, inserting into the extensor tendons of the four medial toes. Occasionally, the muscle may be in spasm or may be hypertrophied and noted as a mass on the dorsolateral aspect of the foot. The muscle needs to be recognized as normal anatomy.[22]

Hagland's Deformity. Hagland's deformity is a prominence of the posterosuperior tuberosity of the calcaneus. It presents as a painful mass just proximal to the insertion of the Achilles tendon. The condition is also referred to as a "pump bump," reflecting the fact that it is caused by chronic pressure from the upper posterior margin of shoe wear. Radiographs may reveal a prominence of the proximal posterior calcaneus. The pain is a result of retrocalcaneal bursal degeneration causing Achilles tendinitis. Occasionally, a resection of a portion of the calcaneus is necessary for relief of symptoms, but this should only be done after very careful consideration.[18, 30]

Stress Fracture of the Metatarsal. A metatarsal stress fracture is not an uncommon condition. It usually presents with pain that is particularly exacerbated by physical activity. The normal biologic response to a stress fracture is to lay down callus, which may present as a mass particularly on the dorsal aspect of the foot. The second and third metatarsals are most frequently affected, but other bones including the calcaneus and the navicular may suffer a stress fracture. The fracture should be recognized by radiograph, although an early stress fracture may need a bone scan to verify its existence. Treatment is symptomatic, but recognition by clinical history and radiologic appearance is mandatory, as biopsy may only further confuse the picture because the histologic appearance of this lesion is not dissimilar to that of an osteosarcoma.[11, 18, 29]

Accessory Navicular Bone. An accessory navicular bone is a congenital anomaly found on the proximal medial aspect of the midfoot. A secondary center of ossification fails to ossify into a single navicular bone. The patient usually presents with a pronated foot with a slightly enlarged painful and tender mass on the medial aspect of the foot. Radiographs reveal the accessory navicular bone. Treatment consists of appropriate physical therapy and shoe inserts; occasionally surgery is required.[18]

Benign Soft Tumor and Tumorlike Tissues of the Foot and Ankle

Gout. Tophaceous gouty deposits may present as a single or multiple masses in the foot. This disease of uric acid metabolism most commonly occurs in middle-aged men and postmenopausal women. Often there is an elevated serum uric acid level. The patient with tophi usually has a long-standing history of poorly controlled gout. The masses are subcutaneous, usually in the area of the Achilles tendon, and may cause skin ulcerations. Aspiration of an involved joint or of the mass itself will reveal needle-shaped crystals showing the typical strongly negative birefringence of monosodium urate. Treatment is primarily medical, although occasional debridement is necessary.[7, 26]

Fibroma. Fibromas are benign fibrous tumors that usually occur subcutaneously. These nontender, discrete, and slow-growing lesions often result from repetitive trauma. They must be carefully distinguished from fibromatosis. If they are a cause of concern, surgical excision will cure the problem.[18]

Plantar Fibromatosis. Plantar fibromatosis is a locally aggressive fibrous tumor found in the area of the plantar fascia in an adolescent and young adult. The lesions are usually firm nodules on the medial plantar aspect of the foot. Fibromatosis may enlarge and cause discomfort; the lesion may be bilateral. Recognition of the disease, reassurance of the patient, and appropriate nonoperative care is recommended. Excision of the fibromatosis should be considered in a few selected situations and can result in a painful plantar scar; additionally there is a possibility of a more aggressive local recurrence.[6, 8, 13, 18]

Neurilemoma (Schwannoma). Neurilemoma is a benign tumor arising from the nerve sheath of peripheral nerves (Fig. 18–1). These tumors are usually small (less than 2 cm) and often occur during middle age, when they become symptomatic as a small mass. The tumors are eccentric intraneural or extraneural tumors but they are encapsulated and can be resected with little damage to the nerve itself.[6, 18, 24]

Neurofibroma. Neurofibromas are benign tumors that arise within the peripheral nerve. They may be solitary or multiple and may represent a part of generalized neurofibromatosis. The skin, subcutis, and peripheral nerves may be involved. Rarely neurofibromatosis may be the cause of macrodactyly. If the neurofibroma involves a peripheral nerve, it is seldom possible to preserve all of the nerve's function with excision. The solitary nerve lesion is excised if symptoms are severe. In generalized neurofibromatosis, the problems of the large weight-bearing bones and the spine are paramount. In the rare cases of gigantism, limited amputation is often the most appropriate treatment.[5, 6, 12, 18]

Lipoma. Lipoma, a common subcutaneous

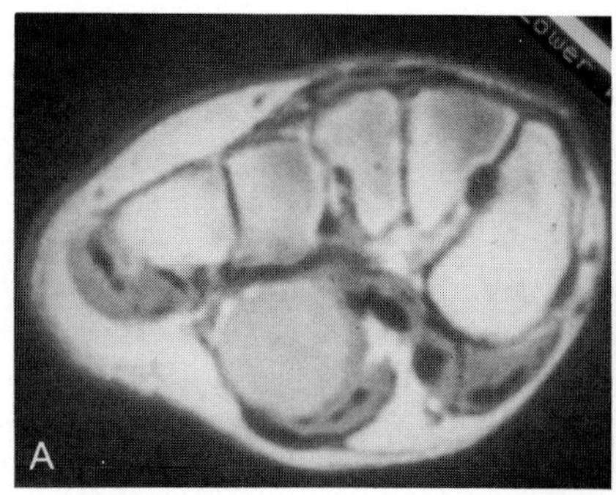

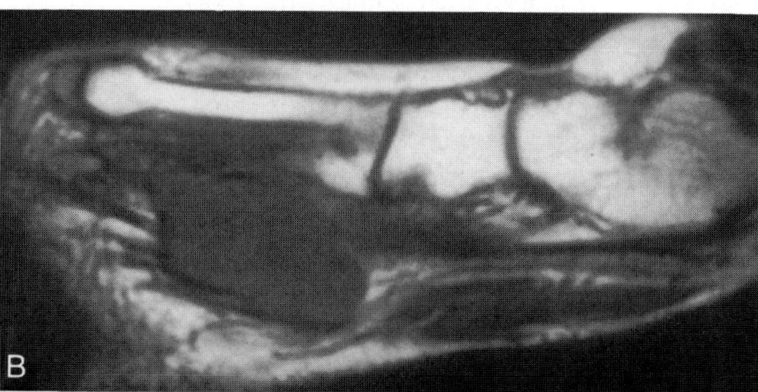

FIGURE 18–1. Plantar schwannoma. A 50-year-old female patient with pain and swelling over the plantar surface. *A, B,* MRI scans reveal homogeneous round fusiform mass. T1 image reveals a relatively low-intensity signal, and T2, a high-signal image.

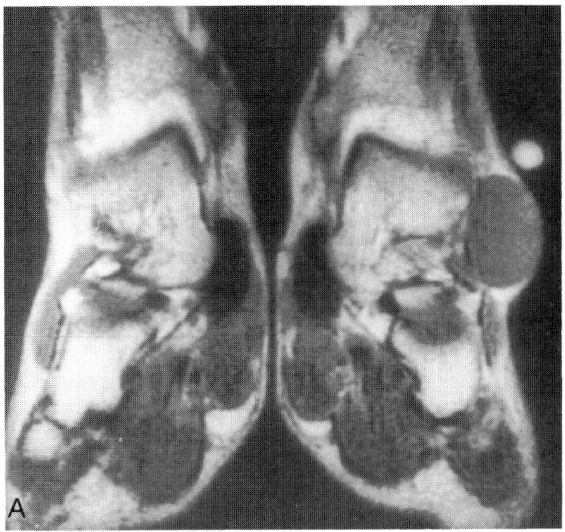

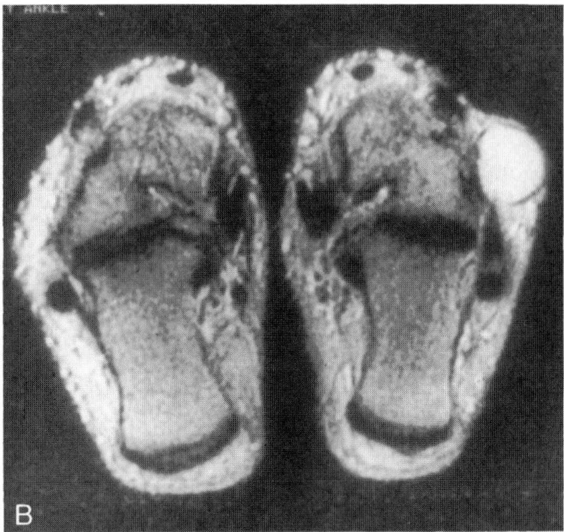

FIGURE 18–2. Ganglion. A 41-year-old male patient with subcutaneous cystic mass over the lateral aspect of the ankle joint. *A, B,* MRI scans reveal homogeneous low-signal in T1 image and a high-intensity signal in T2 image.

tumor, is well-encapsulated, nontender, and readily excised. Histologically the findings are of normal adipose tissue well encased in a fibrous capsule. Treatment is based upon recognition and simple excision.[6, 18]

Ganglion. The ganglion cyst is a common benign mass usually occurring in the foot or hand. It is a well encapsulated, cystic, fluid-filled lesion arising from either joint capsule or tendon sheath (Fig. 18–2). Aspiration will return a clear jellylike fluid. Surgical excision is required if observation and/or aspiration fails to cure the condition.[6, 18]

Pigmented Villonodular Synovitis. Pigmented villonodular synovitis (PVNS) is virtually the same histologic entity as a giant cell tumor of the tendon sheath, although in PVNS the process is diffuse rather than focal. In the case of PVNS the joint has an effusion and synovitis. It occurs most commonly in the knee but is seen in the ankle and rarely in the joints of the foot (Fig. 18–3). Two basic types exist:

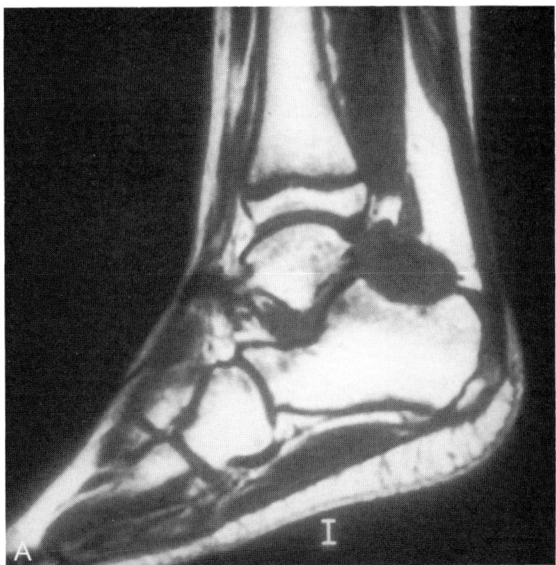

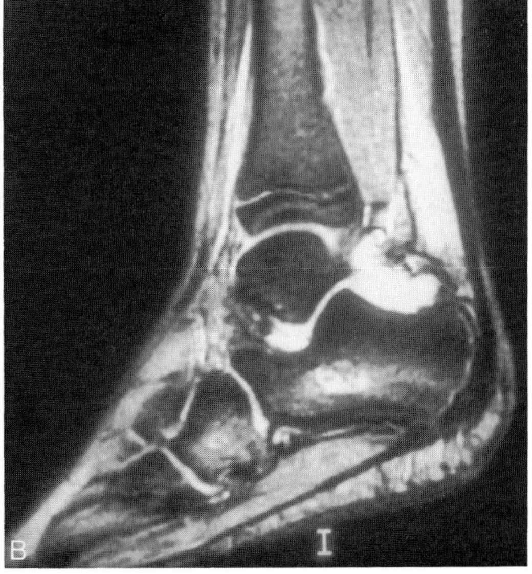

FIGURE 18–3. Pigmented villonodular synovitis. A 12-year-old female patient with a swelling behind the ankle joint. *A, B,* MRI scans reveal low-intensity signal in T1 image, and bright high-intensity signal in T2 image.

an isolated lesion sometimes known as localized nodular synovitis and a more diffuse one. Joint aspiration may return a brownish fluid. Treatment is arthroscopic or open synovectomy. The diffuse lesions recur, but localized nodular synovitis is usually cured by a single excision.[1, 18, 23]

Giant Cell Tumor of the Tendon Sheath. Giant cell tumor of the tendon sheath is a common subcutaneous lesion of the foot and hand that presents as a slowly enlarging mass arising from the synovial tendon sheaths. Histologic features include giant cells and cholesterol-filled histiocytes (foam cells). This pathologic picture is identical to that of pigmented pigmented villonodular synovitis. Needle aspiration is not helpful, but local excision is often done for both diagnostic and therapeutic purposes.[6, 18, 23]

Hemangioma. This benign hamartomatous condition usually presents in childhood as a painless mass with a bluish tint. On examination, the lesion is clearly vascular and compressible. These lesions are benign and rarely require surgical intervention (Fig. 18–4). Larger "cavernous" hemangiomas, involving large dilated thin-walled vessels, are often intermittently painful and do not blush with compression. Radiographs may reveal calcifications (phleboliths) within the cavities. Treatment of symptomatic hemangiomas is surgical.[6, 18]

Glomus Tumor. Pathologically, Masson described a tumor of the neuromyoarterial apparatus, called the glomus. This vascular tumor usually presents as an extremely painful, tender, cold-sensitive, subungual lesion. The nail bed may appear bluish, and there may be ridging of the nail. There is an increase in the number of nerves adjacent to the tumor, which accounts for the lesion's acute sensitivity. Surgical extirpation resolves the problem.[6, 12, 19, 25]

Benign Bone Tumors of the Foot and Ankle

Solitary or Simple Bone Cyst. A simple bone cyst in childhood often is located in the metaphyseal region of long bones as well as in the larger tarsal bones such as the talus and the calcaneus. Radiographs reveal a well-circumscribed, lucent lesion with minimal, if any, expansion (Fig. 18–5). Pathologically, the lesion is fluid filled and lined with a fibrous membrane. Treatment is directed at prevention or fixation of pathologic fractures and any resulting deformities. This includes observation, particularly in younger children (owing

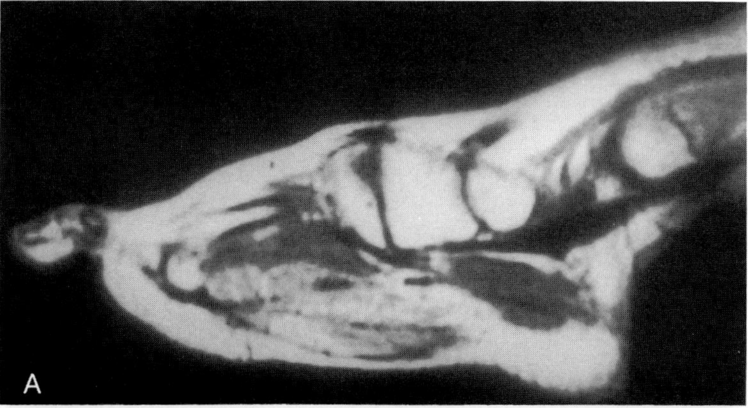

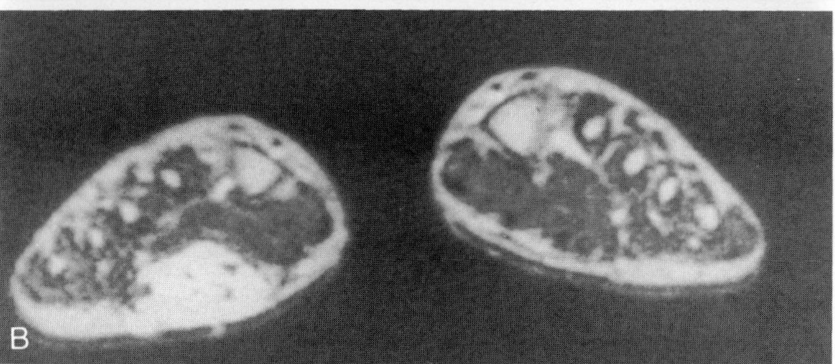

FIGURE 18–4. Plantar hemangioma. A 14-year-old female patient with a painful plantar soft tissue mass. *A, B,* MRI scans reveal heterogeneous ill-defined image; T1 image shows a relatively low-intensity signal and T2 image, a bright signal.

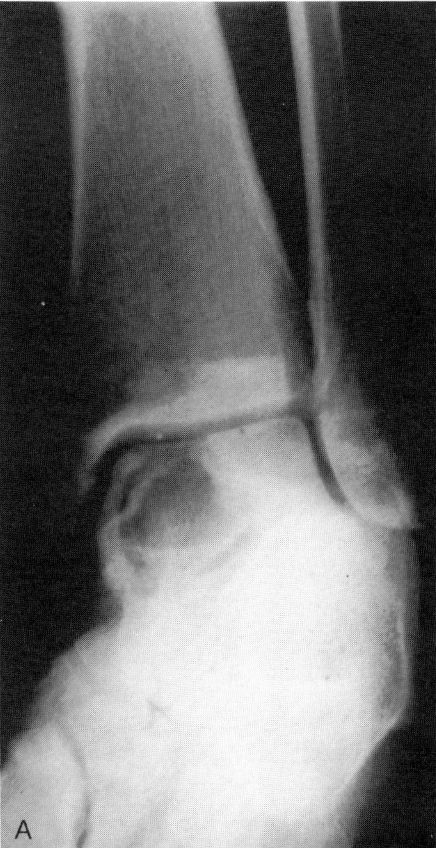

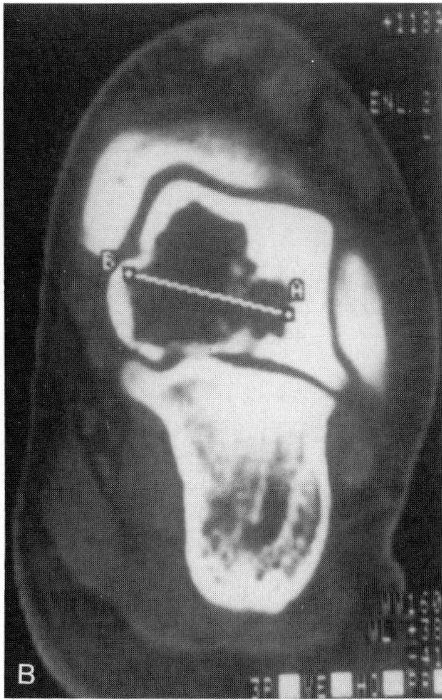

FIGURE 18–5. Bone cyst. A 20-year-old male patient with prolonged history of ankle pain. *A,* Plain film reveals a subchondral cyst over the talus. *B,* CT scan demonstrates the extent of the cavity in the bone.

to a high rate of recurrence), curettage and bone grafting, and multiple steroid injections.[2, 18, 22, 28]

Aneurysmal Bone Cyst. An aneurysmal bone cyst (ABC), a benign lesion, has a predilection for adults in the first and second decades. The lesion is eccentric, lucent, multiloculated, and expansile (Fig. 18–6). At surgery the cyst is blood-filled with a tendency to bleed from its lining when curetted. The histologic appearance is characterized by multiple vascular channels progressing from small vessels to large sinusoids with an incomplete endothelial lining interspersed with a spindle cell stroma containing giant cells. Care must be taken in pathologic examination of the specimens, as an ABC may be associated with a primary neoplasm such as an osteoblastoma or chondroblastoma. Therapy usually consists of thorough curettage and bone grafting.[2, 6, 18]

Epidermoid Cyst. These posttraumatic lesions may rarely present as an intraosseous lucent lesion in the distal terminal phalanx. Pathologically these inclusion cysts are surrounded by keratinizing stratified squamous epithelium with keratin debris within the cyst. Treatment is curettage and bone grafting.[2, 18]

Giant Cell Tumor. Giant cell tumor, a relatively common primary bone tumor found in young adults, has a predilection for long bones but rarely can occur in the foot (Fig. 18–7) and hand. Clinically, patients present with pain and swelling. In the Mayo Clinic series of 429 giant cell tumors, five involved the foot.[4] The radiologic and pathologic findings are summarized in Chapter 2. Treatment requires biopsy, staging based on the radiographs and histologic findings, and appropriate surgical excision.[2, 6]

Osteochondroma (Exostosis). Osteochondromas are common tumors of the long bones, but solitary ones are rarely found in the hands and feet. They are bony protuberances, probably resulting from a herniation of a portion of the growth plate through the periosteum. The lesions continue to grow until skeletal maturity is achieved. In the Mayo Clinic series of 640 osteochondromata, six involved the foot. The radiographic and pathologic findings are summarized in Chapter 2. Treatment consists of observation and/or excision of symp-

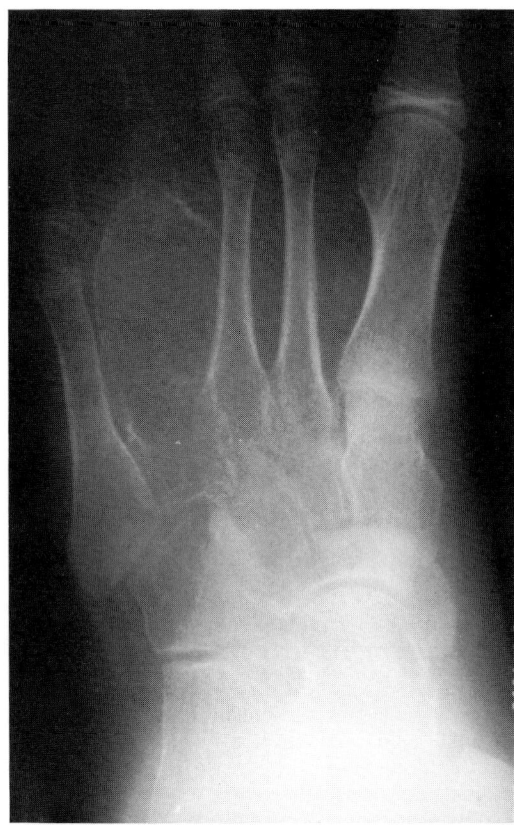

FIGURE 18–6. Aneurysmal bone cyst. Expansile radiolucent lesion occupying the fourth metatarsal.

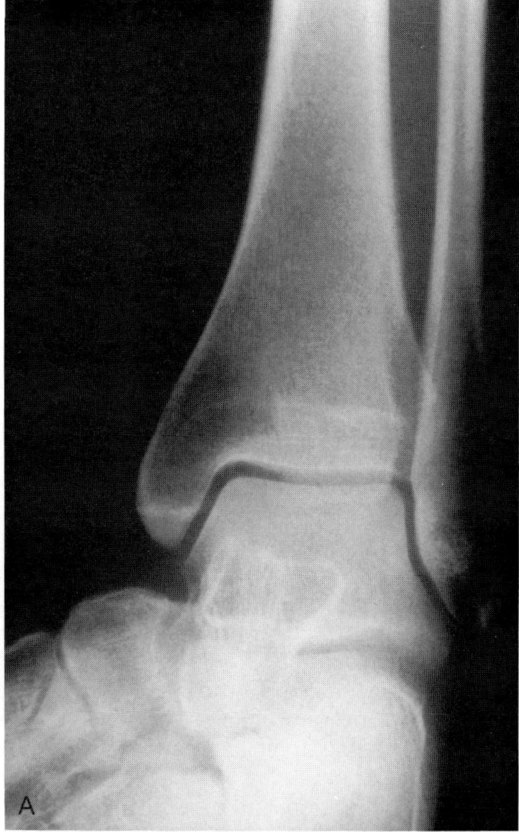

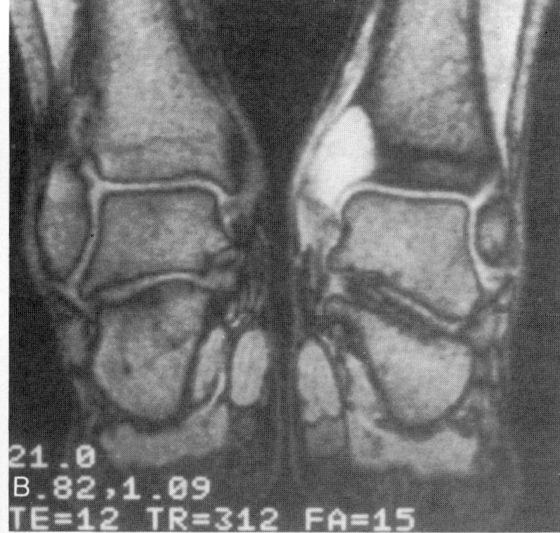

FIGURE 18–7. Giant cell tumor. A 24-year-old female patient with pain over the medial aspect of the ankle joint. *A,* Plain film reveals a radiolucent lytic lesion over the medial malleolus. *B,* MRI T2 image reveals bright high-intensity signal.

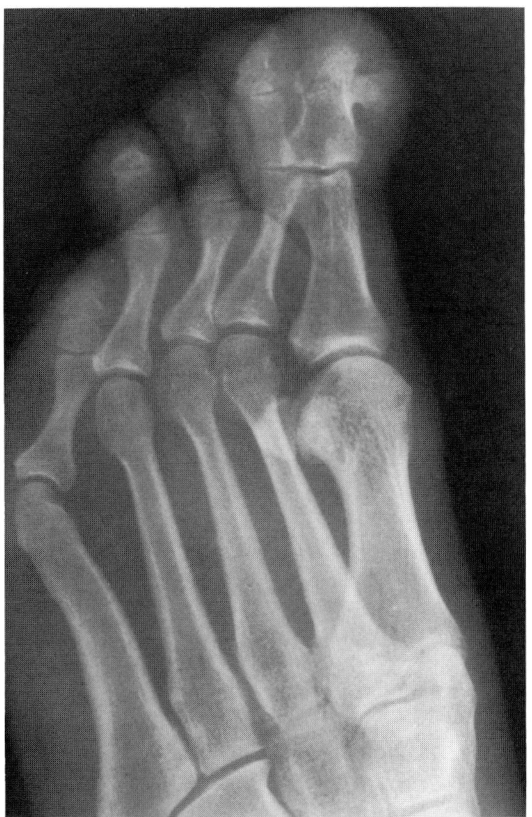

FIGURE 18–8. Ungual exostosis. Subungual bony exostosis is seen in the distal phalanx of the great toe.

tomatic lesions. A low malignant potential exists, but in the syndrome of multiple hereditary exostoses, the malignant potential is much higher, requiring long-term observation.[2, 4, 6, 18]

Subungual Exostosis. This reactive bone spur of the distal phalanx may present with pain or a mass that distorts the toenail (Fig. 18–8). Treatment is surgical excision of the exostosis.[18]

Osteoid Osteoma. The osteoid osteoma is a small lesion (less than 1 cm) commonly found in children. It is characterized by nocturnal pain, which is relieved by aspirin. In the Mayo Clinic's series of 245 osteoid osteomas, 11 involved the foot.[4] The radiologic and pathologic findings are summarized in Chapter 2. Treatment is by surgical excision; operative planning requires precise localization of the lesion, as its position is often obscure at surgery. Radiographs reveal a lucent nidus surrounded by a dense cortical reactive zone (Fig. 18–9). Plain film may be difficult to interpret, and bone scan or computed tomography (CT) may be necessary. Histologically the lesion is characterized by osteoid with prominent osteoblasts and osteoblasts with little vascularization.[2, 6, 18]

Osteoblastoma. An osteoblastoma may be conceptualized as a large osteoid osteoma. These typically painful lesions of young adults have a predilection for the spine but can occur anywhere (Fig. 18–10). In the Mayo Clinic's series of 63 osteoblastomas, two involved the foot.[4] Treatment is by either curettage and bone graft or surgical excision.[2, 3, 6, 18]

Enchondroma. The enchondroma is a common benign intramedullary cartilaginous tumor of the short tubular bones of the feet and hands. The radiologic and pathologic features are summarized in Chapter 2. Rarely a chondrosarcoma may arise from an enchondroma. Treatment often is observation, but symptomatic lesions require curettage and bone grafting.[2, 5, 18]

Chondroblastoma. Chondroblastoma is al-

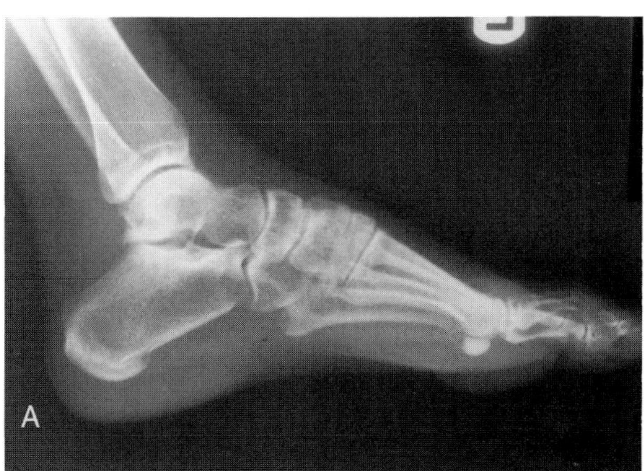

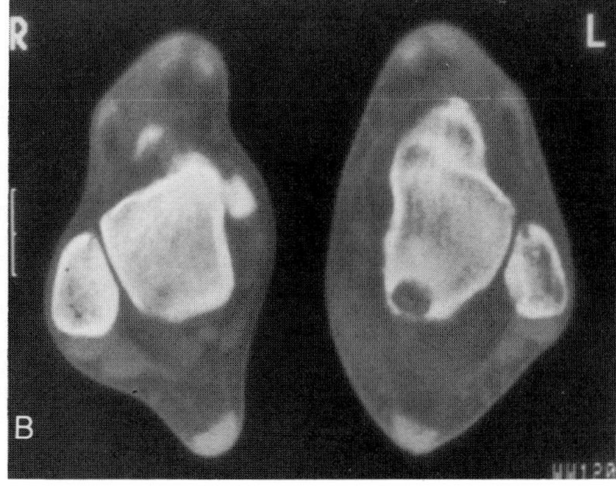

FIGURE 18–9. Osteoid osteoma. A 34-year-old male patient with day and night pain over the ankle joint. *A*, *B*, Radiographs reveal a subchondral nidus surrounded by sclerosis at the posterior aspect of the talus.

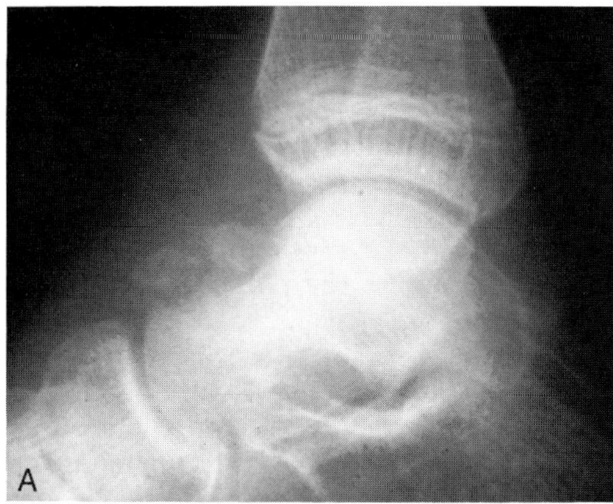

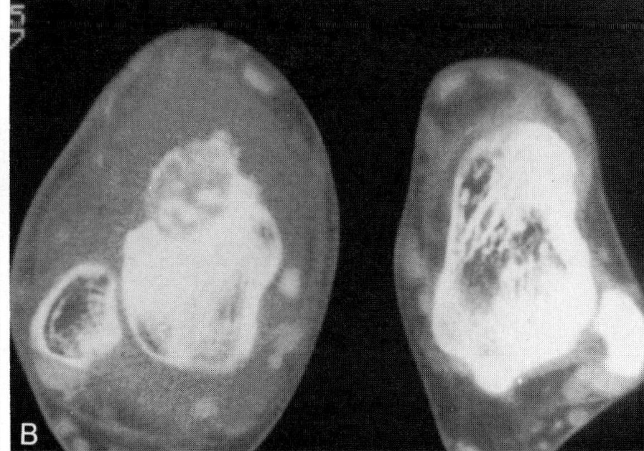

FIGURE 18–10. Osteoblastoma. A 12-year-old female patient with pain over the ankle joint. *A, B,* Radiographs reveal an aggressive lesion over the dorsum of the talus. Cortical erosion associated with soft tissue mass containing focal calcification is also noted.

most always a benign neoplasm, usually seen in the second decade. In the Mayo Clinic's series of 79 chondroblastomas, five involved the foot.[4] The radiologic and histologic features are summarized in Chapter 2. Treatment includes observation (in the young child), curettage and bone grafting, and marginal excisions. Extremely rare pulmonary metastases should be excised surgically.[2, 6, 18]

Fibrous Dysplasia. Monostotic fibrous dysplasia is a relatively common solitary lesion of children and adolescents. Rarely seen in the foot, it accounted for only two of Henry's 50 cases of fibrous dysplasia. The radiologic and histologic features are reviewed in Chapter 2. If the lesion is small, observation alone may be sufficient treatment. However, curettage and bone grafting are usually performed for both therapeutic and diagnostic purposes.[2, 5, 10, 18]

Bone Island. A bone island is a circumscribed focus of mature cortical bone found within trabecular bone radiologically. It is probably a developmental phenomenon and should be recognized as innocuous. Osteopoikilosis is an inherited autosomal dominant condition of multiple bone islands that may sometimes involve the foot and hand.[2]

Osteomyelitis. Osteomyelitis is diagnosed on the basis of direct bone culture or a positive blood culture in the appropriate clinical setting. The initial immune response to infection is an acute inflammatory reaction. Increased pressure in the medullary cavity, secondary to inflammation, results in areas of necrosis that spread to the surrounding cortical bone. In children an elevated subperiosteal bony sleeve or involucrum may be one of the earliest radiologic signs of osteomyelitis. Additionally, if the infection is localized and walled off, a lytic lesion with surrounding sclerosis may be noted (Brodie's abscess). Clinically, acute osteomyelitis presents with pain, swelling, and fever. Treatment requires specific bacteriologic identification, antibiotics, and possibly surgery. Chronic osteomyelitis is a more indolent disease, presenting with pain and perhaps a draining sinus. Therapy involves organism identification, surgical debridement, and antibiotics. Specific to the foot are a number of neuropathic entities that predispose to infection. Most common in the United States is the diabetic foot. Other entities that present with a neuropathic picture include syphilitic neuropathy (tabes dorsalis) and leprosy (Hansen's disease). Treatment is as for other forms of osteomyelitis but should principally be directed at prevention.[2, 18, 21, 31]

Metabolic Bone Diseases

Rickets. Rickets is a childhood disease of vitamin D metabolism. Historically, dietary vitamin D deficiency was the principal cause. In the United States today, the most common cause of rickets is renal tubular dysfunction. Clinically, affected children are listless and hypotonic, and they may be noted to have frontal bosselation, beaded masses of the costochondral junction ("rachitic rosary"), or bulging of the epiphyseal plates at the joint line ("string of pearls"). This latter feature may often be palpated at the distal fibular epiphyseal line. Radiologically a widened epiphyseal plate with cupping of the adjacent metaphyseal bone is noted. Treatment requires accurate diagnosis and understanding of the underlying biochemical abnormalities and appropriate dietary or pharmacologic therapy.[2, 16, 17]

Renal Osteodystrophy. Chronic renal disease leads to characteristic bony changes. In general terms, chronic renal failure has an effect on the metabolism of vitamin D, calcium, phosphate, and parathyroid hormone. Radiologically, evidence of renal osteodystrophy includes osteomalacia, subperiosteal bone resorption of the feet and hands, cystic "brown tumor" areas, resorption of the distal clavicles, osteosclerosis, and soft tissue calcifications. Diagnosis of the underlying disorders is essential, followed by the appropriate therapy.[2, 16, 17]

Hyperparathyroidism. Primary hyperparathyroidism is an overproduction of parathyroid hormones because of the presence of a solitary parathyroid adenoma, multiple adenomata, parathyroid carcinoma, or primary hyperplasia. Secondary hyperparathyroidism is seen in chronic renal failure as a result of hypocalcemia and may have the clinical picture of renal osteodystrophy. The typical patient with primary hyperparathyroidism is middle-aged and has a history of renal stones, peptic ulcers, and vague complaints such as nausea and listlessness.

Diagnosis is suspected when the serum calcium and chloride are elevated and serum phosphate is depressed. Confirmatory measurements of parathyrin show an increase in serum levels. Radiologically, osteopenia may be noted. Characteristic findings in the hands and feet include resorption of the phalangeal tufts, radial subperiosteal erosion of the middle phalanges, and absorption of the pubic and distal clavicles. Lytic "brown tumors" may be present. Histologic evaluation demonstrates an increased osteoblast population with tunneling resorption and paratrabecular marrow fibrosis. Therapy is directed toward the underlying problem and usually involves surgical excision of an adenoma.[2]

Secondary hyperparathyroidism is a more difficult problem, as renal dysfunction is the principal medical concern.[2]

Pseudotumor of Hemophilia. Rarely, in a hemophiliac patient, a mass may develop as a result of chronic bleeding episodes. More often, the hemophiliac is symptomatic as a consequence of intraarticular bleeding with resultant joint destruction.

Osteoporosis. Osteoporosis is a condition of diminished mineralized bone mass per unit volume. Of the many causes of osteoporosis, some show radiologic changes in the foot.[15]

SUDECK'S ATROPHY. This disuse osteoporosis, more commonly called a reflex sympathetic dystrophy, has the radiologic pattern of periarticular osteoporosis. Recognition and appropriate therapy are required for care.

STEROID-INDUCED. The chronic ingestion of corticosteroids can lead to this form of osteoporosis.

SENILE OSTEOPOROSIS. This is the most common cause of osteoporosis and is more frequent in women than men. The etiology is unclear, but a balanced dietary intake during youth seems to be important.

Sarcoidosis. Sarcoidosis is a noncaseating idiopathic granulomatous disease in which the bones (especially of the foot and hand) are involved approximately 10% of the time. Radiographs reveal punched-out cortical erosions from soft tissue lesions or may show centrally lytic lesions of bone. Histologically, in a setting of negative cultures for tuberculosis, brucellosis, fungus, and atypical mycobacteria, noncaseating epithelioid granulomas with a few giant cells are seen.[2, 6, 18]

Ectopic Calcification. This occurs in association with an old injury or in association with a collagen-vascular disease such as scleroderma. Accurate recognition of the entity is important to minimize concern about malignancies (Fig. 18–11).[18]

Malignant Lesions of Soft Tissue and Bone

Synovial Sarcoma. Synovial sarcoma is a rare malignant neoplasm that occurs in the soft tissues around the joints. A mass may be noted particularly in the ankles, heel, or dorsal foot region. In the series of 83 soft tissue tumors of the foot, Kirby and colleagues found five synovial sarcomas.[14] Radiologically, a soft tissue mass, sometimes with calcification and extrinsic bony erosion, may be noted. Histologically, synovial sarcoma demonstrates a biphasic pattern of spindle cells with cuboidal cells. These tumors are highly malignant, and metastases to the lungs are most common. Treatment requires an initial high index of

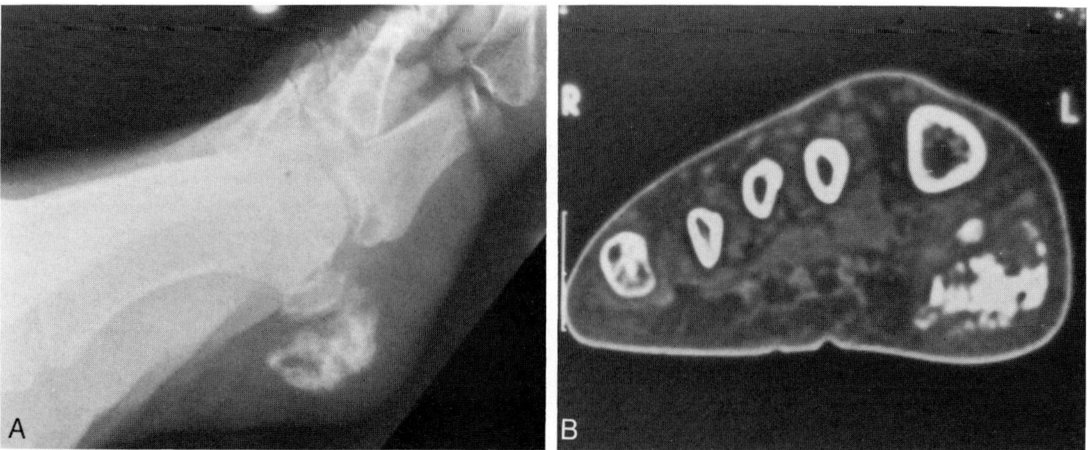

FIGURE 18–11. Ectopic bone fomation. *A, B,* Posttraumatic plantar calcification and bone formation.

suspicion, with subsequent biopsy. Wide surgical excision followed by adjuvant chemotherapy is necessary.[2, 27]

Osteosarcoma. Most osteosarcomas occur in adolescent children in the metaphyseal regions of long bones and rarely in the foot and hand. Clinically the tumor is characterized by an often painful, rapidly enlarging mass. In the Mayo Clinic series of 1274 osteosarcomas, 11 involved the foot. Radiologically the lesion is aggressive and destructive, has a poorly defined border, demonstrates periosteal reaction of (Codman's triangle) and may be radiodense, radiolucent, or mixed (Fig. 18–12). The histologic appearance has been reviewed in Chapter 2. Because these tumors are highly malignant, treatment requires staging, and wide surgical excision in conjunction with adjuvant chemotherapy.[4, 6, 20]

Ewing's Sarcoma. Ewing's sarcoma is a highly malignant tumor of childhood and adolescence. Clinically, a painful, rapidly growing mass is noted, often in the setting of fever and leukocytosis. The tumor usually involves the hematopoietic marrow and may occasionally be seen in the foot or hand. Untreated the course is one of rapid metastases and death. In the Mayo Clinic series of 402 Ewing's tumors, 20 involved the foot. The radiographic and histologic appearance have been reviewed in Chapter 2. As with other malignant tumors, early suspicion and biopsy are mandatory. Treatment usually includes chemotherapy with radiation and surgery, depending on the location.[1, 4, 6]

Chondrosarcoma. Chondrosarcoma is a slow-growing, painless, malignant neoplasm that produces a cartilaginous matrix. Tumors are commonly found in the central skeleton and are rare in the foot. The more proximal lesions are more malignant. In the Mayo Clinic

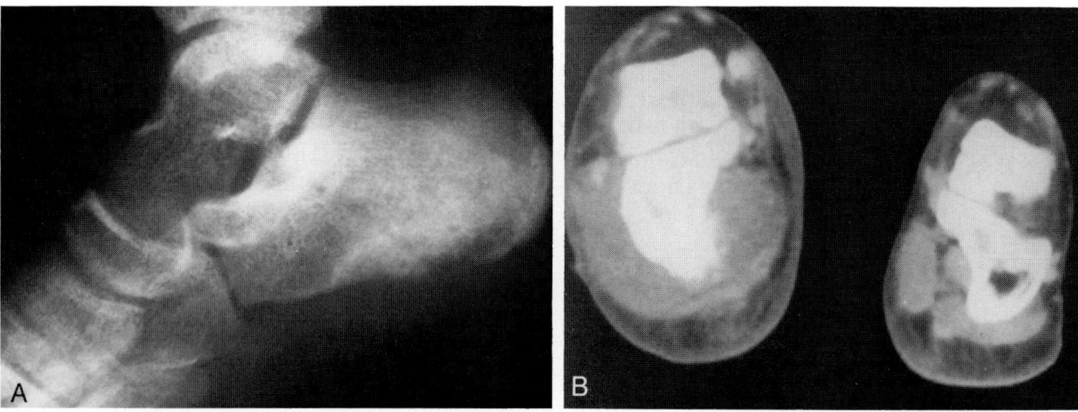

FIGURE 18–12. Osteosarcoma. A 17-year-old male patient with destructive blastic and lytic lesion over the calcaneus (*A*). *B,* CT scan demonstrates the extent of the bone destruction and the surrounding soft tissue mass.

series of 542 chondrosarcomas, seven involved the foot. The radiologic and histologic features have been reviewed in Chapter 2. The high incidence of enchondromas in the foot and hand and the rarity of a chondrosarcoma in these areas require that the pathologic picture be carefully correlated with the radiologic and clinical setting. In general, surgical excision of a chondrosarcoma is the treatment of choice.[4, 6, 7, 20]

Fibrosarcoma. Fibrosarcoma is a rare tumor of bone, occasionally found in the foot. Clinically the lesion can occur at any age and causes pain and swelling. In the Mayo Clinic series of 207 fibrosarcomas, three involved the foot. The radiologic and histologic presentation have been reviewed in Chapter 2. Therapy involves biopsy and radical surgical excision.[2, 4, 6, 7, 20]

Metastatic Tumors. Metastatic cancer is the most common malignant tumor in bone, although it rarely spreads to the foot and hand. Radiologically it appears as a radiolucent or radiodense lesion; the most common lucent metastases are to the lung, kidney, and thyroid. Blastic metastases are usually to the prostate or breast. Treatment depends on whether the site of the primary tumor is known, the anatomic location, and the degree of structural compromise.[2, 9]

References

1. Bogumill GP, Schwamm HA: Orthopaedic Pathology. Philadelphia, WB Saunders, 1984.
2. Bullough PB, Vigorita VJ: Atlas of Orthopaedic Pathology. Philadelphia, JB Lippincott, 1984.
3. Cowie RS: Benign osteoblastoma of the talus. J Bone Joint Surg 48B:582, 1966.
4. Dahlin DC, Unni KK: Bone Tumors: General Aspects and Data on 8542 Cases, 4th ed. Springfield, IL, Charles C Thomas, 1986.
5. DiSomode RE, Berman AT, Schwanter EP: The orthopaedic manifestation of neurofibromatosis. Clin Orthop 230:277–283, 1988.
6. Enneking WF: Musculoskeletal Tumor Surgery. New York, Churchill Livingstone, 1983.
7. Giannestras NJ: Foot disorders. Medical and Surgical Management, 2nd ed. Philadelphia, Lea & Febiger, 1973.
8. Goldner RD, Urbaniak JR: Plantar fibromatosis. *In* The Foot Book. Baltimore, Williams & Wilkins, 1988, pp 325–330.
9. Hattrup SJ, Amado PC, Sim FH, Lombardi RH: Metastatic tumors of the foot and ankle. Foot Ankle 8:243–247, 1988.
10. Henry A: Monostotic fibrous dysplasia. J Bone Joint Surg 51B:300–306, 1969.
11. Hershman EB, Mailly T: Stress fractures. Clin Sports Med 9:183–214, 1990.
12. Kalen V, Burwell DS, Omer GE: Macrodactyly of hands and feet. J Pediatr Orthop 8:311–315, 1988.
13. Keller RB, Baez-Giangreco A: Juvenile aponeurotic fibroma: Report of three cases and a review of the literature. Clin Orthop 106:198, 1975.
14. Kirby EJ, Shereff MJ, Lewis MM: Soft tissue tumors and tumor like lesions of the foot. J Bone Joint Surg 71A:621, 1989.
15. Lane JN, Vigorita VJ: Osteoporosis. J Bone Joint Surg 65A:274, 1983.
16. Mankin HJ: Rickets, osteomalacia, and renal osteodystrophy, part I. J Bone Joint Surg 56A:101, 1974.
17. Mankin HJ: Rickets, osteomalacia, and renal osteodystrophy, part II. J Bone Joint Surg 56A:352, 1974.
18. Mann R: Surgery of the Foot, 5th ed. St Louis, CV Mosby, 1986.
19. Masson P: Le glomus neuromyo-arterial des regions tactiles et ses tumeurs. Lyon Chirurg 21:257–280, 1924.
20. McKenna RJ, Schwann CP, Soong KY, Higinbotham NL: Sarcomatoma of the osteogenic series (osteosarcoma, fibrosarcoma, chondrosarcoma, parosteal osteogenic sarcoma and sarcomata arising in abnormal bone): An analysis of 552 cases. J Bone Joint Surg 48A:1, 1966.
21. Nade S: Acute haematogenous osteomyelitis in infancy and childhood. J Bone Joint Surg 65B:109–119, 1983.
22. Netter FH: The Ciba Collection of Medical Illustrations. Vol 8. Musculoskeletal System. Summit, NJ, Ciba-Geigy Corp, 1987.
23. Rao AS, Vigorita BJ: Pigmented villonodular synovitis (giant cell tumor of tendon sheath and synovial membrane). J Bone Joint Surg 66A:76–94, 1984.
24. Rosai J (ed): Ackerman's Surgical Pathology. St Louis, CV Mosby, 1989.
25. Schugart RR, Soule EH, Johnson EW Jr: Glomus tumors. Surg Gynecol Obstet 117:334–340, 1963.
26. Schumacher HR (ed): Gout. *In* Primer on the Rheumatic Diseases, 9th ed. Atlanta, Arthritis Foundation, 1988.
27. Seale KS, Lange TA, Monson D, Hackbarth DA: Soft tissue tumors of the foot and ankle. Foot Ankle 9:19–27, 1988.
28. Smith RW, Smith CF: Solitary unicameral bone cyst of the calcaneus: A review of twenty cases. J Bone Joint Surg 56A:49, 1974.
29. Sullivan D, Warren RF, Pavlov H, Kelman G: Stress fractures in 52 runners. Clin Orthop 187:188–192, 1984.
30. Taylor GJ: Prominence of the calcaneus: Is operation justified? J Bone Joint Surg 68B:467–470, 1986.
31. Waldvogel FA, Papageorgiou PS: Osteomyelitis: The past decade. N Engl J Med 303:360, 1980.

CHAPTER 19

Reconstructive Techniques in Orthopedic Oncology

CARLIN B. VICKERY
HUBERT WEINBERG
MICHAEL R. HAUSMAN

New reconstructive techniques have greatly facilitated reconstruction of the extremities following resection of a musculoskeletal neoplasm. Refinements in prosthesis, allografts, and large vascularized autografts not only have obviated the need for amputation in many instances, but also permit a remarkable degree of function and improvement in the patient's quality of life.[2, 6, 9, 12, 13, 16, 21, 26, 50–52]

The successful return of a patient to an active high-quality life after treatment of a musculoskeletal tumor requires optimal reconstruction of the operated extremity. Many surgical techniques when performed simultaneously with the tumor resection have the capacity to replace essential resected tissues, resulting in excellent postoperative limb function. Optimal results depend on close collaboration and mutual understanding among the orthopedic, oncologic, and reconstructive teams throughout the planning, operative, and postoperative periods. This collaboration of an ablative surgical team and a reconstructive surgical team provides each patient with an individualized treatment plan that will ensure complete and aggressive tumor control followed by maximal rehabilitation of the extremity.

Successful reconstruction requires adherence to a uniform set of principles prior to selection of a treatment plan. These principles include a medical evaluation of the patient, an assessment of the defect, an understanding of the "ideal" reconstruction, and a review of the possible reconstructive options. Balancing each of these factors, the surgeon then chooses a reconstructive procedure that addresses the specific needs of the patient.

Preoperative Assessment

The initial evaluation of a patient begins with a complete history and general physical examination. The ability of an individual to undergo an extensive resection and a complicated reconstruction must be assessed by evaluating the patient's tumor and any systemic involvement. A patient with local disease or treatable metastatic disease is a candidate for the most sophisticated procedure required to preserve limb function.[9, 13] A patient with a poor prognosis may still require surgery for palliation, but reconstruction must ensure prompt recovery to avoid prolonged hospitalization, although this may preclude maximal preservation of function.[1, 6] The patient's venous and arterial status, any previous surgical sites, and any areas of injury or previous radiation require special attention.[3, 7] Successful microsurgical transfer of tissue necessitates an adequate blood supply; atherosclerosis, previous surgery, injury, or radiation may impair the patient's blood supply and must be evaluated. If microsurgery is being considered, then the arterial and venous supply of the potential donor and recipient sites must be evaluated by physical examination and by angiography and venography when indicated.[48, 49] Finally the projected timing of the surgery should be reviewed. Preoperative adjuvant chemotherapy should be interrupted far enough in advance of the surgery to allow adequate recovery of the hematologic and immune systems.[8]

ASSESSMENT OF THE DEFECT

The exact nature and location of the primary tumor are then evaluated. After the oncologic surgeon has been consulted, the extent of the projected defect—including a list of potential vascular, cutaneous, muscular, osseous, and neural deficits—is estimated. Each structure that is to be resected must then be considered individually so that a prediction of the functional effect of its loss can be made. These structures are then judged as to the necessity and feasibility of their replacement. A successful reconstruction consists of at least two elements: restoration of the structural integrity of the skeleton and of the integument. An inadequate restoration of either will doom the reconstruction. An "ideal" reconstruction would also restore or preserve both sensory and motor nerve function, joint function, and specialized tissue such as pulp tissue of the digits, a thick plantar walking surface, and the potential for growth in the child.[24] Finally the refinement of a reconstruction demands a cosmetically acceptable result.[48]

The limiting factor in limb salvage is the ability to achieve a satisfactory margin without sacrificing a major peripheral nerve. In the lower extremity, resection of either the sciatic nerve or the posterior tibial nerve necessitates amputation, as prosthetic rehabilitation is preferable to preservation of an insensate, functionless limb. In the upper extremity, despite resection of major nerves, preservation of the limb may be preferable for cosmetic reasons.

Today, arterial and venous bypass grafting may preserve an extremity in which sacrifice of the major blood supply has been necessary for control of the tumor. Bypass grafting can be successful utilizing either a prosthesis or autogenous tissue, or both. In extremities in which one of the dominant vessels has been resected, the remaining vessel must be carefully preserved and protected with adequate soft tissue coverage. In addition, if microsurgical tissue transfer is planned for the extremity, the microvascular anastomosis must be performed in an end-to-side fashion for maintenance of vascular integrity of the limb.[54]

Evaluation of the osseous defect and its restoration is made in conjunction with the orthopedic surgeon. Choices for bone replacement include vascularized or nonvascularized autologous bone graft, allograft, prosthetic replacement, or a combination of these techniques. The choice of vascularized or nonvascularized graft is determined by the length of the involved segment; defects longer than 6 cm generally require vascularized bone.[4, 10, 17, 60, 62] In heavily irradiated or scarred beds, shorter segments may necessitate the use of vascularized bone to achieve healing and to provide greater resistance to infection. In a child, resection of a joint or epiphyseal plate requires a prosthetic replacement with the capacity to lengthen as the child grows.[24] All of these skeletal replacements require adequate, stable, soft tissue coverage of the graft or a prosthesis for the successful rehabilitation of the limb. This coverage must be achieved at the time of the bone replacement.[7, 14, 19, 25, 38, 41, 43, 44, 47, 63]

Evaluation of the soft tissue coverage of an extremity is critical to ensure proper design of incisions and flaps planned for final coverage of the underlying structures. The reconstructive surgeon must decide whether durable coverage can be achieved with local skin and muscle or whether the transfer of distant tissue is required. An estimate is made preoperatively of the extent of the skin to be removed and the quality and laxity of the remaining skin.[1, 13]

Previous scars, irradiated skin, and surgically undermined skin must be identified, as these are areas of poor healing potential (Fig. 19–1). If local skin flaps are to be used, exclusion of damaged skin and soft tissue is ideal. Inclusion of compromised areas in a design necessitates a contingency plan in the event that the skin and soft tissue flap are not viable at the time of closure. If local skin flaps are judged inadequate, a decision is made between the transfer of adjacent muscle flaps or a microvascular free tissue transfer. In general, muscle flaps can be used for a defect of moderate size that is adjacent to the muscle to be

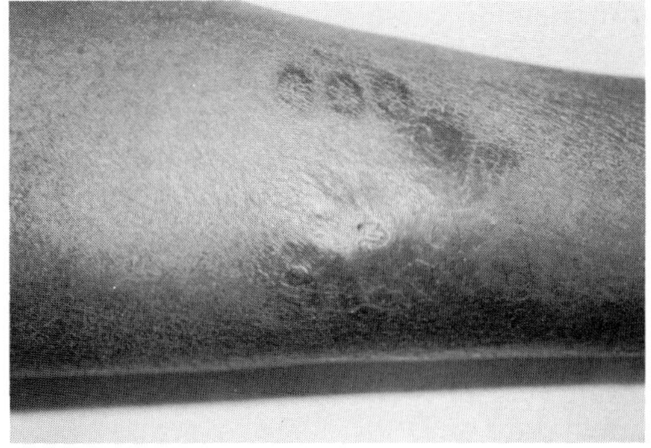

FIGURE 19–1. Large area of involved skin precluding primary closure.

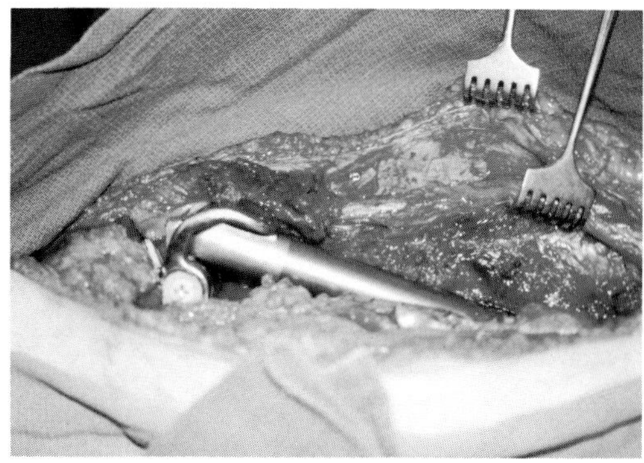

FIGURE 19–2. Primary closure of the wound following musculoskeletal tumor resection.

transferred. However, the use of a local muscle must be balanced against any further restrictions that the loss of the muscle will have on the affected limb. Additionally the transfer of the muscle with division of the musculocutaneous perforators to the overlying skin may result in vascular compromise of remaining skin flaps.[27, 29, 30] In order to avoid these complications, it is often preferable to transfer distant vascularized muscle and skin to avoid further compromise.[55] Free tissue transfer of muscle and skin reliably provides well-vascularized tissue that is capable of closing extensive defects. With the choice of the right donor site, the tissue transferred may vary in length, width, thickness, contour, and type (i.e., skin, muscle, fat, fascia, bone, and nerve potential). Unquestionably, with the advent of microsurgery and the wide range of potential donor sites, the reconstructive surgeon has a vast array of choices in the successful reconstruction of an extremity.[22]

Reconstructive Options

PRIMARY CLOSURE

The simplest method for closure of a wound following musculoskeletal tumor resection is primary closure (Fig. 19–2). However, primary closure should be utilized only when remaining tissue is sufficient to allow primary healing and to provide long-term stable coverage of the underlying structures (Fig. 19–3). Several factors must be considered in the selection of primary closure for coverage: the amount of tension on the skin, preexisting scars, prior tissue radiation, and the viability of the surgically undermined skin (Fig. 19–4). When vital structures or prosthetic implants are being covered, there must be sufficient skin to allow tension-free closure. If, upon closing, the surrounding skin appears blanched with diminished dermal bleeding along skin margins, then primary closure cannot be performed. If there is any question of undue skin tension, it is prudent to transfer new tissue to the area. Necrosis or separation of a primary closure or extrusion of a prosthetic implant under a tight closure with resultant exposure of the underlying vital or prosthetic structures can be catastrophic in the patient with cancer who may have poor healing potential as a result of chemotherapy or radiation and whose immunocompromised state may result in uncontrolled infection. Failures in surgical revision and reconstruction can be avoided if the necessity for additional local or distant tissue is recognized at the time of the initial reconstruction.

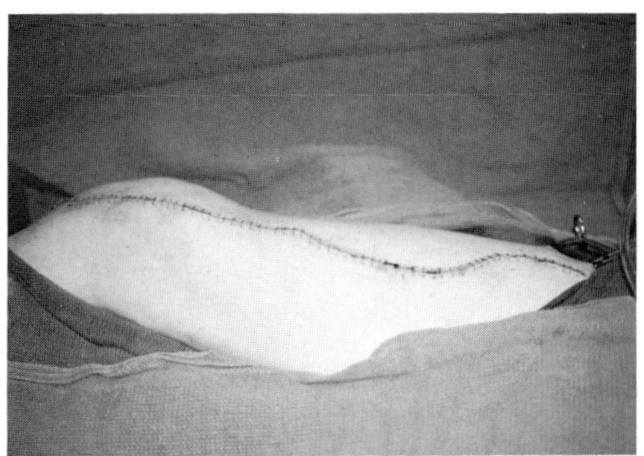

FIGURE 19–3. Sufficient muscle and subcutaneous tissue should be left to allow adequate coverage of the implant without additional tissue.

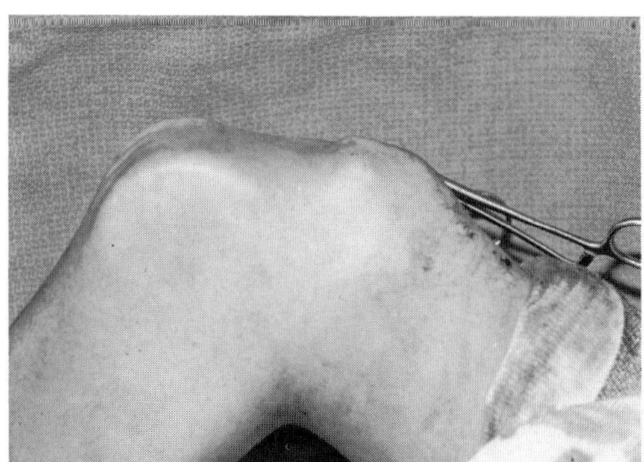

FIGURE 19–4. Tight closure with insufficient protection of implant. Failure to provide additional tissue will result in extrusion of the prosthesis.

SKIN GRAFTS

Skin grafts are the reconstructive option of choice when there is adequate muscle to cover any exposed vital structures or prosthesis but the local remaining skin is not adequate. In these situations, a split-thickness graft may be harvested for coverage of a well-vascularized muscle (Fig. 19–5). Grafts can be utilized over tendons only when the paratenon has been carefully preserved. In specialized areas of the body such as the hands, feet, and joints, full-thickness grafts may be required to avoid flexion contractures and provide thicker coverage with greater durability. It should be emphasized that skin grafting is not a technique for use in a marginal area with poor blood supply of the underlying tissue, as failure of the graft and coverage will result.

A split-thickness graft is a graft that includes part of the donor site's dermal elements. The choice of donor sites can be anywhere on the body, but the most easily harvested usually come from the patient's buttocks and thighs. Harvesting of the graft can be achieved with either the Brown, Reese, or Padgett dermatome; all of these instruments can be callibrated for obtaining a uniform graft of approximately .012 inch in thickness. Grafts can then be expanded by use of a mesher, which creates a net-stocking effect, allowing the graft to cover a larger surface area. The usual choice of meshing is a 1:1.5 ratio; however, if the amount of skin graft in limited, as in a small child, the ratio can be increased to 1:3.

Successful skin grafting is dependent on meticulous preparation of the recipient bed, secure placement of the graft, freedom from infection, and proper postoperative care. The most common cause of skin graft failure in a clean operative wound is a hematoma under a graft, which creates a barrier between the graft and the recipient bed. This can be avoided with careful hemostasis of the recipient site prior to placement of the graft. Of equal importance is the careful placement of a graft into the contours of a defect so that maximal contact between the graft and its bed is ensured. At times it may be necessary to place tacking sutures between the graft and the bed to obliterate dead space and to ensure that the graft will not move postoperatively. Immobilization of a grafted wound is essential for the first 5 days and can be achieved with a combination of the tie-over-bolster–type dressings and/or splinting of an extremity. Postoperatively a grafted area must be protected from shearing forces, dependency, infection, and seroma formation. An extremity should remain elevated for 10 days following grafting and then gradually should be given increasing periods of dependency. Fluid that accumulates under a graft in the early postoperative period can often successfully be aspirated. Infection during the postoperative period is unusual in a clean surgical wound.[46]

After the graft is well vascularized, hyper-

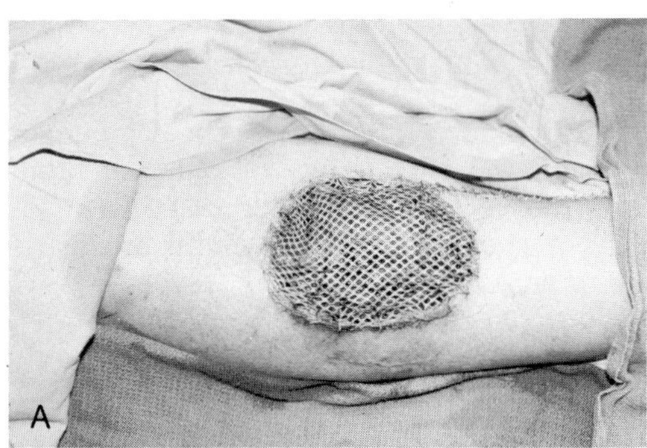

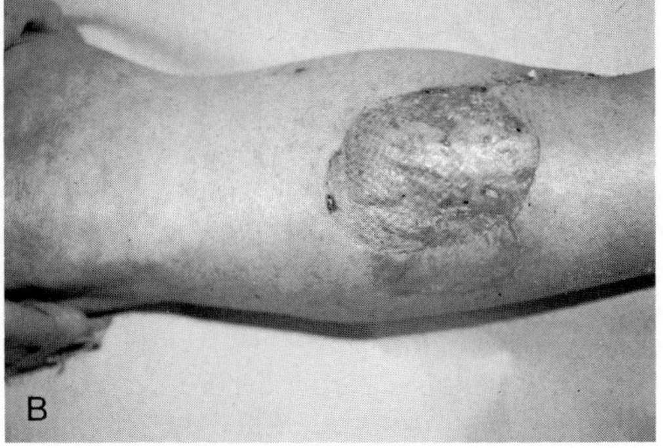

FIGURE 19–5. *A* and *B*, Split-thickness skin grafts over the soleus muscle flap in the mid-tibial region.

trophic scarring can be minimized by the use of a compression garment, especially in children. Donor and graft sites should be lubricated with lanolin and sunscreen for several months postoperatively; skin color changes at these sites continue for at least 1 year.

LOCAL FLAPS

When it has been determined that neither primary closure nor skin grafts will satisfactorily cover a wound, the surgeon may utilize either local flaps or distant tissue transfer. Skin flaps are either "random" flaps (Fig. 19–6*A, B*) or "axial" pattern flaps (Fig. 19–6*C–E*), depending on the anatomy of their blood supply (Fig. 19–7). Axial pattern flaps encompass an anatomically recognizable arteriovenous system coursing along their long axis, whereas random pattern flaps lack a single identifiable vessel in their vascular pattern[35] (Fig. 19–7*A*). "Myocutaneous" flaps are composed of skin, subcutaneous fat, and muscle in which the blood supply to the skin overlying the muscle is provided by perforators that exit through the muscle to the subdermal plexus of the skin (Fig. 19–7*B*). The adequacy of blood supply to the flap determines the predicted survival length when the tissue is transferred (Fig. 19–8). Random cutaneous flaps generally survive a 2:1 length/width ratio. Axial pattern and myocutaneous flaps will survive the length of the axial vessels or muscle perforators together with a distal random pattern flap of 1:1 length/width ratio. Fasciocutaneous flaps are composed of fascia, overlying skin, fat, and a blood supply; when these flaps are elevated with a respect for the microcirculation, transfer of tissue is more reliable than with a randomly designed skin flap.[27–30, 33, 39, 45, 61]

Local random cutaneous flaps are categorized according to the direction in which the

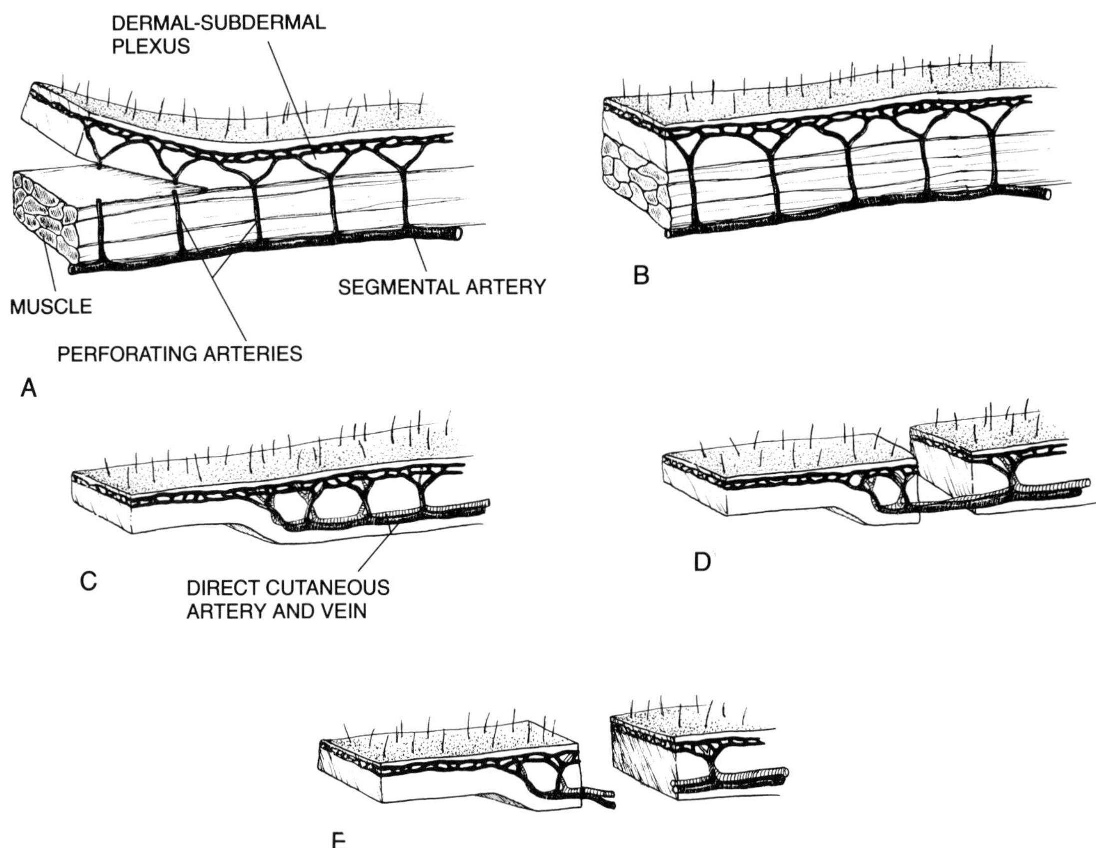

FIGURE 19–6. Skin flaps classified according to the anatomy of the blood supply. *A,* Random cutaneous flap. *B,* Myocutaneous random flap. *C,* Peninsular axial pattern flap. *D,* Island axial pattern flap. *E,* Free flap. (Redrawn from Grabb, WC: Basic techniques of plastic surgery. *In* Grabb WC, Smith JW (eds): Plastic Surgery, 3rd Ed. Boston, Little, Brown & Co., 1979.)

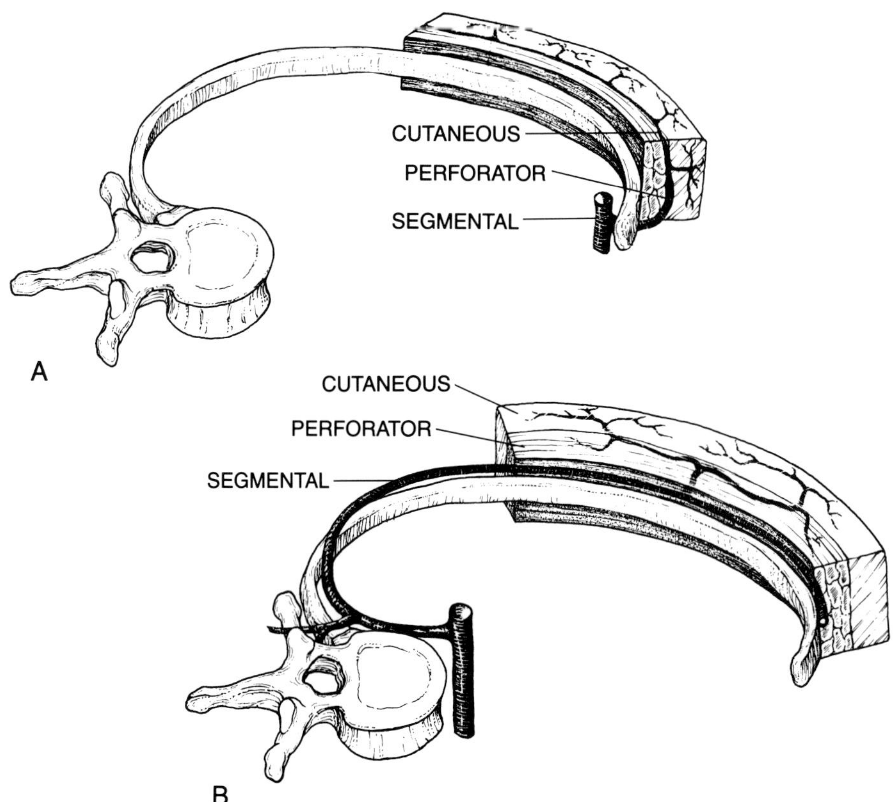

FIGURE 19–7. Schematic drawing of (*A*) direct cutaneous arteries and (*B*) myocutaneous arteries showing perforators to overlying skin.

skin and fat are transferred: advancement flaps (Fig. 19–9*A*), rotation flaps (Fig. 19–9*B*), and transposition flaps (Fig. 19–9*C*). Each of these flaps is useful for small to medium skin defects adjacent to well-vascularized local skin and subcutaneous tissue. They easily cover denuded tendon, bone, or exposed muscle. However, they are rarely used to cover joints, as the motion of the underlying joint creates tension on the random flap, which can jeopardize its viability.

On occasion, axial pattern flaps can be useful in musculoskeletal reconstruction. The two with the greatest potential are the radial forearm flap (Fig. 19–10) and the dorsalis pedis flap (Fig. 19–11). These flaps are designed over their respectively named arteries and veins and can be isolated as an island and rotated and transposed 180 degrees without vascular compromise. In addition, the radial forearm flap can be isolated on its distal pedicle in a reverse fashion for coverage of hand defects. The advantage of this flap is that it can be rapidly raised and provides a thin pliable covering for the hand, elbow, or distal upper arm. However, the donor defect on the distal forearm requires skin grafting for closure, resulting in a significant cosmetic deformity. The donor site of the dorsalis pedis flap likewise requires a skin graft, which does not provide long-term stable coverage of the foot (Fig. 19–12). Thus these flaps should be selected judiciously, balancing the donor site morbidity against the potential surgical benefits. Their greatest applicability is in patients who require a rapid reconstruction and will not tolerate the additional surgery necessary for a distant tissue transfer or in whom the thin tissue available from these flaps is required for reconstruction.[11, 53, 64]

Muscle flaps and musculocutaneous flaps have significantly increased the armamentarium of the reconstructive surgeon in that their dependable vascular supply allows safe transfer of muscle and skin. The flaps may be designed in many shapes and sizes and are capable of restoring large volume and contour deficits; of covering joints with ample, durable, mobile

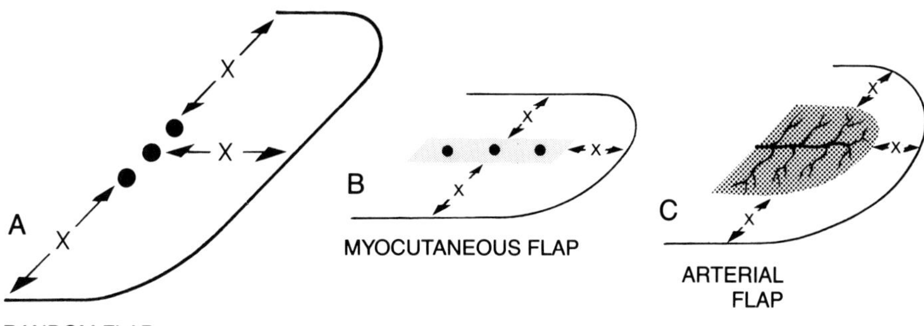

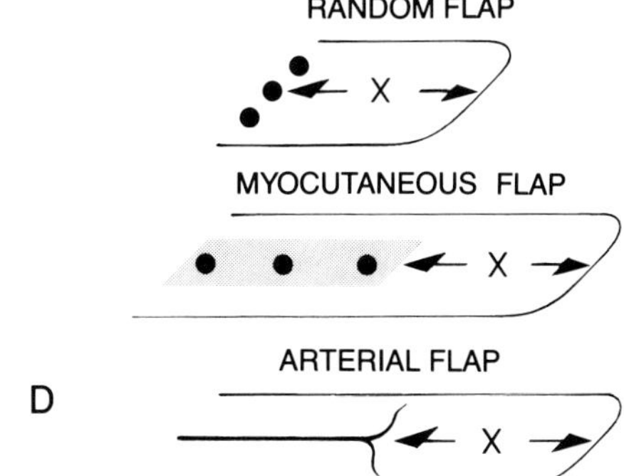

FIGURE 19–8. Schematic drawing depicting the survival patterns of skin flaps. X = the dermal-subdermal plexus. *A,* Perfusion through X determines the survival length of a random cutaneous flap. *B,* The length of the viable muscle included + X = survival length of a myocutaneous flap. *C,* The length of the direct cutaneous artery + X = survival length of an arterial flap. *D,* Similar factors determine the surviving width of the flap. (Redrawn from Daniel RK, Kerrigan CL: Skin flaps: An anatomical and hemodynamic approach. Clin Plast Surg 6:181, 1979.)

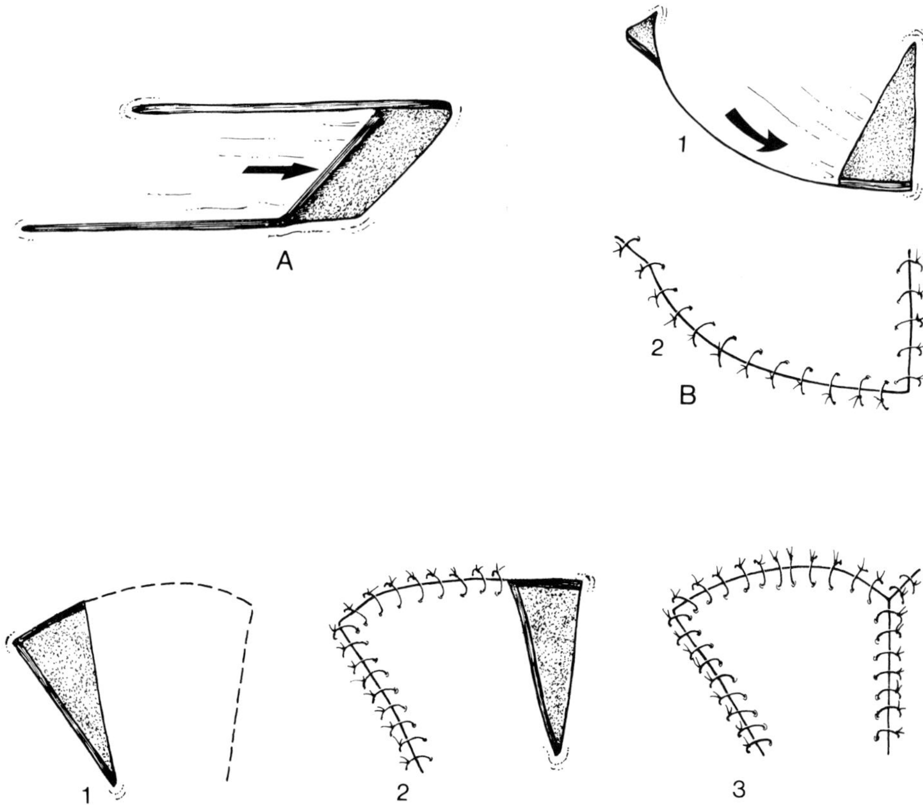

FIGURE 19–9. Diagrammatic representations of (*A*) advancement flap, in which closure of a defect is performed after the skin is undermined; (*B*) transposition flap: (*1*) design, (*2*) resulting defect, and (*3*) V-Y advancement method of closing the secondary defect; (*C*) rotation flap: (*1*) triangle of tissue taken from the base of the flap, and (*2*) rotation accomplished. (Redrawn from Daniel RK, Kerrigan CL: Principles and physiology of skin flap surgery. *In* McCarthy JG, et al: Plastic Surgery. Vol. 1. Philadelphia, WB Saunders, 1990.)

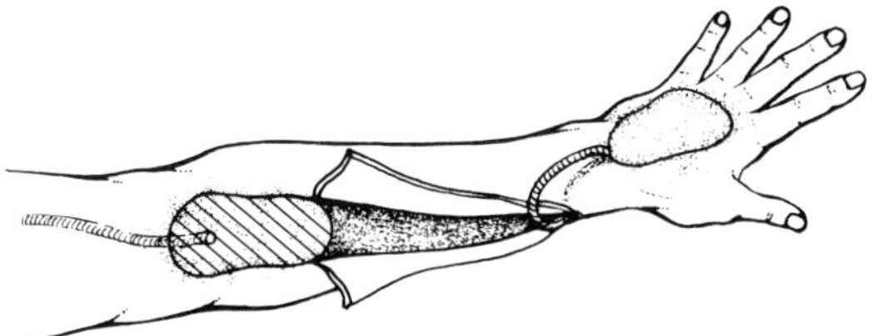

FIGURE 19–10. Drawing of a radial forearm fasciocutaneous flap used as a reverse forearm flap. The solid area denotes skin grafting of the donor site. (Redrawn from Daniel RK, Kerrigan CL: Principles and physiology of skin flap surgery. *In* McCarthy JG, et al: Plastic Surgery, Vol. 1. Philadelphia, WB Saunders, 1990, p. 297.)

tissue that is able to withstand the pressure of the underlying joint; and of providing greater resistance to bacterial infection than random pattern skin flaps. A complete description of each available muscle flap, its blood supply, function, and potential usefulness in reconstructive surgery is provided by Mathes and Nahai.[28] The muscle flaps are classified accord-

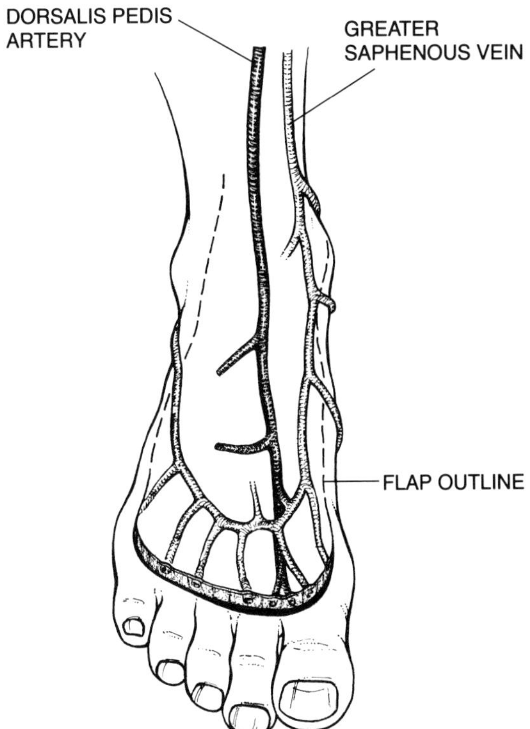

FIGURE 19–11. Dorsalis pedis flap outline showing artery and vein. (Redrawn from Thorne CH, et al: Reconstructive surgery of the lower extremity. *In* McCarthy JG, et al: Plastic Surgery. Vol. 6. Philadelphia, WB Saunders, 1990, p. 4051.)

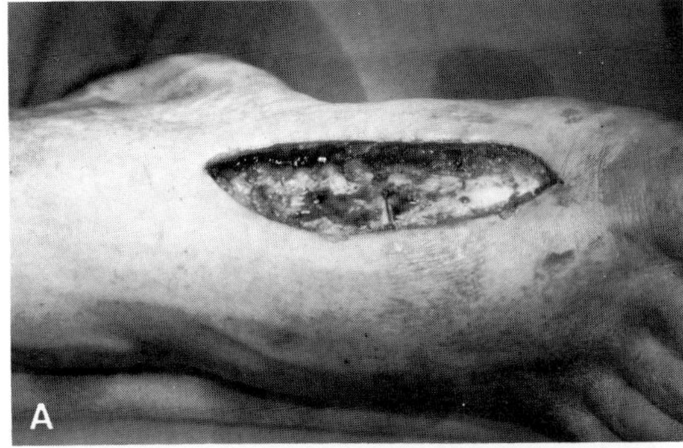

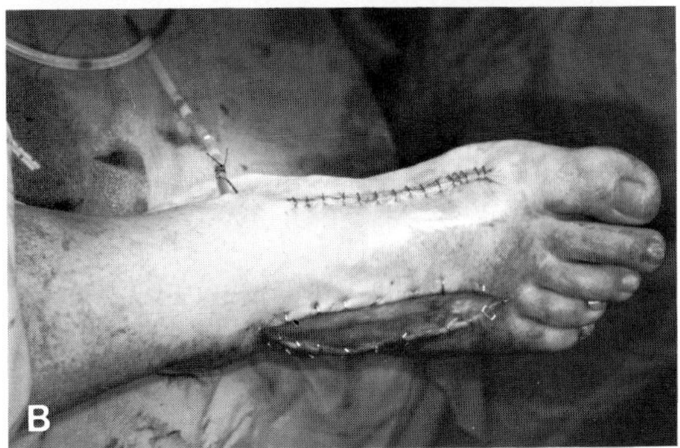

FIGURE 19–12. *A,* A defect of the medial dorsal aspect of the foot closed. *B*, Closure achieved with a bipedicle advancement flap and skin grafting of the adjacent defect.

ing to their patterns of vascular anatomy (Fig. 19–13): type I—one vascular pedicle; type II—dominant pedicle and minor pedicle; type III—two dominant pedicles; type IV—segmental vascular pedicles; and type V—one dominant pedicle and secondary segmental pedicles.

The selection of a muscle or musculocutaneous unit must consider the size of the ablative surgical defect, the size of the donor muscle and skin paddle, and the location of the vascular pedicle. The arc of rotation of the myocutaneous unit without tension on the vascular pedicle must be examined in order to insure coverage of the defect without vascular compromise. Closure of the donor defect must also be planned and the use of any muscle must be balanced against the resulting functional loss. This is particularly true following resection of musculoskeletal tumors of the extremity, when further sacrifice of muscle groups may increase a functional deficit.

The most frequently utilized muscle flaps in lower extremity reconstruction are the gastrocnemius muscle and the soleus muscle flaps (Fig. 19–14). The gastrocnemius muscle is the

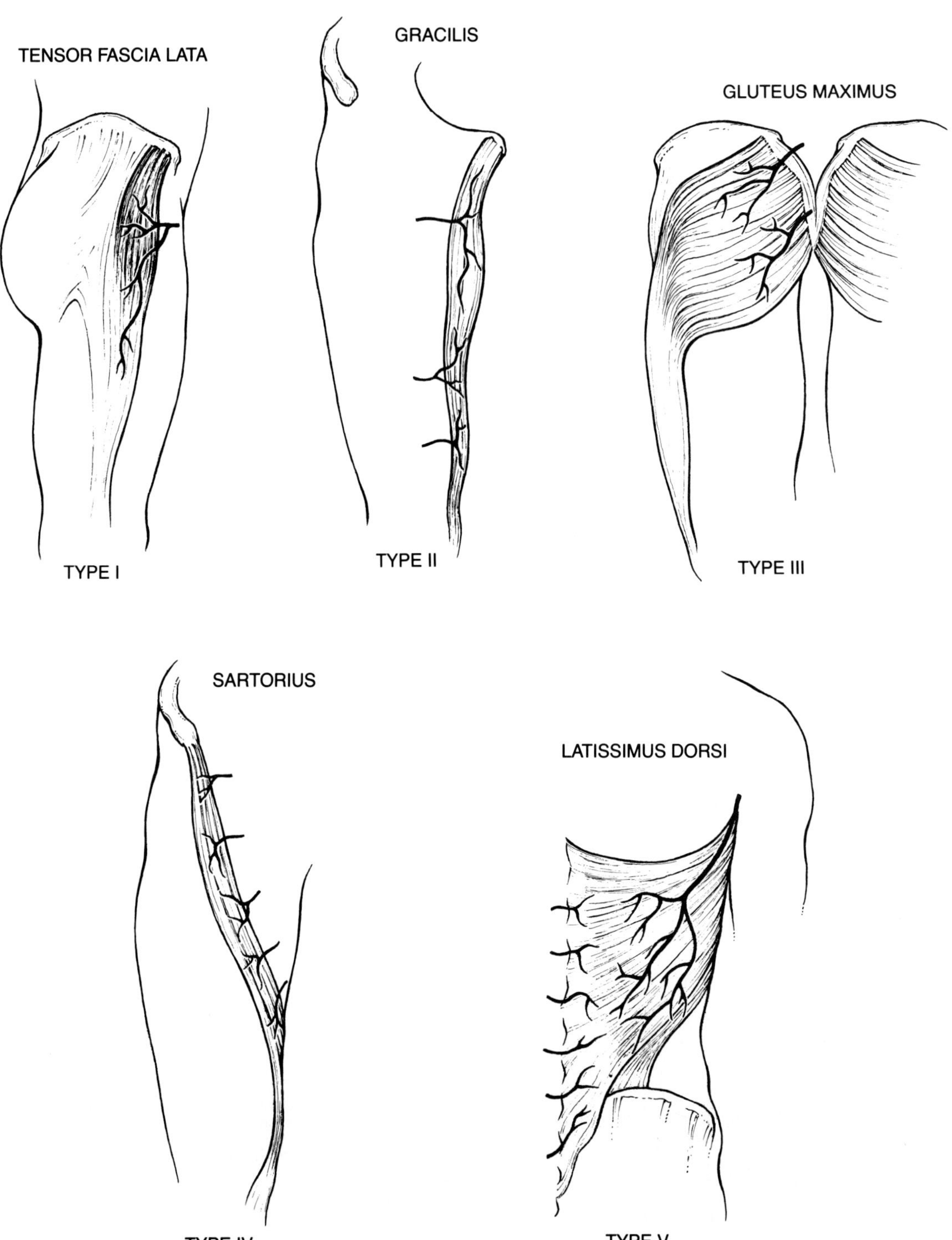

FIGURE 19–13. Drawing of the five patterns of the vascular anatomy of muscle.

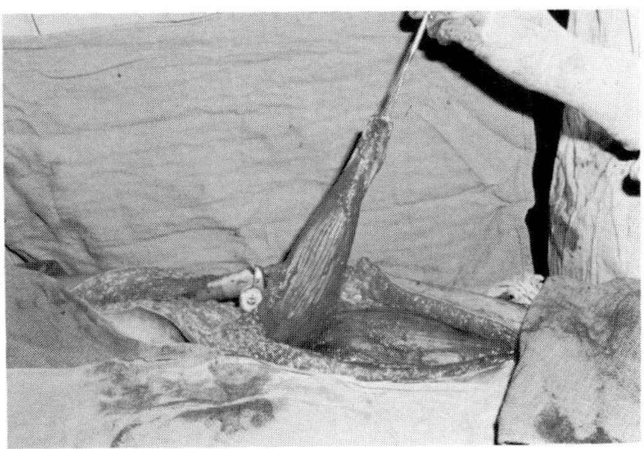

FIGURE 19-14. Rotation of a medial gastrocnemius muscle flap to cover the proximal portion of a tibial prosthesis. The blood supply is provided through the sural artery and vein.

largest and most superficial calf muscle. Of its two heads, the medial is the larger and extends a greater distance inferiorly. The two heads unite, and together with the soleus tendon form the Achilles tendon. The blood supply to the muscle consists of the paired sural arteries off the popliteal artery. The muscle may be raised alone or with a cutaneous unit designed over the muscle belly[23] (Fig. 19-15). Because there are no vascular perforators to the skin over the tendon, any skin raised in these areas must survive as a random skin flap. The medial or lateral head can be raised as an island flap and rotated to cover the upper third of the tibia or the knee (Fig. 19-16). The flap comfortably covers an area measuring 10 × 10 cm below the joint line of the knee. The medial gastrocnemius muscle flap will easily cover the entire width of the tibia (Fig. 19-17). Additionally, when the lateral gastrocnemius muscle is mobilized, care must be taken to protect the peroneal nerve.[3, 15, 27, 34]

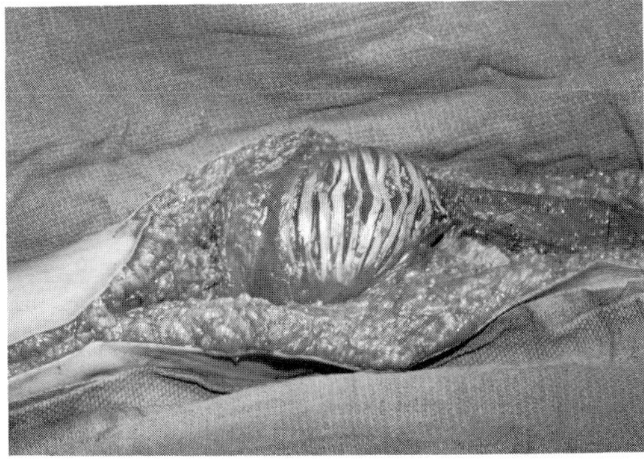

FIGURE 19-15. Fascia over the gastrocnemius muscle has been incised to allow wider draping of the muscle.

The soleus muscle lies immediately below the gastrocnemius muscle. Its muscle fibers extend inferiorly for a greater distance and merge with the tendon of the gastrocnemius muscle. It has a dual proximal blood supply from the peroneal and posterior tibial arteries. In addition, there are several minor branches from the posterior tibial artery to the distal portion of the muscle. This muscle can be raised on its dominant proximal blood supply or, if necessary, on its distal minor blood supply. The distally based soleus flap is not as predictable, owing to the variability of the distal blood supply. This muscle is most useful for midtibial coverage measuring 10 × 10 cm. The substance of this muscle is thinner than the gastrocnemius and will fill defects only a few centimeters deep. Because skin cannot be transferred with the muscle, a skin graft is always required. The gastrocnemius muscle flaps and the soleus muscle flap remain the "workhorse" local flaps of the lower extremity, providing stable, long-term coverage following musculoskeletal tumor resection.[23, 27]

MICROVASCULAR FREE FLAPS

For the patient with a large musculoskeletal tumor who requires both extensive resection of soft tissue and bone for tumor control, the microvascular free flap allows limb preservation by providing sufficient replacement of muscle, skin, and bone from a site distant to the operated extremity. Successful clinical transfer of distant tissue was realized in 1972 by McLean and Buncke following a decade of intensive research and development of microsurgical suture, technique, and operating microscope. A microsurgical free tissue transfer involves the identification and dissection of the dominant artery and vein to a tissue unit (Figs. 19-18 and 19-19). This unit may comprise skin, muscle, fascia, or bone singly or in combination. The vascular pedicle is then divided, and the "free flap" is transferred to the defect or recipient area. With an operating microscope microsurgical anastomoses are then performed between donor and recipient vessels, reestablishing vascular continuity; 9-0 or 10-0 nylon is used. The transferred tissue is then inset to restore any bony or soft tissue defect. Successful reconstruction with microsurgery requires careful preoperative planning and flap selection as well as meticulous microsurgical

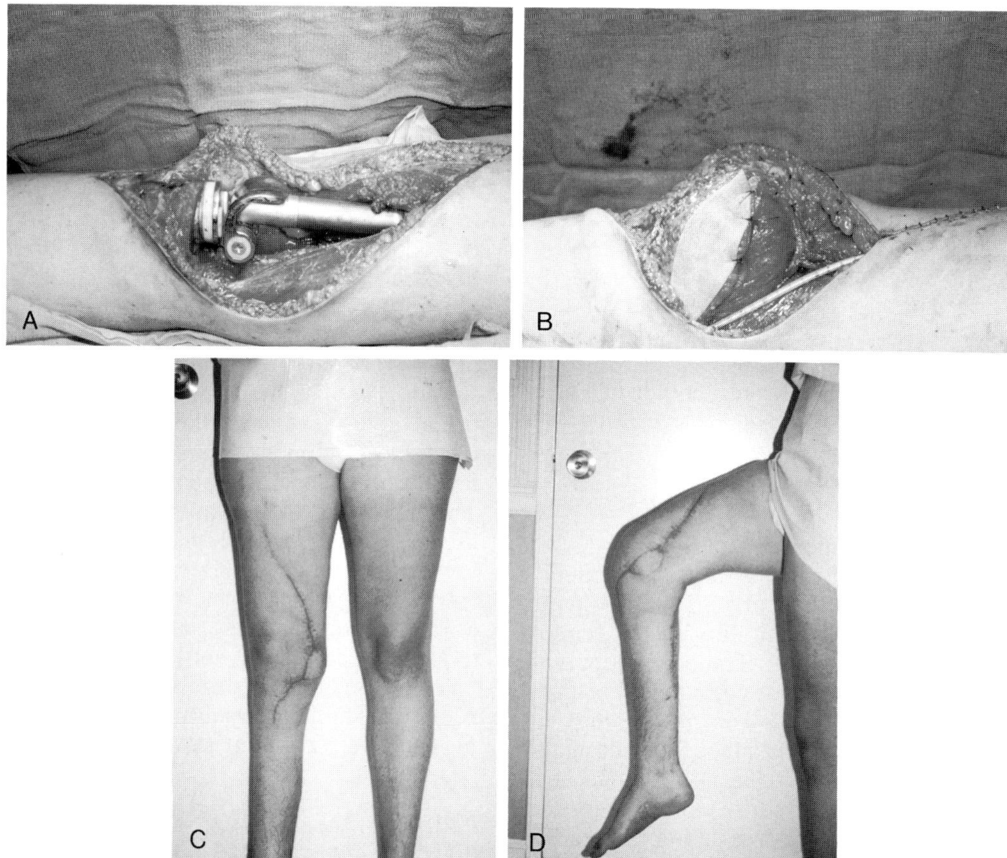

FIGURE 19–16. *A,* Tibial LEAP prosthesis in place following resection of proximal tibia for osteogenic sarcoma. *B,* Medial gastrocnemius myocutaneous rotation flap covering the prosthesis. *C* and *D,* Postoperative healing and function of right leg.

technique. Flap selection should always provide ample tissue to allow proper positioning of the pedicle for vascular anastomosis and a tension-free closure. Bone fixation must be planned to protect the blood supply of the transferred bone as well as to achieve stable fixation. Recipient vessels for anastomosis must also be selected to insure adequate inflow and outflow to the flap as well as preservation of blood supply to the extremity.

Finally, intensive postoperative monitoring through observation of color, temperature, and bleeding of the transferred tissue is required to identify early signs of vascular compromise that may necessitate emergency reexploration. Primary ischemic tissue tolerance is generally thought to be 6 hours, and a secondary ischemic insult resulting from a postoperative thrombosis will not be tolerated even for 6 hours. Identification of vascular compromise and rapid return to the operating room for pedicle revision is thus imperative.

The most widely utilized microvascular free flaps for large soft tissue defects are the latissimus dorsi myocutaneous flaps (Fig. 19–20) and the rectus abdominis myocutaneous flaps (Fig. 19–21). The latissimus dorsi muscle is a large thin muscle with a surface area approximately 500 sq cm.[5, 31, 32] It can be harvested with overlying skin anywhere over its surface, though the usual design allowing primary coverage of the back skin is a skin eclipse that measures 30 × 10 cm. The blood supply to the muscle is the thoracodorsal artery and vein prior to joining the axillary artery and vein. The vascular pedicle to the latissimus is long, measuring 4 to 6 cm and the vessels are reliably 2 mm or greater in diameter. Because of the large size of this flap and the reliability of its vascular pedicle, it can be dependably transferred to cover most defects (Fig. 19–22). The muscle can be wrapped around bone or a prosthesis, and the skin paddle can be used for extra bulk. With atrophy of the muscle

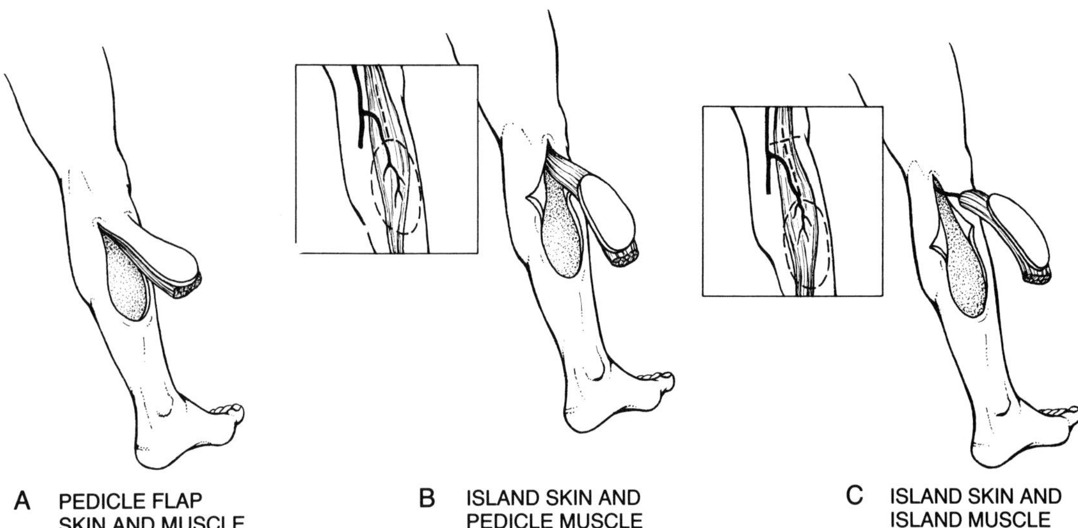

FIGURE 19–17. Drawings of a medial gastrocnemius myocutaneous flap used (*A*) as a pedicle flap with muscle attached, (*B*) as an island skin and pedicle flap, and (*C*) as an island skin and muscle flap attached by a vascular pedicle. (Redrawn from Daniel RK, Kerrigan CL: Principles and physiology of skin flap surgery. *In* McCarthy JG, et al: Plastic Surgery. Vol. 1. Philadelphia, WB Saunders, 1990, p. 302.)

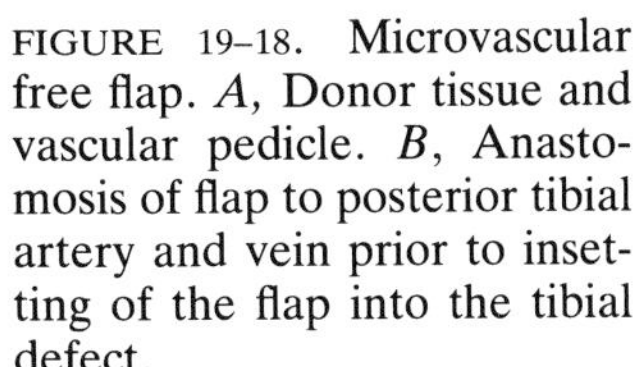

FIGURE 19–18. Microvascular free flap. *A*, Donor tissue and vascular pedicle. *B*, Anastomosis of flap to posterior tibial artery and vein prior to insetting of the flap into the tibial defect.

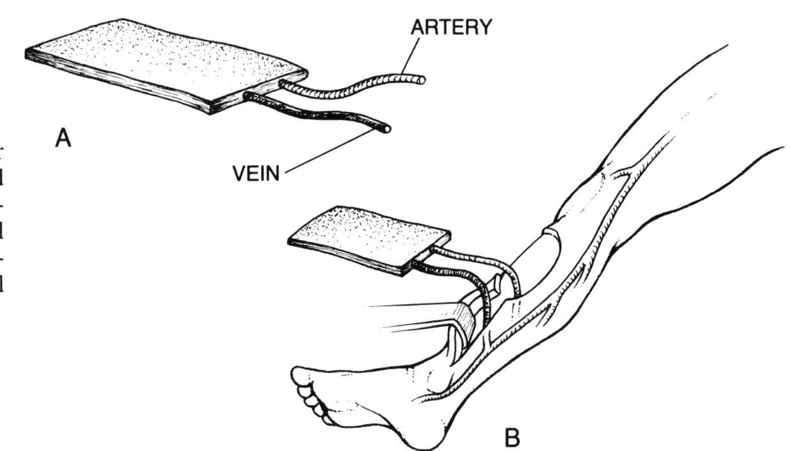

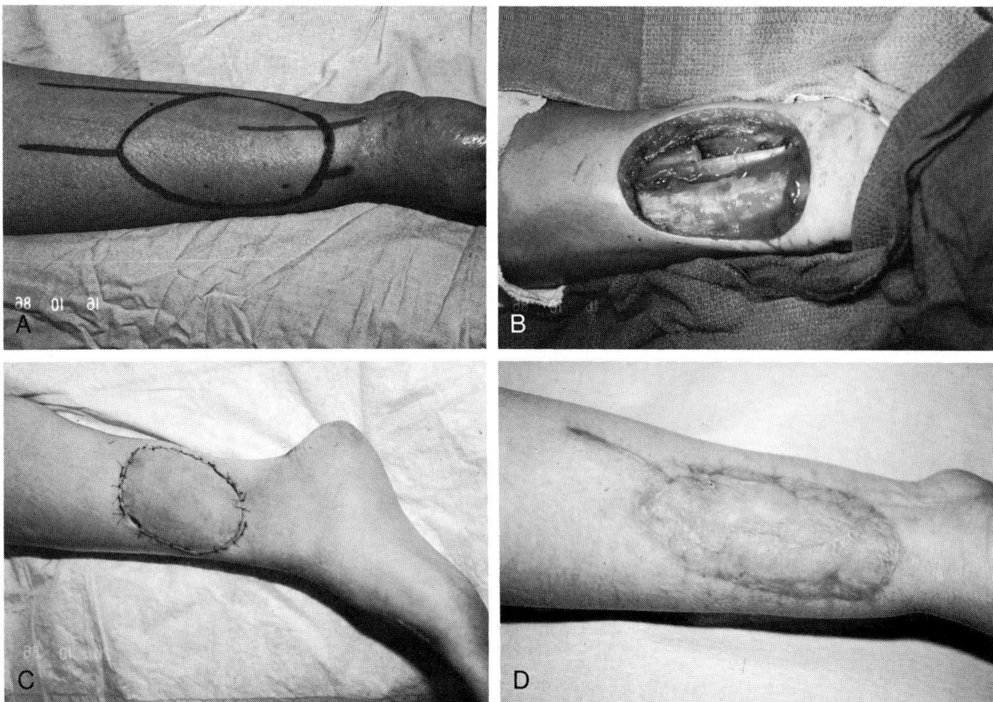

FIGURE 19–19. *A,* Microvascular radial forearm flap outline over distal forearm. *B,* Defect overlying distal one-third of tibia following sarcoma resection. *C,* Coverage of tibial defect following revascularization of radial forearm flap to posterior tibial artery and vein. *D,* Skin-grafted radial forearm donor site.

over time, the volume of the transferred flap will decrease; this may be undesirable if the muscle is covering an underlying prosthesis. If additional padding or soft tissue is desired, the flap can be raised as a myocutaneous flap including muscle and overlying skin. Both the latissimus dorsi and rectus abdominis are excellent myocutaneous flaps, and the skin does not undergo atrophy or contract.

The latissimus dorsi flap can be raised together with the cutaneous scapular flap, which joins the thoracodorsal vessels through the circumflex scapular artery, allowing harvest of both flaps on one pedicle. This dual flap adds an additional 8 × 20 cm skin flap for reconstruction and unquestionably allows coverage of the largest soft tissue defects. The major disadvantage is that harvesting these flaps requires that the patient be turned for exposure of the back.

The rectus abdominis muscle is a long, vertically oriented muscle of the abdominal wall extending from the xiphoid to the pubis. The blood supply is from the dual vessel of the superior and inferior epigastric arteries and veins. The perforators to the overlying skin emerge throughout the length of the muscle, with a preponderance of vessels in the periumbilical area. Microsurgical transfer of this muscle and the overlying skin is performed with harvesting and anastomosis of the inferior epigastric artery and vein. Skin may be oriented vertically along the entire length of the muscle, transversely across the midline, obliquely from the anterior axillary line to the opposite infraumbilical area, and in a combined horizontal and vertical design (Fig. 19–23). Large amounts of skin measuring 18 × 30 cm of skin can be transferred with only a portion of the rectus muscle. Like the latissimus muscle, the vascular pedicle to the rectus muscle is long (8 cm) with vessels at least 2 mm in diameter. In addition, harvesting of the flap is performed in the supine position, thereby avoiding the repositioning of the patient that is required for a latissimus flap. The rectus muscle is extremely useful for reconstruction of soft tissue defects of the lower extremity. In most patients the fat of the abdomen is thicker than the fat of the back, providing greater bulk for coverage of a prosthesis. The muscle will not wrap around a prosthesis as the latissimus muscle will; thus the skin of the rectus flap must provide the majority of the coverage (Fig. 19–24). The

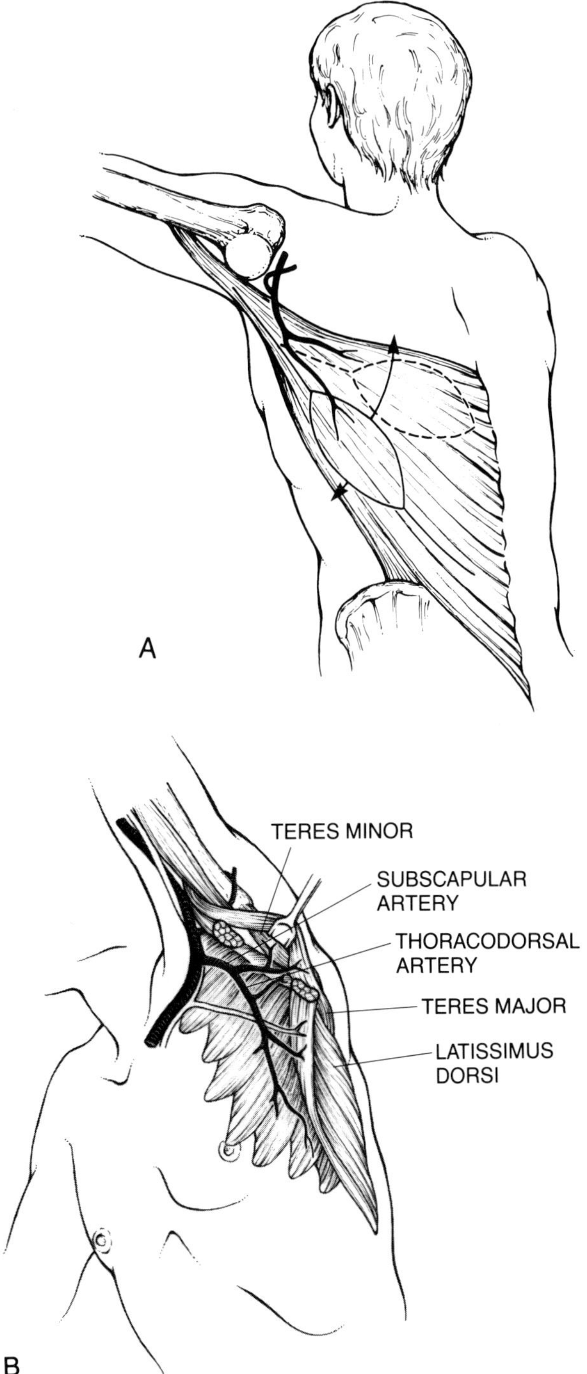

FIGURE 19–20. *A*, Diagram of latissimus dorsi free flap with potential skin paddles. *B*, Blood supply to latissimus dorsi muscle.

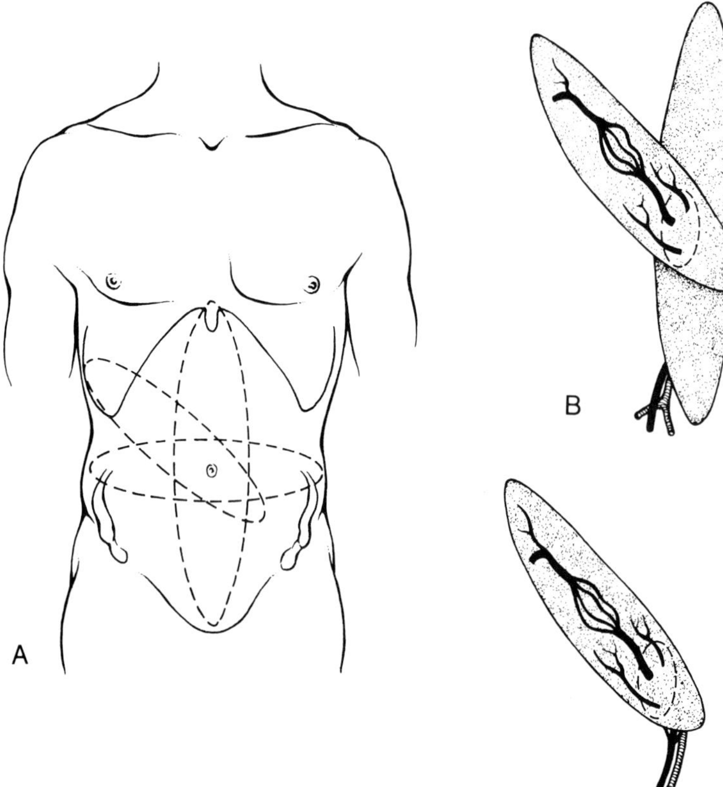

FIGURE 19–21. Diagrams showing the versatility of rectus flaps. *A*, Various tissue combinations can be used for free flap transfer. *B* and *C*, Myocutaneous flap including muscle. (Redrawn from Taylor GI, et al: The versatile deep inferior epigastric inferior rectus abdominis flap. Plast Reconstr Surg 72:751, 1983.)

rectus flap is ideal for large defects of the tibia or the distal femur. In the distal femur area the rectus skin may be largely de-epithelialized and buried for subcutaneous bulk if the distal femur skin flaps remain but are too thin to protect an underlying prosthesis.[18, 42]

When large segments of bone need to be replaced, two sources are available for vascularized transfer: the iliac crest and the fibula. The iliac crest based on the deep circumflex iliac artery and vein can provide 10 cm of bone with the curvature of the crest present.[58, 59] This bone is appropriate for defects measuring 6 to 8 cm. Larger defects would require osteotomies for straightening the curvature of the harvested bone. The iliac crest can be transferred with an overlying elliptical skin paddle measuring 8 × 14 cm and with the internal oblique muscle based on the ascending branch of the deep circumflex artery and vein. This composite flap of skin, muscle, and bone can correct bone defects as well as soft tissue defects. The deep circumflex artery and vein are usually single vessels; however, in 10% of patients they may be a paired system, requiring multiple anastomosis. The donor site requires careful reattachment of the abdominal wall musculature but is well tolerated without functional defects or hernias.

The fibula provides the longest straight segment of bone available for transfer in the human (Fig. 19–25). In an adult fibula of 40 cm, 24 cm can be safely transferred, thereby preserving 8 cm distally for ankle stability and 8 cm proximally for knee stability and peroneal nerve protection. A skin paddle oriented along the length of the fibula and measuring 8 × 20 cm can be harvested with the bone if the perforators to the skin running in the intermuscular septum between the peroneal muscles and the soleus muscles are preserved. The vascular pedicle is variable in length but averages 6 cm, and the vessels average 2 to 3 mm. The peroneal nerve must be carefully protected during the harvesting of this flap, and a syndesmotic screw may be necessary to insure ankle stability if a long segment of bone is harvested. The donor site is otherwise closed primarily.[57]

Following successful microvascular surgery, the vascularized fibular bone flap can replace long segments of tibia or humerus. Healing of the vascularized fibula to the remaining tibia or humerus has been shown to be fracture-

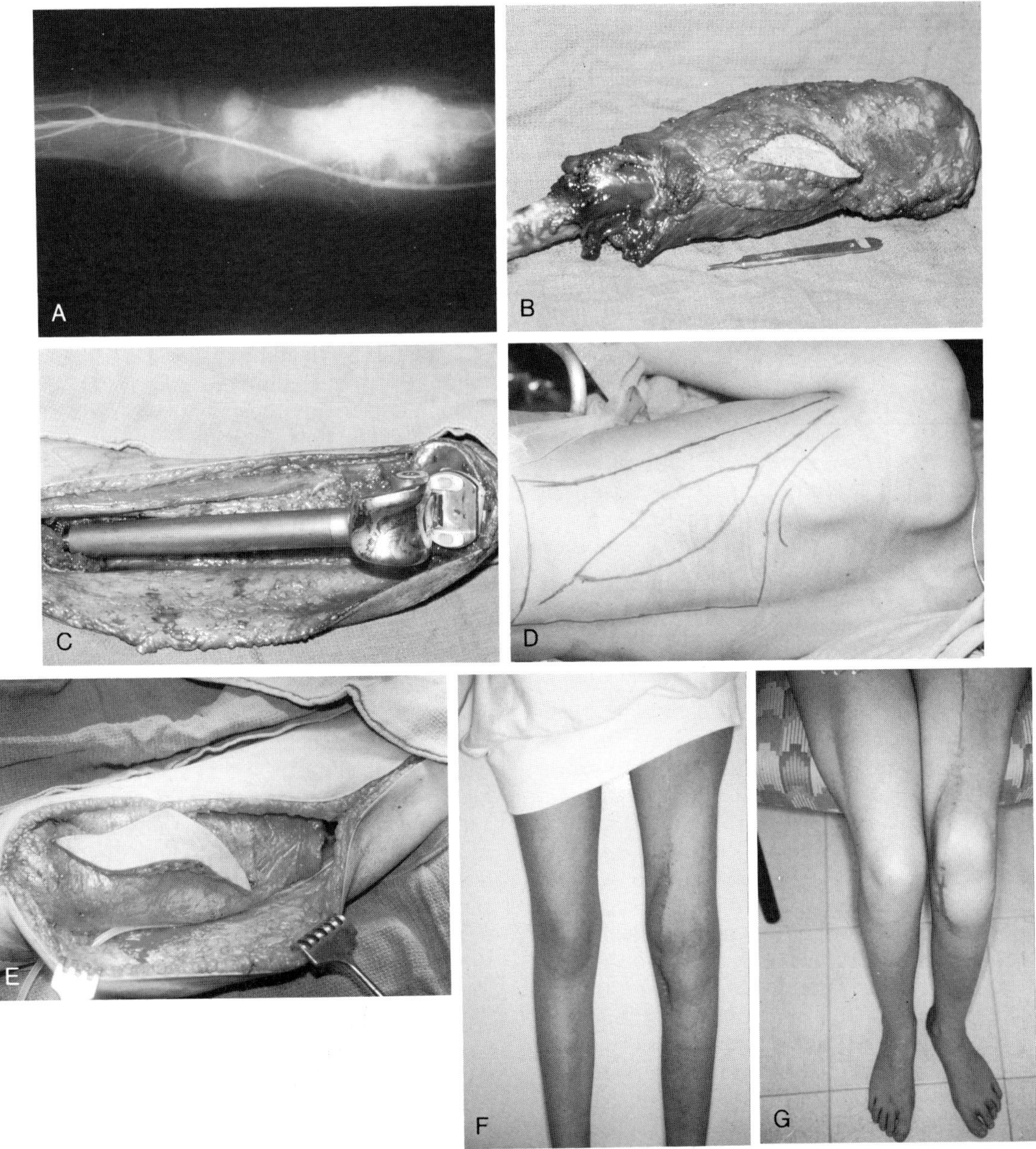

FIGURE 19–22. *A,* Osteogenic sarcoma of distal femur. *B,* Resected specimen of distal femur. *C,* Distal femoral prosthesis in position. *D,* Outline of latissimus dorsi myocutaneous free flap. *E,* Latissimus dorsi myocutaneous free flap revascularized into femoral vessels and sutured into position over prosthesis. *F* and *G,* Stable postoperative coverage of prosthesis.

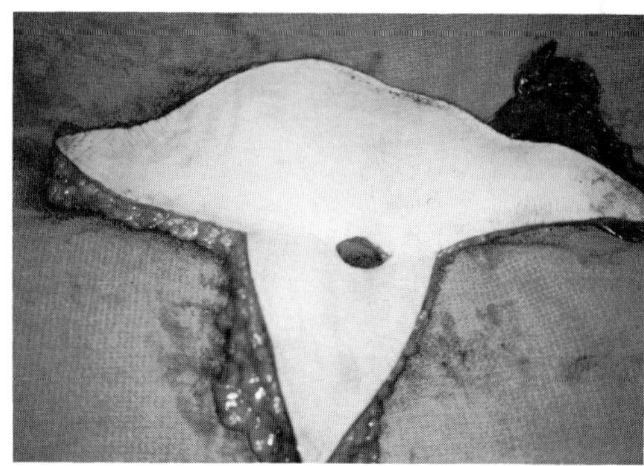

FIGURE 19–23. Rectus myocutaneous flap with large horizontal and vertical components.

type healing, rather than creeping substitution as with nonvascularized bone. With time, hypertrophy of the bone occurs and results in successful weight bearing.[10, 17, 19, 38, 44]

Postoperative Care

The postoperative care of patients following tumor resection and reconstructive surgery must balance the patient's healing requirements with their essential adjuvant chemotherapy or radiotherapy. During the first postoperative week the operated extremity is elevated to reduce swelling and inflammation. The site of closure is observed carefully for signs of hematoma, sepsis, or flap ischemia. Any skin demarcation usually evidenced by dark hemorrhagic tissue is treated aggressively with debridement and closure if it is judged to represent a full-thickness skin loss. Partial loss of skin thickness is treated with topical antibiotic ointment and allowed to epithelialize; however, if several weeks have passed without improvement, it is prudent to re-excise and close the area, as the chemotherapy will cause delayed secondary healing.

If microsurgical free tissue transfer has been performed, the patient must be monitored intensively for the first 72 hours. Hourly monitoring should consist of direct observation of the flap's color, bleeding, and temperature. Probes can be attached to the flap for an accurate assessment of temperature, and this can be compared with a control temperature probe. Once a baseline temperature of the flap and the control are established, they can be observed for any change. An increase in the spread between the control and the flap beyond 2°C may reflect vascular compromise and alerts the staff to examine the flap for arterial occlusion or venous hypertension (Fig. 19–26). The most accurate assessment of vascular compromise is direct needle-stick of the tissue and examination of the color and rate of the bleeding. A healthy, well-vascularized flap has brisk, but not rapid, bleeding of bright red blood. If there is any question, the microvascular surgeon must perform the examination and decide if emergency reexploration is required. The presence of vascular compromise demands rapid return to the operating room in order to avoid prolonged ischemia of the flap tissue and the possibility of the "no-reflow phenomenon" with failure of the flap due to irreversible clotting of the entire vascular system.[40]

Physical therapy of a limb may begin in the first postoperative week on those patients who underwent reconstruction with local tissue. After free tissue transfer, patients are immobilized for 2 weeks in order to protect the vascular anastomosis and to allow intimal healing of the vessels. At 2 weeks there may be sufficient healing and vascular ingrowth of surrounding tissue such that failure of the anastomoses at this time will not result in flap loss. Initial physical therapy should be gradual, and to avoid venous hypertension an operated limb should not remain in a dependent position for longer than 15-minute intervals. The time of dependency is increased over a 2-week period, and a compression wrap is used to avoid edema.

Chemotherapy is generally resumed 2 weeks postoperatively without interference in wound healing. The administration of Adriamycin is delayed as long as possible because of its inhibitory effect on wound healing. Radiation therapy should be delayed, if possible, until primary wound healing has occurred.[8, 12, 13, 56]

Patients with prosthetic implants must be educated so that injury to the reconstructed limb can be avoided and possible sources of infection identified. Small abrasions on the feet

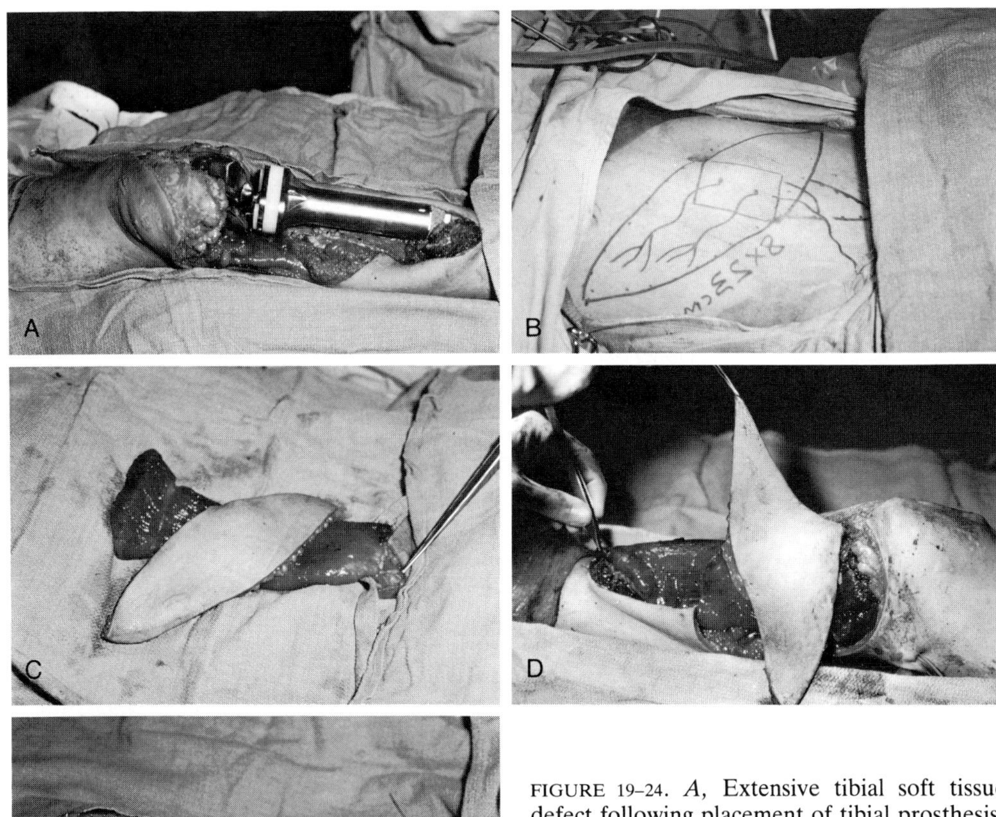

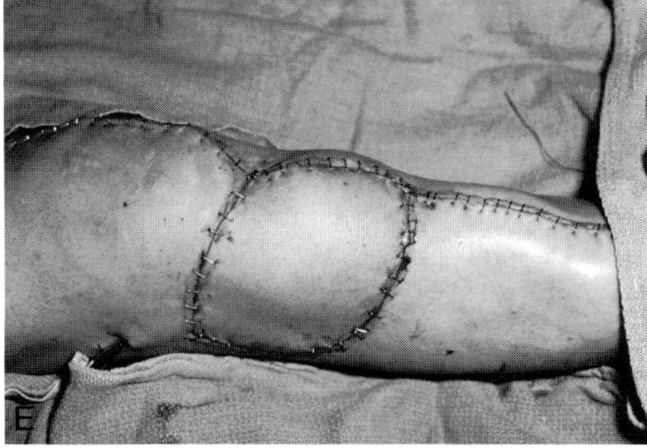

FIGURE 19–24. *A*, Extensive tibial soft tissue defect following placement of tibial prosthesis. *B*, Obliquely oriented skin paddle design over rectus abdominis muscle. Outline of myocutaneous flap and inferior epigastric vessels. *C*, Harvested rectus abdominis myocutaneous flap. *D*, Insetting of flap following revascularization. *E*, Final coverage of tibial prosthesis.

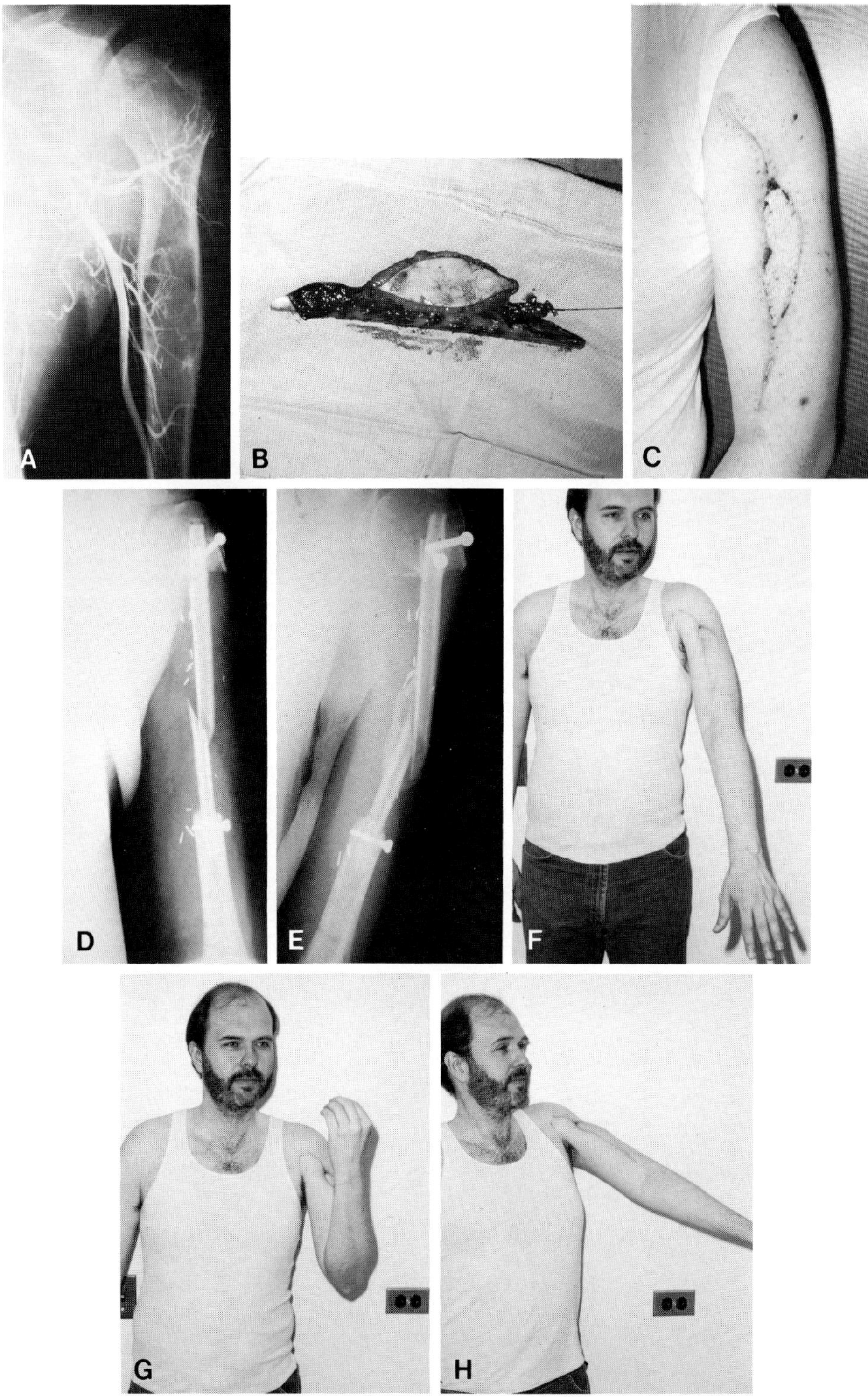

FIGURE 19–25. *A,* Radiograph of extensive chondrosarcoma of humerus. *B,* Free fibula osseocutaneous flap prior to revascularization. *C,* Postoperative healing of cutaneous defect. *D,* Radiograph of stress fracture of fibula graft. *E,* Radiograph showing fracture-type healing with callus formation of vascularized fibula bone graft. *F, G,* and *H,* Flexion and extension of arm following healing of graft.

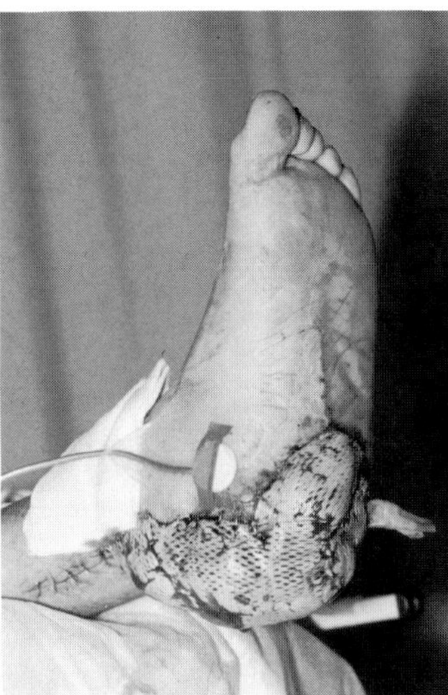

FIGURE 19–26. Venous thrombosis in a muscle flap with skin graft.

or paronychial infections may rapidly progress to cellulitis in the operated limb, potentially infecting the underlying prosthesis. Recognition by the patient of potential sources of infection and rapid treatment with antibiotics will avoid an infected prosthesis.

References

1. Arbeit JM, et al: Wound complications in the multimodality treatment of extremity and superficial truncal sarcomas. J Clin Oncol 5:480, 1987.
2. Arlen M, Marcove RC: Surgical Management of Soft Tissue Sarcomas. Philadelphia, WB Saunders, 1987.
3. Barford B, Pers M: Gastrocnemius-plasty for primary closure of compound injuries of the knee. J Bone Joint Surg 52B:124, 1970.
4. Bergren A, Weiland AJ, Dorfman H: Free vascularized bone grafts: Factors affecting their survival and ability to heal recipient bone defects. Plast Reconstr Surg 69:19, 1982.
5. Bostwick J III, et al: Sixty latissimus dorsi flaps. Plast Reconstr Surg 63:31, 1979.
6. Bryant M, et al: Soft tissue sarcomas of the extremities: Morbidity of combined radiation and limb salvage. Int J Radiat Oncol Biol Phys 11:87, 1985.
7. Burrows HJ, Wilson JN, Scales JT: Excision of tumors of the humerus and femur with restoration by internal prosthesis. J Bone Joint Surg 57B:148, 1975.
8. Chang AE, et al: Adjuvant chemotherapy for patients with high-grade soft tissue sarcomas of the extremities. J Clin Oncol 6:1491, 1988.
9. Collin CH, et al: Localized, operable soft tissue sarcoma of the lower extremity. Arch Surg 121:1425, 1986.
10. Dell PC, Borchardt H, Glowczewskie FP: A roentgenographic, biomechanical and histological evaluation of vascularized and non-vascularized segmental fibular canine autografts. J Bone Joint Surg 67A:105, 1985.
11. Duncan MJ, Zuker RM, Manktelow RT: Resurfacing weight bearing areas of the heel: The role of the dorsalis pedis-innervated free tissue transfer. J Reconstr Microsurg 1:201, 1985.
12. Eckardt JJ, Eilber FR, Dorey FJ, et al: The UCLA experience in limb salvage for malignant tumors. Orthopaedics 8:612, 1985.
13. Eilber FR, et al: Limb salvage for skeletal and soft tissue sarcomas. Cancer 53:2579, 1984.
14. Enneking WF, Eady JL, Burchardt H: Autogenous cortical bone grafts in the reconstruction of segmental skeletal defects. J Bone Joint Surg 62A:1039, 1980.
15. Feldman JJ, Cohen BE, May JW Jr: Medial gastrocnemius myocutaneous flap. Plast Reconstr Surg 61:531, 1978.
16. Gebhart MJ, Lane JM, McCormack RR Jr, Glasser D: Limb salvage in bone sarcomas—Memorial Hospital experience. Orthopaedics 8:626, 1985.
17. Gidumal R, Wood MB, Sim FH, Shives TC: Vascularized bone transfer for limb salvage and reconstruction after resection of aggressive bone lesions. J Reconstr Microvasc Surg 3:183, 1987.
18. Gottlieb ME, et al: Clinical applications of the extended deep inferior epigastric flap. Plast Reconstr Surg 78:782, 1986.
19. Guo F, Ding BF: Vascularized free fibula transfer and the treatment of bone tumors: report of three cases. Arch Orthop Trauma Surg 98:209, 1981.
20. Hausman M: Microvascular applications in limb sparing tumor surgery. Orthop Clin North Am 20:427, 1989.
21. Karakousis CP, et al: Feasibility of limb salvage and survival in soft tissue sarcomas. Cancer 57:484, 1986.
22. Khouri RK, Shaw WW: Reconstruction of the lower extremity with microvascular free flaps: A 10 year experience with 304 consecutive cases. Presented at the 48th Annual Meeting of the Amer. Asso. for the Surgery of Trauma, Newport Beach, CA, October, 1987.
23. Kojima T, Kohno T, Ito T: Muscle flap with simultaneous skin graft for skin defects of the lower leg. J Trauma 19:724, 1979.
24. Lewis MM: The use of an expandable and adjustable prosthesis in the treatment of childhood malignant bone tumors of the extremity. Cancer 57:499, 1986.
25. Lewis MM, Chekofsky KM: Proximal femur replacement for neoplastic disease. Clin Orthop 171:72, 1982.
26. Malawer M: Surgical technique and results of limb sparing surgery for high grade bone sarcomas of the knee and shoulder. Orthopaedics 8:597, 1985.
27. Mathes SJ, McCraw JB, Vasconez LO: Muscle transposition flaps for coverage of lower extremity defects: Anatomical considerations. Surg Clin North Am 54:1337, 1974.
28. Mathes SJ, Nahai F: Muscle flap transposition with function preservation: Technical and clinical considerations. Plast Reconstr Surg 66:242, 1980.
29. Mathes SJ, Nahai F: Clinical Applications for Muscle and Musculocutaneous Flaps. St Louis, CV Mosby, 1982.
30. Mathes SJ, Vasconez LO, Jurkiewicz MJ: Extension and further application of muscle flap transposition. Plast Reconstr Surg 60:6, 1977.
31. Maxwell GP, Manson PN, Hoopes JE: Experience with 13 latissimus dorsi myocutaneous free flaps. Plast Reconstr Surg 64:1, 1979.
32. Maxwell GP, Stueber K, Hoopes JE: A free latissimus dorsi myocutaneous flap. Plast Reconstr Surg 62:462, 1978.
33. McCraw JB, Dibbell DG, Carraway JH: Clinical

definition of independent myocutaneous vascular territories. Plast Reconstr Surg 60:341, 1977.
34. McCraw JB, Fishman JH, Sharzer LA: The versatile gastrocnemius myocutaneous flap. Plast Reconstr Surg 62:15, 1978.
35. McGregor IA, Morgan G: Axial and random pattern flaps. Br J Plast Surg 26:202, 1973.
36. McLean BH, Bunke HJ: Autotransplant of omentum to a large scalp defect with microsurgical revascularization. Plast Reconstr Surg 49:268, 1972.
37. Miller LB, et al: Resection of tumors in irradiated fields with subsequent immediate reconstruction. Arch Surg 122:461, 1987.
38. Moore JR, Weiland AJ, Daniel RK: Use of free vascularized bone grafts in the treatment of bone tumors. Clin Orthop 175:37, 1983.
39. Morrison WA, Crabb DM, O'Brien BM, Jenkins A: The instep of the foot as a fasciocutaneous island and as a free flap for heel defects. Plast Reconstr Surg 72:56, 1983.
40. O'Brien BM, Morrison WA, Gumley GJ: Principles and techniques of microvascular surgery. *In* McCarthy JG (ed): Plastic Surgery. Philadelphia, WB Saunders, 1990, pp 412–473.
41. Okada T, Tsukada S, Obaro K, et al: Free vascularized fibular graft for replacement of the radius after excision of giant cell tumor: Case report. J Microsurg 3:48, 1981.
42. Pennington DG, Lai MF, Pelly AD: The rectus abdominis myocutaneous free flap. Br J Plast Surg 33:277, 1980.
43. Pho RW: Malignant giant cell tumor of the distal end of the radius treated by free vascularized fibular transplant. J Bone Joint Surg 64A:877, 1981.
44. Pho RWH: Free vascularized fibular transplant for replacement of the lower radius. J Bone Joint Surg 61B:362, 1979.
45. Ponten B: The fasciocutaneous flap: Its use in soft tissue defects of the lower leg. Br J Plast Surg 34:215, 1981.
46. Rudolph R, Ballantyne DL: Skin grafts. *In* McCarthy JG (ed): Plastic Surgery. Philadelphia, WB Saunders, 1990, pp 221–274.
47. Salenius P, Santavirta S, Kiviluoto O, Koskinen EV: Application of free autogenous fibular graft in the treatment of aggressive bone tumors of the distal end of the radius. Arch Orthop Trauma Surg 98:285, 1981.
48. Serafin D, Sabatier R, Morris R, et al: Reconstruction of the lower extremity with vascularized composite tissue: Improved tissue survival and specific indication. Plast Reconstr Surg 66:230, 1980.
49. Shaw W, Bahe D, Converse J: Conservation of major leg arteries when used as a recipient supply for a free flap period. Plast Reconstr Surg 63:317, 1979.
50. Sim FH, Bowman WE Jr, Wilkins RN, Chao EY: Limb salvage in primary malignant bone tumor. Orthopaedics 8:574, 1985.
51. Sim FH, Bowman WE Jr, Wilkins RM, et al: Limb salvage in primary malignant bone tumors. Orthopaedics 8:574, 1985.
52. Simon MA, Spanier SS, Enneking WF: Management of adult soft tissue sarcomas of the extremities. Surg Annu 363–402, 1979.
53. Song R, Song R, Song Y, et al: The forearm flap. Clin Plast Surg 9:21, 1982.
54. Steed DL, Petizman AA, Webster MW, et al: Limb sparing operations for sarcomas of the extremities involving critical arterial circulation. Surg Gynecol Obstet 164:493, 1987.
55. Skibber JM, et al: Limb-sparing surgery for soft tissue sarcoma wound-related morbidity in patients undergoing wide local excision. Surgery 102:447, 1987.
56. Suit HD, et al: Conservative surgery and radiation treatment for soft tissue sarcomas of the extremities, torso, and head and neck region. *In* Enneking WF: Limb Salvage in Musculoskeletal Oncology. New York, Churchill Livingstone, 1987.
57. Taylor GI, Miller GDH, Ham FJ: The free vascularized bone grafts, clinical extension of microvascular techniques. Plast Reconstr Surg 55:533, 1975.
58. Taylor GI, Townsend P, Corlett R: Superiority of the deep circumflex iliac vessels as the supply for free groin flaps: Experimental work. Plast Reconstr Surg 64:595, 1979.
59. Taylor GI, Townsend P, Corlett R: Superiority of the deep circumflex iliac vessels as the supply for free groin flaps: Clinical work. Plast Reconstr Surg 64:745, 1979.
60. Tessier J, Bonnel F, Allieu Y: Vascularization, cellular behavior, and union of vascularized bone grafts: Experimental study in the rabbit. Ann Plast Surg 14:494, 1985.
61. Vasconez LO, Bostwick J III, McCraw J: Coverage of exposed bone by muscle transplantation and skin grafting. Plast Reconstr Surg 53:526, 1974.
62. Weiland AJ, Moore JR, Daniel RK: Vascularized bone autografts: Experience with forty-one cases. Clin Orthop 174:87, 1983.
63. Wilson PD Jr, Lance EM: Surgical reconstruction of the skeleton following segmental resection for bone tumors. J Bone Joint Surg 47A:1629, 1965.
64. Zucker RM, Manktelow RT: The dorsalis pedis free flap: Technique of elevation, foot closure, and flap application. Plast Reconstr Surg 77:93, 1986.

CHAPTER 20

Metastatic Disease to Bone

JAMES R. NEFF

Patients presenting with radiographic evidence of skeletal metastases are more common than patients presenting with primary bone tumors. Skeletal metastases are far more common than primary tumors arising within bone. It is estimated that approximately 400,000 people in the United States die each year from cancer, the second leading cause of death, while only slightly more than 1% of these deaths are due to disseminated metastases from primary tumors of bone.[46] The majority of patients dying of malignancy do so as a result of the anatomic compromise of organ systems from metastatic disease.[33]

Metastasis is defined as the transfer of disease from the primary site of origin to another part or organ system of the body. This process and the consequences thereof are the major cause of treatment failure in patients with cancer. Treatment modalities for the primary tumor are reasonably well defined; however, the management of patients with disseminated metastatic disease remains the leading clinical oncologic challenge of the 1990s.

The recognition of skeletal metastases is not new. Metastatic skeletal defects were shown in x-ray films taken of Egyptian mummies and skeletons from the period of 2500 to 1500 BC.[28, 59] Only recently, however, have the cellular processes and the sequence of events been better observed and defined, whereby the pathogenesis of metastasis is now better understood.

Pathogenesis of Metastasis

Most primary tumors metastatic to bone arise in glandular or epithelial tissues. The most common tumors producing metastases to bone are carcinomas of the breast, the lung, the prostate, the kidney, and the thyroid.[60] An estimated 30 to 40% of patients dying from cancer have metastatic disease to bone at the time of death. For those patients dying from carcinoma of the breast, however, approximately 85% have metastases to bone. Even though some tumors have a preferential capacity to produce skeletal metastases, all tumors can metastasize to bone.

Metastasis may occur by direct spread within a body cavity or by hematogenous or lymphatic spread. In the latter two cases, the process of metastasis is a nonrandom, complex, and dynamic sequence of interrelated events, each dependent on the successful completion of others. The process usually begins when the primary tumor is quite small. It has been

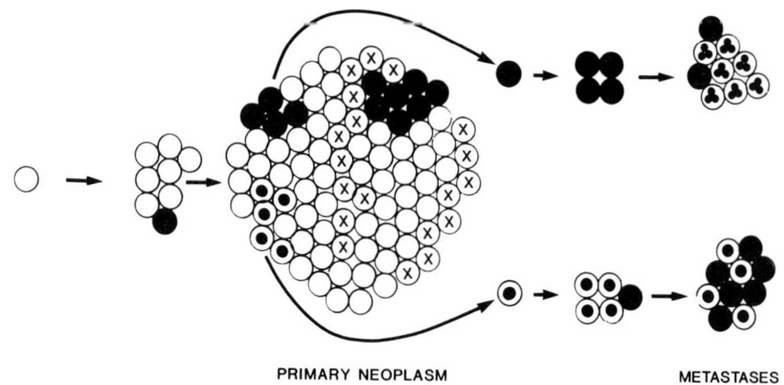

FIGURE 20–1. The development and evaluation of heterogeneous subpopulations of neoplastic cells from the transformed parent cell. The cellular diversity of tumors is attributed to genetic instability, either inherited or acquired. The subpopulations of tumor cells may differ in karyotype, growth range, chemotherapeutic sensitivity, cell surface receptors, and other cell characteristics.

calculated that, for carcinoma of the breast, initiation of metastasis occurs when the primary tumor is less than 0.125 cm^3.[27] Even though the primary neoplastic event may result from the transformation of a single cell, soon the biologic diversity and heterogeneity of tumor cell subpopulations result in the production of highly malignant tumor cells at an early subclinical stage of tumor development[13, 14, 51] (Fig. 20–1).

After tumor initiation occurs (through oncogene activation, carcinogenic insult, or chromosomal rearrangement), the tumor mass rapidly increases in size, mechanically separating the surrounding stromal cells and tissue planes by excessive cellular proliferation (Fig. 20–2). The stromal tissues are composed of supporting cells embedded within the extracellular matrix, consisting of a meshwork of collagen (type I), elastin, proteoglycans, and glycoproteins (laminin and entactin). The supporting stroma serves to form the tissue architecture and acts to isolate one tissue compartment from another.[30] Normally, only motile cells have access through these tissues. The stromal tissues are a natural mechanical barrier to invasion, unless they are traumatized. In general, the stroma is tissue specific and reflects the matrix produced or secreted by the parent tissue.

For the transition from an *in situ* carcinoma to an invasive tumor, the epithelial basal lamina must be penetrated before tumor cells have access to the underlying stromal tissues. Only

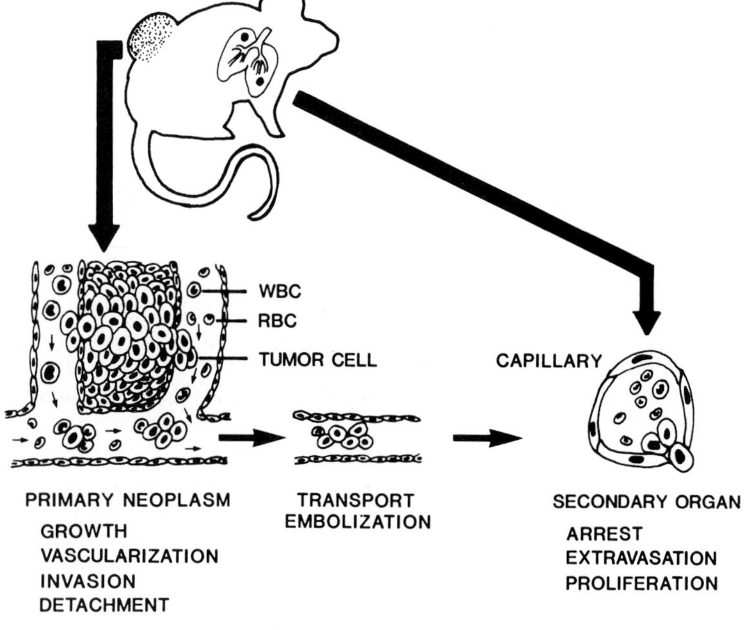

FIGURE 20–2. The metastatic cascade of events, with tumor-host interactions shown on the left. Progression from an *in situ* tumor to invasion of the surrounding stroma and vessels results in circulation and transportation of the tumor emboli. Tumor cells or emboli arrest and adhere to endothelium, followed by extravasation and proliferation. In this case the secondary organ is the lung. WBC, white blood cell; RBC, red blood cell.

after the tumor cells gain access to the stroma do the cells have the opportunity to invade lymphatics and/or small blood vessels.

Tumor cells have been shown to have specific cell surface receptors that bind to extracellular matrix components. Receptors specific for collagen types I, II, III, IV, and V, along with receptors for laminin, fibronectin, fibrin, vitronectin, and others, have been reported.[24, 28, 31] After attachment to the extracellular matrix, the tumor cell secretes proteolytic enzymes capable of locally degrading the matrix and thus providing access to vessels and lymphatics.

Because tumors lack an inherent blood supply, tumor nutrition entails angiogenesis or an ingrowth of new poorly formed vessels about the tumor (neurovascularity). The first factor to be isolated from tumor tissues was a diffusible substance termed tumor angiogenesis factor.[16] A second factor, angiogenin, has also been identified and purified. Both factors recruit new poorly formed thin-walled vessels in and about the tumor, usually beginning when the tumor is no larger than 0.5 cm^3.[16, 19]

Intravasation, or vascular or lymphatic invasion, results from disruption of the luminal subendothelial basement membrane, which is composed of types IV and V collagen, laminin, entactin, fibronectin, and proteoglycans. This is facilitated by the secretion of enzymes by the tumor cell to disrupt the basement membrane, along with the production of tissue inhibitors of metalloproteinases. Tumor cells and surrounding inflammatory cells appear to be capable of secreting enzymes directed at collagen types I, IV, and V; fibronectin; and proteoglycans and thereby facilitate cellular invasion of host stromal tissues.[31] There is also evidence that the *fos* oncogene turns on the gene encoding transin, which disrupts the basement membrane.

Lymphatic channels are usually not present within the tumor and occur only on the invading edge of the tumor. Therefore, lymphatic invasion only occurs on the periphery of the tumor. When lymphatic invasion does occur, the regional draining nodes quickly discharge cells into the adjacent efferent lymphatics, where they enter the systemic venous system through the numerous lymphatic-hematogenous communications. In general, it is believed that the regional nodes do *not* provide a natural or mechanical barrier to tumor dissemination.

After vascular or lymphatic invasion occurs, the cells can either separate and circulate as individual cells or locally proliferate, and then circulate as tumor emboli. Approximately 80% of circulatory tumor cells are in single-cell form, with the remaining cells circulating as tumor emboli. In transit to a secondary site, the cells or emboli are subjected to an extraordinarily hostile environment, including vascular turbulence, the host's immune defense mechanisms (lymphocytes, monocytes, and natural killer cells), and coagulation factors. As a result, it is estimated that less than 0.01% of cells or emboli survive the journey.[43] In general, the process of metastasis is biologically inefficient.

The circulating tumor cells or emboli, usually coated with fibrin and platelets, may embolize in precapillary venules or may adhere directly to exposed vascular endothelium. Within hours, the vascular endothelial cells retract, exposing the subendothelial basement membrane to the tumor cells and then close over the tumor cells, isolating them from further vascular turbulence. The basement membrane is fragmented again by collagen proteolysis (in a process similar to intravasation), producing extravasated tumor cells (extravasation) within the perivascular stroma. Angiogenesis again recruits new poorly formed vessels, usually when the tumor is no larger than 0.5 cm^3.[16] The process of vascular invasion may then proceed again as before and may on occasion lead to secondary metastasis.

Another property of tumor cells is mobility, which facilitates infiltration of stromal tissues and migration through vascular structures. Mobility-stimulating factors produced by tumor cells may provide a chemotactic directional gradient, increasing cellular mobility. These mobility factors also appear to induce the formation of exploratory pseudopodia from the tumor cell rich in matrix protein receptors for laminin and fibronectin, which appear to be essential for cell locomotion.

Preferential Sites of Metastasis

It has been well known since the time of Paget that bone is a preferred site for metastasis. From his autopsy experience, he reasoned that circulating tumor cells bypassed certain organs and were predisposed to spread to specific tissue capillary beds.[40] Ewing later concluded that the process was purely mechanical and was related to blood flow and the first organ encountered by circulating tumor cells in the vascular system.[11] In truth, both theories may be partially accurate in that some metastatic tumors colonize many different tissues, whereas malignant fibrous histiocytoma of bone, neuroblastoma, and Ewing's sarcoma prefer sites in bone, as do metastatic carcinomas of breast, thyroid, kidney, lung, and prostate. Tissues of the skin, muscle, and heart appear either to be protected in some way (related to site specificity or blood flow) and are rarely the site of tumor metastasis.

With the recent identification of numerous growth factors, it is apparent that metastases to specific sites respond preferentially to growth factors found at those sites.[34] Recently, a growth factor was identified in pulmonary tissue that preferentially stimulated the growth of mammary adenosarcoma cells that colonize the lung.[7] The uncontrolled division of cancer cells may be related to excessive growth stimulation or deficient growth inhibition.

Factors may also occur within specific tissues that promote or stimulate growth of tumor cells.[8] Prostate carcinoma cells are known to selectively colonize and grow in bone. A growth factor not found in muscle, skin, lung, and liver, but present in bone, appears to enhance the growth of metastatic prostate carcinoma cells.[8]

Cellular growth can also be controlled by inhibiting factors such as transforming growth factor–beta (TGF-β) and peptides such as macrophage-activated tumor necrosis factor–alpha (TNF-α). These factors are capable of causing cellular death and are found in tissues undergoing macrophage activation. Inhibitors can also be present in specific tissues and may represent a broad class of substances that could regulate the growth of primary tumors. Suramin (Antrypol), originally synthesized in 1916, appears to be capable of blocking the binding of growth factors to their respective receptors. The exact mechanism of action appears to be varied; however, this compound may be useful in the treatment of a variety of malignancies.[47]

Chemotactic factors may also be important and may explain the preferential metastasis to bone of some primary tumors (e.g., breast cancer). It is suggested that bone collagen fragments released during bone remodeling may be chemotactic to certain tumor cells, thereby promoting tumor cell adherence and growth within medullary bone.

Other mechanisms postulated to have a role in preferential metastatic sites suggest that circulating tumor cells respond to chemoattractants produced by certain organs. Evidence also suggests that tumor cells preferentially adhere to specific organ endothelial tissues, whereas other investigators believe that tumor cells adhere equally to all endothelial surfaces but grow preferentially within specific organs.

After dissemination to bone has occurred, however, the tumor cells proliferate and destroy the underlying bone and matrix. The process of bone destruction has been shown to be primarily a cellular event.

Mechanisms of Bone Destruction and Hypercalcemia

Hypercalcemia is a common metabolic complication of cancer and is the most life-threatening associated metabolic disorder. The most frequent clinical symptoms associated with hypercalcemia of malignancy are nausea, vomiting, anorexia, lethargy, confusion, stupor, and coma. These symptoms, even though similar to, should not be confused with the terminal events of cancer. Hypercalcemia is most commonly observed in patients with multiple myeloma and carcinoma of the breast, with approximately 40 to 50% of patients experiencing hypercalcemia at some time during the course of the disease.[37] In contrast, approximately 12% of the patients with squamous cell carcinoma of the lung experience hypercalcemia. The hypercalcemia observed as a secondary effect of malignancy is related to the capacity of the tumor to secrete specific hypercalcemia factors and is not related to increased intestinal absorption of calcium.[37]

Bone resorption associated with neoplasia results in osteolytic metastases and may cause hypercalcemia. Identification of the mechanisms by which tumor cells modify bone cell metabolism has produced a better understanding of the mechanisms of bone destruction. The secondary hypercalcemia may or may not have clinical effects (e.g., on the duration of hypercalcemia or the rate of destruction); however, the resultant bone destruction commonly produces increased morbidity. No one process of altered bone cell metabolism is believed responsible for the bone destruction.

Cytokines

Hematologic malignancies such as multiple myeloma result in either focal or generalized bone destruction produced by activated osteoclasts. Little or no reactive bone can be discerned about these lesions. Cultured myeloma cells were shown to produce a soluble factor that stimulated osteoclasts to resorb bone and was also isolated from lymphoid cells. These factors released by lymphocytes were designated osteoclast-activating factors and constitute a variety of osteoclast-mediated cytokines. Other hematologic malignancies that also produce similar cytokines include lymphomas and Burkitt's lymphoma.

TGFs are released by a variety of hematologic cancer cells. Both TGF-α and TGF-β were shown to be potent inducers of bone resorption.[38] The TGF-α appears quite similar to epidermal growth factor, whereas TGF-β has certain parathyroid hormone (PTH)–like activities.[25] Monocyte-derived interleukin 1 has also been shown to have bone-resorbing properties.

TNFs are also potent inducers of bone resorption *in vitro*.[18] It has also been shown that TNF induces the synthesis of interleukin 1. The exact interactions of the TNFs and tumoral hypercalcemia are not completely understood.

Prostaglandins

Hypercalcemia in patients with carcinoma of the breast is most commonly seen only after widespread bone metastases are discovered. It is observed in approximately 30% of patients. As the process of metastasis occurs, the emboli lodge in the sinusoids of the hematopoietically active bone marrow and migrate to the endosteal surfaces.

The process of bone destruction in this specific solid tumor with bone metastases probably includes several types of cells. The cells involved include tumor cells, osteoclasts, lymphocytes, and monocytes. The osteoclasts are probably primarily responsible for bone destruction; they are stimulated by prostaglandins produced by monocytes and tumor cells and cytokines produced by lymphocytes (i.e., the inflammatory response of the tumor). Tumor cells and monocytes also possess the properties to resorb bone directly.[6] Endogenous prostaglandin release has been implicated in hypercalcemia of malignancy. The E series of prostaglandins (PGE) have potent bone-resorptive properties; however, the serum levels observed in patients with clinical hypercalcemia are probably too low to account for the hypercalcemia observed. The bone-resorptive effects are more than likely due to the local release of prostaglandin from tumor cells stimulated by tumor-derived factors.[54]

Hypercalcemia has also been described in another group of patients with solid tumors but without known metastases. This syndrome has been called the humoral hypercalcemia of cancer. Calcium absorption from the gut and concentrations of 1,25-dihydroxyvitamin D are decreased, thus suggesting that PTH is not the responsible mediator. Many patients do have increased urinary excretion of PGE-M (the primary urinary metabolite of PGE), implicating PGE as a causative local factor of bone resorption. Numerous studies suggest, however, that prostaglandin production alone is insufficient to explain the hypercalcemia seen in humans.

Parathyroid Hormone–like Activity

In general, it is believed that ectopic PTH production cannot be a frequent cause of hypercalcemia in malignancy. Proteins with PTH-like activity are produced by some tumors.[5] Other humoral factors that bind to PTH receptors and can activate PTH-dependent adenylate cyclase have also been described.[49] These findings are important because the hypercalcemia observed might be treated by selectively blocking receptor binding.

Vitamin D

Elevated vitamin D levels have been reported in patients with Hodgkin's disease, multiple myeloma, and other tumors.[23] Additionally, patients with T cell non-Hodgkin's lymphoma have elevated 1,25-dihydroxyvitamin D levels. This is believed to be related to the increased enzymatic conversion of 25-hydroxyvitamin D to 1,25-dihydroxyvitamin D. Resolution of the hypercalcemic state correlates with decreased serum levels of 1,25-dihydroxyvitamin D and generalized control of the disease.

Treatment

PROPHYLAXIS

Prevention of pathologic fractures is achieved through frequent follow-up examinations, including appropriate roentgenograms and bone scintigraphy. Early chemotherapeutic management or radiation therapy can preclude pathologic fracture; however, after sufficient bone destruction has occurred, consideration must be given to prophylactic internal fixation.[41, 42]

General guidelines have been developed regarding the indications for prophylactic internal fixation. In long bones, painful destructive lesions 2.5 cm in diameter or greater or areas of destruction occupying greater than 50% of the circumference of the cortex have been shown to fracture spontaneously or with minimal trauma. In addition, painless lesions occupying more than 50% of the cortical surface fracture with minimal trauma. Patients with defects in long bones satisfying the above criteria should strongly be considered for prophylactic internal fixation (Fig. 20–3).[12, 35, 36] The predictability of failure of the involved bone is sufficiently great to warrant the risks and hazards of prophylactic surgical intervention in most instances.

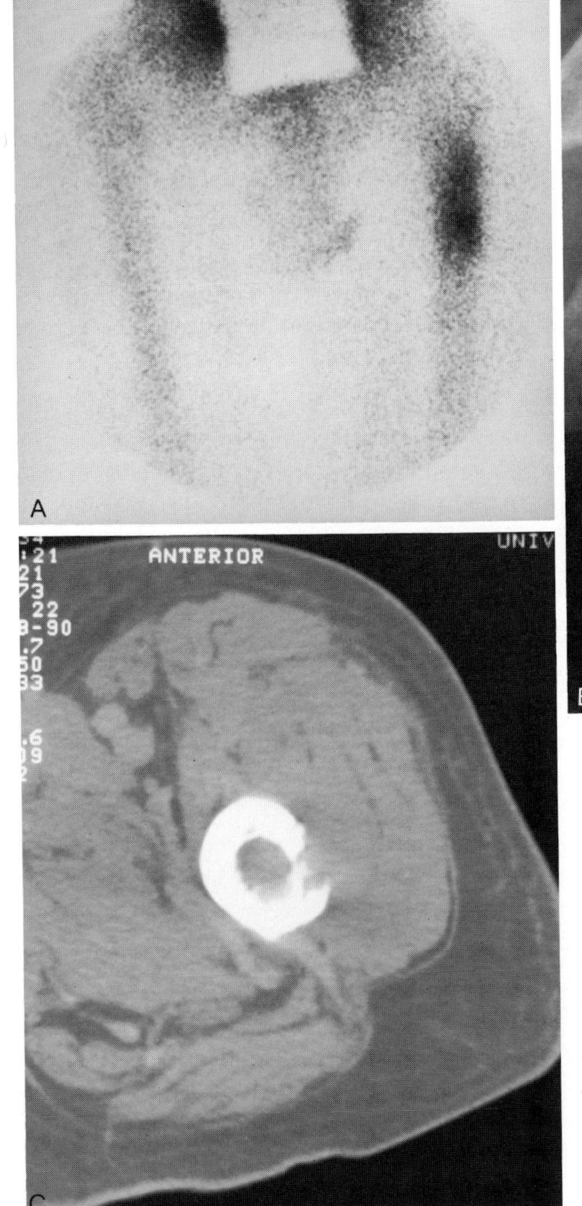

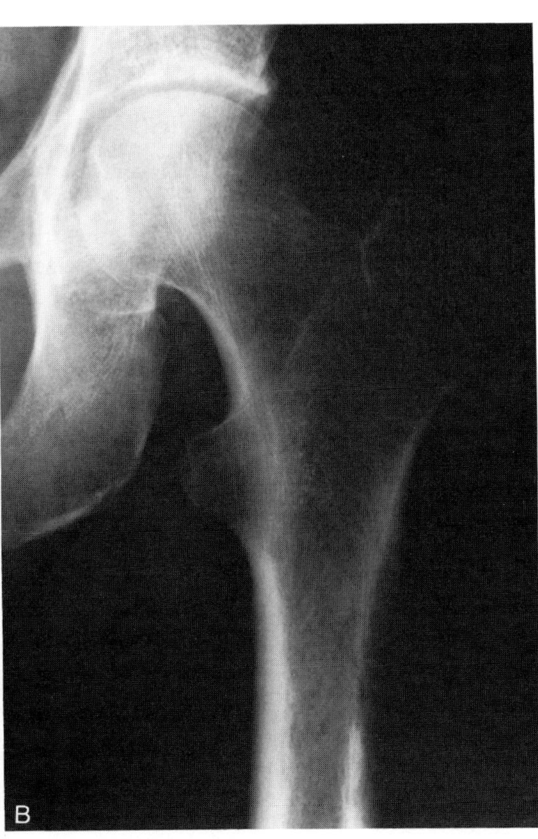

FIGURE 20–3. A 63-year-old male patient experienced pain in the left proximal thigh associated with weight loss. *A*, A bone scan indicated an area of increased uptake within the left subtrochanteric region of the femur, along with several lesions in the posterior ribs. *B*, X-ray film of the left proximal femur shows a lateral cortical defect distal to the lesser trochanter. The position of the cortical defect on the tensile side of the femur predisposes this region to fracture. *C*, Computed tomography (CT) scan through the region clearly shows destruction of at least a third of the cortex. Considering the size and the position of the defect, the patient elected to proceed with prophylactic internal fixation after completion of preoperative external beam radiation therapy (36 Gy).

SKELETAL RECONSTRUCTION

For the purposes of considering reconstruction of pathologic fractures, the skeleton may be subdivided into three separate anatomic areas. The upper extremity may conveniently be addressed as a separate area in that the reconstruction does not necessarily have to be as structurally precise as for lesions within the spine and the lower extremity. The pelvis and the lower extremity are discussed separately to outline better and to demonstrate the unique and numerous techniques available for stabilization and fixation of pathologic fractures in these areas. Reconstruction of the spine and the axial skeleton entails specific techniques.

The majority of surgical implants available for reconstruction of pathologic fractures are adapted from implants used in general orthopedic surgery. They are derived from applications in traumatology and reconstructive surgery. Because of the bone destruction commonly associated with metastases, other space-occupying load-bearing materials are commonly required in conjunction with the use of adapted surgical implants to appropriately reconstruct the skeletal defect.

The use of methyl methacrylate in patients with excessive bone destruction associated with pathologic fractures has been well documented.[20-22] The material may be used in conjunction with a standard implant or with multiple Steinmann pins to produce a composite-like material with multiple points of fixation (e.g., for pelvic and acetabular fractures). The material properties of methyl methacrylate necessitate that it be used to transmit compressive loads for better stress distribution. Methyl methacrylate does not have adhesive properties and therefore should be used only as a complex "filler" in conjunction with a surgical implant to promote fixation and compressive loading of the bone.

Pathologic fractures frequently necessitate therapeutic external beam radiotherapy to curtail continued bone destruction and further loss of fixation. Extensive studies have assessed changes in the material properties of methyl methacrylate after the application of external beam radiation therapy. In general, the structural properties of methyl methacrylate appear unchanged when this material is exposed to greater than therapeutic doses of ionizing radiation.[10, 39]

Upper Extremity Management

HAND AND WRIST

In general, every effort should be made to restore as much function as possible in patients with upper extremity metastases, especially when they are located in the dominant upper extremity[29] (Table 20–1). Digital metastases are best managed by amputation, and limited metacarpal involvement can also be managed by ray amputation (Fig. 20–4). Adjunctive radiation therapy may also be necessary if wide margins of resection are not achieved (the plane of dissection must pass through absolutely normal tissues).

Metastases to the carpus are unusual. In general, the hand and the wrist do not tolerate radiation therapy well; however, radiotherapy may be the treatment of choice if only limited involvement is identified. More extensive involvement of the carpus associated with osseous destruction is generally best managed by a wide amputation above the wrist, where methyl methacrylate and plate reconstruction is not a reasonable option.[17]

FOREARM

Because of the two-bone construction of the forearm and the unlikelihood of simultaneous involvement of both bones at the same location, the majority of lesions involving the forearm lend themselves to some form of therapy short of amputation (Table 20–2). Neoplastic involvement of either bone, whether proximally or distally, necessitates that the integrity of the adjacent joint be preserved if at all possible. Lesions of the distal ulna or the

TABLE 20–1

Treatment of Metastases to Hand and Wrist

Phalanges	Metacarpals	Carpus
1. Amputation (wide)	1. Ray amputation (wide)	1. Radiation
2. Ray amputation	2. Ray amputation + RT	2. Amputation (wide)

*RT, external beam radiation therapy.

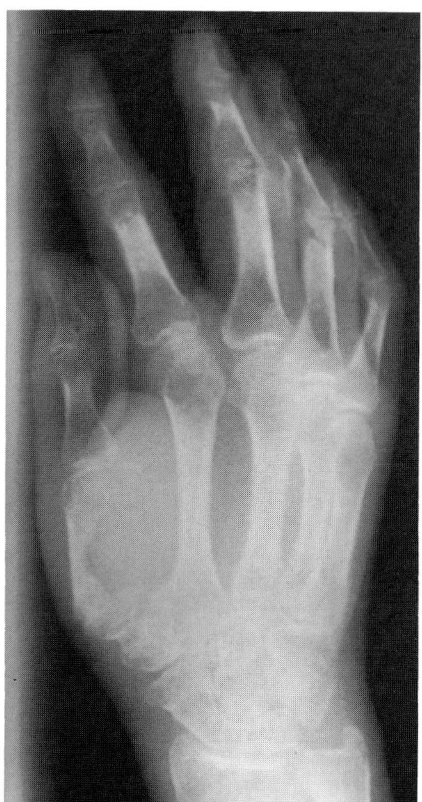

FIGURE 20–4. X-ray film of the right (dominant) hand of a 57-year-old man. The patient had a painful mass within the thenar eminence. The diagnosis of metastatic carcinoma of the lung was made from a chest x-ray film, and external beam radiation therapy was given in an attempt to control the osseous destruction and pain. Three months later, an above-wrist amputation was performed to control persistent pain and an expanding mass.

proximal radius may be excised without major reconstructive efforts or may be alternatively managed by radiation therapy alone. Efforts to retain the architecture and function of the distal radius and the proximal ulna should remain a priority. Uncontrolled destructive lesions, however, may necessitate amputation.

Midshaft lesions in either bone are most often managed by radiation therapy alone (Fig. 20–5). Some fractures may necessitate internal fixation for stabilization and restoration of length; however, most also need methyl methacrylate augmentation. When a below-elbow amputation is necessary for local control and wide margins are achieved, adjunctive external beam radiotherapy may be avoided.

Satisfactory function of the upper extremity can be preserved even with stiffness in the elbow, as long as the hand and limb are maintained in a functional position. Only in patients who are expected to have prolonged survival are elaborate reconstructive efforts justified (e.g., in those with carcinoma of the thyroid).

UPPER ARM

Reconstructive procedures applied to treatment of pathologic fractures of the humerus are structurally and technically demanding (Table 20–3). The upper arm, being a tubular one-bone limb segment, must withstand greater dynamic muscle forces and does not enjoy the shared support observed in the two-bone forearm. Because the humerus is relatively straight and tubular in shape, intramedullary techniques utilized in reconstruction are more demanding than those for the forearm and are frequently incapable of resisting the rotatory forces (torque) commonly observed in the arm.

As in the forearm, every effort should be made to maintain either elbow or shoulder motion short of elaborate reconstructive techniques. In most instances, external beam radiation therapy offers significant relief of pain and allows sufficient healing of the fracture to retain some joint function (Fig. 20–6). If the fracture and periarticular structures do not

TABLE 20–2

Treatment of Metastases to Forearm (Radius and Ulna)

Distal	Midshaft	Proximal
1. Radiation alone	1. Radiation alone	1. Radiation alone
2. RT with or without mm + internal fixation	2. RT with or without mm + internal fixation	2. RT with or without mm + internal fixation
3. RT + excision + allograft	3. Amputation (wide)	3. Excision of proximal radius with prosthesis or synostosis
4. Amputation (wide)		4. Wide disarticulation or AE amputation

AE, above elbow; mm, methyl methacrylate; RT, external beam radiation therapy.

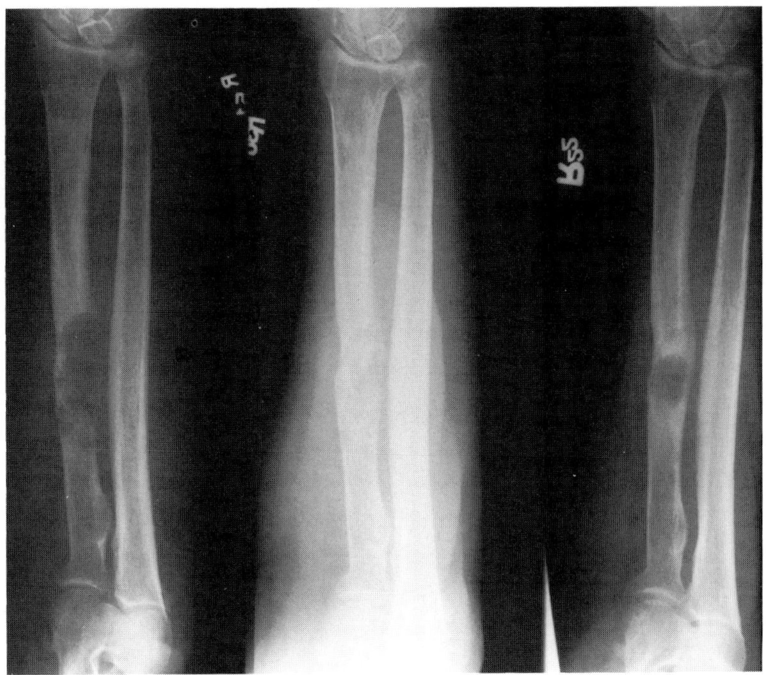

FIGURE 20–5. Three sequential anteroposterior (AP) films of the right (dominant) forearm of a 67-year-old man reveal a destructive process in the radius (left) from metastatic carcinoma of the lung. The ulna was uninvolved and provided structural support of the lesion while external beam radiation therapy (36 Gy) was completed. The middle film shows the healing response 4 months later. The enlarging, locally recurrent lesion can be seen in the film on the right; however, the lesion remained painless until the patient's death 6 months later.

heal, consideration may be given to resection of the involved part with reconstruction using a modular prosthesis, a composite allograft-prosthesis, or an allograft replacement with internal fixation in otherwise healthy patients.

Diaphyseal lesions not amenable to radiotherapy alone may necessitate reconstruction and augmentation using either intramedullary fixation or plate reconstruction and supplementary methyl methacrylate (Fig. 20–7). Most patients with pathologic fractures requiring surgical stabilization benefit from adjunctive preoperative accelerated fractionated radiation therapy, often reducing the overall size of the mass and commonly reducing the anticipated intraoperative blood loss.

Usually, the diaphyseal segment of the humerus is best exposed through an extensile brachialis-splitting anterolateral incision, which provides the option of extending the incision proximally or distally with near-complete exposure of the entire humerus (Fig. 20–8). The anatomic course of the radial nerve frequently complicates the surgical exposure, necessitating excellent surgical technique. This relatively avascular anatomic interval is devoid of neural structures.

SHOULDER

Because the majority of skeletal metastases appearing in the upper extremity develop within the proximal humerus and/or scapula, special attention should be given to patients with pain who have primary tumors known to

TABLE 20–3

Treatment of Metastases to Arm (Humerus)

Distal	Midshaft	Proximal
1. Radiation alone 2. RT with or without mm + internal fixation 3. RT + excision + allograft/ prosthesis or composite 4. Amputation (wide)	1. Radiation alone 2. RT with or without mm + internal fixation 3. RT + excision + allograft/ prosthesis 4. Amputation (wide)	1. Radiation alone 2. RT with or without mm + internal fixation 3. RT + excision + allograft or prosthesis or both 4. Wide disarticulation or forequarter amputation

mm, methyl methacrylate; RT, external beam radiation therapy.

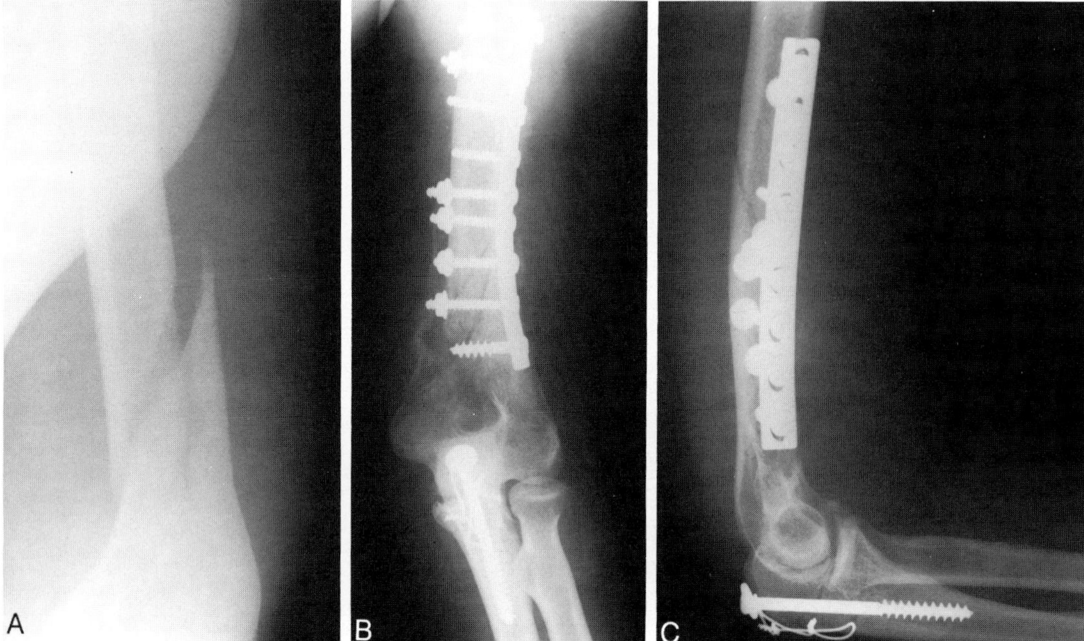

FIGURE 20–6. A comminuted fracture of the distal humerus with moderate displacement was sustained after significant trauma. *A*, AP x-ray film of the left (nondominant) distal humerus after a fall on the outstretched arm. *B*, Open reduction was performed and a frozen section examination of the marrow contents revealed multiple myeloma. Reduction and stabilization were achieved. *C*, Lateral x-ray film shows the reduction achieved. After completing radiation therapy (36 Gy) initiated 4 weeks postoperatively, the fracture healed without complication and with overall excellent function.

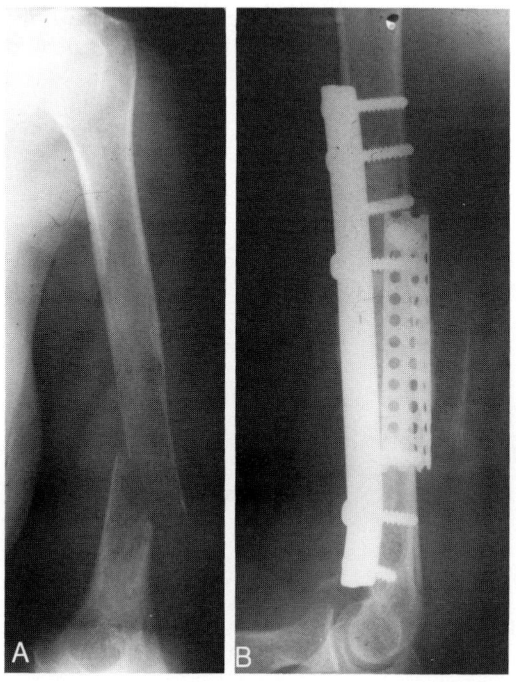

FIGURE 20–7. A 42-year-old black woman with extensive destruction of the distal humerus associated with a pathologic fracture resulting from multiple myeloma. *A*, AP film of the left (nondominant) arm. *B*, Open reduction was performed after 38 Gy of external beam radiation therapy was given. The necrotic tumor was curetted from the medullary canal, and the fracture was stabilized using a preformed bone plate, methyl methacrylate, and titanium mesh.

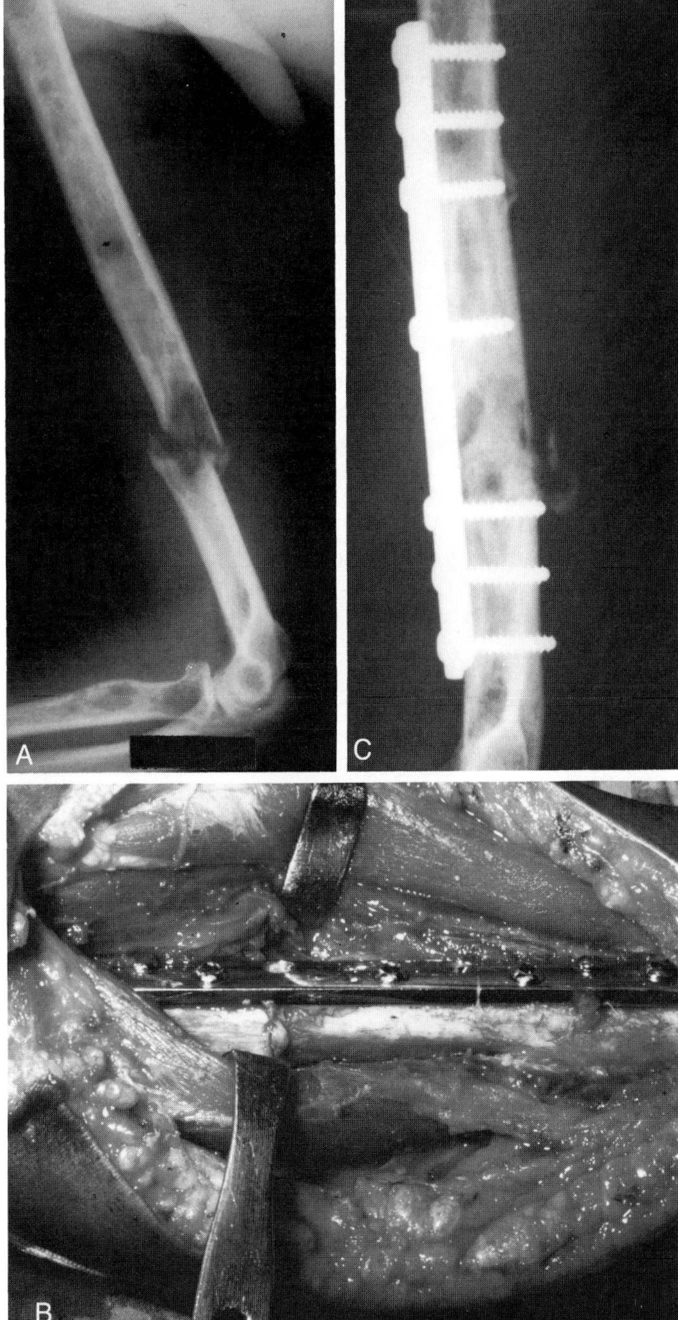

FIGURE 20–8. A 47-year-old black patient with a pathologic fracture of the distal humerus from known multiple myeloma. *A*, Lateral x-ray film of the right (dominant) arm demonstrates the typical punched-out radiographic lesions in both the humerus and the proximal radius. *B*, Intraoperative view of the reconstruction shows the position of the plate after chilled methyl methacrylate was injected into the tumor-associated bone defect and the intramedullary canal before the screws were secured in the plate. *C*, Lateral view of the humerus, showing the radiographic appearance of the reconstruction 6 months postoperatively.

TABLE 20–4

Treatment of Metastases to Shoulder (Scapula)

Glenoid	Body
1. Radiation alone 2. RT + excision + allograft/prosthesis 3. Forequarter amputation	1. Radiation alone 2. Forequarter amputation

RT, external beam radiation therapy.

metastasize to bone. The thick muscle covering the shoulder structures often necessitates special imaging technique for the early recognition and treatment of skeletal metastases in these areas (e.g., bone scintigraphy). Small lesions in the region of the glenoid can often be treated with radiation therapy, whereas other lesions may be managed by more permanent reconstruction techniques (Table 20–4). More extensive lesions not sensitive to nor manageable with radiation therapy may necessitate forequarter amputation for local control.

Pelvis and Lower Extremity Management

Reconstruction techniques for pathologic fractures involving the pelvis and the lower extremity are technically and structurally more demanding. Not only must the extremity be reconstituted for maximal function, but also the structural details and techniques entail considerable preoperative planning to achieve a biomechanically superior result.[1, 50, 58]

PELVIS

Pathologic fractures sustained through an area of the pelvis other than the acetabulum seldom necessitate surgical stabilization. The majority of patients can be managed by radiation therapy. Metastatic lesions associated with pathologic fractures and deformity of the acetabulum are often best managed by preoperative radiation therapy followed by operative reconstruction (Table 20–5). Hip joint function can then be restored by reconstruction using an oversized acetabular cup augmented with methyl methacrylate and multiple Steinmann pins for fixation if necessary. The remainder of the arthroplasty may be performed using a conventional femoral prosthesis and methyl methacrylate. When the fracture is associated with neoplastic involvement of the proximal femur, a long-stem femoral prosthesis may be used in conjunction with a proximal femoral allograft. Fixation may be achieved with methyl methacrylate. Care must be taken to be certain that the cement does not project within the host-graft junction. Interdigitating methyl methacrylate delays or prevents osseous incorporation of the allograft, possibly leading to fatigue failure of the stem of the implant. Single, isolated, late-developing metastases confined to only the acetabulum may be resected using an internal hemipelvectomy or a conventional hemipelvectomy.[48]

THIGH

Similar to the case for the proximal humerus and the scapula, the proximal one-third of the femur and the pelvis is the preferential site of involvement for metastatic lesions in the pelvis and the lower extremity. Pain referred from the hip is most commonly described in the anterior thigh and groin and may be referred to the knee region. The subtrochanteric region of the proximal femur appears to be a preferential site for metastatic disease of the femur (Table 20–6).

A biopsy is necessary to establish a diagnosis of either a primary bone tumor or metastatic disease for patients otherwise free from disease with a lesion in the subtrochanteric region of the proximal femur (Fig. 20–9). A direct approach to the lateral shaft of the proximal femur would in theory contaminate many anatomic planes, making local resection and reconstruction difficult should the lesion represent a primary tumor of bone. Therefore, a limited transtrochanteric approach to the proximal femur using image intensification is recommended for biopsy.

With the patient under regional or general

TABLE 20–5

Treatment of Metastases to Pelvis

Acetabular	Periacetabular (Ilium, Pubis, Ischium)
1. Radiation alone 2. RT + prosthesis 3. RT + allograft-prosthesis composite 4. Internal hemipelvectomy 5. Conventional hemipelvectomy	1. Radiation alone 2. RT + local resection 3. Conventional or radical hemipelvectomy

RT, external beam radiation therapy.

TABLE 20–6

Treatment of Metastases to Thigh (Femur)

Distal	Midshaft	Proximal
1. Radiation alone 2. RT with or without mm + internal fixation 3. RT + allograft/prosthesis 4. Wide amputation	1. Radiation alone 2. RT with or without mm + internal fixation 3. RT + allograft/prosthesis 4. Wide amputation	1. Radiation alone 2. RT with/without mm + internal fixation 3. RT + allograft/prosthesis 4. Wide disarticulation or modified hemipelvectomy

mm, methyl methacrylate; RT, external beam radiation therapy.

anesthesia and in the lateral decubitus position and with the involved leg draped free, a limited exposure can be made to the tip of the greater trochanter through the gluteus medius tendon. A small osseous window can then be made in the top of the greater trochanter and a bone biopsy trochar introduced within the medullary canal and radiographically directed to the area in question. Multiple biopsy and culture specimens can be obtained with only minimal soft tissue contamination using a long pituitary rongeur. After the diagnosis is established, appropriate treatment can be instituted. If the lesion represents metastasis, the entry point is appropriate for the immediate insertion of a Zickle nail.[61] If a conventional intramedullary nail design is used, the entry point is relocated more medially and posteriorly (Fig. 20–10).

Because of the anatomic varus shape of the proximal femur and the bending moment associated with muscle forces and weight bearing, lesions in this region often require prophylactic internal fixation with or without supplementary methyl methacrylate. Destructive lesions with a pathologic fracture at the base of the femoral neck that are manageable with a hip screw-plate combination often are treated by removal of the necrotic tumor and bone and supplementation with methyl methacrylate. The methyl methacrylate acts to fill the osseous void so that the bone-methyl methacrylate interface continues to transmit compressive loads across the bone and down the shaft of the femur. In this instance, the hip screw-plate may even act as a tension band, reducing the bending moment across the screw-plate combination.

In some instances, pathologic fractures may be expected to heal after radiation therapy. Properly fractionated radiotherapy of 38 Gy or less commonly allows osseous union. Fractures associated with radiosensitive lesions such as multiple myeloma often heal with proper immobilization (Fig. 20–11).

Midshaft femoral metastases are often best managed by intramedullary fixation and adjunctive methyl methacrylate after preoperative radiation therapy.[26] The design of the nail should be nearly anatomic with an anterior bow to assist in placing the largest-diameter nail possible within the femur. Biomechanically, the strength of the nail in bending at the fracture site increases as the square of the diameter of the nail. Methyl methacrylate may be used to fill associated osseous defects; however, if considerable length is to be restored or the fracture site appears unstable in rotation, a nail with interlocking capability should be considered to enhance fixation.

Fortunately, metastases to the region of the distal femur are uncommon. Lesions arising within the distal metaphysis commonly necessitate an interlocking intramedullary nail or either single- or double-plate reconstruction with methyl methacrylate. Some distal lesions necessitate a blade-plate or a screw-plate combination with adjunctive methyl methacrylate. Very destructive lesions may be resected, with reconstruction using an osteoarticular allograft, an allograft-prosthesis composite, or a modular prosthesis. Other large destructive lesions may require amputation with wide margins for local tumor management in an effort to rehabilitate the patient with the least overall morbidity.

LEG

Metastatic deposits in the tibia are uncommon. When identified early, the majority of the proximal lesions can be managed by radiation therapy alone (Table 20–7). More destructive lesions may necessitate joint surface reconstruction using similar modalities as discussed for management of distal femoral involvement. Metaphyseal lesions can be reconstructed using either single- or double-plate reconstruction with methyl methacrylate after radiation therapy (Fig. 20–12). However, wound closure

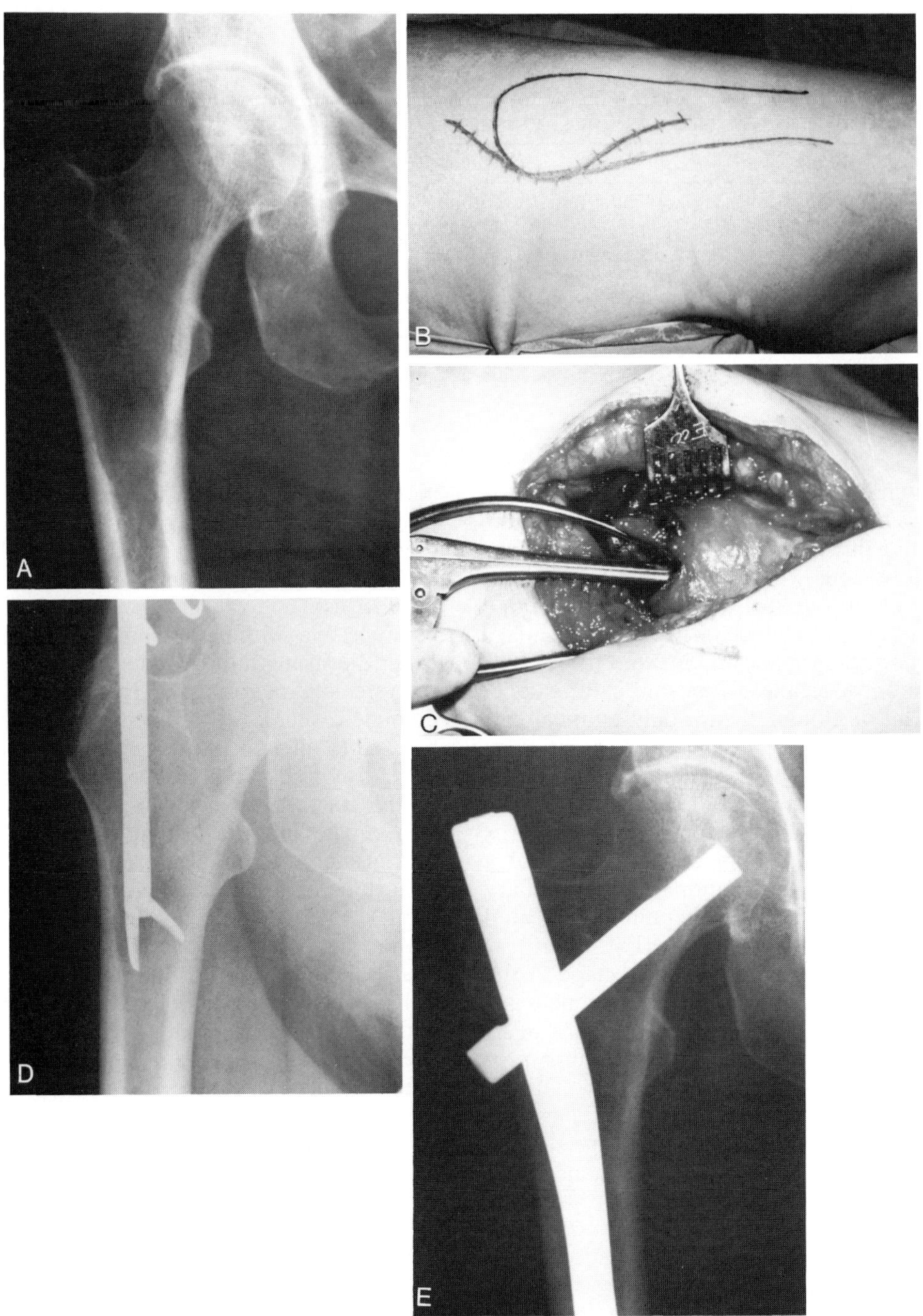

FIGURE 20–9. A 73-year-old man experienced pain in the right anterior thigh and groin. *A*, X-ray film of the right proximal femur revealed a loss of trabeculation within the subtrochanteric region. A bone scan did not reveal other osseous sites of concern, and a CT scan of the chest and abdomen did not reveal any specific abnormalities. *B*, An open biopsy was done to establish a diagnosis of either a primary bone tumor or metastatic disease. To minimize soft tissue contamination, a limited exposure to the upper aspect of the greater trochanter was planned to obtain tissue from within the intramedullary canal. The patient was in the left lateral position with intraoperative image intensification available. *C*, Intraoperative photograph shows the limited exposure through the tip of the greater trochanter, revealing the intramedullary canal. A pituitary rongeur was used to obtain tissue for diagnostic examination. *D*, Intraoperative x-ray film shows the position of the pituitary forceps within the region of concern. A diagnosis of metastatic adenocarcinoma was made. *E*, After the diagnosis was established, an intramedullary guide wire was inserted. The medullary canal was then progressively reamed to accept the insertion of a 13-mm Zickle nail. After appropriate wound healing (5 weeks), the entire femur and skin incision was treated with external beam radiotherapy (38 Gy).

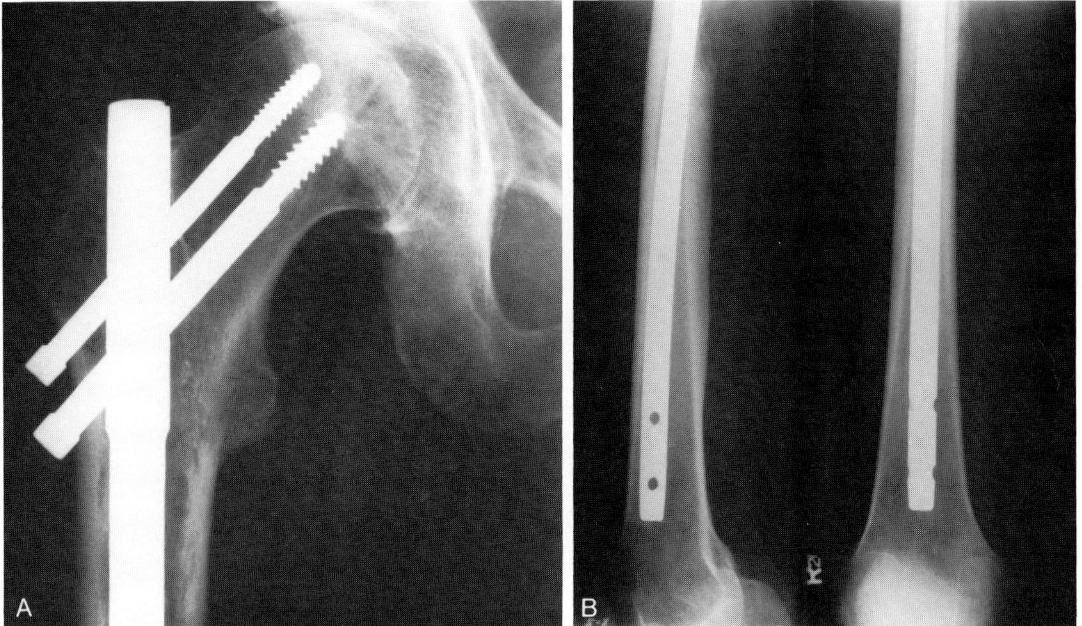

FIGURE 20–10. *A*, This AP x-ray film shows the postoperative result when the right proximal femur was prophylactically nailed with a Russell-Taylor intramedullary nail for an impending pathologic fracture from multiple myeloma. The preoperative pain was relieved with internal fixation. *B*, Distal interlocking screws were not used in this case but may be used when attempting to unload the area of destruction proximally and for controlling rotatory forces. Note that the insertion point at the base of the femoral neck is more medial and posterior than the insertion point required for the Zickle nail.

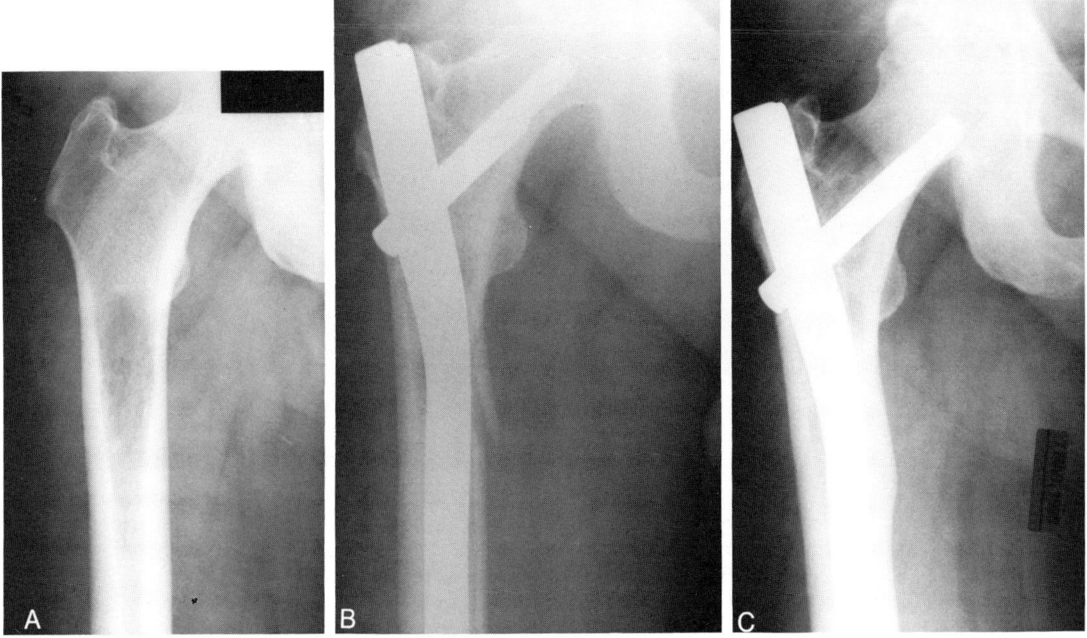

FIGURE 20–11. A 47-year-old man was examined for pain about his right hip. *A*, A diagnosis of multiple myeloma was made from a serum protein electrophoresis. Because the patient continued to experience pain in his right hip after completing radiotherapy, it was elected to proceed with prophylactic internal fixation. *B*, A 15-mm Zickle nail was inserted with intraoperative disruption of the medial femoral cortex. The postoperative course was uncomplicated, with the patient using crutches for 6 weeks. Progressive weight bearing was allowed, with full weight bearing at 10 weeks. *C*, AP x-ray film of the proximal femur taken 33 months postoperatively shows complete healing of the fracture with remodeling.

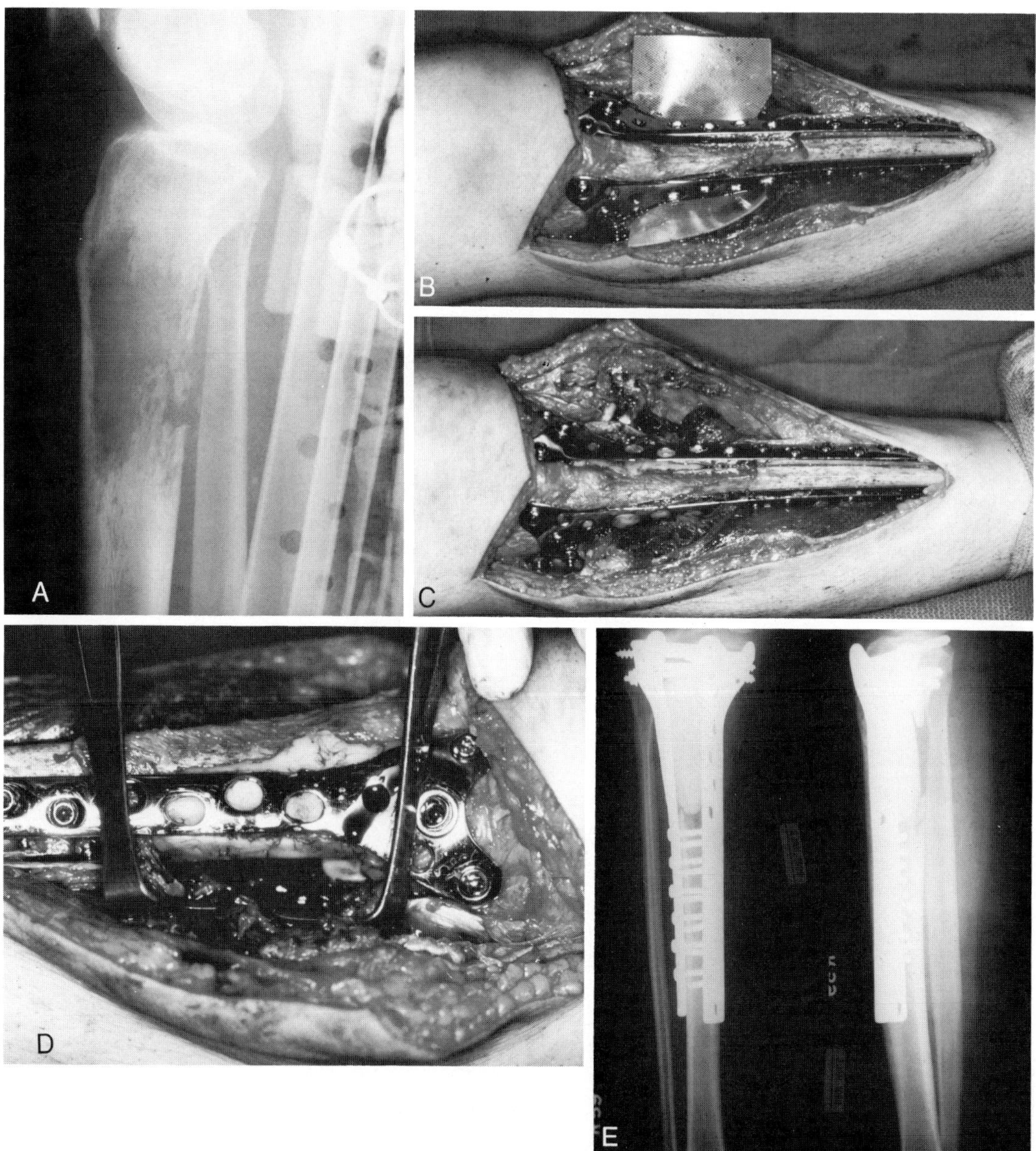

FIGURE 20–12. A 42-year-old woman sustained a pathologic fracture of the right proximal tibia attributable to metastases from pancreatic carcinoma. *A*, Radiographic appearance. *B*, Tibial reconstruction after completion of a 36-Gy course of radiotherapy was selected. Circumferential exposure was achieved about the proximal tibia, with reconstruction using opposing bone plates. Methyl methacrylate was required to augment the reconstruction. A silicone (Silastic) dam placed posterior to the tibia was used to control the flow of the methyl methacrylate. *C*, Intraoperative photograph shows the reconstruction using opposing plates and methyl methacrylate. The reconstruction was stable on intraoperative testing. *D*, Lateral photograph shows the posterior aspect of the methyl methacrylate reconstruction, demonstrating the ability of the silicone (Silastic) dam to model and retain the material during the curing phase. *E*, Postoperative x-ray film shows the overall excellent result and reconstruction of the proximal tibia. Some patients would have elected an above-knee amputation.

TABLE 20–7

Treatment of Metastases to Leg (Tibia and Fibula)

Distal	Midshaft	Proximal
1. Radiation alone 2. RT with or without mm + internal fixation 3. BK amputation (wide)	1. Radiation alone 2. RT with or without mm + internal fixation 3. RT + excision of fibula only (wide) 4. BK amputation (wide)	1. Radiation alone 2. RT with or without mm + internal fixation 3. RT + excision of fibula only (wide) 4. RT + allograft/prosthesis 5. Wide disarticulation or AK amputation

AK, above knee; BK, below knee; mm, methyl methacrylate; RT, external beam radiation therapy.

complications occur because of the limited soft tissues available in the leg. A medial or lateral gastrocnemius muscle flap and split-thickness skin graft may be required for wound closure.

Midshaft lesions may necessitate prophylactic fixation using either open or closed intramedullary nailing techniques to provide sufficient strength to prevent a pathologic fracture. Most oncologic surgeons prefer to consider closed intramedullary nailing only after accelerated fractionated radiation therapy to prevent tumor contamination of the entire intramedullary canal.

Distal tibial lesions may occasionally be managed by radiation therapy alone, but the majority necessitate the addition of a plate and methyl methacrylate fixation. Some patients may require a below-knee amputation and immediate prosthetic fitting.[17] The absence of good muscle coverage and the limited soft tissues available for wound closure prohibit major reconstructive efforts in the distal leg in most patients.

FOOT AND ANKLE

The foot, unlike the hand, can readily be replaced with a reliable prosthesis with predictable overall excellent function (Table 20–8). Therefore, efforts to preserve the foot or the ankle involved with metastatic disease are less often attempted.[29] Small lesions in the os calcis may be managed by radiation therapy alone, whereas lesions associated with painful pathologic fractures are often best managed by amputation and immediate prosthetic fitting.

Metastatic disease to the metatarsals can be managed by ray amputation, as in the hand. Postoperative radiation therapy may be required if the margins are not free from disease. Metastases to the phalanges are best managed by amputation.

Management of Spine

Spinal cord and cauda equina compression most commonly results from tumor involvement of the vertebral column and only rarely from intradural metastases.[2] Experimentally, with gradual compression of the cord, decompression can be delayed and the patient can still retain neurologic function, whereas rapid compression necessitates immediate decompression to retain neurologic function.[52, 53] The use of dexamethasone to reduce vasogenic edema has also been well established.[56, 57] Systemic dexamethasone may result in transient clinical improvement until operative decompression can be performed.

The anatomic distribution of metastases to the spine is approximately 10% for cervical,

TABLE 20–8

Treatment of Metastases to Foot and Ankle

Phalanges	Metatarsals	Tarsus
1. Amputation (wide) 2. Ray amputation	1. Ray amputation (wide) 2. Ray amputation, RT	1. Radiation 2. Amputation (wide) a) Syme b) BK

AK, above knee; BK, below knee; mm, methyl methacrylate; RT, external beam radiation therapy.

70% for thoracic, and 20% for lumbosacral spine. The distribution appears to be related to the total number of vertebrae in each anatomic segment rather than a preferred anatomic site.[55] The skeleton is the second most frequent site of metastasis in the human body, with the vertebral column being the most commonly affected region.[9, 32] Experimental studies on the pathogenesis of vertebral metastasis suggest that tumor cells lodge and grow within the hematopoietic bone marrow and invade the spinal canal through the vertebral vein foramina. Experimentally, tumor cell lines growing as compact tumors commonly form an extradural tumor mass anteriorly, compressing the cord anteriorly, while cell lines growing in an infiltrating fashion tend to migrate posteriorly, producing posterior compression. Of interest was the observation that the tumor cells invade the extradural space through the venous foramina and not by cortical bone destruction.[2]

The majority of patients with metastasis to the spine have pain as their major presenting symptom. Plain films of the spine may show loss of definition of a pedicle or a compression deformity; however, they are frequently interpreted as "normal." Bone scintigraphy remains the major diagnostic aid to identifying the area or areas of concern and is considered to be the most sensitive and inexpensive skeletal radiographic survey method (96% sensitivity) for the majority of metastases. Actual "cold" scans have been reported in patients with multiple myeloma, making the skeletal radiographic survey the most effective method for radiographic follow-up in patients with myeloma and histiocytic lesions.

Computed tomography (CT) of the spine often shows evidence of bone destruction and, on occasion, an adjacent soft tissue mass, whereas conventional polytomography may demonstrate only cortical destruction of a pedicle or a portion of the body of the vertebra. Magnetic resonance imaging (MRI) has essentially replaced myelography as the method of demonstrating the level and the degree of vertebral collapse and extradural compression. The MRI may also show other sites of vertebral marrow replacement. If the lesion remains untreated, a neurologic deficit commonly follows.

The majority of patients recognized to have vertebral metastases but without a neurologic deficit should have preoperative radiation therapy before operative decompression and stabilization is considered (Table 20–9). Patients with a slow but progressive compromise of neurologic function should be given systemic dexamethasone before the initiation of radiation therapy, whereas patients with a rapidly progressive neurologic deficit should have immediate decompression and a stabilization procedure.

The primary region of the vertebral body destruction is often best demonstrated by CT and MRI using both sagittal and cross-sectional reconstruction. Patients with posterior column disease but without cord compression are often best managed by radiation therapy alone. Pa-

TABLE 20–9

Treatment of Metastases to Spine

Anterior Column	Middle Column	Posterior Column
1. Radiation alone 2. RT, pedicle fixation, posterior instrumentation (prevent collapse) 3. RT, anterior decompression and stabilization with body replacement (thoracic spine with limited posterior involvement) 4. RT, pedicle fixation, posterior instrumentation, total laminectomy (stage I); anterior decompression and stabilization with body replacement (stage 2) (anterior and posterior involvement)	1. Radiation alone 2. RT, pedicle fixation, posterior instrumentation, total laminectomy with transpedicular decompression	1. Radiation alone 2. RT, total laminectomy (facets intact) 3. RT, pedicle fixation, posterior instrumentation, total laminectomy with transpedicular decompression (facets and pedicles involved)

RT, external beam radiation therapy.

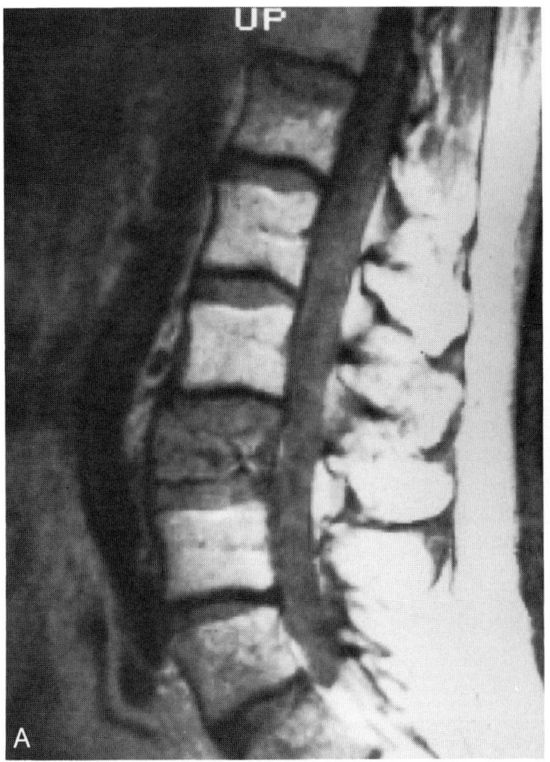

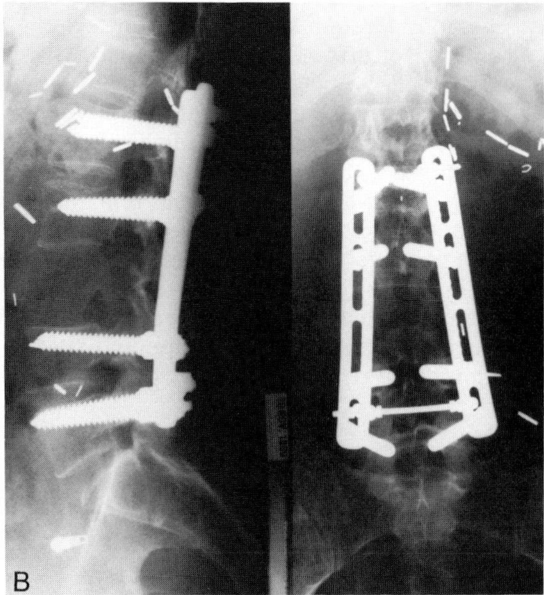

FIGURE 20–13. A marrow-replacing lesion in the body of L3 with little compromise of the neural canal. *A*, T1 sagittal magnetic resonance imaging (MRI) view of the lumbar spine. A nephrectomy for renal cell carcinoma was performed previously. After completion of radiotherapy, decompression of the region of L3 and stabilization of the spine using pedicle screw fixation and plates was elected. *B*, AP and lateral films of the lumbar spine taken 18 months later reveal complete replacement of the body of L3 without loss of fixation. The patient remained ambulatory and experienced only minor pain and no neurologic deficit until the time of his death at age 47.

tients with evidence of posterior cord compression may require posterior decompression without internal stabilization if the facet joints remain intact. If the facet joints are either unilaterally or bilaterally involved or destroyed, pedicle screw fixation and stabilization above and below the involved segment is indicated.

Patients with primary involvement of the middle column often have neurologic compromise. Occasionally, radiation therapy alone suffices for treatment, especially for metastases in the lumbar spine below the level of the conus. Most often, however, the patient requires stabilization above and below the involved vertebrae with pedicle screw fixation followed by a complete laminectomy and removal of the involved pedicle and decompression of the tumor mass (Fig. 20–13).

Most patients with anterior column involvement have an anterior compression deformity and evidence of an anterior extradural tumor mass on MRI. Many of these patients require either an anterior procedure alone or a combined anteroposterior procedure and stabilization.[44, 45] If possible, the lesion should be treated with external beam radiation therapy before the intended operative procedure. In patients with markedly compromised health, preoperative radiation therapy followed by posterior decompression *with reduction* of the compression deformity and posterior stabilization using pedicle fixation may produce superior results with minimal, acceptable postoperative morbidity[4, 15] (Fig. 20–14).

TREATMENT OF LATE METASTASES

Some patients, notably those with a renal or a gastrointestinal primary tumor, may develop only a single isolated metastasis 18 to 24 months after surgical therapy for the primary tumor. If restaging studies, including bone scintigraphy, routine chest radiography, and CT of the abdomen and chest, indicate that the patient remains otherwise free of disease, careful consideration should be given to radical surgical efforts to rid the patient of disease.

Cellular kinetics suggest that, if only one lesion is radiographically identifiable 2 years after removal of the primary lesion, the lesion seen may be the only metastasis remaining. Consideration should be given to treating the lesion aggressively for cure rather than palliation (Fig. 20–15); in reality, only some of these patients are cured. However, even if the procedure is not curative, most patients experience improved overall survival.[3, 48]

Survival

Survival after pathological fracture varies with the type of the primary tumor. Patients with carcinoma of the lung rarely survive longer than 1 year and often do not survive 6 months, whereas patients with carcinoma of the thyroid commonly live 5 years or longer. In general, approximately 50% of patients sustaining a pathologic fracture survive longer than 6 months and approximately 30% survive 1 year.[33] As the ability to manage the primary tumor through the use of chemotherapy, radiation therapy, and surgery improves, a corresponding increase in postfracture survival time necessitates improved surgical methods and the development of implants to better manage these patients.

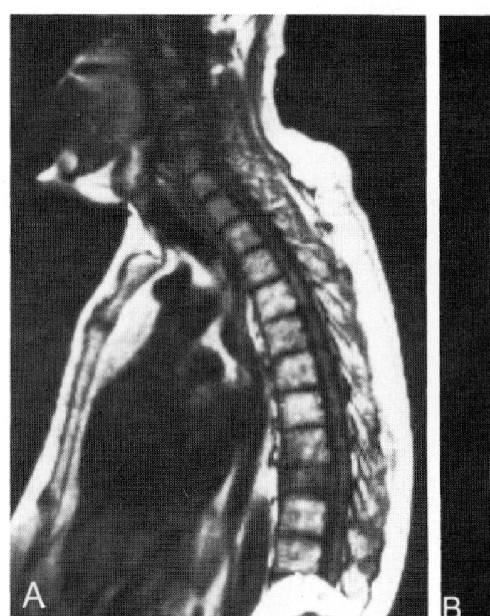

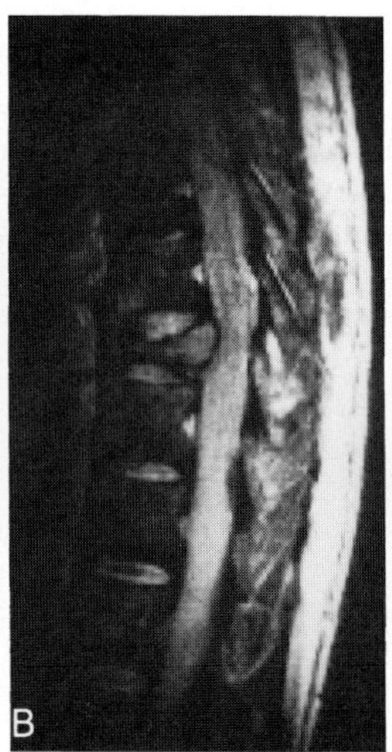

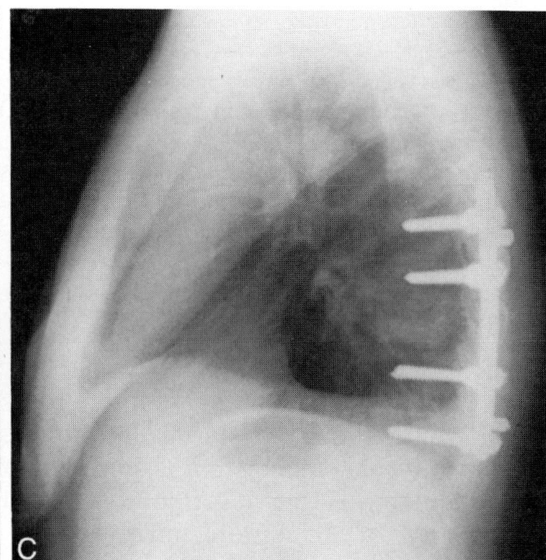

FIGURE 20–14. A 56-year-old man with known carcinoma of the lung. *A*, T1 sagittal reconstruction of the MRI scan shows complete marrow replacement of the body of T10 with slight posterior displacement. The patient had no neurologic deficit. *B*, The T2-weighted image shows some loss of anatomic detail as expected; however, the posterior protrusion of a portion of the body of T10 can be seen. *C*, Because of other evidence of metastatic disease and advancing pulmonary compromise, the patient elected to avoid a transpleural approach to the body of T10 and to proceed with a posterior decompression, reduction, and pedicle screw and plate fixation. The patient remained without pain and was without neurologic complications until his death 8 months later.

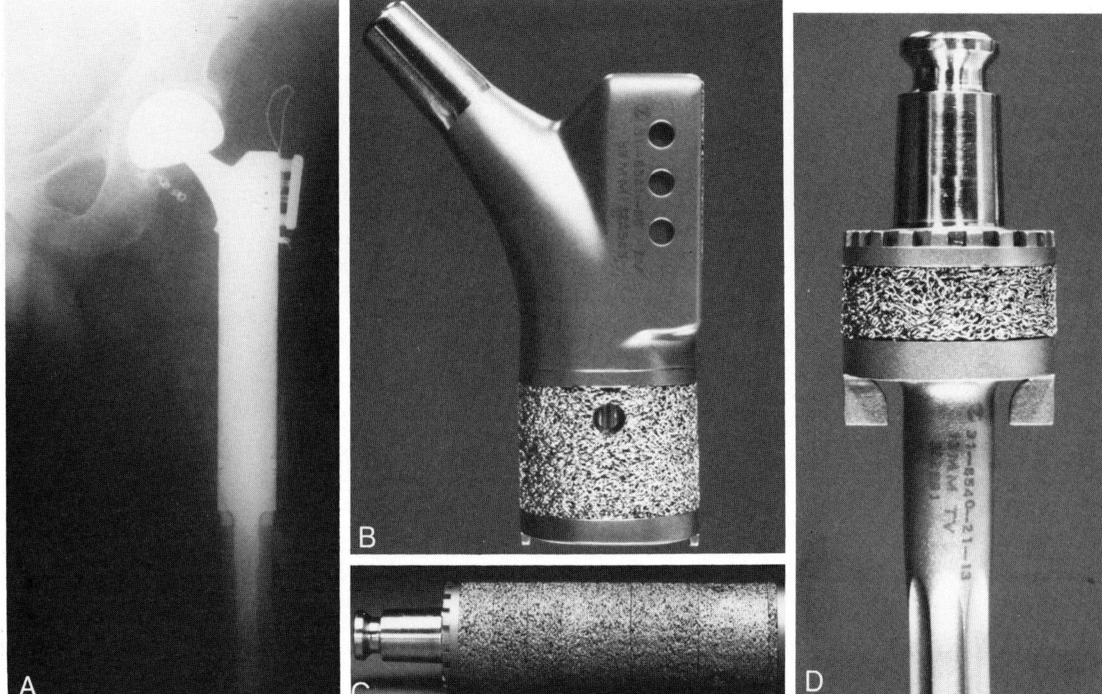

FIGURE 20–15. A 53-year-old man developed pain in his left hip 3 years after a left nephrectomy for renal cell carcinoma. A bone scan, plain films of the chest, and a CT scan of the chest and abdomen revealed no other areas of potential metastasis. *A*, After preoperative radiation therapy and angiographic embolization, 185 mm of the proximal femur was radically resected and reconstructed using a modular titanium femoral prosthesis. The abductor musculature was reattached to a laterally placed fiber-metal pad in the region of the greater trochanter with a titanium clamp as shown. *B*, The modular portion of the titanium femoral prosthesis, which accommodates varying sizes of prosthetic femoral heads and acetabular cups. *C*, Modular titanium spacers with mechanically attached fiber-metal of different lengths may be interconnected to the other modular components with a 4-degree conical couple and locking screws. The conical couple provides the structural integrity and allows modulation of the design. *D*, An intramedullary stem (available in various diameters) accommodates the diameter of the femoral intramedullary canal and is secured using methyl methacrylate. A coronally positioned keel is provided to resist rotatory forces. The patient remained otherwise free of disease 18 months after reconstruction and used a cane in his right upper extremity.

Conclusion

The treatment of patients with pathologic fractures has progressed significantly over the past 15 years with the addition of better supportive and occasionally curative chemotherapy, radiation therapy, and surgery. A significant improvement has been realized through the use of better biomaterials, implant design and construction, and their application. The use of methyl methacrylate has provided better fixation and stress distribution to previously inoperable fractures. The philosophy of early management of impending pathologic fractures using radiotherapy either alone or with surgery and more frequent follow-up has reduced the pain and morbidity commonly associated with the management of these patients.

References

1. Anderson JT, Erickson JM, Thompson RC Jr, Chao EY: Pathologic femoral shaft fractures comparing fixation techniques using cement. Clin Orthop 131:273, 1978.
2. Arguello F, Baggs RB, Duerst RE, Johnstone L, McQueen K, Frantz CN: Pathogenesis of vertebral metastasis and epidural spinal cord compression. Cancer 65:98–106, 1990.
3. Bowers TA, Murray JA, Charnsangavej C, Soo C-S, Chuang VP, Wallace S: Bone metastases from renal carcinoma. J Bone Joint Surg 64A:749–754, 1982.
4. Bridwell KH, Jenny AB, Saul T, Rich KM, Grubb RL: Posterior segmental spinal instrumentation (PSSI) with posterolateral decompression and debulking for metastatic thoracic and lumbar spine disease. Limitations of the technique. Spine 13:1383–1394, 1989.
5. Burtis WJ, Brady TG, Orloff JJ, Ersbak JB, Warrell RP, Olson BR, Wu TL, Mitnick ME, Broadus AE, Stewart AF: Immunochemical characterization of circulating parathyroid hormone–related protein in patients with humoral hypercalcemia of cancer. N Engl J Med 322:1106–1112, 1990.
6. Calo L, Cantaro S, Bertzarro L, Vianello A, Vido L, Borsatti I: Synthesis and catabolism of PGE_2 by a neuroblastoma associated with hypercalcemia without bone metastases. Cancer 54:635, 1984.
7. Cavanough PG, Nicolson GL: Purification and some properties of a lung-derived growth factor that differentially stimulates the growth of tumor cells metastatic to the lung. Cancer Res 49:3928–3933, 1989.
8. Chackal-Roy M, Niemeyer C, Moore M, Zetter BR: Stimulation of human prostatic carcinoma cell growth by factors present in human bone marrow. J Clin Invest 84:43–50, 1989.
9. Clark CR, Keggi KJ, Panjabi MM: Methylmethacrylate stabilization of the cervical spine. J Bone Joint Surg 66A:40–46, 1984.
10. Eftekhar NS, Thurston CW: Effect of irradiation on acrylic cement with special reference to fixation of pathological fractures. J Biomech 8:53, 1975.
11. Ewing J: A Treatise on Tumors, 3rd ed. Philadelphia, WB Saunders Co, 1928.
12. Fidler M: Prophylactic internal fixation of secondary neoplastic deposits in long bones. Br Med J 1:341, 1973.
13. Fidler IJ, Hart IR: Biological diversity in metastatic neoplasms: Origins and implications. Science 217:998, 1982.
14. Fidler IJ, Kripke ML: Metastasis results from preexisting variant cells within a malignant tumor. Science 197:893, 1977.
15. Flatley TJ, Anderson MH, Anast GT: Spinal instability due to malignant disease. Treatment by segmental spinal stabilization. J Bone Joint Surg 66A:47–52, 1984.
16. Folkman J: Tumor angiogenesis. Adv Cancer Res 43:175, 1985.
17. Francis KC: The role of amputation in the treatment of metastatic bone cancer. Clin Orthop 73:61, 1970.
18. Garrett IR, Durie BGM, Edwin GE, et al: Production of lymphotoxin, a bone-resorbing cytokine by cultured human myeloma cells. N Engl J Med 317:526–532, 1987.
19. Gullino PM, Grantham F: The vascular space of growing tumors. Cancer Res 24:1727, 1964.
20. Harrington KD: Current concepts review. Metastatic disease of the spine. J Bone Joint Surg 68A:110–1115, 1986.
21. Harrington KD, Johnston JO, Turner RH, Green DL: The use of methylmethacrylate as an adjunct in the internal fixation of malignant neoplastic fractures. J Bone Joint Surg 54A:1665, 1972.
22. Harrington KD, Sim FH, Enis JE, Johnston JO, Dick HM, Gristina AG: Methylmethacrylate as an adjunct in internal fixation of pathological fractures. J Bone Joint Surg 58A:1047, 1976.
23. Helikson MA, Hrvey AD, Zerwekh JE, et al: Plasma cell granuloma producing calcitriol and hypercalcemia. Ann Intern Med 105:379–381, 1986.
24. Hynes RO: Integrins: A family of cell surface receptors. Cell 48:549, 1987.
25. Insogna KL, Weir EC, Wu TL, et al: Co-purification of transforming growth factor beta–like activity with PTH-like and bone-resorbing activities from a tumor associated with hypercalcemia of malignancy. Endocrinology 120:2183–2185, 1987.
26. Janssen HF, Robertson WW, Berlin S: Venous drainage of the femur permits passage of 100-μm particles. J Orthop Res 6:671–675, 1988.
27. Koscielny S, Tubiana M, Valleron A-J: A simulation model of the natural history of human breast cancer. Br J Cancer 52:515, 1985.
28. Lagier R, Baud CA, Arnaud G, Arnaud S, Menk R: Lesions characteristic of infection or malignant tumour in Paleo-Eskimo skulls. Virchows Arch (Pathol Anat) 395:237–243, 1982.
29. Leeson MC, Makley JT, Carter JR: Metastatic disease distal to the elbow and knee. Clin Orthop 206:94–99, 1986.
30. Liotta LA: Tumor invasion and metastases: Role of the extracellular matrix. Rhoads Memorial Award Lecture. Cancer Res 46:1, 1986.
31. Liotta LA, Thorgeirsson UP, Garbisa S: Role of collagenases in tumor cell invasion. Cancer Metastasis Rev 1:277, 1982.
32. Manabe S, Tateishi A, Abe M, Ohno T: Surgical treatment of metastatic tumors of the spine. Spine 14:41–47, 1989.
33. Marcove RC, Yang D-J: Survival times after treatment of pathologic fractures. Cancer 20:2154, 1967.
34. Marx JL: Cell growth control takes balance. Res News 239:975–976, 1988.
35. McBroom RJ, Cheal EJ, Hayes WC: Strength reductions from metastatic cortical defects in long bones. J Orthop Res 6:369–378, 1988.
36. Menck H, Schulze S, Larsen E: Metastasis size in pathologic femoral fractures. Acta Orthop Scand 59:151–154, 1988.
37. Mundy GR, Martin TJ: The hypercalcemia of malignancy: Pathogenesis and management. Metabolism 31:1247, 1982.
38. Mundy GR, Ibbotson KJ, D'Souza M, Simpson EL, Jacobs JW, Martin TJ: The hypercalcemia of cancer: Clinical implications and pathogenic mechanisms. N Engl J Med 310:1718, 1984.
39. Murray JA, Bruels MC, Lindberg RD: Irradiation of polymethylmethacrylate. *In vitro* gamma radiation effect. J Bone Joint Surg 56A:311, 1974.
40. Paget S: The distribution of secondary growths in cancer of the breast. Lancet 1:571–573, 1889.
41. Parrish FF, Murray JA: Surgical treatment for secondary neoplastic fractures. J Bone Joint Surg 52A:665, 1970.
42. Ryan JR, Rowe DE, Salciccioli GG: Prophylactic

internal fixation of the femur for neoplastic lesions. J Bone Joint Surg 58A:1071, 1976.
43. Schirrmacher V: Cancer metastasis: Experimental approaches, theoretical concepts, and impacts of treatment strategies. Adv Cancer Res 43:1, 1985.
44. Siegal T: Vertebral body resection of epidural compression by malignant tumors. Results of forty-seven consecutive operative procedures. J Bone Joint Surg 67A:375–382, 1985.
45. Siegal T, Siegal T: Current considerations in the management of neoplastic spinal cord compression. Spine 14:223–228, 1989.
46. Silverberg E, Boring CC, Squires TS: Cancer Statistics, 1990. CA 40:9–25, 1990.
47. Stein CA, LaRocca R, Myers C: Suramin: An old compound with new biology. Prin Pract Oncol 4:1–12, 1990.
48. Stener B, Henriksson C, Johansson S, Gunterberg B, Pettersson S: Surgical removal of bone and muscle metastases of renal cancer. Acta Orthop Scand 55:491–500, 1984.
49. Stewart AF, Wu TL, Burtis WJ, et al: The relative potency of a human tumor-derived PTH-like adenylate cyclase–stimulating preparation in three bioassays. J Bone Miner Res 2:37–43, 1987.
50. Stubbs BE, Matthews LS, Sonstegard DA: Experimental fixation of fractures of the femur with methylmethacrylate. J Bone Joint Surg 57A:317–321, 1975.
51. Sutherland RM: Cell and environment interactions in tumor microregions. The multicell spheroid model. Science 240:177–240, 1988.
52. Tarlov IM: Spinal cord compression studies. III Time limits for recovery after gradual compression in dogs. Arch Neurol Psychiatry 71:588, 1954.
53. Tarlov IM, Klinger H: Spinal cord compression studies, II. Time limits for recovery after acute compression in dogs. Arch Neurol Psychiatry 71:271, 1954.
54. Tashjian AH, Voelkel EF, Lazzaro M, et al: Alpha and beta transforming growth factors stimulating prostaglandin production and bone resorption in cultured mouse calvaria. Proc Natl Acad Sci USA 82:4535–4538, 1985.
55. Torma T: Malignant tumors of the spine and the spinal epidural space. A study based on 250 histologically verified cases. Acta Chir Scand 225:1, 1957.
56. Ushio Y, Posner R, Kim J, et al: Treatment of experimental spinal cord compression caused by extradural neoplasms. J Neurosurg 47:380, 1977.
57. Ushio Y, Posner R, Posner JB, Shapior WR: Experimental spinal cord compression by epidural neoplasms. Neurology 27:422, 1977.
58. Wang G-J, Reger SI, Maffeo C, McLaughlin RE, Stamp WG: The strength of metal reinforced methylmethacrylate fixation of pathologic fractures. Clin Orthop 135:287, 1978.
59. Wells C: Ancient Egyptian pathology. J Laryngol Otol 77:261–265, 1963.
60. Wirth CR: Metastatic bone cancer. Curr Probl Cancer 3:3, 1979.
61. Zickel RE, Mouradian WH: Intramedullary fixation of pathological fractures and lesions of the subtrochanteric region of the femur. J Bone Joint Surg 58A:1061, 1976.

CHAPTER 21

Metabolic Mimickers of Tumor

MARK S. BROMSON
THOMAS A. EINHORN

Under certain circumstances, metabolic bone disease may simulate neoplasia. Although it is usually noticed incidentally as generalized osteopenia, metabolic bone disease may first appear as focal or multifocal bone lesions, which are radiographically difficult to distinguish from primary or metastatic bone tumors. Although misdiagnosis may lead only to a delay in proper treatment, it may also eventuate in unnecessary limb salvage procedures or even amputations. It is therefore crucial for the orthopedic surgeon to be familiar with those bone diseases, metabolic or otherwise, that may mimic bone tumors. This familiarity prevents unnecessary biopsies, inappropriate therapy, and unjustified anguish for the patient.

This chapter does not provide a comprehensive overview of the variety of metabolic conditions. Rather, it concentrates on those aspects of commonly occurring metabolic diseases that may simulate bone neoplasms.

Osteoporosis

Osteoporosis can be defined pathologically as "an absolute decrease in the amount of bone, leading to fracture after minimal trauma."[21] It is the most prevalent metabolic bone disease, causing approximately 1.2 million fractures per year in the United States. These fractures are distributed as follows: the vertebrae, 538,000 cases per year; the hip, 227,000 cases per year; the distal radius, 172,000 cases per year; and other sites in the extremities, 283,000 cases per year.[13]

Two distinct syndromes of involutional osteoporosis have been identified.[20] Type I, known as postmenopausal osteoporosis, occurs most commonly 15 to 20 years after menopause in women. It mainly affects trabecular bone and is clinically associated with vertebral crush fractures and distal radial fractures. Type II, known as senile osteoporosis, occurs in men and women older than age 70 years, with a female/male ratio of 2:1. It affects cortical and trabecular bone equally and is clinically associated with vertebral wedge fractures, femoral neck fractures, and intertrochanteric hip fractures.[7]

Osteoporotic fractures may mimic destructive neoplasms such as metastatic carcinoma or multiple myeloma. Casey and colleagues reported a series of 8 women with 12 parasymphyseal insufficiency fractures of the os pubis.[1] Even though the fractures had a benign cause, radiographs revealed deceptively destructive

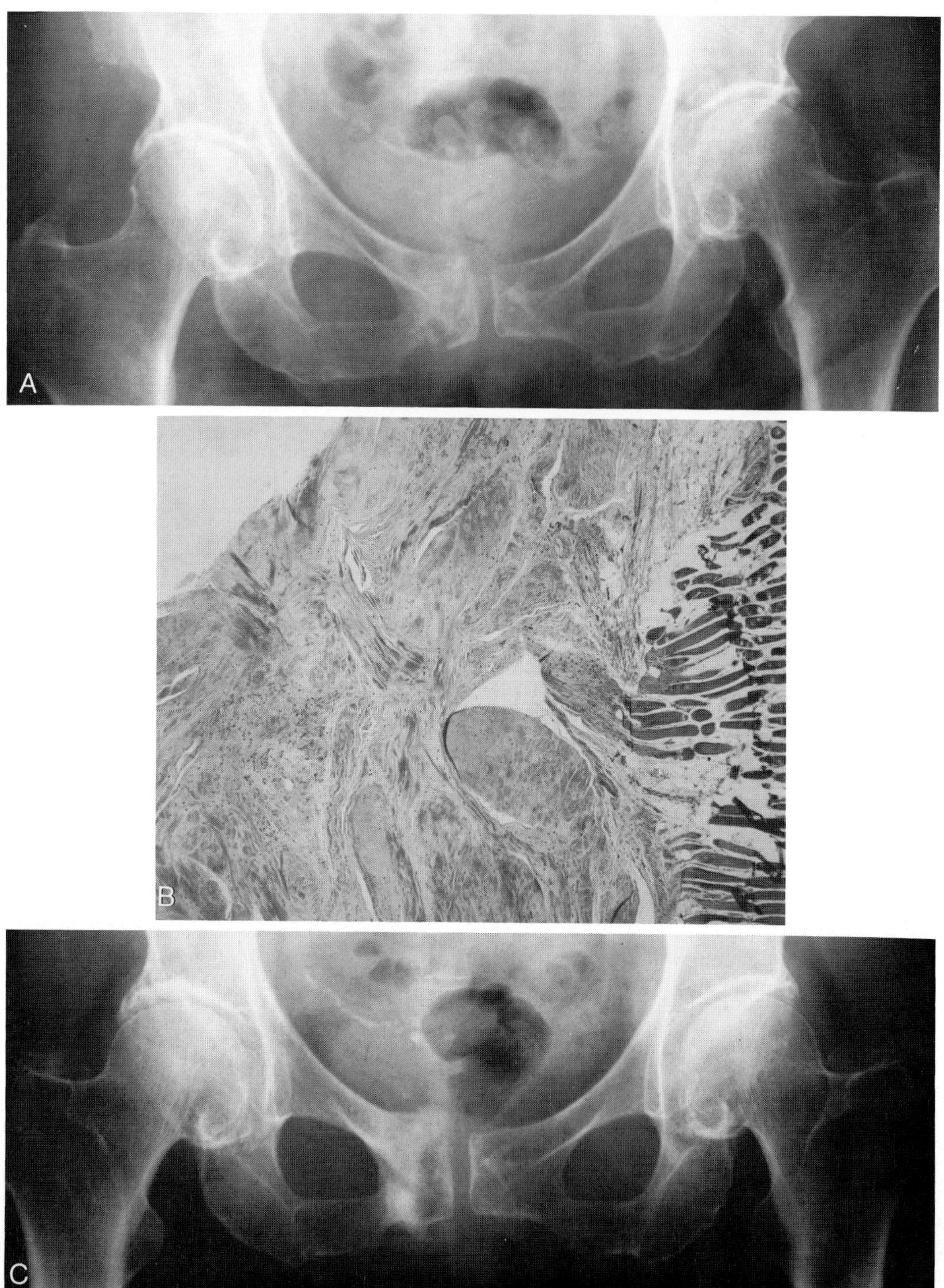

FIGURE 21–1. Parasymphyseal insufficiency fracture of the os pubis. *A,* Radiograph of the pubic symphysis of a 78-year-old white woman with spontaneous onset of pelvic pain. Note the presence of a lytic lesion of the right pubis and the associated fracture. *B,* Biopsy was performed to rule out primary neoplasm or metastatic disease. The tissue was found to consist of normal fibrocartilage with no evidence of tumor. *C,* Follow-up radiograph 1 year later showed sclerosis and healing of the fracture.

and malignant-appearing lesions because the patients were seen initially during the healing phase, when there are varying degrees of lysis and callus formation (a typical presentation is shown in Figure 21–1). Bone scan was performed in three patients and revealed localized increased uptake. Six patients underwent biopsy (two underwent biopsy twice). One patient even had a radical excision of the left pubic bone for what was a preliminary diagnosis of chondrosarcoma. Gacetta and Yandow reported a case of a 61-year-old woman after total abdominal hysterectomy, bilateral salpingo-oophorectomy, and postoperative irradiation for stage V-1B leiomyosarcoma of the uterus, who had sacrococcygeal pain and was thought to have metastatic leiomyosarcoma.[8] Radiographs revealed osteopenia without evidence of fracture. A bone scan showed an H-shaped pattern of activity over the sacrum, which is highly characteristic of osteoporotic sacral fractures.[19] Computed tomography scan confirmed the presence of a sacral fracture.

The patients in these examples were all postmenopausal women older than age 50 years whose osteopenia was evidenced on radiographs. The presence of these factors should alert the physician to the possibility of osteoporotic fractures and prevent unnecessary surgery.

Disuse Osteoporosis

Disuse osteoporosis may occur after immobilization (posttraumatic) or voluntary limitation of use. In 1969, Jones described four different radiologic patterns of disuse osteoporosis[9]: generalized, or diffuse; speckled, or "spotty"; linear translucent bands; and cortical changes. In certain individuals these changes may "produce a very striking roentgen pattern of their medullary bone which may simulate neoplastic bone replacement."[12]

Joyce and Keats reported six cases of disuse osteoporosis characterized by diffuse and/or spotty medullary bone demineralization and cortical bone loss involving any of three layers—endosteal, intracortical, and subperiosteal[10] (Fig. 21–2). Kattapuram and associates reported 11 patients with posttraumatic osteoporosis of the humerus characterized by a permeative, moth-eaten pattern with cortical tunneling and endosteal scalloping.[11] Such lesions may be confused with malignant neoplasms unless the physician pays careful attention to the history and is aware of the radiographic patterns in disuse osteoporosis.

Osteomalacia

Osteomalacia can be defined as an accumulation of unmineralized osteoid on bone trabeculae as a result of impaired deposition of minerals.[7] It may be caused by vitamin D deficiency (owing to diet, malabsorption, or insufficient sunlight), impaired vitamin D synthesis (owing to liver disease, renal disease, or anticonvulsant therapy), hypophosphatasia, hypophosphatemia, and tumors.[7, 26] Clinically, the diagnosis is often difficult to make. Patients may have vague, generalized bone pain; multiple fractures; thoracic kyphosis; and deformity of the lower limbs.[4] Laboratory screening tests usually reveal elevated serum alkaline phosphatase activity and decreased calcium and phosphate levels. Radiographic examination reveals generalized osteopenia of both cortical and trabecular bone, with loss of the secondary trabeculae, prominence of the remaining primary trabeculae, and indistinct cortical margins. Pseudofractures (Milkman's pseudofractures, Looser's lines or zones) are pathognomonic of osteomalacia and appear as ribbon-like radiolucencies extending through one cortex and part of the medullary canal of long bones with some adjacent sclerosis.[18] These are typically symmetric and are usually seen in the axillary border of the scapula, the femoral neck and subtrochanteric region, the pubic and ischial rami, the ilium, and the ribs.[18, 26] Histologically, they represent unmineralized osteoid seams. Bone scans usually demonstrate generalized increased skeletal uptake, increased periarticular accumulations, prominent costochondral junctions, and symmetric bilateral focal uptake in the pseudofractures.[25] However, osteomalacia may mimic neoplastic disease on bone scans. There are case reports of patients with osteomalacia whose bone scans exhibited multiple areas of asymmetric focal uptake suggestive of skeletal metastases[25, 26] (Fig. 21–3). In these cases, however, radiographs demonstrated multiple pseudofractures, and the clinical history and laboratory screening test results were consistent with the diagnosis of osteomalacia.

Paget's Disease

Paget's disease (osteitis deformans) is a skeletal disorder of unknown cause and slight male

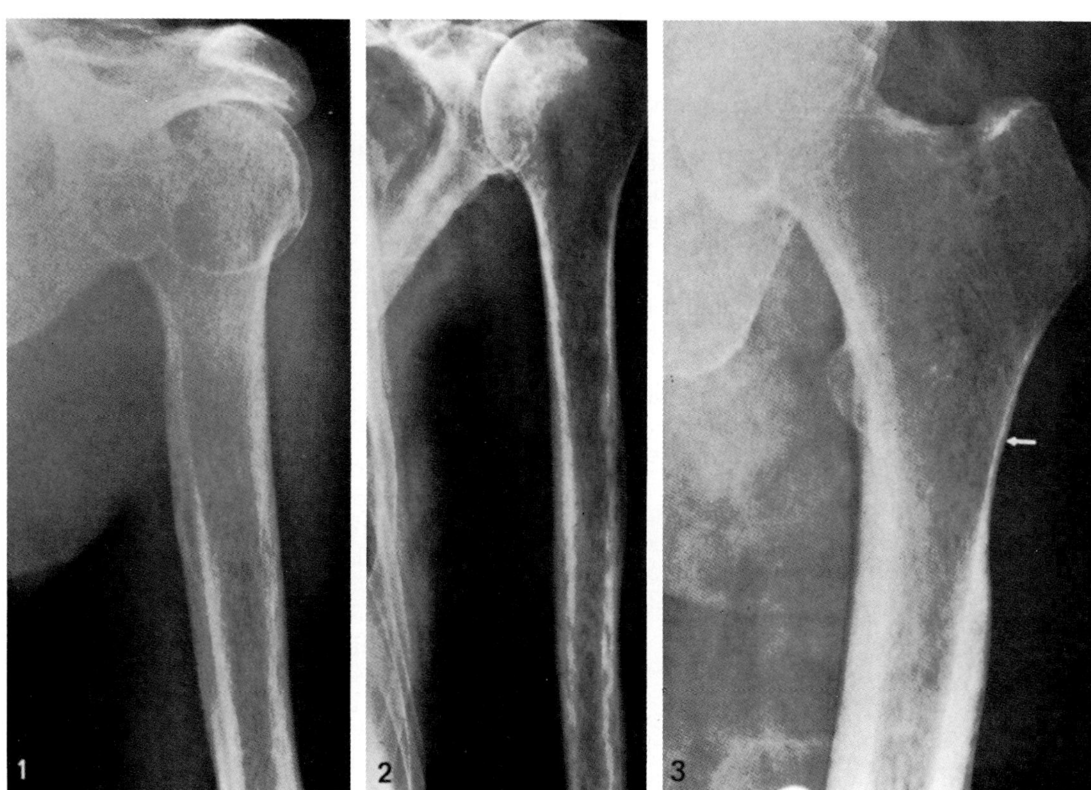

FIGURE 21–2. Disuse osteoporosis. *1,* Proximal humerus of a 58-year-old man with an 8-month history of left shoulder pain treated by immobilization, showing diffuse medullary demineralization, endosteal resorption, and intracortical tunneling. *2,* Proximal humerus of a 69-year-old man with left shoulder pain and restricted motion. The radiograph shows diffuse and spotty demineralization of the medullary bone and cortical resorption. *3,* Proximal femur of a 66-year-old man with left lower extremity weakness resulting from a stroke 2 years earlier. The radiograph reveals diffuse and spotty osteoporosis with cortical resorption of the proximal femur. Note the thinned cortex inferior to the greater trochanter (*arrow*). (From Joyce JM, Keats TE: Disuse osteoporosis: Mimic of neoplastic disease. Skeletal Radiol 15:130, 1986.)

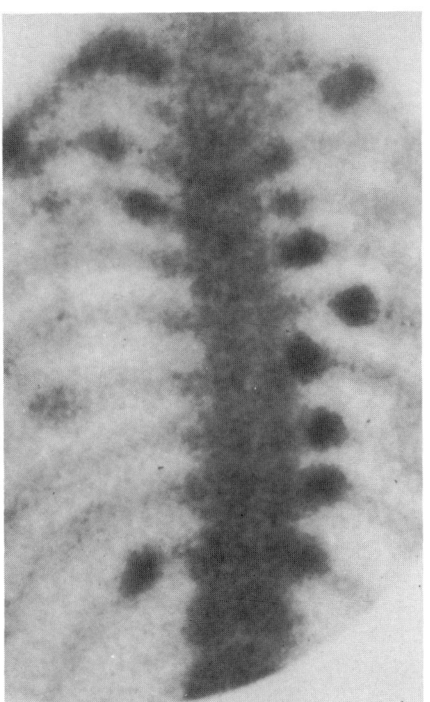

FIGURE 21–3. Bone scan of a patient with osteomalacia, demonstrating multiple asymmetric, abnormal focal areas of increased radionuclide accumulation. These sites correspond to pseudofractures in the ribs, mimicking skeletal metastases.

preponderance, which is found in 1 to 3% of elderly individuals.[3, 15, 22] The disease is usually mild or asymptomatic, although in severe cases it may produce intense pain.

Paget's disease may be monostotic or polyostotic. The monostotic form generally involves the tibia. The polyostotic form usually affects the sacrum and spine, followed in frequency by the femur, the skull, the sternum, the pelvis, the clavicle, the tibia, the ribs, and the scapula.[15] The primary abnormality is excessive bone resorption. Lesions progress through three phases: (1) an initial osteolytic phase, (2) a mixed osteolytic and osteoblastic phase, and (3) the inactive or osteoblastic sclerotic phase.[15, 22] Histologically, there are irregular broad trabeculae, multinucleated osteoclasts, irregular reversal or cement lines, and fibrous vascular connective tissue between the trabeculae. The resultant tilelike or mosaic pattern is characteristic of active Paget's disease.[2, 22]

Clinically, the most common symptoms are bone pain, deformity, and increased skin temperature. Pathologic fractures, arthritis, neural compression, and high-output congestive heart failure may also occur. The serum alkaline phosphatase activity and 24-hour urinary hydroxyproline levels may be elevated in polyostotic Paget's disease; in monostotic disease, these values are usually normal.[15]

Radiologically, Paget's disease may mimic neoplastic disease. In the early lytic phase, resorption of bone is prominent, and the resultant, well-demarcated areas may simulate primary tumors of bone (Fig. 21–4). On bone scan, the lesions appear "hot."[14] Although these lesions occur most commonly in the skull, where they are known as osteoporosis circumscripta, they may also be present elsewhere, where they can be misdiagnosed. The mixed phase is characterized by bone sclerosis and osseous demineralization, resulting in trabecular prominence, cortical thickening, and increased overall bone size and mass. In the final phase, homogeneous sclerosis is pro-

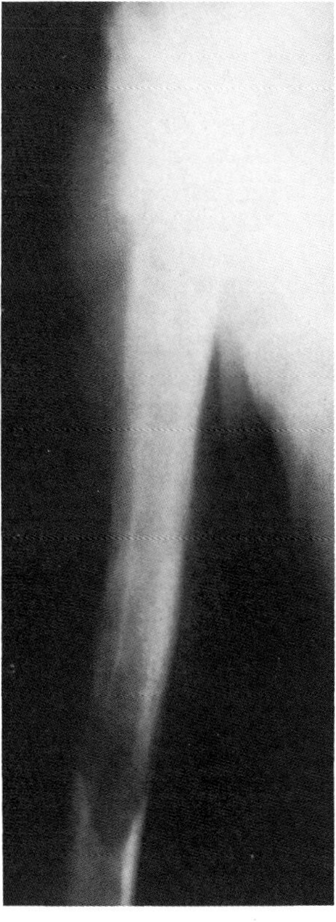

FIGURE 21–4. Radiograph of a humerus, demonstrating an advancing flame-shaped osteolytic wedge characteristic of early Paget's disease. (From Merkow RL, Lane JM: Current concepts of Paget's disease of bone. Orthop Clin North Am 15:749, 1984.)

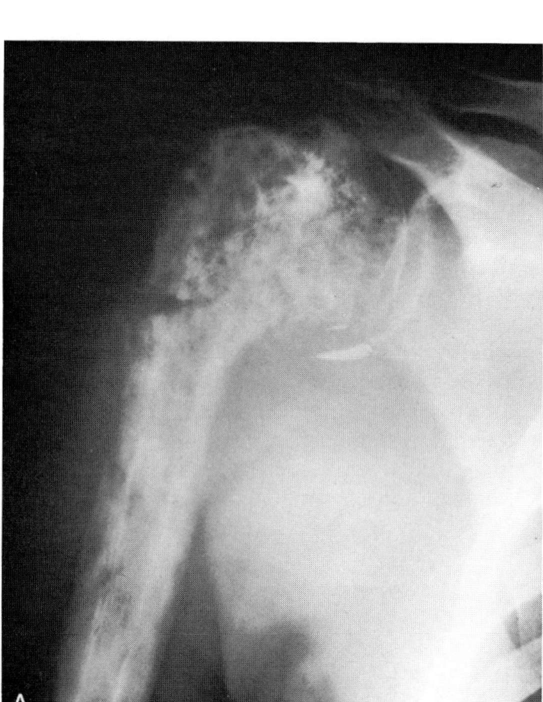

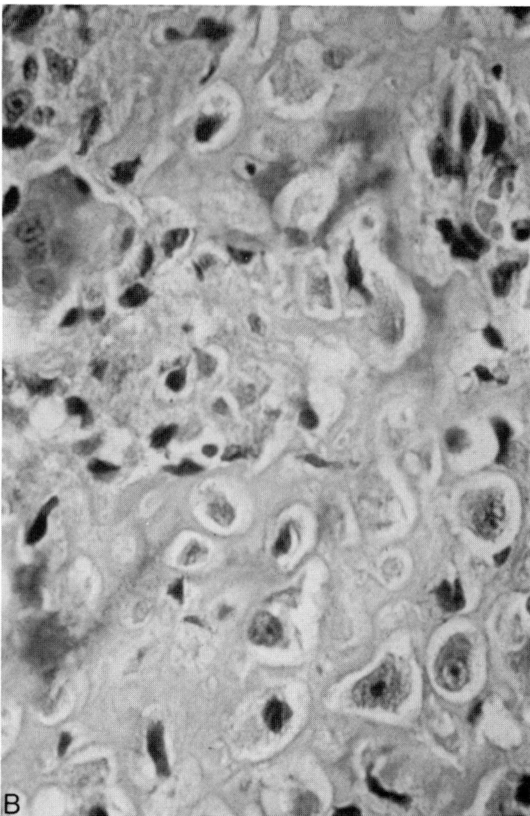

FIGURE 21–5. Paget's sarcoma. *A,* Radiograph of the proximal humerus of a 79-year-old man with long-standing Paget's disease. Two weeks before presentation, he had significantly increasing pain in the arm without antecedent trauma. Radiograph revealed a pathologic fracture. *B,* Photomicrograph of the biopsy specimen taken from this patient, demonstrating the marked cellularity, anaplastic fibrous tissue, giant cells, and osteoid trabeculae formation found in Paget's sarcoma.

nounced.[15] With diffuse involvement of the skeleton, differentiation of Paget's disease from osteoblastic metastases may be difficult. Enlargement of the affected bone is, however, strong evidence that the sclerosing lesion is a manifestation of Paget's disease.[2, 24]

Sometimes the radiologic picture is complicated by the development of bone sarcomas, which occur in less than 1% of all cases. Paget's sarcoma is characterized by increased pain, pathologic fracture, and radiographic evidence of cortical destruction, often associated with a soft tissue mass[23] (Fig. 21–5). The extensive changes induced by Paget's disease may, however, obscure the early signs of a superimposed malignancy. Florid cases of Paget's disease may, in turn, mimic Paget's sarcoma via excessive proliferation of benign periosteal new bone, producing a large soft tissue mass, which is often associated with an underlying pathologic fracture and radiographic evidence of bone destruction and spiculation[16] (Fig. 21–6). In such cases, biopsy is necessary to establish the diagnosis.

Hyperparathyroidism

Hyperparathyroidism, whether primary or secondary, can cause progressive resorption and destruction of bone. The incidence of bone lesions in this disease is reported to range from 10 to 15%[22] to as high as 30 to 40%.[5] Pathologically, the osseous lesions can be characterized as "a relative excess of osteoclastic over osteoblastic activity accompanied by fibrous replacement of the marrow."[22] In advanced cases, pronounced local resorption may lead to the formation of cystlike lesions called brown tumors, an unfortunate misnomer because these lesions are nonneoplastic.

Brown tumors appear grossly as well-demar-

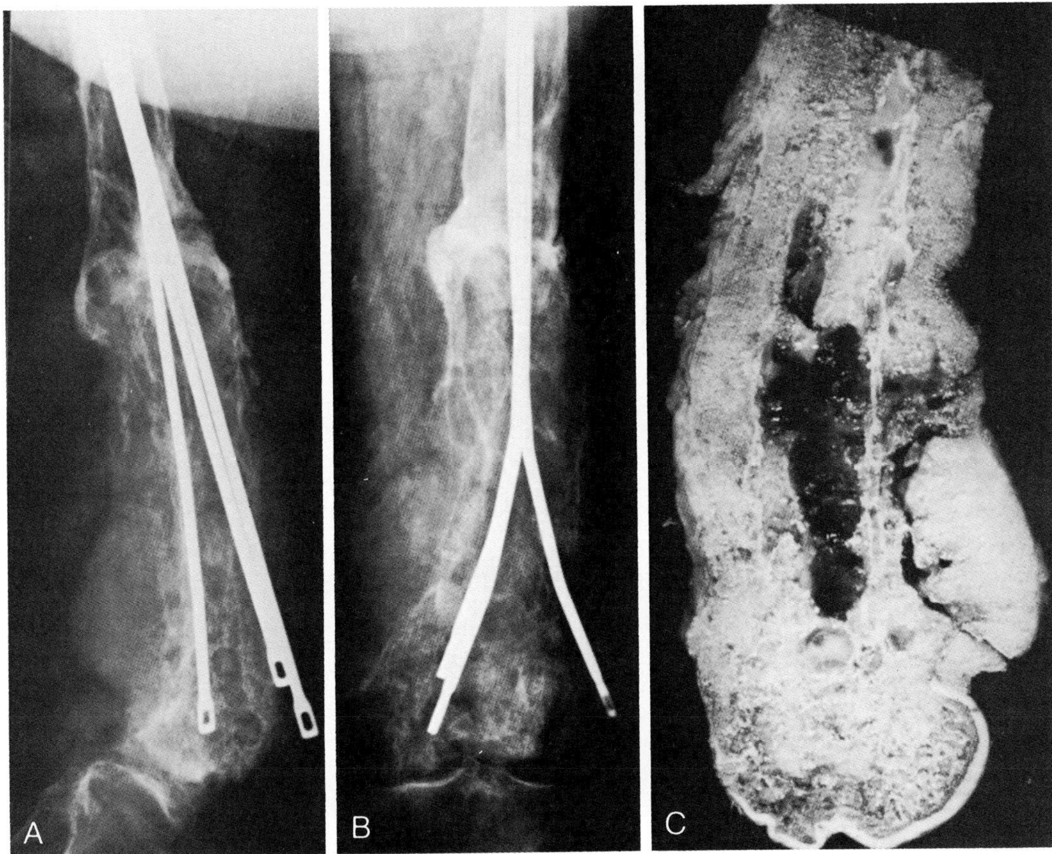

FIGURE 21–6. A 71-year-old man with Paget's disease and a pathologic fracture of the femoral diaphysis, which was treated successfully with Ender rods. Two years later, he was seen because of a gradual but marked increase in pain around the knee and thigh. *A, B,* Radiographs demonstrate a large soft tissue mass arising posteriorly from the distal metaphysis. Cortical destruction is present medially in the distal diaphysis and metaphysis. *C,* Photograph of a sagittal section of the surgical specimen, which was removed because of chronically disabling pain. Abundant formation of pagetic bone is present anterior and posterior to the original cortices without evidence of sarcomatous degeneration. (From Monson DK, et al: Pseudosarcoma in Paget disease of bone. A case report. J Bone Joint Surg 71A:454, 1989.)

cated, reddish-brown, soft masses with both hemorrhagic and cystic areas. Radiographically, brown tumors may mimic primary bone neoplasms, presenting as solitary or multifocal osteolytic lesions with generally indistinct margins and striations, often accompanied by cortical expansion and narrowing (Fig. 21–7*A*). They may be located in the diaphysis, the metaphysis, or rarely the epiphysis and can occur throughout the body, although the mandible, the pelvis, the ribs, and the femurs are most frequently affected.[6] More widespread involvement of the skeleton by hyperparathyroidism may simulate carcinomatosis or multiple myeloma.

Histologically, these lesions represent foci of hemorrhage, possibly caused by microfractures, that contain hemosiderin and an accumulation of macrophages, fibroblasts, and osteoclastic giant cells[22] (Fig. 21–7*B*). They may be difficult to distinguish from true giant cell tumors of bone, although the fibrous nature of the lesion or an atypical skeletal location should guide the pathologist to the correct diagnosis.[24]

Differentiating the skeletal lesions of hyperparathyroidism from other entities can be difficult if one does not suspect the correct diagnosis. In primary hyperparathyroidism, other radiographic findings are present, including subperiosteal resorption (most commonly in the distal phalanges of the hands and the inferolateral clavicle), generalized osteopenia, and chondrocalcinosis. Laboratory screening tests show increased serum calcium, alkaline phosphatase, and parathyroid hormone levels;

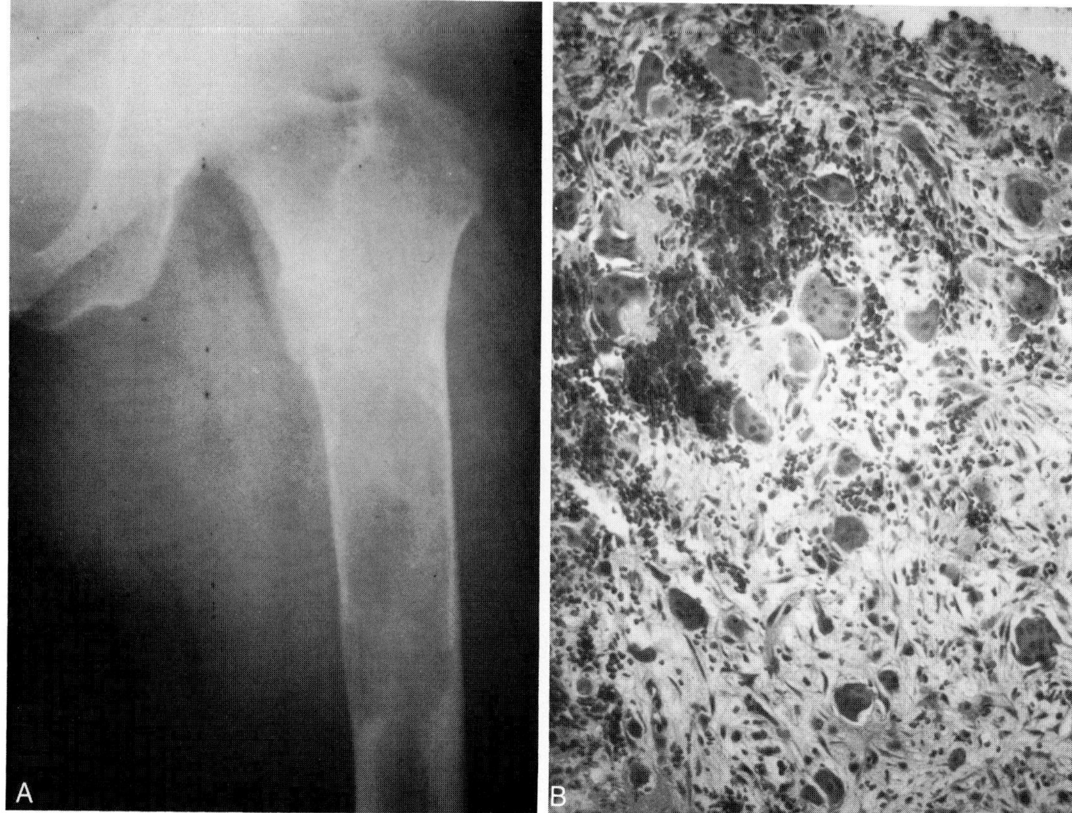

FIGURE 21-7. A 38-year-old woman with a history of parathyroid adenoma and recent onset of left thigh pain. At the time of parathyroidectomy, prophylactic intramedullary nailing of the femur was performed. *A,* Radiograph of the proximal femur revealed a central osteolytic lesion with cortical erosion. *B,* Biopsy specimen demonstrated foci of hemorrhage and large, multinucleated, osteoclastic giant cells embedded in a stroma of fibrous connective tissue. The fibrous background helps differentiate this lesion from giant cell tumor.

decreased serum phosphate levels; and increased urinary calcium excretion. In secondary hyperparathyroidism, similar radiographic findings are present, along with prominent areas of bone sclerosis, especially in the spine (rugger jersey pattern).[17] Laboratory screening tests show high levels of serum alkaline phosphatase and parathyroid hormone, low urinary calcium excretion, and usually a high serum phosphate level. The presence of these other findings can establish a definitive diagnosis, avoiding a biopsy.

Summary

Metabolic bone disease may produce a clinical picture easily confused with that of a malignant process. It is crucial for the physician to remain cognizant of this potential for mimicry to allow prompt and proper diagnosis, correct treatment, and the avoidance of unnecessary procedures with potentially tragic consequences.

References

1. Casey D, Mirra J, Staple TW: Parasymphyseal insufficiency fractures of the os pubis. Am J Radiol 142:581–586, 1984.
2. Dahlin DC, Unni KK: Bone Tumors: General Aspects and Data on 8,542 Cases, 4th ed. Springfield, IL, Charles C Thomas, 1986.
3. Dalinka MK, Aronchick JM, Haddad JG Jr: Paget's disease. Orthop Clin North Am 14:3–19, 1983.
4. Doppelt SH: Vitamin D, rickets, and osteomalacia. Orthop Clin North Am 15:671–686, 1984.
5. Edeiken J: Roentgen Diagnosis of Diseases of Bone, 3rd ed. Baltimore, Williams & Wilkins, 1981.
6. Ehrlich GW, Genant HK, Kolb FO: Secondary hyperparathyroidism and brown tumors in a patient with gluten enteropathy. Am J Radiol 141:381–383, 1983.

7. Einhorn TA: Evaluation and treatment methods in metabolic bone disease. Contemp Orthop 149:21–34, 1987.
8. Gacetta DJ, Yandow DR: Computed tomography of spontaneous osteoporotic sacral fractures. J Comput Assist Tomogr 8:1190–1191, 1984.
9. Jones G: Radiological appearances of disuse osteoporosis. Clin Radiol 20:345–353, 1969.
10. Joyce JM, Keats TE: Disuse osteoporosis: Mimic of neoplastic disease. Skeletal Radiol 15:129–132, 1986.
11. Kattapuram SV, Khurana JS, Ehara S, Ragozzino M: Aggressive posttraumatic osteoporosis of the humerus simulating a malignant neoplasm. Cancer 62:2525–2527, 1988.
12. Keats TE, Harrison RB: A pattern of post-traumatic demineralization of bone simulating permeative neoplastic replacement: A potential source of misinterpretation. Skeletal Radiol 3:113–114, 1978.
13. Kelsey JL: Osteoporosis: Prevalence and incidence. *In* Proceedings of the NIH Consensus Development Conference, April 2–4, 1984, pp 25–28.
14. Krane SM: Paget's disease of bone. Clin Orthop 127:24–36, 1977.
15. Merkow RL, Lane JM: Current concepts of Paget's disease of bone. Orthop Clin North Am 15:747–763, 1984.
16. Monson DK, Finn HA, Dawson PJ, Simon MA: Pseudosarcoma in Paget disease of bone. A case report. J Bone Joint Surg 71A:453–455, 1989.
17. Pitt M: Osteopenic bone disease. Orthop Clin North Am 14:65–80, 1983.
18. Reynolds WA, Karo JJ: Radiologic diagnosis of metabolic bone disease. Orthop Clin North Am 3:521–543, 1972.
19. Ries T: Detection of osteoporotic sacral fractures with radionuclides. Radiology 146:783–785, 1983.
20. Riggs BL, Melton LJ III: Evidence for two distinct syndromes of involutional osteoporosis. Am J Med 6:899, 1983.
21. Riggs BL, Melton LJ III: Involutional osteoporosis. N Engl J Med 314:1676, 1986.
22. Robbins SL, Cotran RS, Kumar V: Pathologic Basis of Disease, 3rd ed. Philadelphia, WB Saunders Company, 1984.
23. Schajowicz F, Araujo ES, Berenstein M: Sarcoma complicating Paget's disease of bone. A clinicopathological study of 62 cases. J Bone Joint Surg 65B:299–307, 1983.
24. Shives TC, Cooper KL, Wold LE: Lesions simulating tumors of bone. *In* Sim FH: Diagnosis and Treatment of Bone Tumors: A Team Approach. Thorofare, NJ, Slack, 1983, pp 153–189.
25. Singh BN, Kesala BA, Mehta SP, Quinn JL III: Osteomalacia on bone scan simulating skeletal metastases. Clin Nucl Med 5:181–183, 1977.
26. Velchik MG, Makler PT Jr, Alavi A: Osteomalacia. An impostor of osseous metastasis. Clin Nucl Med 10:783–785, 1985.

CHAPTER 22

Soft Tissue Sarcomas and Limb Sparing

CONSTANTINE P. KARAKOUSIS

The management of soft tissue sarcomas has undergone a dramatic change in the past 15 years. Before this time, surgical treatment was relied on exclusively for the treatment of localized sarcomas. Wide surgical margins were necessary to avoid local recurrence and often amputation was resorted to. In the period 1965 to 1975, at Roswell Park Memorial Institute (RPMI), 251 patients with localized soft tissue sarcomas were treated with surgery alone. Of the patients with extremity sarcomas, 40% underwent an amputation. The incidence of local recurrence at 5 years was 65% with local excision, 36% with wide excision, and 8% with amputation. The 5-year survival rate was 45% for lesions in all anatomic locations and 50% for the extremity sarcomas.[1]

In a report by Shiu and associates, reflecting the experience at Memorial Sloan-Kettering Cancer Center, the incidence of local recurrence after wide excision was 28% and the rate of amputation was about 50%.[19]

With compartmental resection, the rate of local recurrence could be reduced to 2%, whereas the local recurrence rate was 100% when inadequate margins were obtained.[21] However, compartmental resection is applicable primarily in the thigh.

In the mid-1970s, the results obtainable with surgical treatment alone were fairly standardized. There was a need to improve local control and to reduce the rate of amputations. Simultaneously, the concept of combination of modalities was becoming accepted. In theory, it contained the solution to this problem. Surgical excision could eliminate the macroscopic bulk of the tumor, while the adjuvant modality would destroy microscopic residual in the surrounding tissues. Such combination of modalities would permit more conservative surgery and therefore would increase the rate of limb salvage.

In fact, these expectations regarding limb salvage have been largely fulfilled. Limb preservation is now possible in about 95% of extremity sarcomas, with local control exceeding 90%.[11, 12] This has been achieved with the preoperative administration of intraarterial chemotherapy and radiation,[2, 3] radiation alone,[20] or the postoperative use of adjuvant radiation.[15] Preoperative administration of adjuvant modalities is justified on the rationale of decreasing the tumor mass, thereby rendering previously unresectable tumors resectable. Potential disadvantages of this approach are that wound-healing problems occasionally occur in a previously radiated field and that the decision to employ a combination of modalities has to be made preoperatively on the basis of the somewhat limited information provided by the physical and radiologic examination results alone.

Postoperative use of adjuvant modalities leaves the burden of resection of a large tumor, undiminished in size, to the surgeon, but has the advantage that wound-healing problems are decreased. In addition, the tissue planes remain distinct, the decision to use adjuvant treatment can be based on pathologic examination of the specimen and accurate evaluation of margins, and postoperative radiation can include a boost to the area of narrowest margins. For these reasons, the author prefers the postoperative use of adjuvant treatments. In the author's experience, the size of the tumor is not an important determinant of its resectability. With the exception of tumors involving the suprarenal aorta and the inferior vena cava or the spinal column, most tumors are resectable with the use of appropriate incisions, exposure, and technique of dissection.

The surgical treatment in the context of limb salvage has undergone an evolution. The attempt to perform *en bloc* resection is tempered by the need to preserve important functions of the extremity.

The surgical approach to limb salvage in various anatomic regions, as it has evolved at RPMI during the past 12 years, is described below.

Technical Aspects

Soft tissue sarcomas are most often noticed as a swelling by the patient, although pain or other symptoms of the increasing mass also appear not infrequently.

Given the known propensity of these tumors to metastasize preferentially to the lungs, a chest x-ray film is advisable. Computed tomography (CT) or magnetic resonance imaging (MRI) defines the extent and location of the lesion at the primary site. When the lesion is close to major vessels, an arteriogram may be desirable to define the relation of the tumor to the vessels, possible encroachment of the latter, and any major feeding branches supplying the tumor.

If the pathologist is experienced, a needle biopsy specimen may be sufficient in establishing the diagnosis. Often, an open, incisional biopsy is required to identify the specific histologic type and grade of the tumor. The biopsy incision, in the extremities, is usually longitudinal because it thus conforms with and can be easily encompassed in the incision of the definitive operation. The incision is usually placed over the most protuberant portion of the tumor. Care is taken not to expose major vessels or nerves because they thus become part of the contaminated biopsy track. The incision is deepened through the underlying tissues until the tumor is encountered, and a generous biopsy specimen is obtained. No flaps should be raised, so that the biopsy track can be easily encompassed and removed during the definitive procedure. Examination of frozen section of the biopsy specimen is advisable to ensure that representative, diagnostic tissue has been obtained.

In the definitive procedure, an elliptic incision is made around the biopsy incision and is extended for the full length of the corresponding compartment. Flaps are raised to beyond the palpable extent of the tumor. The CT scan, the MRI image, and palpation during the procedure provide good guidance as to how extensive the flaps should be. For a tumor apparently confined in a muscular compartment, the thin flaps are raised for a short distance only, sufficient to gain enough distance from the biopsy track, dissection thereafter continuing on the surface of the deep fascia.

An *en bloc* resection should always be performed. The specimen should be one piece, including the biopsy incision and track and the surrounding tissues with the tumor in the center.

Entry into the tumor or spillage should be scrupulously avoided. A wide margin in all directions around the tumor, in which the tissues can be removed without serious functional impairment, should be obtained. Certainly this applies to adipose tissue around the biopsy incision and tumor. Owing to overlapping in their activity and a remarkable functional reserve, muscles around the tumor can often be resected without substantial impairment in the function of the extremity. If a portion of a muscle is resected, a procedure that invalidates the function of this muscle, one might as well obtain extra margin without extra morbidity by removing the muscle from origin to insertion. Owing to the shape of the extremities and the orientation of their muscles, longitudinal incisions are preferable because they provide greater exposure and they interrupt fewer lymphatics (which also follow a longitudinal course in the subcutaneous fat of the extremity).

Discussion of sarcomas of the pelvic wall

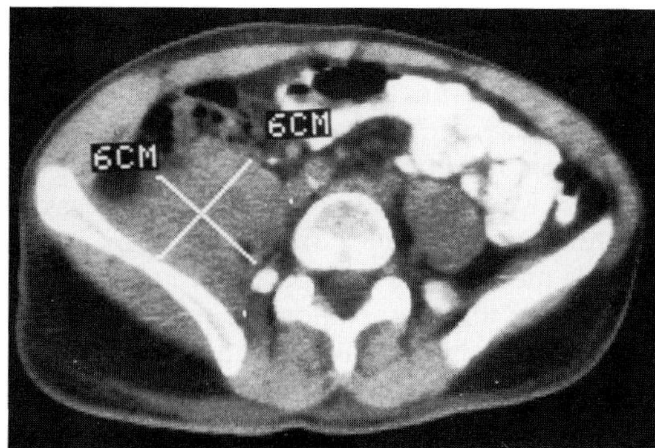

FIGURE 22–1. Malignant fibrohistiocytoma in the area of the right iliopsoas muscle. On one previous exploration this sarcoma was considered to be unresectable, and on another exploration it was considered to require hemipelvectomy.

and shoulder girdle is also included because these areas anatomically belong to the extremity and can be managed, if necessary, with a hemipelvectomy or forequarter amputation, respectively.

LOWER EXTREMITY

Pelvis and Groin

Soft tissue sarcomas in the area of the iliopsoas, the external iliac vessels, and the wall of the lesser pelvis (between the obturator nerve and the external iliac vein) and those involving by extension the pubic bone (Figs. 22–1 to 22–3) cannot be removed easily through the conventional abdominal incisions. These are often declared unresectable or they are managed with hemipelvectomy. Sarcomas in the groin, also owing to the frequent involvement of the vessels and the need often to resect a portion of the lower abdominal wall including the inguinal ligament, were also routinely believed in the past to necessitate an amputation.[21]

The reason for the "unresectability" of these tumors and the frequent need for hemipelvectomy in the past was the lack of effective techniques of exposure. The abdominoinguinal incision provided the answer for the exposure of the majority of the tumors in that area.[6, 7] This incision consists of a lower midline incision, which is then extended transversely from the pubic symphysis to the midinguinal point and then vertically for a few centimeters over the femoral vessels. The rectus abdominis muscle is transected from the pubic crest; the inguinal ligament is divided from the pubic tubercle and dissected from the femoral vessels by ligating and dividing the inferior epigastric vessels, its lateral third being dissected further from the iliac fascia. This incision provides an incontinuity exposure of the abdominal cavity with the groin on the affected side, including an incontinuity exposure of the iliac and femoral vessels. The iliopsoas muscle may be removed in its entirety. The femoral nerve is easily dissected lateral to the femoral artery and its relation to the tumor is defined (Fig. 22–4). The vessels may be included in an *en bloc* resection and replaced with vascular grafts (Fig. 22–5). The pubic bone may be resected *en bloc* with any soft tissue extension (Fig. 22–6). A defect in the lower abdominal wall, including the inguinal ligament, may be replaced with a mesh; one should interpose the mobilized sartorius or other muscle so that there is no direct contact between the mesh and the vessels to avoid possible erosion and bleeding from the latter. When there is a

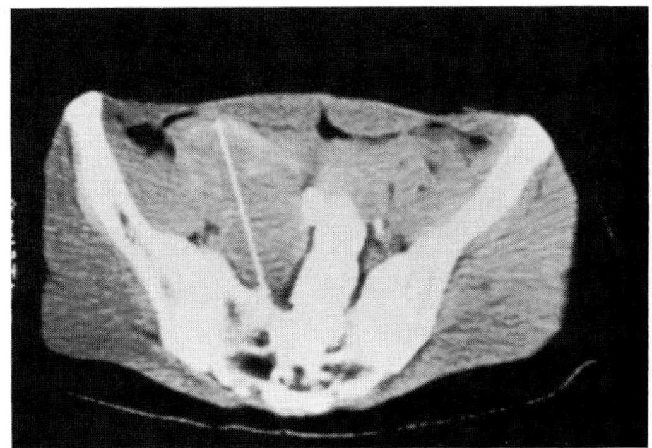

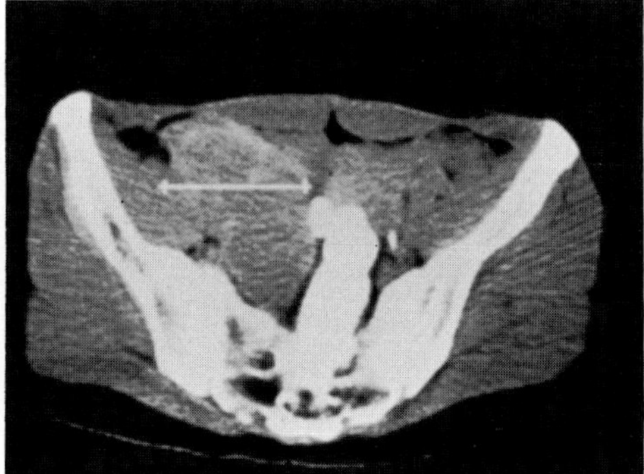

FIGURE 22–2. Fibrosarcoma involving the wall of the lesser pelvis, the right iliac artery, and the right ureter: it was declared unresectable on a previous exploration.

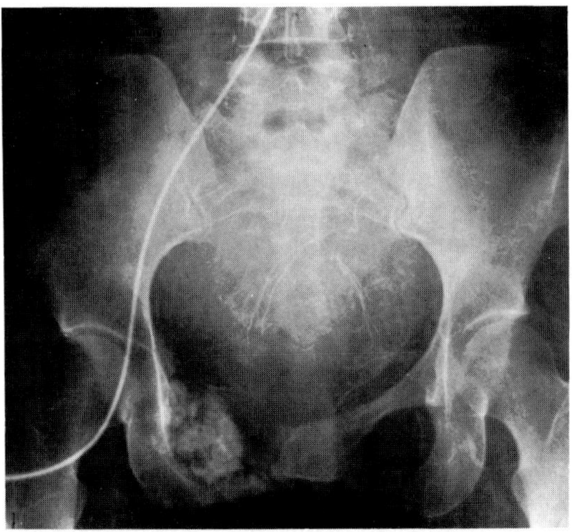

FIGURE 22–3. Recurrent chondrosarcoma in the right pubic bone.

concomitant skin defect, the contralateral rectus abdominis muscle with the posterior sheath, based on the inferior epigastric vessels, may be rotated to cover the defect with immediate application of a skin graft.

For soft tissue sarcomas involving by extension the iliac bone and possibly the acetabulum, internal hemipelvectomy (i.e., resection of the involved bone and soft tissues with preservation of the extremity) may be performed, as long as the blood supply and the two major nerves (i.e., sciatic and femoral) can be preserved[8] (Fig. 22–7). When the acetabulum is resected also, traction of the leg for about 3 weeks is required to avoid excessive shortening. Avoidance of weight bearing for about 3 months and then partial weight bearing for 3 more months is allowed, to be followed by full weight bearing. The leg becomes shorter by about 3 cm, necessitating the use of a shoe-lift (Fig. 22–8). There is normal movement at the ankle and knee joints, but no hip movement, and crutches are needed for ambulation on a permanent basis. When the iliac bone is removed above the acetabulum, no traction is required postoperatively, weight bearing is allowed more rapidly, and despite some shortening of the extremity, nearly normal ambulation is finally achieved without any external support.

Thigh and Buttock

In treating sarcomas of the anterior compartment, it is usually possible to preserve a small portion of the quadriceps muscle, this being often the distal third of the vastus medialis with intact nerve supply. In these cases, it is

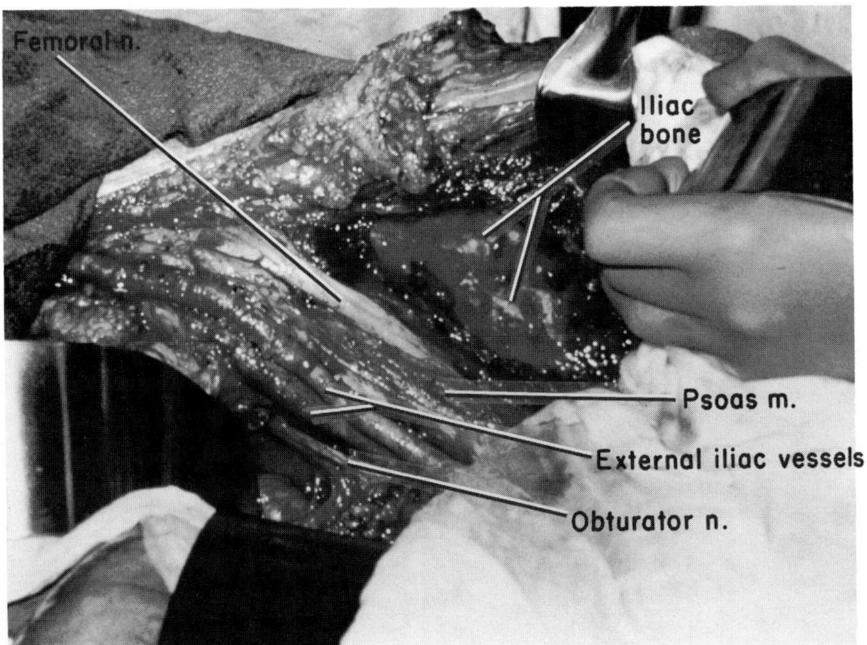

FIGURE 22–4. Operative field after resection of the sarcoma shown in Figure 22–1. The iliofemoral vessels and the femoral nerve are visible. The patient is well 6 years later.

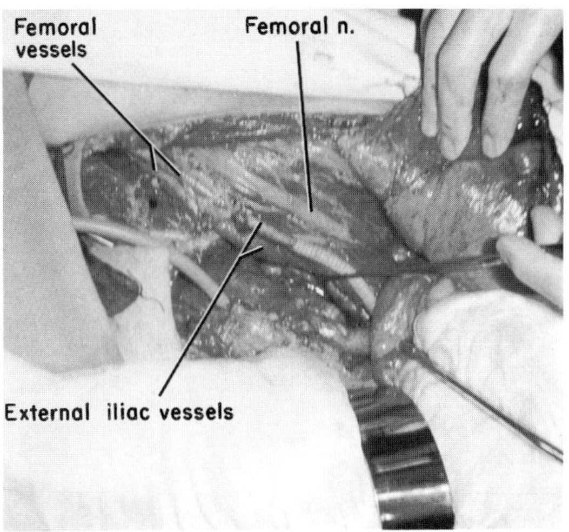

FIGURE 22–5. Operative field after resection of the tumor shown in Figure 22–2. The right iliac artery has been replaced with a polyester fiber (Dacron) graft.

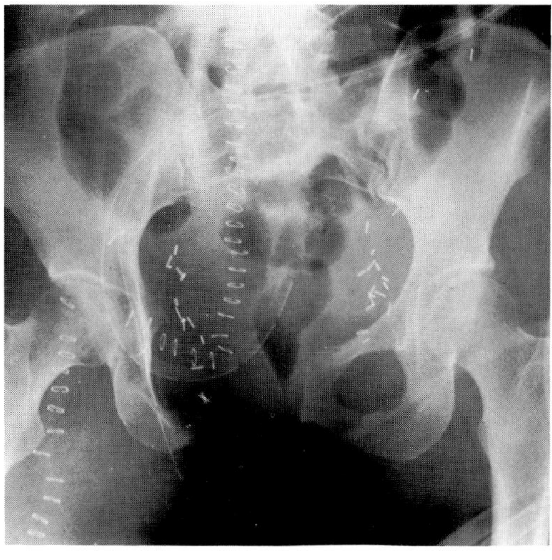

FIGURE 22–6. Postoperative x-ray film after resection of the right pubic bone. The defect was replaced with a polypropylene mesh. The patient is well 7 years later.

important to expose proximally the femoral vessels and nerve. It is also necessary to trace the superficial femoral vessels, in Hunter's canal, to the adductor hiatus. The profunda femoris vessels are exposed and the branches supplying the quadriceps are ligated and divided as they are about to course underneath the tendon of origin of the rectus femoris. The femoral nerve is dissected underneath the inguinal ligament. It gives off a few sensory branches to the skin of the anterior thigh: a sensory branch, the saphenous nerve, courses along the femoral vessels; a long, slender motor branch courses in the interspace between the vessels and the quadriceps to the distal third of the thigh, where it enters underneath the fascia covering the distal portion of vastus medialis and supplies this muscle. A smaller branch of this nerve supplies the proximal portion of the vastus medialis. The bulk of the femoral nerve deviates laterally about 5 cm below the inguinal ligament and courses under the tendon of origin of the rectus femoris, along with the profunda vessels, dividing further into branches for the rectus femoris, the vastus intermedius, and the vastus lateralis.

FIGURE 22–7. X-ray film of the pelvis after internal hemipelvectomy.

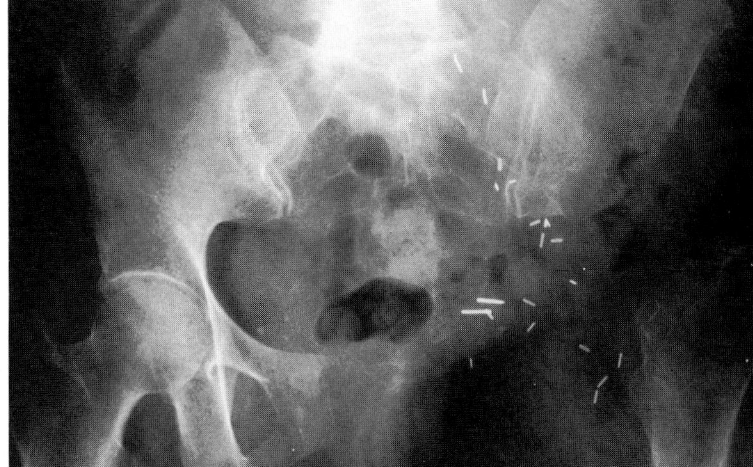

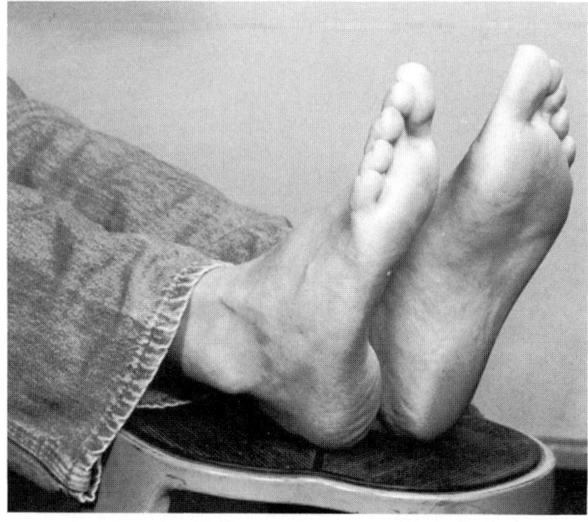

FIGURE 22–8. Shortening of the operated extremity by 3 cm occurs after internal hemipelvectomy if it includes resection of the acetabulum.

The heads of the quadriceps to be removed are resected from origin to insertion. For a deep-seated tumor, the periosteum is peeled from the femur with a periosteal elevator to obtain the maximal margin. In most cases, it is possible to preserve the distal third of the vastus medialis muscle with intact innervation (Figs. 22–9, 22–10). The corresponding edge of this muscle is sutured to the stump of the quadriceps tendon for a direct effect on the patellar tendon when this muscle contracts.

Occasionally, for a tumor located in the vastus medialis, the vastus lateralis may be preserved with intact innervation. It is thus possible, in most patients with anterior compartment sarcomas, to preserve a portion of the quadriceps with intact innervation. This facilitates rehabilitation markedly, so that in 4 to 6 weeks the patients may walk freely without any support.

In three patients referred with extensive, recurrent soft tissue sarcomas, after repeated operations and radiation elsewhere, the author resected the entire quadriceps muscle (Fig. 22–11). In these patients, rehabilitation was slow. They required use of crutches and then a cane for 6 months after the operation. Subsequently, they managed to walk without external support, but the gait was slow and cautious, and occasionally, they were liable to trip and fall. Apparently, the hip flexion during ambulation allows a passive extension of the knee in these patients.

Anatomically, the sartorius muscle belongs

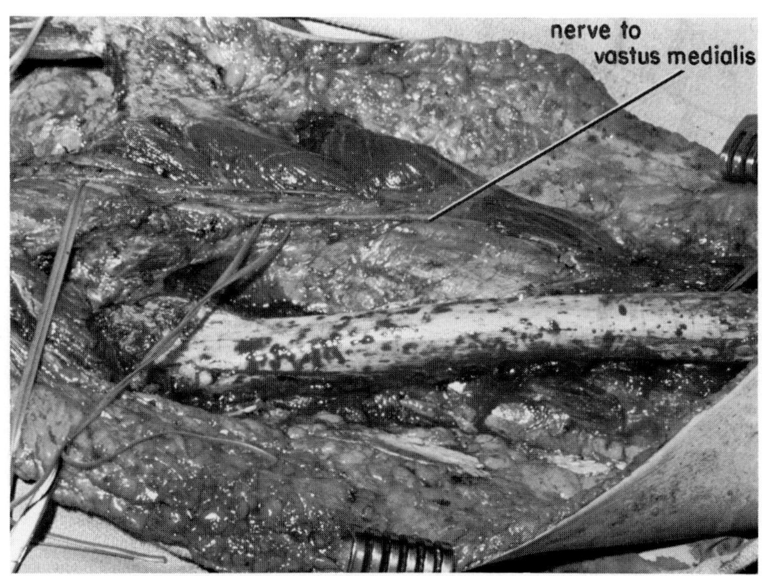

FIGURE 22–9. Anterior compartment resection of the right thigh with preservation of the distal third of the vastus medialis muscle and its innervation.

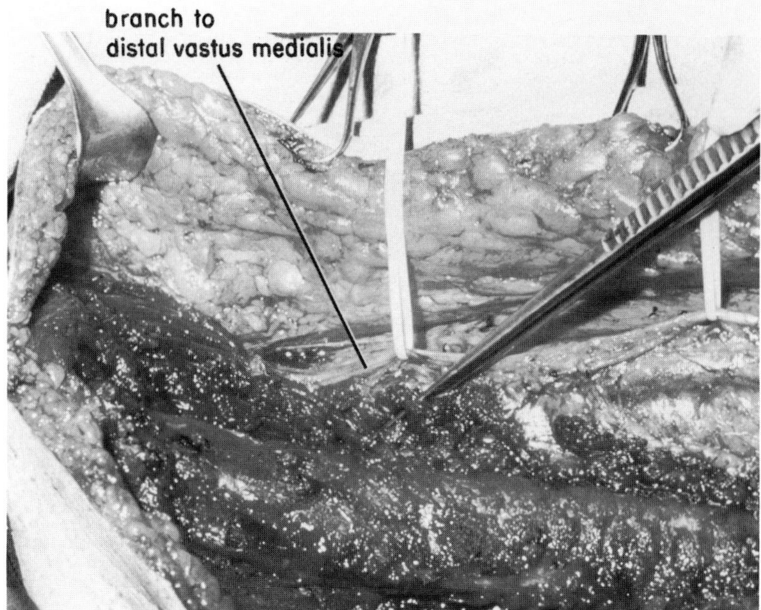

FIGURE 22–10. Operative field after anterior compartment resection of the left thigh. In this close-up view, the nerve branch to the distal portion of the vastus medialis muscle (indicated by the forceps point) is surrounded by two vessel loops.

to the anterior compartment. Depending on the location of the tumor, this muscle may or may not have to be removed. When it is to be removed, it is divided proximally near its origin and distally at the level of the adductor hiatus. It is dissected laterally toward the quadriceps, and small branches from the femoral artery supplying this portion are ligated and divided. When it is to be preserved, it is dissected and retracted medially so that the superficial femoral vessels can be exposed and dissected from the anterior compartment.

For sarcomas of the medial compartment of the thigh, it is best for all but the smallest tumors to resect the entire medial compartment (Fig. 22–12). This exposes posteriorly

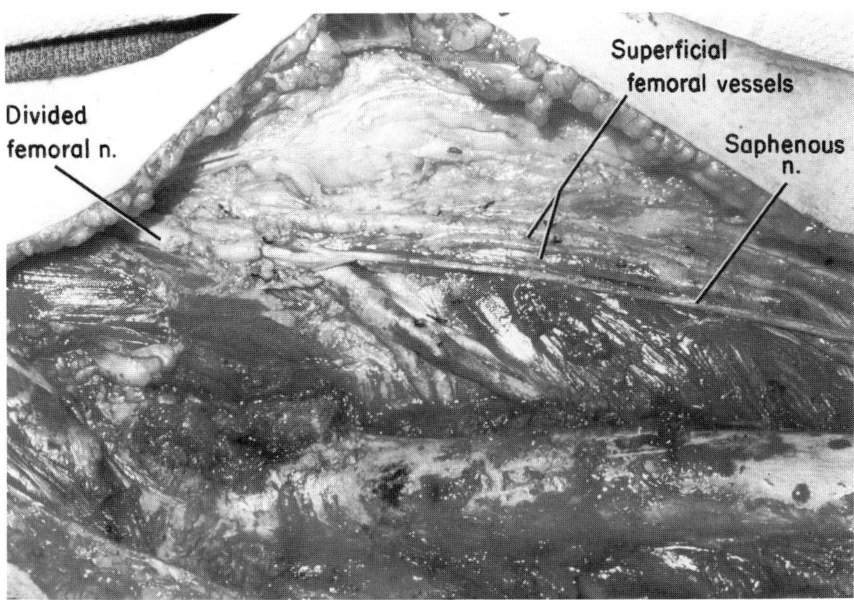

FIGURE 22–11. Anterior compartment resection of the thigh; in this patient it was not possible to preserve any portion of the femoral nerve.

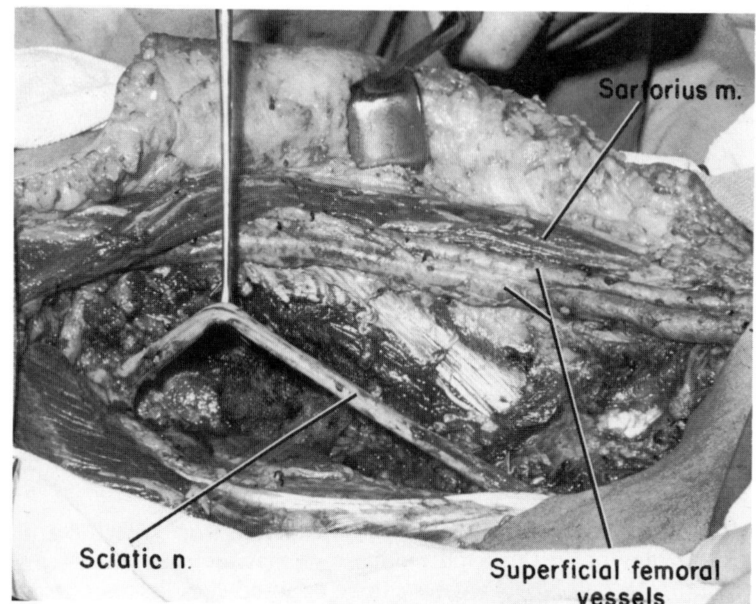

FIGURE 22–12. Medial compartment resection of the right thigh. The femoral vessels are visible. The sciatic nerve is shown retracted.

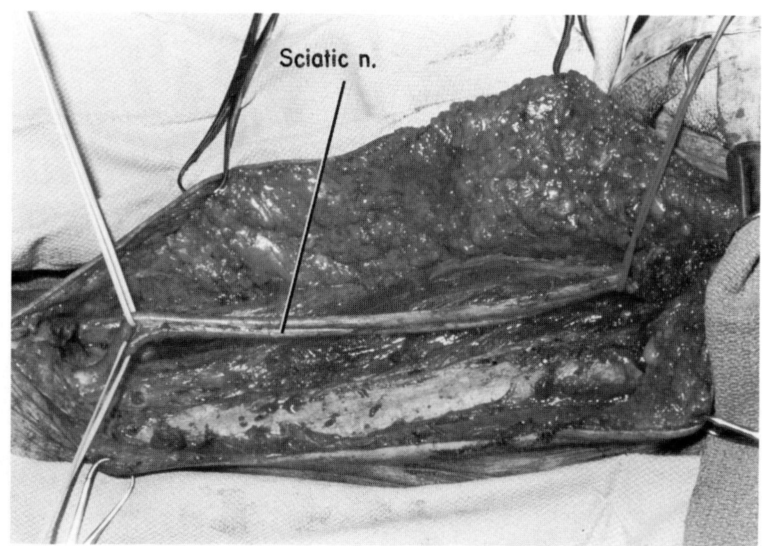

FIGURE 22–13. Posterior compartment resection of the thigh. The sciatic nerve and its bifurcation in the popliteal fossa are clearly shown.

the sciatic nerve, which normally lies behind the adductor magnus muscle. Proximally, the obturator externus muscle should be exposed. The adductor muscles are divided at their origin from the pubic bone and at their insertion in the linea aspera. Removal of the entire medial compartment does not cause any observable deficit in ambulation or other ordinary activities.

For sarcomas of the posterior compartment, it is advisable to remove the muscles of this compartment from their common origin at the ischial tuberosity to their insertions (Fig. 22–13). The patients are still able to flex their knee after this operation, apparently owing to the action of gastrocnemius and sartorius-gracilis muscles. In most situations, the sciatic nerve is merely displaced and is separable through a clean fascial plane from the tumor contained in the hamstring muscles. When the tumor, however, arises in the sciatic nerve (as in a neurogenic sarcoma) or invades or circumferentially envelops this nerve, it is best to resect *en bloc* a sufficient portion of this nerve, along with the posterior compartment. The functional result is far superior to that after an amputation. After division of the sciatic nerve at the level of the buttock, the patient has no sensation at the back of the leg or the foot, but has sensation in the front of the leg through the saphenous branch of the femoral nerve. The patient can extend the knee because the femoral nerve is intact but can also flex it against gravity, apparently through the effect of sartorius and gracilis muscles (Fig. 22–14). There is no movement in the ankle joint, but the net effect during ambulation is that of the footdrop. The patients have the characteristic gait of the common peroneal nerve palsy. This is corrected, however, with the use of a light orthotic device with a horizontal part that fits in the shoe and a vertical part that supports the calf and maintains the foot in a right-angled position to the leg (Fig. 22–15).

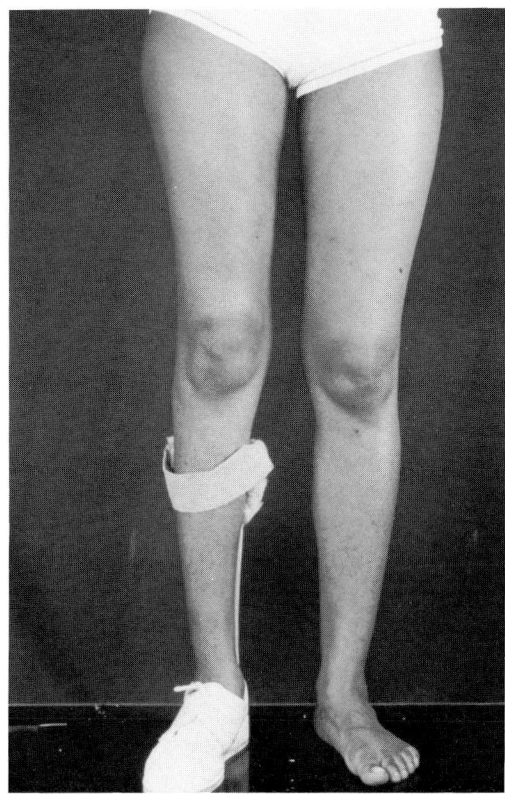

FIGURE 22–15. Anterior view of the same patient as in Figure 22–14. With the use of an orthotic device, the footdrop is eliminated during ambulation.

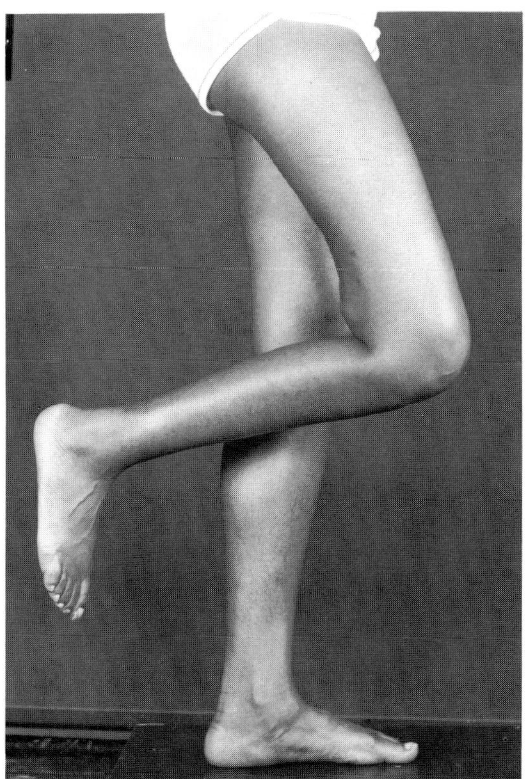

FIGURE 22–14. The patient is able to flex her knee after posterior compartment resection of the right thigh, including the sciatic nerve.

Sarcomas over the lateral aspect of the thigh may be treated with resection of the vastus lateralis (possibly also rectus femoris and vastus intermedius) and biceps femoris muscles. Sarcomas over the anteromedial aspect of the

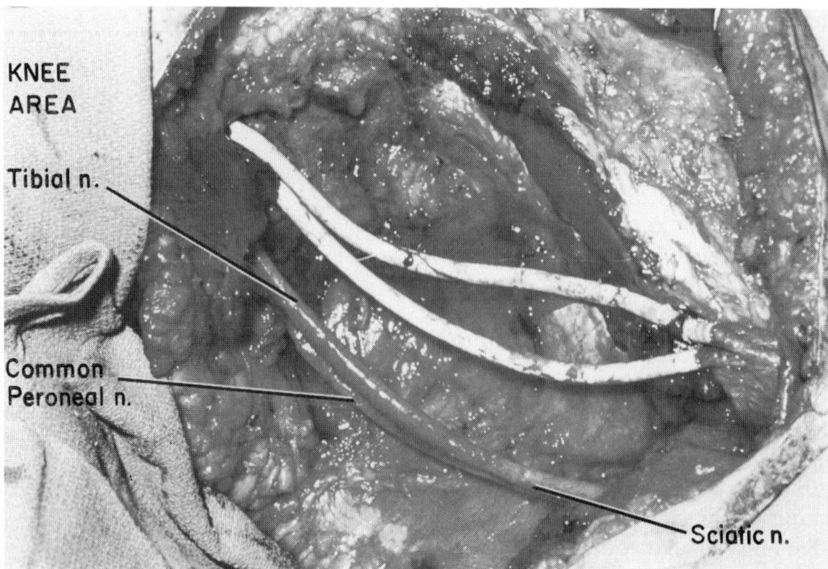

FIGURE 22–16. Operative field after resection of the distal portion of the superficial femoral vessels and replacement with vascular grafts. The sciatic nerve is seen posteriorly.

thigh may necessitate resection of the vessels and replacement with vascular grafts (Fig. 22–16).

Sarcomas involving both medial and posterior compartments (Fig. 22–17) pose the need for exposure and dissection of the femoral vessels (approached anteriorly) and of the sciatic nerve (approached usually through a posterior incision). The solution to this quandary is a long anteromedial incision, which allows the dissection and retraction of the femoral vessels and, after division of the adductor muscles at the linea aspera, permits the identification of the sciatic nerve immediately behind adductor magnus (Fig. 22–18). This is an anterior approach to the sciatic nerve worth remembering in suitable cases.

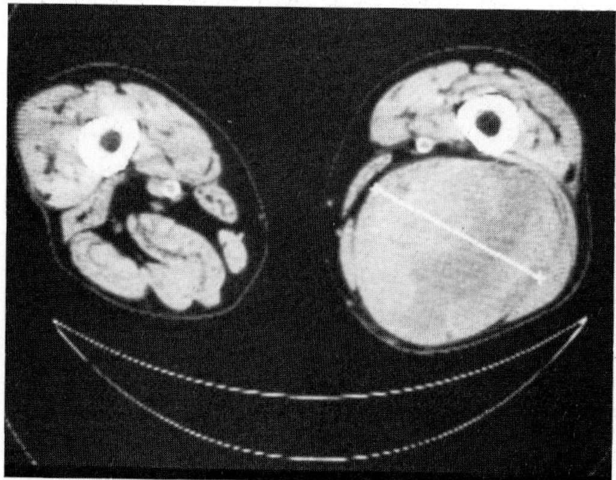

FIGURE 22–17. Large soft tissue sarcoma involving the medial and posterior compartments of the left thigh.

Some authors have described the use of transverse incisions in the area of the buttock.[22] However, longitudinal incisions are much better because (1) they can be much longer, allowing the development of wide flaps and permitting the resection of gluteus maximus (and when necessary the other gluteal muscles) from origin to insertion; and (2) by extending the incision below the gluteal fold, the sciatic nerve can be identified and dissected there, permitting a more deliberate and safe resection of the gluteal muscles as the nerve is gradually traced proximally, along with the removal of these muscles.

Knee

For small tumors in the area of the knee, a simple excision with or without a skin graft followed by radiation has provided good local control in the author's patients. For larger tumors anteriorly, the patella may have to be resected along with the overlying skin, exposing the joint. In one patient with this problem, a myocutaneous flap of the vastus lateralis based on genicular branches distally was rotated. The muscle tendon was used to bridge the defect in the quadriceps tendon. Part of

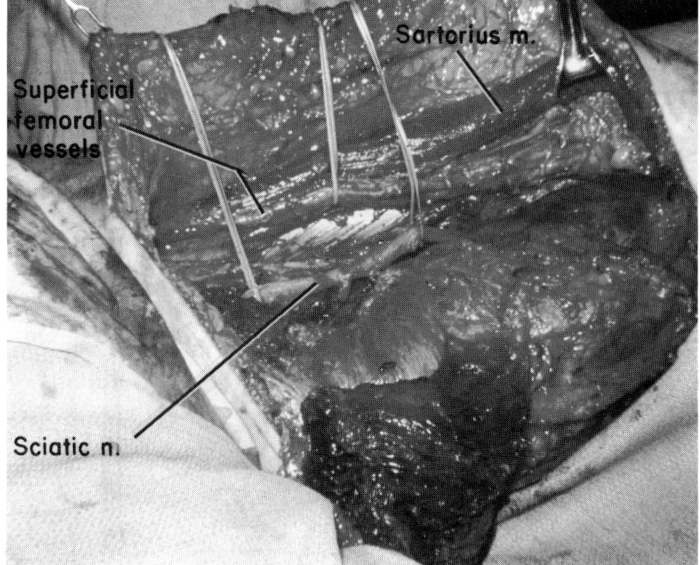

FIGURE 22–18. Same patient as in Figure 22–17. The superficial femoral vessels have been dissected anteriorly. After division of the insertion of the adductor muscles at the linea aspera, the sciatic nerve was identified and retracted with two vessel loops.

the skin was lost distally, but the muscle remained viable and was later successfully skin grafted. Free flaps or rotation flaps from the posterior thigh compartment and from the gastrocnemius and a lower posterolateral thigh flap[13] have been used to cover anterior knee skin defects exposing the joint.

A sarcoma in the popliteal fossa may be resected by modifying the technique of popliteal node dissection[5] to suit the particular tumor. A skin defect in that area may be dealt with by dividing the tendons of insertion of one or more of the hamstring muscles (semitendinosus, semimembranosus, or biceps femoris). The semimembranosus is bulkier near its insertion and more suitable for this maneuver, when it is available. This allows medial displacement of the muscles in the center of the popliteal fossa to cover the vessels and nerves and to provide the bed for the application of a split-thickness skin graft.

For large tumors in the popliteal fossa, it may be necessary to sacrifice a major nerve, but usually it is only one of two (i.e., common peroneal or tibial). A deliberate dissection and decision is made by exposing the nerves both proximal and distal to the tumor and by carefully dissecting inside the sheath that envelops the nerves. In cases of neurofibromatosis associated with neurogenic sarcoma, extra margin around the malignant portion of the tumor is attained by removing the adjacent neurofibromas. A nerve stimulator is useful in differentiating between the sensory and the motor component of a nerve and in helping to plan the extent of resection.

Leg

Sarcomas in the anterior compartment, when small, may be resected by removing only one of the muscles or portions around the tumor from the adjacent muscles of this compartment in the manner of a wide resection. For large tumors, the entire compartment may have to be resected. When the tumor is adjacent to the fibula, a combined anterior and lateral compartment resection with fibulectomy may be necessary. When a portion of the anterior compartment can be preserved, dissection of the common peroneal nerve on the medial side of the biceps femoris tendon and along its course around the neck of the fibula is essential to determine its relation to the tumor and the feasibility of its preservation. In cases of footdrop after resection of the common peroneal nerve, the orthotic device described above (after resections of the sciatic nerve) may be used. After resection of large soft tissue sarcomas of the anterior compartment extensively involving the skin, the exposed tibia may be covered proximally by rotating the distal portion of the medial head of the gastrocnemius (based on its proximal supply), while distally the bone is covered by mobilizing the soleus muscle without transecting its continuity with the Achilles tendon. A skin graft may then be applied directly on these muscles (Fig. 22–19).

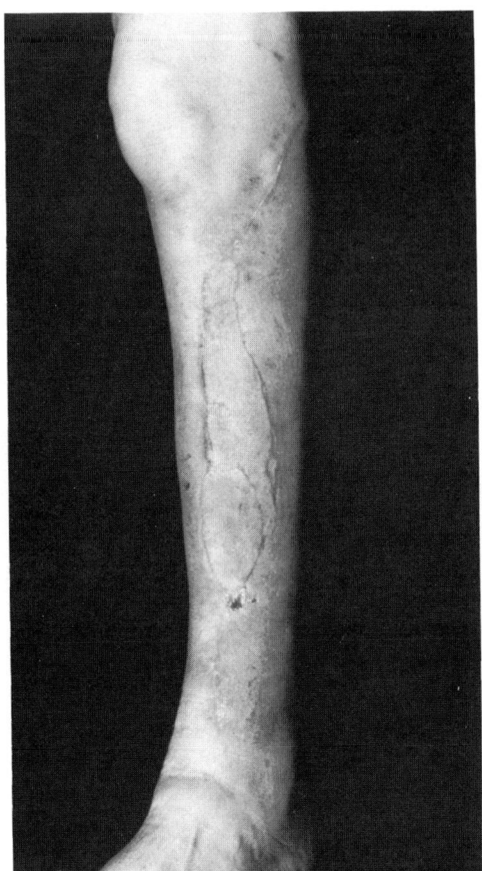

FIGURE 22–19. Appearance after anterior compartment resection of the left leg for a recurrent liposarcoma that extensively involved the skin overlaying the compartment. A skin graft was applied over the rotated lateral head of the gastrocnemius and the mobilized soleus muscles.

Owing to the bulk of the involved muscles in the posterior compartment of the leg, it is usually possible to perform a satisfactory resection and yet preserve some of the muscles. A small portion of the gastrocnemius or the soleus muscle may be preserved intact with its innervation and continuity with the Achilles tendon. In a complete posterior compartment resection, the plantar surface of the foot is anesthetic, there is no longer the "lifting" effect on walking provided by the contraction of these muscles, and the foot maintains a right-angled position to the leg during ambulation, which is carried efficiently without support, albeit in the manner one moves with a below-knee prosthesis. In complete anterior or posterior compartment resections of the leg, in addition to sacrifice of the common peroneal or the tibial nerve, the anterior or the posterior tibial artery, respectively, is sacrificed also. The viability of the foot remains intact with preservation of one of these branches if the foot's circulation is not compromised with atherosclerotic disease.

In the area of the ankle or the dorsum of the foot, it is difficult to obtain a wide margin. Usually, resection with a clean margin of a few millimeters is obtained, requiring the use of adjuvant modalities to improve the rate of local control.

For sarcomas that are somewhat superficial in the plantar aspect of the foot, an adequate resection may be obtained with the *en bloc* removal of the appropriate portion of the skin, the plantar aponeurosis, and the short flexors of the foot. A skin graft may be applied directly on the surface of the second layer (long flexors) (Fig. 22–20). No pain on ambulation results from the operation, and most patients are pain free after this procedure. However, one of the author's patients treated postoperatively with radiation developed pain later, which appeared only during weight bearing on the foot, although she has remained disease free for 12 years.

UPPER EXTREMITY

A sarcoma in the lower neck may be treated with simple excision. Because of the proximity of the cervical spine, the carotid artery, and the brachial plexus, wide margins are usually

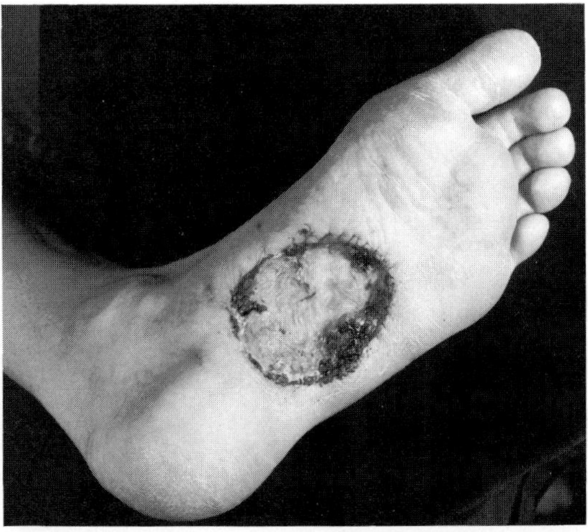

FIGURE 22–20. Appearance after resection of a sarcoma in the plantar aspect of the foot; resection involves skin, plantar fascia, and the first layer of muscles.

not possible and therefore adjuvant postoperative radiation is often required.

When the tumor extends below the clavicle, claviculectomy is essential to provide the exposure needed. In two of the author's patients, the subclavian artery and vein were resected and replaced with Gore-Tex grafts. Claviculectomy, along with division of the origin or resection of the pectoralis major muscle, provides an improved exposure, which may be necessary for the removal of soft tissue sarcomas in this area. Through this approach, one may resect a tumor as posteriorly located as the subscapularis muscle.

Sarcomas near the tip of the scapula may be resected with partial scapulectomy (i.e., resection of the scapula below its spine with preservation of the glenoid), which, when feasible, retains a great deal of shoulder function. For large tumors, total scapulectomy and, if necessary, resection of the head of the humerus *en bloc* with the involved soft tissues may be performed, a procedure known as the Tikhoff-Linberg operation.[16]

Sarcomas in the posterior compartment of the arm can often be managed with wide resection, permitting the preservation of one of the heads of the triceps and the radial nerve. Because it winds around the humerus, the radial nerve is usually not involved by the tumor. If the radial nerve is invaded or surrounded by the tumor, it may be sacrificed, in preference to an amputation if a satisfactory resection can be obtained. The mere presence of the tumor close to the radial or any other major nerve, in the author's experience, is not an indication to sacrifice that nerve if a clean plane can be developed between the nerve and the tumor. One, of course, may have to rely on adjuvant postoperative radiation for the control of any microscopic residual in these cases.

Sarcomas in the anterior compartment of the arm can often be managed in the manner of a wide excision. The biceps and/or the brachialis muscles may be resected along with the tumor. One should be familiar with the anatomy of the musculocutaneous nerve, which courses between the two muscles, so that the remaining muscle will have intact innervation. Occasionally, both muscles of the anterior compartment may have to be resected (Fig. 22–21); in this situation, weak flexion of the elbow is still possible through the action of the brachioradialis muscle with the forearm in a neutral position between pronation and supination.

In the flexor compartment of the forearm, wide excision is often possible (Figs. 22–22, 22–23). It is important to be familiar with the course of the median nerve and to preserve it when possible. Similarly, the extensor compartment of the forearm permits only local or wide resection.

In the wrist and hand, only simple, local excision is possible and should always be fol-

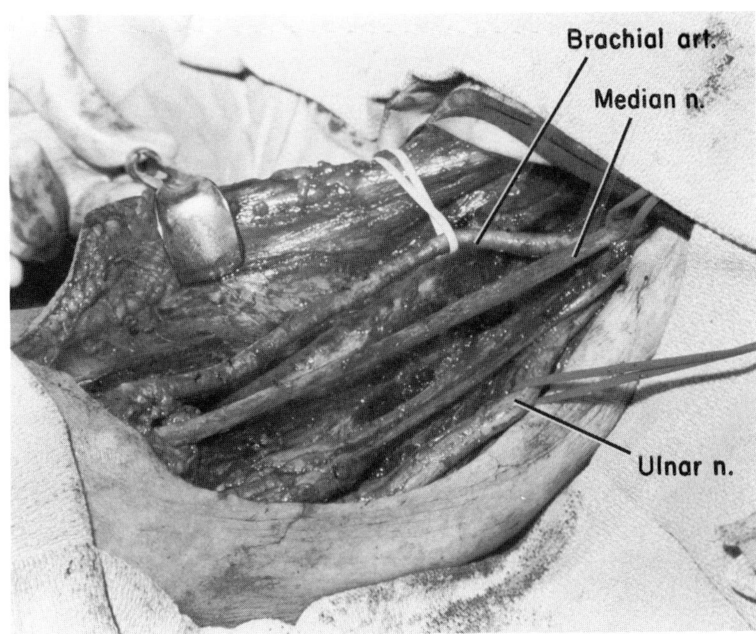

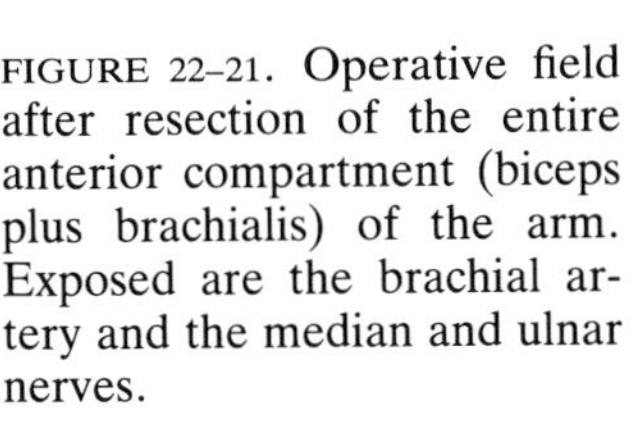

FIGURE 22–21. Operative field after resection of the entire anterior compartment (biceps plus brachialis) of the arm. Exposed are the brachial artery and the median and ulnar nerves.

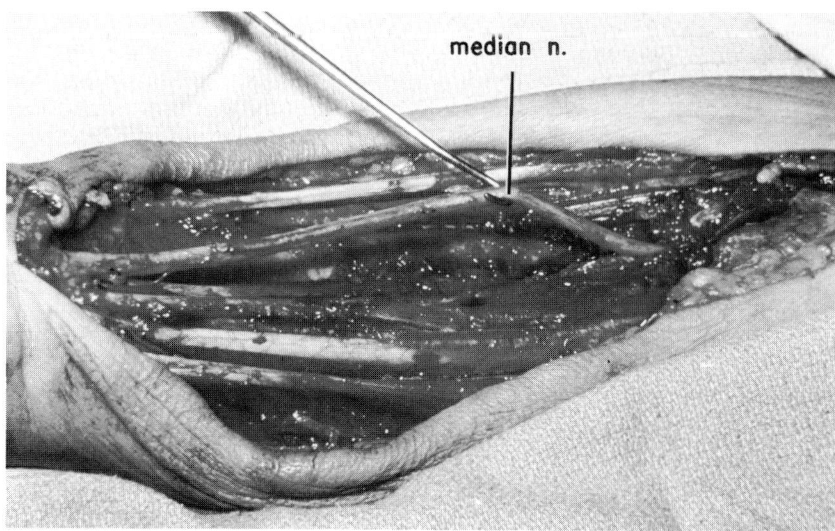

FIGURE 22–22. Operative field after resection of a liposarcoma of the flexor compartment of the forearm. Retracted is the median nerve.

lowed by adjuvant radiation (Figs. 22–24, 22–25). The results of this approach are encouraging in the author's series: of eight patients with soft tissue sarcomas in the area of the hand, only one has experienced local relapse outside the field of previous radiation on long-term follow-up.

MAJOR AMPUTATIONS

The current rate of limb preservation is 95% for all patients referred to RPMI with a primary or locally recurrent soft tissue sarcoma of the extremity.[11, 12] However, in patients with extensive involvement of the soft tissues, including bone or joint, that precludes an *en bloc* resection with a functionally adequate extremity, amputation may be the only choice. Involvement of major vessels is not an indication for amputation because they can be resected *en bloc* with the tumor and replaced with vascular grafts.

For tumors in the iliac fossa, the groin, or the wall of the lesser pelvis necessitating amputation, hemipelvectomy with a posterior flap is performed. To guarantee the viability of the posterior flap, one should preserve and leave

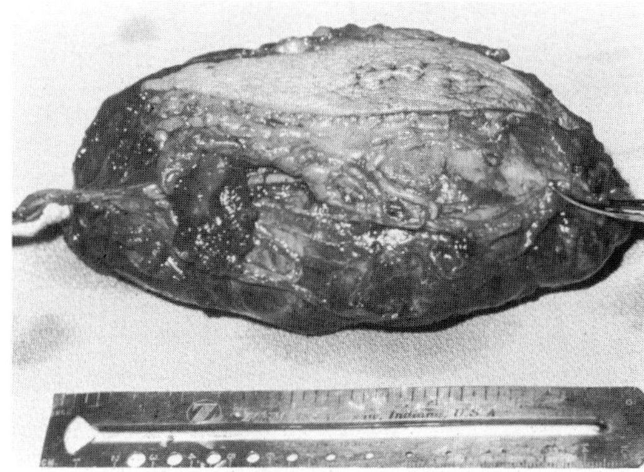

FIGURE 22–23. The specimen removed from the patient in Figure 22–22. The clamps on each side of the specimen are on the radial artery, which had to be resected with the tumor.

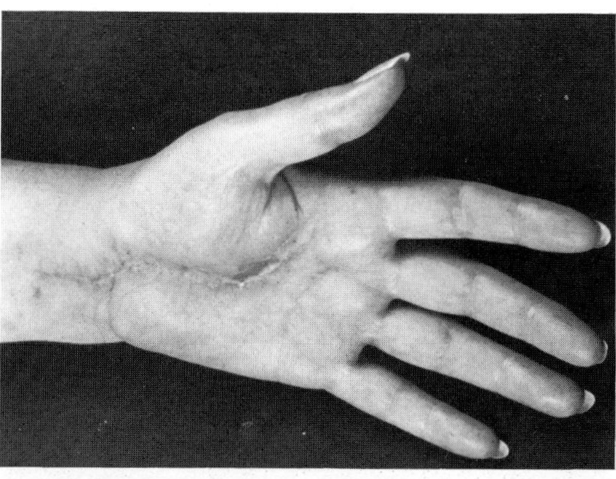

FIGURE 22–24. Appearance after treatment of synovial sarcoma of the wrist by simple excision and adjuvant postoperative radiation. The patient is well 12 years later.

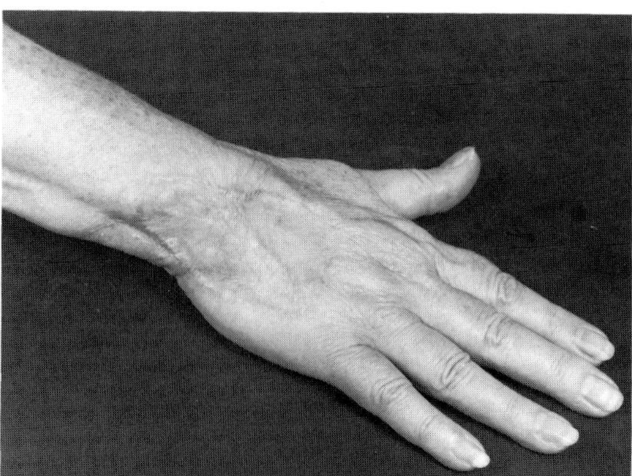

FIGURE 22–25. Appearance after treatment of a recurrent sarcoma of the dorsum of the hand by simple excision and postoperative radiation.

the gluteus maximus attached to the flap. It makes no difference whether the vessels are divided at the common iliac or the external iliac level. A posterior flap, thus constructed, can be long and reach to the level of the umbilicus. This is occasionally necessary after resection of the lower part of the abdominal wall, particularly for involvement following radiation.

For large sarcomas of the buttock involving the sciatic nerve and underlying bone or joint posteriorly, an anterior flap hemipelvectomy is required. The anterior flap may consist of a large and long flap centered over the superficial femoral vessels, consisting of skin, subcutaneous fat, fascia lata, and the femoral vessels attached to and supplying the flap.[10] When a particularly wide and more lateral flap is required, it is preferable to preserve at least a portion of the quadriceps femoris attached to the flap with its blood supply intact from the profunda femoris vessels.[23]

In forequarter amputations, the subclavian vessels may be divided early in the procedure after division of the medial portion of the clavicle and the underlying subclavius muscle. However, when the area has been radiated or when the tumor extends high toward the neck, it is preferable to complete the dissection all the way around and divide the vessels as the last step in the procedure. For tumors involving the medial wall of the axilla, particularly when there is a probable need for rib resection, a deltoid flap consisting of skin, subcutaneous fat, and fascia, is helpful in covering the resulting defect.[9]

Prognostic Indicators and Staging

It is well known that the histologic type influences survival. Synovial sarcomas, rhabdomyosarcomas, and leiomyosarcomas have worse prognosis generally compared with fibrosarcomas and liposarcomas.[1] Currently, the most common variety is liposarcoma, followed by malignant fibrous histiocytoma, and then leiomyosarcoma in the author's series (Table 22–1). Apart from a varying tendency to hematogenously metastasize, the different histologic types show a varying tendency for lymphogenous spread. Although the latter tendency is low overall, some histologic types, such as synovial sarcomas and malignant fibrous histiocytomas, demonstrate metastases to the regional lymph nodes in 20 to 30% of cases.[26]

However, the grade of the tumor has assumed overriding importance both because of its prognostic significance and because it has made the comparison of the results of various series of soft tissue sarcomas more rational and has permitted the identification of high-risk groups for possible adjuvant therapy. Currently three grades are distinguished: grade I, the low-grade tumors; grade II, intermediate grade; grade III, the high-grade tumors. Grades correspond to survival. In the American Joint Committee on Cancer staging sys-

TABLE 22–1

Histology of Soft Tissue Tumors*

Tumor Histology	Number of Patients	Percentage
Rhabdomyosarcoma	5	3
Leiomysarcoma	18	11
Liposarcoma	50	29
Synovial sarcoma	13	8
Fibrosarcoma	11	6
Malignant fibrohistiocytoma	33	19
Malignant schwannoma	3	2
Hemangiopericytoma	4	2
Malignant mesenchymoma	1	1
Epithelioid sarcoma	3	2
Neurogenic sarcoma	7	4
Unclassified	10	6
Extraosseous sarcoma	2	1
Other	11	6

*Patients at Roswell Park Memorial Institute, 1977 to 1986.

TABLE 22–2

Grade or Stage of Sarcoma and Survival*

	Number of Patients	Median Survival (months)	5-Year Survival
Grade I	50	>108	70%
Grade II	38	>106	78%
Grade III	78	63	53%
Stage I	41	>108	74%
Stage II	33	>106	77%
Stage III	59	67	56%
Stage IVa	33	>44	†

*Patients at RPMI, 1977 to 1986.
†Longest follow-up is 44 months.

tem, stages I through III correspond to grades I through III with subdivision to a and b for each stage according to the size of the tumor (less than or greater than 5 cm, respectively). Stage IIIc indicates involvement of the regional nodes; stage IVa designates invasion of adjacent major vessels, nerve, or bone; and stage IVb is disseminated disease.[18]

Some authors find that the identification of an intermediate grade corresponding to intermediate survival is difficult and prefer the use of a two-grade system (i.e., low and high grade).[4] The author's results support this view (Table 22–2).

The anatomic location of the tumor also influences survival, with lesions in the extremities being associated with longer survival than for those in intraabdominal locations (Table 22–3).

Local recurrence in the absence of metastatic disease should be managed aggressively, with resection plus adjuvant radiation if necessary. A significant proportion of these patients (approaching the proportion for primary sarcomas) attain 5-year disease-free survival.[1]

Results of Treatment

Among 171 patients (144 with extremity tumors) referred to RPMI from 1977 through 1986, only about 10% were admitted with an intact, unbiopsied tumor. In the remaining patients, the tumor bed had been biopsied in 28%, partially resected in 16%, and "completely" resected in 26%, and it was locally recurrent in 20%. Interestingly, 31% of the patients referred with "complete resection" at reoperation at RPMI had residual macroscopic or microscopic disease, a finding suggesting that these rare tumors are best managed in a referral center. Ninety-seven (57%) of these patients with a minimal resection margin of 2 cm or greater had no other therapy locally. The minimal margin was restricted only in a small area adjacent to major nerve or bone, whereas satisfactory 10- to 20-cm margins were procured in most areas around the tumor.

Seventy-four (43%) of the patients with minimal margin less than 2 cm were given adjuvant postoperative radiation, starting up to 3 weeks after the procedure, except in the presence of

TABLE 22–3

Location of Tumor and Survival*

Location	Number of Patients	Median Survival (months)	5-Year Survival
Upper extremity	30	>118	77%
Lower extremity	102	89	69%
Trunk	12	41	40%
Intraabdominal	20	46	37%
Head and neck	2†	—	—

*Patients at RPMI, 1977 to 1986.
†Alive and well at 38 and 65 months.

a skin graft, when it was delayed to longer than 5 weeks from the operation. Using a fractionation schedule of 2 Gy per day (10 Gy per week), 40 Gy to the whole operative field was given; to a smaller area, corresponding to the site of narrowest margin, further radiation to a total of 45 to 60 Gy was given over 4½ to 6 weeks. For extremity sarcomas, the dose was usually carried to 60 Gy. For pelvic sarcomas, the dose was limited to 45 to 50 Gy.

Of 144 patients with extremity sarcomas, only 8 (6%) were treated with amputation. Amputation became necessary in these patients because of concomitant, extensive involvement of bone or joint. In the RPMI experience, major nerve or vessel involvement is not an indication for amputation. However, at the National Institutes of Health Consensus Development Conference on Limb-Sparing Treatment of Adult Soft Tissue Sarcomas and Osteosarcomas, involvement of a major nerve or vessel was still considered an indication for amputation.[14]

For lesions of all anatomic locations, the estimated 5-year survival rate was 64%, whereas the local recurrence rate for those treated with surgical resection alone was 7%, and for those treated with resection plus adjuvant radiation, it was 8%. For the 144 patients with extremity sarcomas, the 5-year survival rate was 71%, whereas the 5-year local recurrence was 6%, for both those with surgical resection alone and those with narrower margins treated with resection and radiation. None of 11 patients with resection of iliac, femoral, or subclavian vessels manifested local recurrence.

Although an inappropriately placed biopsy incision at a primary care center complicates the definitive operation, none of the patients at RPMI required an amputation for this reason.

Similar local control rates were achieved in extremity soft tissue sarcomas by Eilber and colleagues, using preoperative intraarterial infusion of doxorubicin (Adriamycin) plus radiation followed by resection.[2, 3] Local recurrence rates in other series ranged from 13%[24] to 22.3%[15] with the use of combination therapy.

At RPMI, a conscientious effort is made to minimize potential microscopic residual. Compartment resections are advisable for all sarcomas of the medial and posterior compartments of the thigh, whereas a modified anterior compartment resection (described above) is usually performed in the anterior thigh. In most other areas of the extremities, a wide resection is performed, in which satisfactory margins from 5 to 20 cm are obtained in most directions around the tumor, but the margins are restricted in the vicinity of a major structure (e.g., a major nerve or bone), provided a clean plane can be developed between the specimen and the structure to be preserved. If a muscle is removed, it is removed from origin to insertion. Surgery in the context of combination therapy is discriminating in that wide margins are sought and procured in most directions around the tumor concerning tissues that are relatively dispensable, but narrow margins are accepted in the vicinity of a functionally major structure. Thorough knowledge of the regional and functional anatomy is required. Generally, a remarkable amount of functional reserve exists in the musculature of an extremity, which is available for the extremes of action, but unnecessary for most ordinary activities.

At RPMI, postoperative rather than preoperative radiation is preferred because one can better judge which patients need radiation. One may also avoid some of the wound problems associated with preoperative radiation. The need to shrink a large tumor (cited in favor of preoperative radiation) is not a significant factor, because with appropriate incision and exposure, the size of the tumor becomes a negligible variable in its resectability.

At present, the various therapeutic techniques (namely, preoperative intraarterial infusion plus radiation, preoperative radiation alone, the "sandwich" technique using a portion of the radiation preoperatively and the remainder postoperatively, and postoperative radiation) are combined with resection to provide effective local control in soft tissue sarcomas. It is not yet clear whether any of these techniques is superior to others in terms of improved results or decreased incidence of complications.

The role of adjuvant chemotherapy is still unclear. One prospectively randomized study showed significant improvement in the survival of patients with extremity soft tissue sarcomas,[17] but other studies present equivocal or negative results, and therefore the role of adjuvant chemotherapy in high-grade sarcomas remains investigational.

Other than local recurrence, relapse most commonly involves the lungs, which often are the only site of metastatic involvement. In addition to chemotherapy, wedge resections of pulmonary metastases in patients with a small number of lesions and long disease-free intervals provide 5-year survival rates ranging from 20 to 30%.[23]

Conclusions

Soft tissue sarcomas are uncommon, manifesting themselves most frequently as a mass.

Radiologic investigations clarify the location and extent of the mass. Unless there is a clear explanation for its occurrence, such a mass should be biopsied at a referral center.

After a positive biopsy finding and identification of the histologic type, resection of the mass should be undertaken with an effort to obtain the maximal margin around the tumor consistent with a functionally acceptable result. Involvement of major vessels is uncommon and may be treated by resection and replacement with grafts. Direct invasion or circumferential involvement of a major nerve is best managed with *en bloc* resection of the nerve in preference to an amputation, if satisfactory margins can be obtained.

Improvement in surgical techniques of exposure and knowledge of the functional anatomy has increased resectability and the rate of limb preservation to about 95%, with improved function for the extremity.

Selective use of combination therapy in the RPMI series, with the use of postoperative radiation for narrow margins, reduced the 5-year local recurrence rate to 6% for extremity sarcomas, while the 5-year survival rate was 71%.

References

1. Abbas JS, Holyoke ED, Moore R, Karakousis CP: The surgical treatment and outcome of soft-tissue sarcoma. Arch Surg 116:765–769, 1981.
2. Eilber FR, Giuliamo AE, Huth JR, Mirra JJ, Morton DL: High grade soft tissue sarcomas of the extremity: UCLA experience with limb salvage. *In* Wagener DJT (ed): Primary Chemotherapy in Cancer Medicine. New York, Alan R. Liss, 1985, pp 59–74.
3. Eilber FR, Mirra JJ, Grant TT, Weisenburger T, Morton DL: Is amputation necessary for sarcomas? A seven-year experience with limb salvage. Ann Surg 192:431–437, 1980.
4. Hajdu SI: Histologic grade of sarcoma. *In* Hajdu SI (ed): Differential Diagnosis of Soft Tissue and Bone Tumors. Philadelphia, Lea & Febiger, 1986, pp 402–404.
5. Karakousis CP: The technique of popliteal lymph node dissection. Surg Gynecol Obstet 151:420–423, 1980.
6. Karakousis CP: Exposure and reconstruction in the lower portions of the retroperitoneum and abdominal wall. Arch Surg 117:840–844, 1982.
7. Karakousis CP: The abdominoinguinal incision in limb salvage and resection of pelvic tumors. Cancer 54:2543–2548, 1984.
8. Karakousis CP: Internal hemipelvectomy. Surg Gynecol Obstet 158:279–282, 1984.
9. Karakousis CP: Variants of forequarter amputation. *In* Karakousis CP: Atlas of Operations in Soft Tissue Tumors. New York, McGraw-Hill, 1985, pp 115–121.
10. Karakousis CP, Vezeridis MP: Variants of hemipelvectomy. Am J Surg 145:273–277, 1983.
11. Karakousis CP, Emrich LJ, Rao U, Khalil M: Selective combination of modalities in soft tissue sarcomas: Limb salvage and survival. Semin Surg Oncol 4:78–81, 1988.
12. Karakousis CP, Emrich LJ, Rao U, Krishnamsetty RM: Feasibility of limb salvage and survival in soft tissue sarcomas. Cancer 57:484–491, 1986.
13. Laitung JKG: The lower posterolateral thigh flap. Br J Plast Surg 42:133–139, 1989.
14. Lawrence W Jr: Concepts in limb-sparing treatment of adult soft tissue sarcomas. Semin Surg Oncol 4:73–77, 1988.
15. Lindberg RD, Martin RG, Romsdahl MM, Barkley HT: Conservative surgery and postoperative radiotherapy in 300 adults with soft tissue sarcomas. Cancer 47:2391–2397, 1981.
16. Marcove RC, Lewis MM, Huvos AG: *En bloc* humeral interscapulo-thoracic resection. The Tikhoff-Linberg procedure. Clin Orthop 124:219–228, 1977.
17. Rosenberg SA, Tepper J, Glatstein E, et al: The treatment of soft-tissue sarcomas of the extremities: Prospective randomized evaluation of 1) limb-sparing surgery plus radiation therapy compared with amputation and 2) the role of adjuvant chemotherapy. Ann Surg 196:305–315, 1982.
18. Russell WO, Cohen J, Enzinger F, et al: A clinical and pathological staging system for soft tissue sarcomas. Cancer 57:484–491, 1986.
19. Shiu MH, Castro EB, Hajdu SI, Fortner JC: Surgical treatment of 297 soft tissue sarcomas of the lower extremity. Ann Surg 182:597–602, 1975.
20. Sim FH, Pritchard DJ, Reiman HM, Edmonson JH, Schray MF: Soft-tissue sarcomas: Mayo Clinic experience. Semin Surg Oncol 4:38–44, 1988.
21. Simon MA, Enneking WF: The management of soft-tissue sarcomas of the extremities. J Bone Joint Surg 58A:1317–1327, 1976.
22. Sugarbaker PH, Chretien PA: A surgical technique for buttockectomy. Surgery 91:104–107, 1982.
23. Sugarbaker PH, Chretien PA: Hemipelvectomy for buttock tumors utilizing an anterior myocutaneous flap of quadriceps femoris muscle. Ann Surg 197:106–115, 1983.
24. Suit HD, Russell WO, Martin RG: Sarcoma of soft tissue: Clinical and histopathologic parameters and response to treatment. Cancer 35:1478–1483, 1975.
25. Takita H, Edgerton F, Karakousis C, Douglass HO Jr, Vincent RG, Beckley S: Surgical management of metastases to the lung. Surg Gynecol Obstet 152:191–194, 1981.
26. Weiss SW, Enzinger FM: Malignant fibrous histiocytoma. An analysis of 200 cases. Cancer 41:2250–2266, 1978.

CHAPTER 23

Rehabilitation of Patients with Physical Disabilities Caused by Tumors of the Musculoskeletal System

KRISTJAN T. RAGNARSSON

Diagnosis and treatment of malignant tumors affecting the musculoskeletal system have markedly changed during the past decade. No longer does the definitive treatment of malignant primary tumors in the limbs automatically entail limb amputation nor does metastatic bone disease indicate certain imminent death. New reconstructive surgical procedures that use cadaveric bone allografts or metallic prostheses to replace diseased bone allow sparing of many limbs. When the procedures are combined with effective chemotherapy and/or radiotherapy, tumor recurrence and appearance of metastases can be markedly delayed, or avoided. Even though the new surgical approaches have improved functional prognosis, variable disability usually results from limb-saving procedures. Thus, early and continued aggressive rehabilitation interventions (i.e., physical and occupational therapy) are required. Yet for certain patients, the treatment of choice for primary malignant limb tumors continues to be amputation, and some patients who have initially undergone reconstruction ultimately require amputation.

Despite improved oncologic management and control of cancer, the most common type of musculoskeletal tumor continues to be metastatic cancer to bones, primarily to the spinal column, the pelvis, the ribs, and the long bones of the extremities. Metastases often cause pathologic fractures, neurologic deficits, and pain. Application of rehabilitation techniques often results in quick functional improvements and reduction in subjective complaints even in certain patients whose prognosis for life is considered poor. Modern diagnostic techniques and effective treatment of malignant disease, which have improved the prognosis, have also made it more difficult to accurately predict life expectancy. A patient with metastatic disease to the bones, therefore, should not be denied the benefits of aggressive management, including appropriate surgical intervention, chemotherapy, radiation, and comprehensive rehabilitation treatment. These interventions, when offered in combination, prolong life, reduce pain, protect the nervous system, maximize self-care skills and ambulatory function, and thereby provide dignity and quality of life for the cancer patient.

Successful rehabilitation of patients disabled by tumors of the musculoskeletal system depends on early referral and good communication among the surgeon, the oncologist, the physiatrist, and the other members of the rehabilitation team. Success is further facilitated by a comprehensive rehabilitation approach that simultaneously addresses the physical, psychologic, and social problems caused by the disease and consequent disability. Most important for success, however, is the patients' motivation to apply themselves to the demands of the rehabilitation program and to pursue the rehabilitation goals with the firm support of family and close friends.

Rehabilitation Concepts and Cancer Management

Most cancer patients with physical disabilities can be significantly helped by rehabilitation services. Cancer rehabilitation can be defined, by modifying Rusk's definition of rehabilitation medicine, as the maximal restoration of physical, psychologic, social, vocational, recreational, and economic function within the limits imposed by the malignant disease and its treatment.[29a] Quite clearly, to effectively address such a variety of functions and needs, a multidisciplinary cancer rehabilitation team must provide an organized cancer rehabilitation program (Table 23–1). Unfortunately, referrals of cancer patients to rehabilitation services are often made late. This may reflect a certain reluctance on the part of the primary care physician and the rehabilitation staff, who expect a different outcome for cancer patients when they are compared with patients disabled by trauma or relatively static medical disorders. However, with improving prognosis for many types of cancer and increased optimism with respect to outcome, the demand for rehabilitation services for disabled cancer patients has grown. Primary care physicians have become aware that, to meet the multiple needs of cancer patients, involvement of a multidisciplinary rehabilitation team is required. Although goal-oriented rehabilitation of cancer patients can be cost effective,[7] rehabilitation is a time-consuming and costly process, with great personnel demands. It may therefore be argued that comprehensive rehabilitation services are most economically provided for disabled cancer patients whose disease is considered cured or controlled. However, even for those who have a poorer prognosis, short-term rehabilitation goals should be established and aggressively pursued.

The annual incidence of cancer in the United States, including nonmelanoma skin cancer and carcinoma in situ, is reported to be 1,000,000 and the prevalence rate to be 7,000,000.[5a] About half of these individuals have a major or minor, but distinct, physical disability, which is amenable to rehabilitation intervention.

The physical disability associated with cancer may result from tissue destruction caused by the cancer itself, prolonged bed rest or inactivity, or definitive treatment (i.e., surgery, radiotherapy, or chemotherapy). The exact nature of the disability may vary, but in essence the range of disabilities is no different from those not caused by cancer that are managed by the rehabilitation team. A specific rehabilitation goal must be established for each patient and an individualized program prescribed, which is designed to obtain measurable, early results. The primary rehabilitation goals for physically disabled people are (1) to obtain maximal function in the activities of daily living (ADL) (Table 23–2) allowed by the disability, and (2) to obtain independent ambulation with or without assistive devices (e.g., wheelchairs, prostheses, orthoses, crutches, and canes). To obtain these goals, the rehabilitation therapy includes physical exercises to increase muscle strength, endurance,

TABLE 23–1

Multidisciplinary Cancer Rehabilitation Team

Physician
Rehabilitation oncology nurse
Physical therapist
Occupational therapist
Prosthetist-orthotist
Nutritionist
Speech pathologist
Social worker
Psychologist or psychiatrist
Chaplain
Vocational counselor
Recreational therapist

TABLE 23–2

Activities of Daily Living

Eating and drinking
Dressing and undressing
Bathing and grooming
Toileting
Managing bladder and bowel functions
Manipulating small objects
Caring for health and fitness
Moving in bed
Changing position
Walking
Climbing stairs
Performing general wheelchair skills
Using a manual wheelchair
Using an electric wheelchair

Adapted from Diller, et al.[7a]

joint range of motion, and self-care skills, as well as the application of physical modalities to reduce pain and swelling. Prescription, fabrication, and fitting of prosthetic and orthotic devices, followed by training in their use, is essential for most amputees and individuals with significant weakness, paralysis, or unstable skeletal structures.

Rehabilitation interventions that are directed at the psychologic, social, and vocational consequences of the cancer and the resulting physical disability help the patient and the family to cope with these problems, which are often profound. Optimally, psychosocial and vocational difficulties should be addressed at the time of initial diagnosis and treatment. The goal of cancer treatment is not only to eradicate the disease and keep the patient alive, but also to maintain or reestablish a quality of life. Although fatal or physically disabling sequelae of cancer are well recognized and usually well attended to by the hospital staff, the psychologic, social, and vocational consequences of cancer, which commonly become more evident after the patient is discharged from the hospital, frequently are unnoticed and therefore untreated. Consequently, the psychosocial and vocational difficulties may become more disabling than the physical disability.

The rehabilitation goals for cancer patients may be classified in a fashion that parallels the different stages of the disease:[18]

1. *Preventive rehabilitation* therapy is started early after diagnosis of cancer (i.e., before or immediately after surgery, radiotherapy, and/or chemotherapy). At this stage no significant disability may exist, but therapy is started to prevent disability.

2. *Restorative rehabilitation* therapy aims at the comprehensive restoration of maximal function for patients whose disease is considered cured or controlled but who have a residual disability.

3. *Supportive rehabilitation* therapy is geared toward increasing the self-sufficiency of the cancer patient with progressive disability and growing cancer by using quick, effective methods (e.g., providing appropriate assistive devices and teaching simple techniques for self-care). Supportive rehabilitation therapy includes physical exercises to prevent the effects of immobilization (e.g., joint contractures, muscle atrophy, weakness, and pressure sores). Frequently, this type of quick mobilization serves the additional purpose of reducing mental depression. These interventions may be thought of as an effort "to do something" in the presence of poor prognosis, but on the other hand, they have few negative side effects and may increase the patient's sense of well-being.

4. *Palliative rehabilitation* therapy seeks to increase or maintain the comfort and function of patients with terminal cancer by using physical modalities, orthotic devices, and various equipment to control pain, treat joint contractures and pressure sores, and provide at least a degree of greater self-sufficiency.

Cancer Rehabilitation and Adaptation Team

Organized cancer rehabilitation programs have significant and measurable benefits in relation to such established goals as restoration of physical function and community reintegration.[7, 17] Multidisciplinary cancer rehabilitation and adaptation teams are utilized by most cancer rehabilitation programs (see Table 23–1). Many different health care professions may be represented on these teams. The composition of the team may vary considerably, depending on the program's philosophy and size, the type of institution, and the range of disabilities encountered. The team is led by a physician, either an oncologist or, more commonly, a physiatrist.[17] Oncology nurses, social workers, psychologists, physical and occupational therapists, vocational counselors, chaplains, and nutritionists are present on most such teams.[17] Other rehabilitation professionals may contribute in an important way to the rehabilitation of cancer patients, depending on the specific disability (e.g., prosthetist, orthotist, speech pathologist, driver's trainer, and recreational therapist).

Physician. The physician who directs the rehabilitation team, usually a physiatrist, needs to be knowledgeable and experienced both in oncology and in the field of physical medicine and rehabilitation. The physician is the team's primary link with other treating physicians—the surgeon, the oncologist and/or the radiotherapist. To establish realistic goals and prescribe or design an appropriate and comprehensive rehabilitation program, the physiatrist needs to know (1) the exact cancer diagnosis with organ site, histologic type, and grade of anaplasia; (2) the cancer's anatomic staging (primary site only, involvement of regional lymph nodes, or metastases); (3) the patient's prognosis for life (cured or controlled, or the anticipated rapidity of the cancer's progression); and (4) the specific treatment plan for the cancer (timing of surgery, chemotherapy, and/or radiation) and the anticipated efficacy and potential side effects of treatment. The physiatrist shares with and explains this information to the team members for each to develop a specific and realistic plan of action (preventive, restorative, supportive, or palliative). The physiatrist introduces the patient and the family to the goals of the cancer rehabilitation team and meets regularly with the team as well as with the patient and the family to direct and coordinate their efforts while taking into account the patient's progress and changing needs.

Rehabilitation Oncology Nurse. The rehabilitation oncology nurse functions primarily as an easily accessible resource person both for the nursing staff who care for the cancer patient and for the patient and the family. The nurse assesses the patient's nursing needs; plans the care; assists in obtaining nursing supplies; teaches nursing care techniques to other nurses, the patient, and the family; educates them about treatment; facilitates patient and family self-management; evaluates discharge plans; and assists the patient and the family in the discharge process.

Physical Therapist. The physical therapist instructs the patient to perform specific exercises to strengthen muscles, to increase general endurance, and to improve joint range of motion. The physical therapist teaches balancing and coordination activities, as well as functional tasks such as transfers into and out of bed, wheelchair mobility, ambulation with or without assistive devices, the most effective gait patterns, and techniques for ascending and descending stairs and curbs. Various physical modalities may be used by the therapist to reduce pain (e.g., application of heat or cold, transcutaneous electrical nerve stimulation [TENS], and massage), but heat and massage are contraindicated directly over and in the vicinity of a tumor site. Physical exercise, which has long been given little consideration by physicians as a therapeutic modality, may have a distinct value in both prevention and management of cancer. For example, regular endurance exercise influences hormonal production, possibly reducing the risk of cancer of the female reproductive organs and breasts.[14] In addition, exercise reduces obesity and constipation, both of which are well-known risk factors for certain types of cancer, and it promotes better health habits with respect to smoking, alcohol consumption, and diet. Although the beneficial effects of exercise on mental health are well known, less well investigated are the potential beneficial effects on the body's immune system. Chronic pain is often reduced by exercise through several different mechanisms—by stronger muscles supporting pathologically affected body parts; by better joint mobility; by increased production of endorphins; by stimulation of proprioceptive nerve fibers, which might block painful stimuli from reaching consciousness according to the gate theory; and finally by improved self-image and mental outlook.

Occupational Therapist. The role of the occupational therapist overlaps to some extent with that of the physical therapist. The activities of the occupational therapist, however, are more focused on upper extremity exercises and self-care. The occupational therapist works with the patient with impaired function of the arms and hands to improve strength and coordination, as well as to teach and train her or him in the various ADL. The therapist provides the patient with different adaptive equipment to facilitate self-care and work-related activities. The occupational therapist is capable of making relatively simple orthotic devices (e.g., hand splints for joint immobilization or support of weak muscles). Additionally, the occupational therapist often performs a gross assessment of cognitive and visual perceptual skills and initiates therapy to compensate for deficits in these areas. The occupational therapist works with the disabled patient and the family to make the home and the workplace more accessible and more conducive to complete self-sufficiency and greater productivity. The occupational therapist, independently or working with a recreational therapist, strives to make resumption of leisure time activities easier for the patient.

Prosthetist-Orthotist. The primary role of the prosthetist or orthotist is to fabricate the optimal artificial limb (prosthesis) or brace (orthosis) for patients in need of such devices. The prosthetist or orthotist should assist the physician and the therapist in the evaluation of the patient's needs and the selection of the most appropriate components and materials for the device and the technology to be employed in its fabrication on the basis of the pathologic changes and the biomechanics involved. On delivery of the prosthesis or orthosis, the physician evaluates its comfort and fit, but the prosthetist or orthotist modifies and services the equipment as long as it remains in use.

Nutritionist. The nutritionist assesses the patient's nutritional status, determines the additional metabolic demands that the cancer places on the body, and designs the most appropriate diet with respect to the specific clinical problems, caloric intake, food ingredients of choice, optimal consistency for easy swallowing, and individual taste or choice. The nutritionist may assess food intake by calorie counting and assists in facilitating oral intake in the presence of poor appetite or swallowing disorders. The nutritionist should educate the patient and the family about general and specific dietary guidelines and consult with the clinical staff about the optimal parenteral nutrition, if needed.

Speech Pathologist. The speech pathologist evaluates and provides therapy for deficient oral communication, but also works closely with the occupational therapist and the nutritionist in the evaluation and management of swallowing disorders.

Social Worker. Social workers play an important role in the rehabilitation of the cancer patient in many respects, but in particular their role relates to continuity of care, discharge planning, smooth transition from the hospital to the community, and provision of appropriate follow-up services after discharge from the hospital. The social worker assists the patient in securing financial resources, including health insurance coverage, Social Security benefits, and disability compensation, and in obtaining authorization and payment for necessary equipment. Furthermore, the social worker should help in arranging, before hospital discharge, for transportation, attendant care, home modifications, and other appropriate posthospital services. This sometimes involves placement in and transfer to other health care institutions. The social worker may act as a liaison among the patient, the family members, and the various physicians involved in the patient's care, as well as the other professionals on the multidisciplinary rehabilitation team.

Psychologist or Psychiatrist. The rehabilitation psychologist or psychiatrist evaluates the patient's psychologic functioning, including intelligence; personality (e.g., ideational, emotional, behavioral, and characterologic patterns); past personal history; motivation; reaction to disability; and coping skills. Frequently, after the diagnosis of cancer and development of a disability, both the patient and family members experience reactive depression or grief, which often is expressed in diverse ways (e.g., denial, anger, anxiety, panic, fear, dependent behavior, depression, and unmasking of previously controlled psychopathologic conditions). A major role of the psychologist or psychiatrist is to assist the patient and the family in coping, as well as to counsel and consult with the rehabilitation team members in managing the patient.

Chaplain. A chaplain is frequently a member of the cancer rehabilitation team. The chaplain may be able to relate to the patient and the family in a way that can aid them to use their faith to adapt to the illness and disability.

Vocational Counselor. A vocational counselor should be enrolled in the care of all physically disabled cancer patients with even the slightest potential of returning to work. The vocational counselor should interview the patient while at the hospital and continue to see the patient on an outpatient basis. The vocational intervention, which may include evaluations, counseling, testing, exploring career options, and educational planning, proceeds to the extent and at a pace that is sensitive to the patient's needs and readiness to become involved vocationally. At the appropriate time, the counselor initiates job or school site visits and consults with employers and teachers to ease the transition from disability to productivity as a worker or a student. For school-aged children who are unable to attend school regularly, home tutoring may have to be arranged. Skills can be taught to solve problems and to seek jobs successfully. An office of vocational rehabilitation (OVR) exists in each state and can be a source of funding for various vocational rehabilitation services, such as certain aspects of rehabilitation, education, training, job placement, equipment, and environmental modifications, if these enable the patient eventually to return to school or work. The vocational counselor makes the initial referral to OVR and maintains a close cooperative and effective relationship with the OVR representatives.

Recreational Therapist. The recreational

therapist designs a program to meet the varied needs and interests of disabled individuals through various activities both inside and outside the hospital (e.g., engaging in art or music therapy, attending performances or sporting events, and going to restaurants and shops). Family and friends are encouraged to join the recreational activities to stimulate socialization, encourage more leisure time activities, and support positive attitudes. The trips into the community may facilitate the eventual discharge process for a physically disabled person and the reintegration into community life.

Functional Assessment

The outcome of rehabilitation treatment is not measured as in other medical disciplines, for example, by whether the patient lives or dies and whether the fever is down, the stitches are out, or even if the pain is diminished. The effectiveness of rehabilitation services is evaluated by how functional the disabled person becomes after the rehabilitation intervention. The ability to perform the various ADL skills (see Table 23–2) and the quality of life are measured and documented; improvement justifies the continuation of treatment. Currently, it is relatively easy to measure function in gross terms (e.g., if the patient is able to walk and perform self-care), but numerical assessment of subtle progress in the fine motor skills and in the quality of life is still difficult. Accurate comprehensive functional assessment requires collection of a great number of diverse data. The simpler functional assessment scales (e.g., PULSES profile, Barthel Index, and functional independence measure [FIM]) are simple and easy to use but provide incomplete information. The newer and more comprehensive scales (e.g., rehabilitation indicators and ESCROW functional scale) address hundreds of variables and require the use of computers. These scales assess not only performance of the various self-care skills but also the quality of life with respect to diverse aspects of role functioning: employment, income, education, participation in family and social activities, living arrangements, transportation, and so on. Performance is rated with regard to the amount of assistance required in each skill area. The performance data are collected by physical examination and direct observation, review of records, and reports from the various members of the rehabilitation team, as well as information collected directly from the patient and the family. An appropriately programmed computer can subsequently plot changing performance for each skill and the overall performance of the patient, and thus document progress during both inpatient and outpatient rehabilitation.

Rehabilitation Management of Musculoskeletal Tumors

TUMORS OF SPINE

Primary bone tumors of the spine are uncommon, the most frequently seen being multiple myeloma. Metastatic disease involving the spinal column, on the other hand, is common. At least 5% of patients with systemic cancer at autopsy have evidence of spinal cord compression,[1] usually from an anterior epidural mass that involves bone. Although the histologic features and response to treatment are quite different for multiple myeloma than for metastases to the spine, the symptoms, signs, and therapeutic principles are quite similar, which allows the clinical findings and the rehabilitation management of these two conditions to be addressed simultaneously.

Symptoms and Signs

Pain is by far the most frequent initial symptom of a tumor of the spine. The pain may be diffuse, localized, or radicular. It is typically made worse by movement and by the Valsalva maneuver. Unlike back pain from more benign conditions, the pain caused by tumors tends to be persistent, present or even worse at night, and not relieved by rest.

Neurologic dysfunction may occur gradually or suddenly, depending on the tumor's rate of growth and its location or on the occurrence of a sudden pathologic fracture. Slowly progressive neurologic loss is often seen with tumors of the lumbosacral spine encroaching on the cauda equina, whereas tumors of the thoracic spine may quickly cause collapse of the vertebral body with direct compression of the spinal cord or its blood supply. Although only 50% of all tumors of the spine are in the thoracic region, these are the cause of 70% of all spinal cord compressions that result in paraplegia. Paraplegia can be neurologically complete, with total paralysis and sensory loss below the level of the lesion. More commonly, the neurologic lesion is incomplete, with some sensation and motor function preserved. Disturbances of bladder and bowel control initially may present clinically as urinary urgency or hesitancy, but with progressive cord compression, urinary retention or bowel and bladder incontinence may occur.

Treatment

Appropriate rehabilitation management depends on accurate diagnosis and staging of the tumor, just as does the medical and surgical management. Most patients can and should be managed nonsurgically with chemotherapy, irradiation, and orthotic stabilization of the spine, as radiotherapy alone of most spinal metastases provides equal or better results than surgery that is followed by radiotherapy.[13] Generally, decompression solely by laminectomy has been of limited use compared with radiation, because the compressive lesion is usually located anteriorly and the procedure itself contributes to spinal instability. However, severe neurologic loss, especially when occurring rapidly, may warrant decompression surgery, which should be done preferably by an anterior approach, followed by surgical stabilization. Decompression, unfortunately, is not effective after the patient has become paraplegic. Surgical stabilization may also be indicated in the presence of gross spinal instability, as best judged by destruction of two of the three columns of the spine (anterior, middle, and posterior).[9] The extent of stabilization procedures varies with the patient's anticipated life expectancy. Patients with a relatively poor prognosis (survival for less than 1 year) benefit most from a simple procedure employing methyl methacrylate, which allows instantaneous stability and rapid mobilization of the patient, whereas patients with a more favorable prognosis may be better served with instrumentation and bone fusion in conjunction with methyl methacrylate.[9]

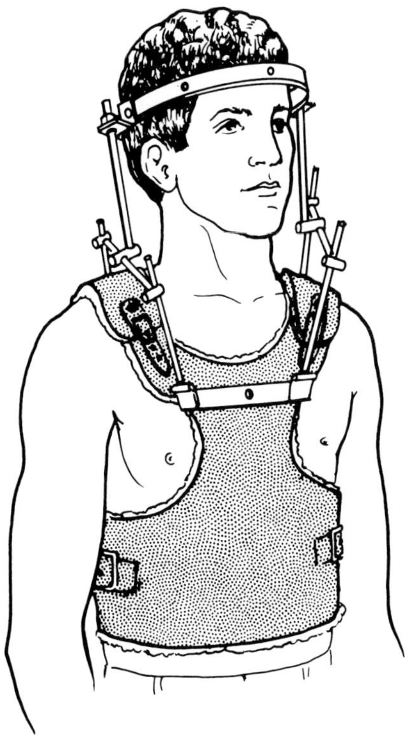

FIGURE 23–1. Halo-orthosis. (Reproduced by permission from Ragnarsson KT: Orthotics and Shoes. *In* DeLisa JA (ed): Rehabilitation Medicine: Principles and Practice. Philadelphia, JB Lippincott, 1988.)

Spinal metastases and myelomatous lesions, even when accompanied by compression fractures and minor or modest spinal instability, can be well managed by spinal orthotic support (body brace) and radiotherapy, both of which may significantly reduce pain. Such lesions in the cervical spine are best immobilized by a halo brace (Fig. 23–1) or even by sternal-occipital-mandibular immobilizer (SOMI) brace (Fig. 23–2). When lesions of this type are present in the upper thoracic spine, orthotic devices may not be of much value, as this part of the spine is stabilized inherently by the rib cage. Lesions in the more mobile lower thoracic spine and in the lumbar spine are often accompanied by severe pain. A simple ready-made but adjustable thoracolumbosacral (TLS) corset (Fig. 23–3) with posterior stays may provide adequate support for less severe lesions, reduce pain, and give the patient increased mobility. The soft anterior portion of the corset (the apron) should fit snugly over the entire abdomen, thus generating a liquid column that spreads the weight over a large area. More severe lesions and postoperative conditions may warrant fabrication of a custom-molded TLS bivalved plastic brace (body jacket) (Fig. 23–4), which firmly holds the pelvis below and the chest above.

When neurologic deficits are present, the rehabilitation interventions have to be carefully individualized, taking into consideration the extent of the neurologic loss, the general medical condition, and the patient's life expectancy. Severe spinal cord dysfunction with severe or complete paralysis and sensory loss, as well as loss of bowel and bladder control, necessitates a comprehensive but relatively short-term rehabilitation program, which involves all members of the rehabilitation team or as many as is judged appropriate by the

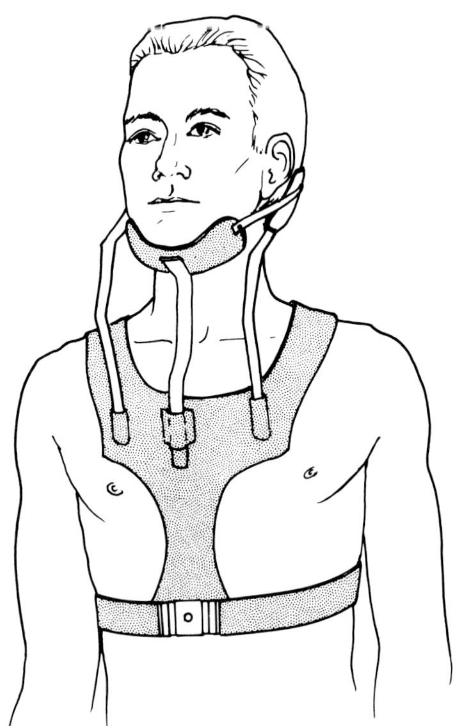

FIGURE 23–2. Sternal-occipital-mandibular immobilizer (SOMI orthosis). (Reproduced by permission from Ragnarsson KT: Orthotics and Shoes. *In* DeLisa JA (ed): Rehabilitation Medicine: Principles and Practice. Philadelphia, JB Lippincott, 1988.)

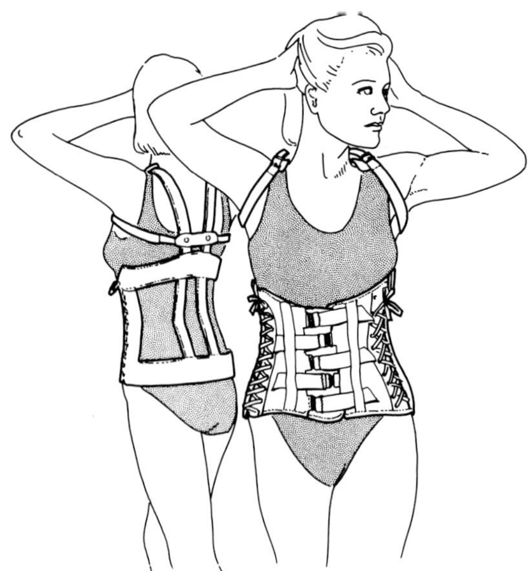

FIGURE 23–3. Thoracolumbosacral orthosis (TLSO, Knight-Taylor brace).

physiatrist. The rehabilitation interventions should address each of the multitude of clinical complications and conditions customarily seen in persons with spinal cord dysfunction of traumatic origin (Table 23–3). Immediate intervention should include bedside physical and occupational therapy, initiation of bowel and bladder training programs, and the application of nursing principles to prevent complications such as bedsores and joint contractures, which often prolong the subsequent rehabilitation period. Proper positioning of the patient in bed and turning the patient at least every 2 hours is of paramount importance in this regard. The patient and the family are given psychologic support and are educated in the medical aspects of spinal cord dysfunction and its management. If life expectancy is short (less than 6 months), the patient is best instructed in the ADL that he or she can readily learn to accomplish; is provided with necessary assistive devices, nursing supplies, and personal assistance; and is discharged from the hospital as soon as medically appropriate to the home or a nursing facility. When the life expectancy is greater (longer than 1 year), the medical or surgical condition is stable, and no major medical complications exist, the paraplegic patient is best transferred to an inpatient rehabilitation unit for a more comprehensive and intensive rehabilitation program.

The inpatient rehabilitation unit should be in a hospital with an inhouse physician on call and the various medical and surgical consultation services continuously available (around the clock). On the inpatient rehabilitation unit,

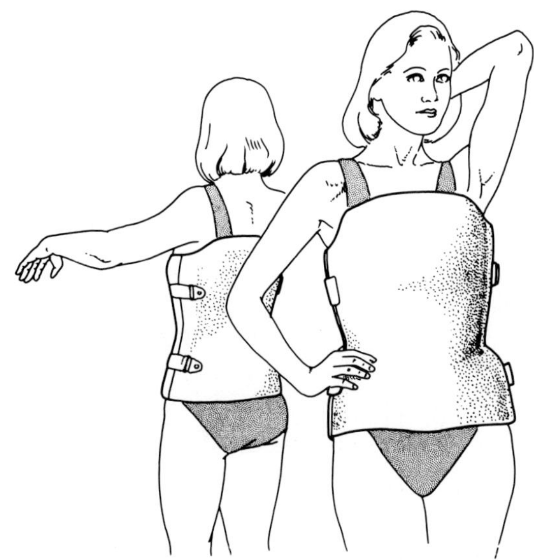

FIGURE 23–4. Custom-molded thoracolumbosacral orthosis (TLSO), a two-piece removable plastic orthosis (body jacket).

TABLE 23–3

Conditions and Complications Associated with Spinal Cord Dysfunction

Loss of motor power
Loss of sensation
Pressure sores
Urinary dysfunction
Bowel dysfunction
Sexual dysfunction
Autonomic dysfunction
Pain
Spasticity
Joint contractures
Heterotopic ossification
Metabolic and hormonal disturbances
Circulatory disorders
Respiratory insufficiency
Psychological problems
Social and vocational problems

the paraplegic patient is again examined by the physiatrist, who obtains a detailed medical and social history and assesses the general medical condition and the precise neurologic status to determine the level and completeness of spinal cord lesion, as well as the current functional ability. The physiatrist writes the customary medical orders (e.g., nursing instructions, administration of medications, and specific diagnostic tests—urologic evaluation, pulmonary function tests for high-level cord lesions, appropriate radiologic and electrodiagnostic studies, blood and urine tests, and so on). The physiatrist sets the general rehabilitation goals for the patient and prescribes detailed evaluation, which is then followed by interventions by the various members of the multidisciplinary rehabilitation team. The physiatrist prescribes the specific exercises and training methods to be given by physical and occupational therapists, as well as the interventions by the psychologist or psychiatrist and the vocational counselor, when those are needed.

The rehabilitation program starts immediately after the transfer to the rehabilitation unit. During the first days the actual participation of the patients is often impeded by their physical deconditioning or by special evaluations and tests, but thereafter they generally spend 4 to 6 hours daily in an active therapy program in addition to their ward activities (e.g., bowel and bladder management, self-care training, education, and recreational activities). When serious medical complications arise during the course of rehabilitation and interfere with the patient's ability to attend the rehabilitation program for at least 3 hours a day, for more than 3 consecutive days, the patient should be transferred to the appropriate medical or surgical service for definitive care.

An initial team conference is usually held within 1 or 2 weeks of admission, during which the patient's medical, neurologic, functional, psychologic, social, and vocational status, as well as the rehabilitation potential and prognosis, are presented and discussed. More specific rehabilitation goals are set, equipment needs are assessed, and a discharge date is predicted. Shortly after this conference, the physiatrist meets with the patient and the family, together or separately, to discuss these issues and answer questions regarding the patient's medical condition and rehabilitation program. Team rehabilitation conferences are usually held biweekly to discuss the patient's progress and plans for discharge. Communication among rehabilitation members, a most critical component, is facilitated through informal meetings, during which the medical, psychologic, social, and other specific concerns that any member of the team may have about any patients are shared and discussed. When the patient is discharged from the hospital, it is most important to ensure that necessary equipment and supplies have been obtained, family members or home health care aides have been instructed and trained in the patient's care, follow-up by a visiting nurse service has been arranged, and referrals have been made for continuing therapy and visits with the various physicians (e.g., oncologist, surgeon, physiatrist, and family physician).

TUMORS OF LIMBS

The treatment of primary malignant limb tumors is usually surgical. The main goal is to remove the tumor by an excision with wide margins through a site well clear of any neoplastic tissue or, when indicated, by a radical resection (i.e., the removal of the entire compartment involved by the tumor). The secondary surgical goal is to reconstruct the resulting defect for optimal function and cosmesis. Previously, the standard and most widely accepted surgical method was limb amputation, but during the past decade, limb preservation by local resection and reconstruction often has become the treatment of choice. The period of disease-free life and the survival rate for both types of surgical approaches have improved in recent years owing to the use of chemotherapy and/or radiotherapy. The return to optimal function can best be assured by the cooperative efforts of a multidisciplinary team, which includes the orthopedic surgeon, the radiation therapist, the medical oncologist, the physiatrist, and personnel from allied health care professions.

Preoperative Care

As soon as diagnosis of the primary limb tumor is confirmed, rehabilitation efforts should be initiated. Regardless of whether amputation or limb-sparing reconstructive surgery is planned for tumor removal, or whether chemotherapy and/or radiotherapy is to be instituted preoperatively or postoperatively, the patient and the family should be counseled regarding the implications of surgery and the postoperative course. At the same time, an appropriate physical exercise program should be started. The initiation of these interventions during the highly emotional and stressful preoperative days can be valuable aids in easing the patient's adjustment and reaction to the postoperative course. Emotional support is best given by acknowledging the patient's anxiety and by providing practical information and explicit factual instructions that can be easily grasped and followed. Although it is important that the positive aspects of the procedure be explained (for instance, that it is a life-saving technique and that modern technology and training allow significant restoration of function), it is still considered best for the physician to resist overly optimistic predictions and to discourage fanciful aspirations until certain postoperative success has been obtained. Nonetheless, pessimistic predictions of what the patient will never be capable of doing are needless and usually inaccurate. A timetable should be given for postoperative rehabilitation phases and possible return to different functional activities, taking into account the type of surgery and the patient's general physical and mental status, age, athletic ability, life style, and so on. Peer counseling by a successfully rehabilitated patient may further help the patient to anticipate postoperative events and function.

When limb-sparing surgery or amputation is planned, the surgical approach or the exact level of amputation should be chosen carefully, considering not only the location and type of the tumor, but also the probability of good healing and the successful fitting of a prosthesis when required. It is thus useful for the surgeon to consult with the physiatrist and the prosthetist. The preoperative exercise program should focus on muscle-strengthening exercises for the uninvolved extremities, the trunk, and the muscles to be spared in the affected limb. For example, the patient should be taught isometric exercises for the quadriceps and gluteal muscles. Isotonic strengthening exercises with progressive resistance should be started for all the unaffected limbs, emphasizing specifically shoulder depressors and elbow extensors, which are critical for ambulation with crutches or walkers. Trunk strengthening and balancing exercises further facilitate postoperative ambulation success. Ambulation with a walker or crutches, with avoidance of weight bearing on the affected limb, should be taught preoperatively, while the patient is not fearful of falling because of lack of limb support and is not affected by incision pain, medications, or postoperative complications. These preoperative interventions not only help the patient to succeed quickly postoperatively in ambulation and self-care activities, but also speed restoration of function, which greatly eases the psychologic adjustment to the disability and social reintegration.

Amputation

There are approximately 45,000 amputations performed yearly in the United States, but neoplasms account for only 5 to 10% of these. In the past, amputation for cancer was discouraged, as it was believed that life expectancy did not justify the procedure and the aftercare. However, a retrospective study of 199 amputations performed for cancer at the Mayo Clinic between 1965 and 1969 showed that 5-year survival was 49% for these patients, a favorable outcome compared with that for patients with amputations done on ischemic limbs.[33] Functional skills of cancer amputees were shown to be superior to those of amputees for other causes.[20]

Until a decade ago, amputations for cancer were radical and infrequently left any residual limb (stump), except in the case of the most distal limb tumors. Lower extremity amputations for malignancies thus were done frequently by a hip disarticulation or hemipelvectomy, and upper limb amputations, by shoulder disarticulation or interscapulothoracic (forequarter) amputations. These extensive limb ablations were thought to be necessary because of the high incidence of metastases, especially metastases to the lungs, and concern about local recurrence. New diagnostic techniques, such as magnetic resonance imaging, improved computer tomography, and radionuclide bone scanning, now can verify the presence or absence of metastasis with a great degree of accuracy. A recent survey found that metastases apparently are not as common as was previously thought.[12] Therefore, when indicated, most oncologic surgeons now employ less extensive amputation techniques, typically cross-bone amputations. This type of surgery results in greater residual limb length and consequently better functional outcome for most patients. Thus, if an amputation is considered the best surgical treatment, a malignant primary tumor in the distal femur would now be treated by an amputation through the proximal femur; a tumor in the proximal tibia, by amputation in the midfemur or even the distal femur; and tumor in the distal tibia, by a below-knee amputation (BKA). Analogous amputation levels would be appropriately considered for tumors of the upper limbs.

Although maximal preservation of limb length compatible with appropriate tumor eradication is desirable, certain levels of amputation result in stumps that are difficult to fit and therefore are best avoided (e.g., the hindfoot, the distal third of the leg, and the femoral supracondylar region). The preservation of the knee joint, whenever possible, is critical with respect to smoothness of gait, lower energy expenditure, and better function. Preferably 12 to 18 cm of tibia should be preserved for optimal prosthetic fitting, but even a short BKA with as little as 2.54 cm of tibia preserved is better than an above-knee level. The fibula, if preserved, should be slightly shorter than the tibia. Knee disarticulation is also preferable to above-knee amputation (AKA), as it provides a wide weight-bearing surface, long lever arm, and some proprioception. AKA should be at least 10 cm above the knee joint for prosthetic purposes but otherwise should provide a stump as long as possible. An AKA that preserves less than 8 cm measured from the greater trochanter functions poorly; in general, hip disarticulation is preferable to an amputation at or above the level of the lesser trochanter. Hip disarticulation and hemipelvectomy[8] should have a long posterior flap whenever possible to provide adequate seating for the prosthesis. Hemicorporectomies (translumbar amputations) have been performed on only a few patients with widespread cancer of the pelvis but absent metastasis above.

Most malignant tumors of the upper limbs unfortunately are located in the proximal humerus, and therefore when amputation is indicated, shoulder disarticulation or interscapulothoracic amputation is most commonly performed. In the former approach, retention of the humeral head results in better prosthetic fitting and function, but in either approach, it is important to retain normal skin and as much muscle mass as possible.

The surgical techniques of amputation[3] are of enormous significance for prosthetic success. It is not sufficient just to retain maximal length of the stump, although this is important for leverage, and a large total contact area for weight bearing. A good stump needs to be firm and tapered or cylindric in shape, with all bone ends well padded. The skin should be nonadherent, without sensitive scars, but with good innervation and blood supply. The surgical handling of each tissue (i.e., skin, fascia, muscles, bone, nerves, and blood vessels) is of great concern to the physiatrist who needs to be familiar with the techniques used and to communicate openly with the orthopedic surgeon on this matter both preoperatively and postoperatively to ensure success. Owing to recent improvements in prosthetic techniques, the exact placement of the scar is not of as great importance. The skin should be closed carefully edge to edge without tension. Muscles should be cut cleanly to avoid maceration. Stabilization of sectioned muscles to opposing muscles or to bone by myoplasty or myodesis is traditionally done, although in recent years this technique has become somewhat controversial and is believed to be of limited long-term benefit. The nerves should be ligated high and cut with a sharp knife and allowed to retract. When the bone is cut, the periosteum is elevated about 1.5 to 3 cm above the cut end. Careful rounding of the edges with a sharp file should be done. When chemotherapy or radiotherapy is to follow surgery, appropriate suture material should be used at all depths. A Penrose through-and-through drain or even a suction drain is usually placed.

Postoperative care should aim for uneventful wound healing, reduction of swelling, and prevention of stump edema and joint contractures, as well as increased muscle strength and function. Early stump care focuses on appropriate dressing and application of external pressure by a variety of means. Methods of postoperative stump dressing were compared by Katz and Wu,[19] taking into account several factors of importance in stump care, including immobilization of soft tissue for more rapid healing; prevention of edema, trauma, excessive moisture collection, and pressure sore formation; spread of stump shrinkage; ease of inspection of wound; and the stump response to weight bearing. Soft sterile dressings covered with snugly wrapped elastic (Ace) bandages still may be the most commonly employed dressing technique, but this approach was inferior to the more rigid dressings with respect to most of the above-mentioned factors. Stump wrapping with elastic bandages needs to be done carefully and frequently reapplied to provide maximal pressure and to avoid a tourniquet effect. Various forms of semirigid dressings have been used, both nonremovable and removable (e.g., Unna paste dressing, custom-made elastic stump socks, plastic film, and inflatable air splints, each of which has different advantages and disadvantages). The inflatable air splints have gained some popularity. These are made of clear plastic, which allows easy inspection, and have a zipper for easy donning and doffing.

Immediate postsurgical fitting (IPSF)[2] is a more rigid form of dressing, which may effectively reduce edema, postoperative pain, and mental depression. This technique seems to be of particular benefit to young victims of limb tumors, but for various reasons discussed below it is not widely employed. The surgical skin incision should be covered with a silk or nylon dressing, which is soaked in saline with a ¾-inch absorbent gauze on top. A three-ply stump sock is then rolled over the gauze. Bony prominences are relieved with felt pads as necessary to generate a weight-bearing surface. An elastic plaster bandage is then used to form a plaster socket, carefully avoiding a tourniquet effect proximally. A prosthetic pylon and foot may be attached to the plaster to allow standing with minimal weight bearing as early as 1 or 2 days postoperatively. This is followed by progressive ambulation and increasing weight bearing, with full weight bearing possible 3 to 4 weeks postoperatively. Several studies showed the benefits of this technique in terms of reduction of edema, pain, mental depression, and postoperative morbidity and mortality and perhaps more rapid functional restoration.[25] Several disadvantages account for its low popularity. The wound cannot be readily examined and may heal more slowly owing to the recommended early end-weight bearing and the resulting pressure on the incision line. Suspension is relatively easy for a below-knee stump but difficult for an above-knee stump. Most important, the regularly scheduled or emergency cast changes are time consuming and in practice mean that an experienced person needs to be available continuously. These disadvantages, while recognizing the shaping and shrinking benefits of end pressure on the stump from a rigid dressing, led to the development of a modified and removable rigid dressing (RRD), which allows for easy stump inspection, dressing change, adjustment for progressive stump shrinkage, and even attachment of a temporary adjustable prosthesis. The RRD may be made of plaster[36, 37] in a similar fashion as for IPSF or of fiberglass or plastic[16] and have attachments for a pylon-foot unit.

POSTOPERATIVE EXERCISE PROGRAM

Postoperatively, physical and occupational therapy should be started as soon as the patient is medically stable. The specific exercises initiated preoperatively are resumed for general and specific muscle strengthening effect, as well as for joint range of motion to prevent contractures that often develop easily (e.g., knee flexion contractures for the BKA and hip flexion and abduction contractures for the AKA). Mobilization is started first in bed and, 1 or 2 days postoperatively, out of bed by transferring to a wheelchair and starting ambulation in parallel bars or with a walker. The amputee progresses to ambulation with two crutches and eventually to a cane when a prosthesis has been obtained. Various types of ready-made or prefabricated temporary prosthetic devices exist (e.g., a pneumatic adjustable prosthesis made of transparent plastic, which allows early weight bearing). A custom-fitted provisional prosthesis should be made as soon as skin healing has occurred. This prosthesis is worn for several months until most of the stump shrinking and shaping has occurred. When applicable, proper stump wrapping techniques are taught. An occupational therapist reviews performance in ADL and provides training as needed. The amputee may be discharged from the hospital when he or she is ambulating safely without a prosthesis and can independently perform ADL. Transfer to an inpatient rehabilitation service can occur at anytime before those two goals are reached if the amputee is otherwise medically stable.

PROSTHETIC PRESCRIPTION

Multiple factors in addition to the amputation level and stump condition need to be considered carefully when a prosthesis is prescribed. These include associated medical conditions and other physical disabilities, life expectancy, coordination, muscle strength, endurance, motivation, learning ability, emotional adjustment, and various personal and life style factors (e.g., age, weight, family support, recreational activities, geography, home environment, ordinary daily demands, and occupation). Functional outcome can be predicted with some accuracy on the basis of an initial evaluation, as each symptomatic medical defect lowers functional expectations. Ability to ambulate with a walker or a pair of crutches or with a temporary inflatable prosthesis may further clarify the patient's candidacy for a prosthesis. By considering all the factors above, the physician prescribing the prosthesis must select between relatively greater safety with stability versus higher function with great mobility as well as durability and lightness of weight, besides considering differences in cosmetic appearance and cost. Even the skill and expertise of the prosthetist should be considered and the distance between the prosthetic facility and the patient's home needs to be taken into account when prosthetic components are chosen.

No prosthesis can ever function as well, or look as natural, as a healthy limb, although it may present significant improvement over an unhealthy limb. Today, most prostheses are fabricated from metals and plastics, but rarely of wood. The most common lower limb prostheses prescribed for cancer amputees are below-knee, above-knee, hip disarticulation, and hemipelvectomy prostheses. The traditional below-knee prosthesis consists of a socket and shank and foot components as well as a suspension system. The socket generally should have a patellar tendon–bearing (PTB) design and total contact with the stump for greater distribution of pressure. Occasionally, supracondylar/suprapatellar PTB socket (PTS SC/SP) may be indicated. Soft liners inside the socket may increase comfort by shock absorption and several-ply stump socks may have to be worn to accommodate a shrinking stump. The shank may be of an endoskeletal design with an internal metal pylon covered with foam, or a plastic-laminated exoskeletal structure. The foot is usually of the solid ankle cushion heel (SACH) design. This simple, durable, lightweight, and still cosmetic foot has many advantages over other older designs (e.g., the single-axis or multiple-axes feet). Supracondylar cuff suspension is most commonly prescribed, but other alternatives include a rubber or neoprene sleeve, a medial supracondylar wedge, PTS SC/SP design, and a laced thigh corset with a waist belt. The old-fashioned open-ended socket with a PTB area, a laced thigh corset, and side knee joints is now rarely seen, but still can be considered for amputees with short or tender stumps, patients with unstable or fused knees, or those subject to great physical demands.

The patient with AKA most commonly receives a prosthesis with a rigid quadrilateral socket with a posterior ischial seat for weight bearing, as most of these amputees poorly tolerate end-weight bearing. The anterior socket wall is slightly higher and concaved to provide a posteriorly directed force to keep the ischial tuberosity on its "seat." A single-axis knee joint with constant friction is simple, durable, and most popular. Polycentric or hydraulic knee units may provide superior function for young physically active amputees but are costly and have been prone to mechanical problems. Posterior placement of the knee axis increases stability during stance but makes initiation of knee flexion more difficult. Automatic knee locks activated by weight bearing can be added for safety, but manual locks are simpler and lighter. Suspension for the AKA prosthesis ideally is provided by total suction, but partial suction with a Silesian bandage and a pelvic band with a lateral hip joint represent frequently considered alternatives. An endoskeletal pylon connects the knee unit above to a SACH foot below.

The amputee with hip disarticulation invariably is fitted with the Canadian-type prosthesis, which has a plastic-laminated socket encircling the pelvis. It uses the ischial tuberosity for weight bearing and the iliac crest for suspension. The hemipelvectomy patient uses the same type of prosthesis with an extension to the rib cage for weight bearing. Placement of the hip joint results in excellent stability, while permitting free hip and knee motion.

Upper limb amputations for malignant tumors usually result in shoulder disarticulation or interscapulothoracic amputation. Fitting with a functional, body-powered prosthesis is difficult with the former and almost impossible with the latter. Externally powered or myoelectrically controlled prostheses have provided these patients with some gross function. A plastic-laminated socket covering the chest and the shoulder blade is secured by a chest harness. A flexion-abduction shoulder joint unit connects the socket to an artificial arm, which has an alternating internal locking elbow unit. A wrist unit allows passive positioning and an interchangeable terminal device, which may be a body-powered hook or functional hand, passive cosmetic hand, or alternatively an externally powered hook or hand. Externally powered devices usually use electrical batteries and are activated by myoelectric signals. These are relatively expensive and heavy and require more frequent maintenance than body-powered prostheses. Nonetheless, myoelectric prostheses have gained wide acceptance, particularly in Europe.

RECENT ADVANCES IN LOWER LIMB PROSTHETICS

Prosthetic technology has advanced greatly during the last decade.[32] Evaluation of the amputation stump for socket fit has been facilitated by the use of diagnostic transparent check sockets, biostereometric techniques, xeroradiography, magnetic resonance imaging, and computer-aided design–computer-aided manufacturing (CAD-CAM),[11] supplementing the traditional subjective methods of the user's self-assessment and reliance on the prosthetist's judgment and experience. New methods to make cast impressions of the stump by stage or by vacuum casting and controlled pressure application resulted in more accurate replication of the stump for socket shaping as well as in better fit and comfort.[22] The CAD-CAM system may result in improved socket fitting and reduce fabrication time. Using this method, stump measurements are fed into a computer, which designs a socket model that can be modified on the screen in the same manner as a cast. The digital information of the final model is transmitted to a computerized machine, which automatically carves an actual stump model, which in turn is used to fabricate a prosthetic socket in a relatively conventional way.

Socket design has changed dramatically with the introduction of new concepts. The contoured adducted trochanteric–controlled alignment method (CAT-CAM)[30] for AKAs follows the anatomic shape of the stump and allows the femur to be in its normal adducted position in contrast to the quadrilateral socket design. It allows the ischial tuberosity to sit inside the socket to generate a three-point pressure system through the ischial tuberosity, the greater trochanter, and the entire shaft of the femur, thus offering stability to the abductor muscles and the pelvis in relation to the femoral adduction. Recently, this method has been referred to as ischial-ramal containment (IRC) socket rather than CAT-CAM, which is easily confused with CAD-CAM. Another new concept is the use of flexible wall sockets as an interface between the stump and the outer hard socket, which in turn may have fenestrations cut out in strategic locations to reduce weight and improve sensory feedback without compromising support. The inner flexible sockets are made of transparent thermoplastic materials, mostly polyethylene or Surlyn. The rigid outer socket may be made of ultralight materials (e.g., carbon graphite laminates). The flexible socket design, initially introduced in Scandinavia, has been used mostly for AKA prostheses, but recently also for BKA prostheses. It has resulted in improved fit and suspension by suction and has generally met enthusiastic patient response (Icelandic–Swedish–New York [ISNY] prosthesis, Scandinavian flexible socket, total flexible socket [TFS], Icelandic roll on suction socket [Iceross]). Multidurometer socket liners made of lightweight washable thermoplastic foams of different densities (e.g., Pelite and Aliplast) can be laminated together both to improve support and to provide pressure relief.

Endoskeletal modular pylons covered with foam have been successfully used for many years, but recently introduced alignment systems that are added to the pylon have made it much easier to establish the optimal linear and angular relationships between the socket and the foot for maximal comfort and function.

Knee units have changed relatively little during the past few years, although improved hydraulic systems (e.g., Henschke-Mauch unit) have enhanced knee control during stance and resulted in smoother, more energy efficient gait patterns.

New designs in prosthetic feet have improved both their looks and function. Energy-storing feet, which are made of lightweight materials, have gained popularity, especially among physically vigorous amputees, as they seem to diminish energy cost and increase endurance during walking and running, although they are not necessarily lighter than the SACH foot. The Carbon Copy II foot is a modification of the SACH foot with a long flexible nylon lever arm reaching from the prosthetic hindfoot to the toes to provide "spring" action. The Flex-Foot is a composite structure made of carbon and graphite with an anterior leaf spring configuration and a posterior heel extension, both of which are capable of storing energy and aiding forward propulsion. Perhaps best known is the Seattle foot, which incorporates a keel made of high-strength nylon. The keel stores energy through compression at midstance to heel-off and transmits it back during the push-off phase of the gait cycle.[4] The SAFE foot has a flexible inner keel with a strong plantar band, which provides considerable adaptability to rugged, uneven terrain.[5]

Most of these feet as well as shanks may be covered with cosmetic outer layers to simulate the appearance of a real foot. New finishing techniques (e.g. mirror imaging[6] and cosmetic skin covering[24]) are time consuming and expensive, but result in superb appearance.

PROSTHETIC TRAINING AND WEAR

During the final stages of prosthetic fabrication, the patient needs to visit the prosthetist several times to ensure optimal fit. The rehabilitation goals are that the prosthesis provides maximal function and comfort and that the amputee learns to use the prosthesis to her or his greatest advantage. After delivery of the prosthesis, the prescribing physician needs to evaluate the prosthesis for proper fit and comfort, stability of the socket, joint motions, appropriate functions, and appearance. Monthly reevaluations are recommended for the next 3 months, but thereafter visits every 3 to 6 months are usually sufficient. Prosthetic training with physical and occupational therapies focus primarily on gait instruction for the lower extremity amputees with or without gait aids, such as canes and crutches; proper donning and doffing techniques; continued muscle-strengthening and joint range of motion exercises; balancing techniques; and instructions for postural symmetry. For the upper extremity amputee, therapy focuses on learning to open and close the terminal device, positioning the arm, manipulating objects, and training in self-care. Initially, the prosthesis can only be worn comfortably for 15 to 30 minutes at a time, with frequent rest periods between wearing, and therapy sessions are therefore necessarily short. The skin should be carefully examined after each use for signs of excessive pressure or poor socket fit. The eventual acceptance and use of the prosthesis reflects the amputee's opinion about its benefits and shortcomings.

Early on, prosthetic usage can produce many potentially confrontational situations between the amputee and the health care professionals. Initial discomfort is unavoidable both at the prosthesis-user interface and in other body parts that are subjected to new and increased demands. A common reaction of the amputee is to feel somewhat disappointed with the final appearance, weight, ease of wear, level of comfort, and functional limitations of the device. The rehabilitation team needs to understand the adjustment process and help the amputee to work through this period with encouragement, attention to legitimate complaints, and appropriate and careful adjustments of the prosthesis. Inadequate communication may lead the amputee to start "shopping around" and end up with another prosthesis and similar complaints.

A multitude of gait deviations may occur with lower limb prosthetic use. These are caused by numerous factors, including those due to medical conditions, poor prosthetic design or adjustment, emotional reactions, and inadequate training. The gait deviations need to be carefully evaluated.[27] After the prosthetic factors disturbing gait have been identified, the device can be adjusted.

The energy expenditure of patients during ambulation with a prosthesis is significantly increased when compared with that of nondisabled persons.[10, 15, 34, 35] Depending on stump length, the BKA patient expends 10 to 40% more oxygen than normal at the same walking speed and the AKA patient expends 65% more. However, to conserve energy most amputees in real life slow down their ambulation speed to 2.0 to 2.5 mph for BKA and 1.0 to 1.5 mph for AKA, compared with the normal speed of 3 to 4 mph for nonamputees. The difference in energy expenditure and speed of ambulation between BKA and AKA patients vividly demonstrates the importance of saving the knee joint, if possible.

AMPUTATIONS IN CHILDREN AND ADOLESCENTS

Although most amputees are elderly, 10 to 15% of new amputees are younger than 21 years of age. Although most are due to congenital limb deficiencies, malignant tumors account for 30% of acquired amputations in young people and are the most frequent cause of amputation within the age range of 10 to 19 years.[28] Treatment principles for young amputees are similar to those used for adults, although in the growing child any possible preservation of epiphyses is beneficial to allow maximal growth of the residual limb. Bone overgrowth is relatively common and may cause symptomatic skin pressure. This may require skin traction, but if it proves unsuccessful, bone resection may be advised. Children with amputations should be fitted with a prosthesis as soon as they are developmentally able to sit alone. Although lower limb amputees require little training to learn to ambulate, children should be carefully instructed in the use of upper limb prostheses to prevent poor habits that may interfere with future control and function. Training of young children may be a difficult and frustrating task, as their attention span is short. Parents should be instructed on how to put on and remove the prosthesis and how to promote maximal wear and optimal use. Without the parents' compliance, acceptance, and encouragement, an upper limb prosthesis is likely to be rejected by the child. Children's prostheses require greater maintenance and more frequent repair than those of adults, owing to greater wear and tear, and more frequent refabrication because of children's limb growth.

MEDICAL PROBLEMS RELATING TO AMPUTATIONS

Various problems may be specifically related to the amputation and prosthetic wear, including pain, skin lesions, stump swelling, joint contractures, and mental depression. Phantom pain is experienced by approximately 5% of all amputees in contrast to the more common phantom sensation (i.e., a painless awareness of the amputated limb), which is usually felt by most. These phenomena can be interpreted as false information from afferent nerve endings to the brain, which still has not adjusted to neurologic silence. Phantom pain may be perceived as burning, crushing, cramping, or shooting sensations in the amputated phantom. These are not in the stump, but may be aggravated by stump contact or different physical activities. The cause of phantom pain remains unknown, and most patients have no detectable stump abnormality or premorbid neurotic behavior. Preventive efforts include careful preoperative explanations of the nature of the phantom, optimal surgical techniques, postoperative regular examinations, and manual handling and good care of the stump, as well as vigorous treatment of infections if they occur and early provision of a functional prosthesis. Treatment is difficult but should aim at restoring a relatively normal situation (e.g., ambulation with a prosthesis) as soon as possible. The amputee should be encouraged to inspect and handle the stump himself or herself. Additional interventions that may be helpful include application of superficial heat or cold, deep heating with ultrasound, massage, vibration, TENS, imaginary exercises of the phantom limb, active exercises of the contralateral normal limb, local anesthesia of the stump, and psychologic interventions, such as emotional support, hypnosis, distraction, relaxation, biofeedback, or even psychotherapy. Nerve blocks, rhizotomies, and neurosurgical procedures on the spinal cord may be indicated for persistent burning pain related to reflex sympathetic dystrophy, but these procedures usually provide only brief relief. Analgesics are of little value, but amitriptyline and other central acting agents may be helpful.

Stump pain is common, especially early after the amputation and may be due to a variety of factors, including infection, adherent scar, bursitis, synovitis, arthritis, neuroma, periostitis, muscle spasm, and poor socket fit. Additionally, pain may be referred by more central lesions to the stump or to the phantom.

Meticulous care is required to protect the health of the stump skin. The stump should be washed with soap and water and thoroughly dried. The socket should be cleaned with a damp soapy cloth, and if stump socks are worn, these should be washed and rinsed immediately after removal. The washing should be done each evening, rather than in the morning to ensure thorough drying before wearing. The stump should be frequently exposed to air for drying. Sweating and any trauma, even trivial, should be minimized to prevent maceration. Talcum powder makes the skin dry and smooth, but cocoa butter, lanolin, or silicone creams are helpful to lubricate the scar. Porous materials, cotton stump socks, and antiperspirants help to reduce sweating and maceration of the skin. Regular prosthetic use gradually toughens the skin and fewer skin problems arise as time passes. However, it is indeed common initially to experience skin maceration, tearing of adhesions, abrasions, blisters, and infected hair follicles and sweat glands, each of which necessitates specific interventions. Fungal skin infections can be treated with antifungal creams. When skin lesions are open, draining, or painful, prosthetic wear should be halted until healing occurs and prosthetic fit has been carefully assessed.

EMOTIONAL REACTION

The cancer amputee reacts to his or her new disability with the usual symptoms of depression or grief. These symptoms are aggravated by the uncertain prognosis. The psychologic adjustment indeed may be more difficult for the cancer patient than for other amputees.[28] Early restoration of function and emotional support given by the entire health care team are of greatest value to counteract these psychologic symptoms, but psychiatric treatment may occasionally be indicated. Various psychologic factors, such as impairment of self-esteem, body image, and sense of masculinity or femininity, may combine with physical factors to affect sexual functioning, which has been found to be decreased after amputation.[29]

Limb-Sparing Reconstructive Surgery

It has been demonstrated repeatedly that local resection of a malignant tumor with limb-sparing reconstruction can result in survival rates and disease-free periods that equal those achieved with amputation[31] and in function that is often superior to that with amputation. However, it is not always possible to resect the tumor through normal tissues well clear of neoplastic growth while preserving nerves and vessels, nor is it always possible to reconstruct a functional limb after the necessary wide resection. Amputation thus may still have to be the primary treatment for certain patients.

The surgical reconstruction of a limb after tumor resection may be a complex procedure. The resected bone or even an entire joint removed *en bloc* can be replaced by a fresh frozen cadaveric allograft transplantation,[26] an autogenous bone graft, or more commonly a synthetic metallic prosthetic implant. Although prosthetic joints may be used frequently, an arthrodesis of a joint may be preferred to an implant. Growing children, especially those younger than 10 years of age, have until recently fared better with an amputation than with limb-saving reconstruction because of the unavoidable limb length discrepancy, but the newly designed expandable and adjustable prosthesis has provided an excellent alternative.[23] Another alternative to a high AKA in children is the turn-about procedure, which optimally functions as a BKA with a reversed ankle joint substituting for a knee.[21] Regardless of the exact reconstruction methods, limb-saving surgery should be undertaken only if it will predictably restore lasting and better limb function than would be possible with amputation with subsequent prosthetic fitting and training. This is often hard to determine, especially given the additional pressure from the patient and the family in favor of limb preservation, for the obvious cosmetic and emotional reasons. The current trend thus appears to be away from amputation and toward limb-saving surgery.

The rehabilitation staff, the physiatrist, and the therapists need to know and understand the surgical approach employed to plan a safe and effective rehabilitation program for the patient. Of particular importance is to know what muscles or muscle parts were resected, which nerves were sacrificed, what type of graft or prosthesis was inserted, and especially whether a local rotational tissue flap or a free vascularized muscle flap was done for closure.

Preoperatively, all patients undergoing limb-saving surgery should be carefully counseled regarding their expectations for function. As noted above, physical or occupational therapists should provide instructions for the specific postoperative exercises, emphasizing joint range of motion and muscle-strengthening exercises for the uninvolved limbs and joints, as well as active exercises of the intact joints of the involved limb. Precautions are given regarding proper joint positioning, weight bearing, and activity level after surgery.

After lower limb-saving surgery (Table 23–4), the patient may begin exercises for the uninvolved limbs on the first postoperative day, as well as active exercises for the ankle on the involved side, if it is not immobilized by an orthosis to protect a surgical flap, graft site, or arthrodesis. Initiation and pace of further rehabilitation therapy with active joint motions on the involved side and weight bearing depend on the mode of reconstruction employed and the postoperative course. In general, reconstruction by allografts or autografts may require 6 to 8 weeks of immobilization to allow healing before protected weight bearing can be safely resumed, whereas reconstruction by metallic implants generally allows weight bearing within 2 weeks. Patients who have had a local rotational tissue flap with metallic prosthesis inserted generally can begin using a continuous passive motion (CPM) machine to increase knee range of motion on the sixth postoperative day for 8 to 12 hours daily, increasing the motion range by 5 to 10 degrees per day. These patients may start active or active-assistive exercises for all joints of the involved limb as well as ambulation with a walker or crutches and weight bearing as tolerated on the seventh postoperative day. Frequently, an adjustable temporary orthosis is required at this time to support the weak or painful knee (e.g., knee immobilizer). A prefabricated ankle-foot orthosis, with or without spring action, may be used to support the ankle

TABLE 23–4

Physical Therapy After Lower-Limb Sparing Surgery with Muscle Flap and Metallic Prostheses

Preoperative days

Active and resistive exercises for uninvolved limbs. Crutch walking with PWB on affected limb. Appropriate precautions for patients with hip replacement.

Postoperative days

POD 1–5: Active and resistive exercises for uninvolved limbs. Active ankle motions if not immobilized. Precautions given. Nurses to reinforce exercises.

POD 6–7: On physicians order, CPM machine is used for passively exercising the knee on the involved limb for patients with local rotational flap (*not* with free vascularized muscle flap). The CPM is set at 0–30° of knee flexion initially and increased as tolerated by 5–10° per day. CPM is to be used for 8–10 hours daily. Patient, family, and nurses are instructed in use of CPM.

POD 8–9: Patients with rotational flap start ambulation with a walker or pair of crutches, weight bearing as tolerated. Isometric, active-assistive, and active exercises for all muscles and joints of the involved limb including glut and quad sets and active motion of hip, knee, and ankle. Orthotic need is assessed.

POD 10–12: On physicians order, CPM is used as above for patients with free vascularized muscle flap.

POD 12–14: Ambulation started as above for patients with free flap. Orthotic need is assessed.

From Abrams J, Ryniker D: Rehabilitation protocols after limb sparing procedure with muscle flap. Mount Sinai Hospital, Department of Rehabilitation Medicine, New York, NY, 1987.

or compensate for weak muscles. Those who have had surgery with free vascularized muscle flap usually can start using the CPM machine on the tenth postoperative day and begin ambulating on the twelfth postoperative day. Occupational therapy is started at the same time as ambulation to ensure maximal self-sufficiency before discharge from the hospital. When the hip joint has been replaced, certain precautions regarding joint positioning need to be given (e.g., to avoid excessive flexion, adduction, and rotation). The patient is usually maintained on bed rest with abduction slings and lateral leg supports to resist the tendency for external rotation until ambulation is started. Wound infection and neurovascular compromise of the flap contraindicate the use of a CPM machine and flexion exercises for the knee and/or the hip. Other postoperative complications and symptoms (pain, anemia, increased bleeding tendency, and side effects from medications, chemotherapy, and/or radiotherapy) obviously may affect performance and rehabilitation goals.

Most upper limb-sparing procedures are done proximally at the shoulder. In most cases this leaves a well-functioning hand and forearm but causes weakness or extensive paralysis at the shoulder, depending on the location and the exact mode of reconstruction. A variety of orthotic devices may be required postoperatively for a variable length of time to provide immobilization for healing; these include a sling, a shoulder abduction orthosis (airplane splint), an elbow immobilizer, and a wrist-hand orthosis. The use of allografts or autografts generally necessitates many weeks of complete segmental immobilization for healing. On the first postoperative day, active hand exercises are started with opening and closing of the palm, often using a piece of clay to manipulate. Otherwise, the rehabilitation program varies depending on the nature of the procedure. Following curettage of a relatively benign bone tumor and autogenous bone grafting, immobilization is required for 4 to 6 weeks, after which active and active-assistive exercises of adjacent joints may begin, whereas allografts necessitate weeks of immobilization before union becomes evident and such exercises can cautiously begin. After total resection of the scapula or the clavicle, a sling and swathe are applied for 2 weeks before graded active or active-assistive exercises are started, followed by resistive exercises when tolerated. The Tikhoff-Linberg procedure for malignant tumors of the proximal humerus or of the scapula may be an alternative to forequarter amputation. This procedure involves resection of the proximal humerus, the shoulder joint, and part or all of the scapula along with the deltoid muscle and part of several other muscles traversing this region. Postoperative immobilization is required for 2 to 3 weeks, after which gentle passive range of motion exercises are initiated. Early isometric exercises for the residual shoulder muscles and active exercises for elbow and hand should be started early, followed by resistive exercises as tolerated 2 to 3 weeks postoperatively. Resection of the humeral shaft, with or without the elbow joint, necessitates 2 to 8 weeks of immobilization of the surgical site, depending on the type of implant used, before active or passive elbow exercises can be started. Bone tumors in the forearm are usually confined to either the radius or the ulna. The affected bone is resected and reconstruction done by different means, depending on the extent of resection. Often no grafting is necessary, in which case immobilization period is brief, 1 to 2 weeks postoperatively.

Depending on the type of surgery, patients with an uncomplicated course can be discharged from the hospital 2 to 3 weeks after surgery. Before the patient is discharged from the hospital, the patient and the family receive instructions and precautions regarding permissible activities and use of devices. Ambulation techniques, both for walking on level surfaces and for climbing and descending stairs and curbs, and safety are explained. Instructions are given in the use and care of the CPM machine and assistive devices, and a home exercise program is written. Changes in sensation and motor function are discussed, and instructions are given for simple intervention techniques (e.g., massage, TENS, splinting, and use of proper footwear). At this time, a decision is made regarding the need for a more permanent orthosis, a prescription is written when indicated, and a referral is made to an orthotist for fabrication. Continued therapy after discharge from the hospital is arranged through home health care agencies or at an outpatient rehabilitation facility. The social worker assists the patient and the family in obtaining attendant or nursing care at home, if needed. Appointments are made for follow-up visits with the treating physicians (e.g., orthopedic surgeon, oncologist, and physiatrist), as may be appropriate in each case.

Conclusion

New techniques in preoperative, operative, postoperative, and nonoperative care of patients with tumors of the musculoskeletal system have contributed to the increased length of survival and to improved quality of life for these patients. Cancer has wide-ranging effects on the patient and the family. These effects may be organ specific or systemic and directly resulting from either the neoplastic growth or the various forms of treatment. The disabilities resulting from these tumors may be treated by diverse means. Thus, there is a great need for a well-coordinated multidisciplinary rehabilitation team effort. When such a philosophy is applied early in the course of cancer treatment, many complications may be avoided and the rehabilitation process is facilitated, enabling the patient to achieve a higher level of function and greater community reintegration, which may last for the remainder of his or her life.

References

1. Barron KD, Hirano A, Araki S, Ferry RD: Experiences with metastatic neoplasms involving the spinal cord. Neurology 9:91–106, 1959.
2. Burgess EM, Romano RL: Management of lower extremity amputees using immediate postsurgical prosthesis. Clin Orthop 57:137–146, 1968.
3. Burgess EM, Zettl JH: Amputations below the knee. Artif Limbs 13:1–12, 1969.
4. Burgess E, Henberger D, Forsgren S, Lindh D: The Seattle foot. Orthot Prosthet 37:25–31, 1983.
5. Campbell J, Childs C: The SAFE foot. Orthot Prosthet 34:3–16, 1980.

5a. Cancer Facts and Figures—1991. American Cancer Society, Inc. 1599 Clifton Rd. NE, Atlanta, GA 30329.

6. Childs C: The Mirror Image Finishing Technique (Teaching Manual). UCLA Prosthetics Education Program, Advanced Below Knee Prosthetics Saturation Seminar, October 1984.
7. Dietz JH Jr: Rehabilitation Oncology. New York, John Wiley & Sons, 1981, pp 69–75.

7a. Diller L, Fordyce W, Jacobs D, Brown M, et al: Final Report, Rehabilitation Indicators Project, 1983. NIHR, U.S. Dept. of Education.

8. Enneking WF, Dunhaus WK: Resection and reconstruction for primary neoplasms involving the innominate bone. J Bone Joint Surg 60A:731–746, 1978.
9. Errico TJ, Kostuik JP: Diagnosis and treatment of metastatic disease of the spinal column: A review. Contemp Orthop 13:15–26, 1986.
10. Fisher SV, Gullickson G: Energy costs of ambulation: Review of the literature. Arch Phys Med Rehabil 59:124–133, 1978.
11. Foort J, Davies R, Lawrence R: Construction methods and materials for external prosthesis—present and future. J Int Rehabil Med 6:72–78, 1984.
12. Gebhardt MC, Mankin HJ: Osteosarcomas: The treatment controversy—part II. Surgical Rounds for Orthopaedics 2(7):25–42, 1988.
13. Gilbert RW, Kim JH, Posner JB: Epidural spinal cord compression from metastatic tumor. Diagnosis and treatment. Ann Neurol 3:40–51, 1978.
14. Goldsmith MF: Will exercise keep women away from oncologists—or obstetricians? Medical news and perspectives. JAMA 259:1769–1770, 1988.
15. Gonzales EG, Corcoran PJ, Reyes RL: Energy expenditure in below knee amputees: Correlation with stump length. Arch Phys Med Rehabil 55:111–119, 1974.
16. Gottschalk F, Mooney V, McClellan B, Carlton A: Early fitting of the amputee with a plastic temporary

adjustable below knee prosthesis. Contemp Orthop 13:15–18, 1986.

17. Harvey RF, Jellinek HM, Haback RV: Cancer rehabilitation: Analysis of 36 program approaches. JAMA 247:2127–2131, 1982.
18. Hinterbuchner C: Rehabilitation of physical disability in cancer. NY State J Med 78:1066–1069, 1978.
19. Katz RT, Wu Y: Postoperative and preprosthetic management of the below knee amputee. Contemp Orthop 10:53–63, 1985.
20. Kegel B, Carpenter ML, Burgess EM: Functional capabilities of lower extremity amputees. Arch Phys Med Rehabil 59:109–120, 1978.
21. Kotz R, Salzer M: Rotation plasty for childhood osteosarcoma of the distal part of the femur. J Bone Joint Surg 64A:959–969, 1982.
22. Krouskop TA, Muilenberg AL, Doughterty DR, Winningham DJ: Computer aided design of prosthetic socket for an AKA. J Rehabil Res Development 24:31–38, 1987.
23. Lewis MM: The use of an expandable and adjustable prosthesis in the treatment of childhood malignant tumors of the extremities. Cancer 57:499–502, 1986.
24. Lundt J, Staats T: The USMC prosthetic skin. Orthot Prosthet 37:59–61, 1983.
25. Malone J, Moore W, Leal JM, Childers SJ: Rehabilitation for lower extremity amputation. Arch Surg 116:93–98, 1981.
26. Mankin HJ, Gebhardt MC: Allografts in the management of bone tumors: Part II. Surgical Rounds for Orthopaedics 2:24–40, 1988.
27. New York University Postgraduate Medical School: Lower Limb Prosthetics, Prosthetics and Orthotics, New York University, New York, 1981 Revision.
28. Reinstein L: Rehabilitation of the lower extremity cancer amputee. Md State Med J 29:85–87, 1980.
29. Reinstein L, Ashley J, Miller K: Sexual adjustment after lower extremity amputation. Arch Phys Med Rehabil 59:501–404, 1978.

29a. Rusk HA: Preventive medicine, curative medicine—then rehabilitation. New Phys 13:165–167, 1964.

30. Sabolich J: Contoured adducted trochanteric–controlled alignment method (CAT-CAM): Introduction and basic principles. Clin Prosthet Orthot 9:15–31, 1985.
31. Simon MA, Aschliman MA, Thomas N, Markin HJ: Limb-salvage treatment versus amputation for osteosarcoma of the distal end of the femur. J Bone Joint Surg 68A:1331–1337, 1986.
32. Staats TB: Advanced prosthetic techniques for below knee amputations. Orthopedics 8:249–258, 1985.
33. Subbarao JV, McPhee MC: Prosthetic rehabilitation: Comparison of the outcome in patients with cancer, and vascular amputations of the extremities. Orthop Rev 11:43–51, 1982.
34. Traugh GH, Corcoran PJ, Reyes RL: Energy expenditure of ambulation in patients with above-knee amputations. Arch Phys Med Rehabil 56:67–71, 1975.
35. Waters RL, Perry J, Antonelli D, Hislop H: Energy cost of walking of amputees: Influence of level of amputation. J Bone Joint Surg 58A:42–46, 1976.
36. Wu Y, Flanagan DP: Rehabilitation of the lower extremity amputee with emphasis on a removable below knee rigid dressing. *In* Bergan JJ, Yao JST (eds): Gangrene and Severe Ischemia of the Lower Extremity. New York, Grune & Stratton, 1978, pp 435–453.
37. Wu Y, Keagy RD, Krick HJ, Stratigos JS, Betts HB: An innovative removable rigid dressing technique for below-the-knee amputation. J Bone Joint Surg 61A:724–729, 1979.

CHAPTER 24

Behavioral Medicine and Cancer: A Clinical Guide

BARRY R. SNOW
PAUL GUSMORINO
ISAAC PINTER

Despite continuing advances in medical and surgical treatment of cancer, the diagnosis of cancer continues to convey to many patients and their families an ominous warning of prolonged suffering and eventual death. This message is strongly reinforced by emphasis in the mass media on potential carcinogens in food and the environment and their dangers. Moreover, the scientific literature inadvertently reinforces this message of danger. An informal survey of behavioral medicine, liaison psychiatry, and health psychology texts shows few chapters dealing exclusively with the psychosocial issues relating to cancer. This information was rather more typically presented in chapters dealing with death and dying or with depression in the medically ill. Those texts that include specific information on the role of behavioral medicine treatment techniques are often not encountered by oncologic specialists in their routine readings.

This chapter reviews specific clinical areas in which behavioral medicine principles can be effectively used by the physician in the treatment of patients with cancer. Specific issues that arise in each phase of the clinical progression of the illness are identified. Special attention is given to the impact of cancer on children and adolescents, who experience a large proportion of bone tumors. The chapter concludes with an overview of guidelines for the treatment of pain, treatment-related side effects, and emotional distress, three key problem areas for cancer patients. Both pharmacologic and behavioral treatment approaches are considered.

Clinical Progression of Illness

PREDIAGNOSTIC PHASE

The experiences of the cancer patient and the need for a comprehensive approach to both the physical and the psychologic response of the cancer patient and the family can best be understood by following the cancer patient through the various stages of the diagnostic and treatment course.[2, 10, 11, 40] Cancer patients typically enter the health care system with a visit to their primary care physician for evaluation of an unremitting symptom. This symptom may be as dramatic as a lump in the breast, a bloody discharge, or a rapidly growing mole, or may be a more nagging symptom such as constant pain or unexplained weight loss. For some of these patients, the current publicity regarding the need for early detection has made them think, albeit fleetingly, of the possibility of cancer. Other individuals may have become extremely sensitized to the widespread information about the danger signs of cancer and seek reassurance for any bodily symptom that appears, regardless of its severity. At the other extreme are patients who either deny the presence of disease or delay seeking diagnosis because they fear the consequences. The latter group may mention the symptom of interest in a rather offhand manner during a "routine" medical check-up.

The physician encountering these different types of patients must struggle with how much to inform the patient at the different stages of the work-up. The physician must provide the patient with emotional support and at the same time arrange for the expeditious conduct of tests either to confirm or to refute his or her clinical impression. Frequently, the orthopedist or the oncologist becomes involved at this point in performing a specific examination or supervising further diagnostic work-up.

DIAGNOSTIC PHASE

The specialist examining the patient should be aware of the attitudes that patients may have about their own health. These attitudes may be directly challenged by the specialist's specific questions as to family history of cancer or referral for specific and often extensive laboratory examinations. The principal guide for the physician at this point is to follow rather than lead the patient in exploring the diagnostic and treatment possibilities. By their choice of words and questions, patients often provide important clues about their readiness for information. Euphemisms such as mass, rapidly growing tissue, or unusual growth may be used by the physician in the early stages of discussion to delay temporarily the use of the word cancer, which usually evokes the image of an inevitable fatal outcome. At the same time, the physician must provide enough information for the patient to recognize the nature of the illness and to give informed consent to any treatment regimen that is decided on.[38]

Patients may react to the initial diagnosis with shock and disbelief. They may call again several hours later and inquire as to the diagnosis, as if they had never been given this information. Schmale suggests that the physician schedule a second visit within several days after first telling the patient of the diagnosis.[29] This pause allows the patient to think through various questions and concerns. This follow-up visit also enables the patient the opportunity to discuss her or his condition with others before committing to a course of treatment. This additional time may be especially important for the adolescent patient who is confronted with the cancer diagnosis during a critical developmental stage. The parents of a child with cancer can also use this second visit to bring along important family members who may be involved in the care of the patient. Such time spent before beginning treatment may be of fundamental importance in building the supportive network that helps the youngster deal with the various demands of cancer treatment.

The physician should be aware of several emotional issues that are often raised when cancer is diagnosed in a child.[15, 20, 21] Some parents, for example, question whether they are at fault for providing their child with a harmful environment or diet or whether the disorder is related to hereditary factors, accident, or trauma at birth. They may also blame themselves for a delay in the diagnosis and wonder whether this delay will have an impact on the patient's outcome. Parents also need to be informed that relatives, particularly grandparents, may reject the diagnosis and insist that the parent stop considering the child as ill. Such family opposition may make the job of the physician more difficult.

The physician needs to be aware of different approaches that may be beneficial for adolescents and younger children. The former group often benefit from a private, truthful relationship with the surgeon. This relationship recognizes the increasing maturity of the adolescent and helps secure his or her compliance. Children, on the other hand, need to be addressed at their appropriate developmental level. In general, all children need to be truthfully informed that they are "sick" and that the disease and the uncomfortable treatments they will be receiving are not punishments for their behavior. Specific information about the treatments and side effects should be given, but not enough to produce more anxiety than the illness itself.

The physician will ultimately make the work easier by ensuring that the parents feel involved throughout the treatment planning. Often, a course of hospitalization and postoperative rehabilitation signals parents that they have little to contribute to the care of the child. This signal can disrupt strong family ties that may otherwise have helped the patient's recovery. Parents who feel excluded, moreover, may reflect nonverbal signals of anxiety and distress onto their child. The child's expectation of discomfort and distress often results in heightened complaints of pain and distress in the postoperative phase.

INITIAL TREATMENT

Modern techniques for treatment of many forms of bone tumor involve a planned sequence of treatments that may include chemotherapy, radiotherapy, and surgery. Each of these treatments produces a strong set of emotional responses that need to be anticipated and dealt with. These responses may come from the direct effects of these treatments, the setting and conditions under which these treatments are given, and the loss of normal routines experienced by patients undergoing these treatments. Each of these concerns needs to be dealt with in a straightforward manner.

Chemotherapy

A primary source of concern for patients undergoing chemotherapy is the side effects of these treatments.[25, 27] These side effects may include such physical responses as nausea, vomiting, lethargy, hair loss, gastrointestinal distress, and changes in taste acuity and appetite. These effects are linked to the physiologic toxicity of the chemotherapeutic agents and typically begin 1 to 2 hours after the injection and can persist for 2 to 24 hours or longer. Such effects directly interfere with the patient's functional ability and quality of life. Many patients also report a distressing pattern of anticipatory nausea and/or vomiting. For these individuals, the sight or smell of the room and procedures associated with their therapy induce a learned response of anxiety, nausea, and vomiting before or during subsequent treatments. These effects typically appear after the fourth or fifth treatment session and escalate in severity during subsequent treatments. These effects may hamper the patient's cooperation with the treatment process. In addition, side effects from chemotherapy may increase noncompliance, ranging from delay in treatment scheduling to outright treatment refusal. These concerns are especially heightened for adolescents, who are typically concerned about their appearance and keeping up with their peers.

Patients undergoing chemotherapy may also experience distress relating to their lack of understanding of the different treatment protocols or their discomfort with the injection of potent substances into their body. These fears may be expressed as repeated questions as to the potential harmful effects of these drugs on their personality or their cognitive abilities. These concerns need to be addressed directly. Lack of clear information may also promote patient noncompliance.[35]

The physician should also consider any adverse effects that may be attributed to encountering other patients with various states of disease and disability. For example, scheduling the sickest patients at the beginning or the end of the day, when the facility is least congested, may be an easily accomplished intervention that could significantly reduce this distress. Certain individuals may also find it difficult to wait extended periods of time for their treatment. These individuals would also benefit from attention to scheduling appointments. This increase in distress may be especially strong for young cancer patients in the early stages of their disease.

Radiotherapy

Patients receiving radiation therapy are often confused as to the nature of the treatments that they are receiving.[9, 23, 37] This confusion may result from the invisible nature of x-rays, the extended duration of a treatment schedule, and the general caution most individuals have about undergoing x-ray treatment. These fears may present as questions regarding the potential risk of being "burned," sterility, or additional cancer sites due to the therapy. Patients may also experience such side effects as fatigue, anorexia, nausea, and vomiting. Local treatment reactions may also occur. In addition, patients may experience claustrophobic reactions to the confined quarters of the scanning equipment. This reaction may not be limited to patients with a previous history of anxiety disorders. Rather, these reactions may be a reflection of the patients' increasing health concern and sense of isolation. An accurate description of the treatment area and the therapeutic suggestion that the patient will probably have to draw on coping skills and resources during the isolating experience of treatment may help prepare the patient for successfully dealing with this event.

Surgery

Patients facing surgery often have mixed feelings.[19, 39] On one hand, surgery causes a great amount of immediate discomfort and disability as well as frequently resulting in permanent disfigurement. These changes may include loss of normal body functions, significant change in appearance, and significant changes in sexual functioning. Surgery may also be viewed as a direct challenge to the vitality and self-worth of the individual. This is especially true when the organ lost (e.g., a leg) plays a major role in the growth and development of younger patients and in the mobility and functioning of all individuals. On the other hand, surgery is viewed by many individuals as a more complete form of treatment for cancer. This completeness may help the patient accept the important body changes that are experienced. A frank discussion of these issues may help the patient adjust to the novel demands of the postoperative period. The surgeon may also communicate directly to key family members a concern regarding the patient's postoperative recovery as well as specific information on the impact of surgery on the patient's life style. This information may make the postoperative recovery period and its demands more tolerable. Although the orthopedic surgeon may believe that this task should best be left to the patient's primary care physician, clergyperson or spiritual leader, or another health care professional, the surgeon should note the heightened expectation with which patients regard their visits. This expectation enhances the impact of any therapeutic behavior and suggestions that the surgeon provides.

The problem of stump pain and phantom limb pain after amputation must also be addressed. The former type of pain is often caused by the formation of neuromas in the amputated area. Phantom limb pain, on the other hand, is experienced in the body part that is no longer there; the pain is usually characterized as severe and burning or throbbing. In some cases, the phantom pain becomes distorted or grotesque, and the patient feels as if the limb is being held in an unnatural position or in an unusual state of tension. Many patients report that phantom pain tends to fade with time, gradually telescoping itself into the stump. A substantial number of patients, especially those with higher-level amputations, however, report persistence of phantom pain at a steady level for many years after the surgery. These patients need to be assured that the lingering pain is not a sign that they are decompensating but rather a direct effect of the body's delayed sensory processing of traumatic surgery. When patients are given this introduction, a referral for pain management is often appreciated.

The effects of the treatment setting (discussed above) may be especially difficult for children with bone tumors. These individuals often do not feel sick and are confronted by strangers who insist on performing painful and invasive procedures. These procedures may be performed without the presence of a comforting parent or, in a small percentage of cases, in the presence of a parent who heightens the child's anxiety. The occurrence of the tumor and its treatment may occur in developmentally significant periods of an individual's life. For example, during adolescence, the child is struggling to achieve independence from her or his parents, but is forced to rely on parents and health care givers because of his or her illness. Occasionally, this reliance produces regression by both parents and children to earlier modes of mutual dependency. Patients may show extreme anxiety when separated for even brief periods. Because the behavior is not, however, age appropriate, parents and children may interact in a hostile manner when they are together and pose problems for the treatment staff. These behaviors often continue even when the cancer is in remission.

A specific example of treatment-associated distress is school phobia. This behavior, which appears in a significant minority of school-aged children, is characterized by somatic complaints, refusal to attend school, and fear of separation from the parents. School phobias typically develop with a childhood complaint of headaches or abdominal pain and parental agreement for the child to skip school for a period of time. During this time, the child clings to the parent and misses the learning and the social interaction that is a crucial part of development. School phobias are often related to the parents' intense fears that the child will die or experience severe crisis if separated from the parent. The parent may also show a decided ambivalence toward school and harbor the inner thought regarding the worthlessness of educating a child who will die young. Resolution of these problems is often facilitated by appropriate referral to a mental health professional.

FOLLOW-UP

The surgeon's responsibility to the patient traditionally ends at the successful conclusion of the course of treatment. The patient usually returns to the primary care physician or the oncologist who made the original referral. Physicians should note, however, that many patients have encountered numerous specialists during diagnostic work-up and treatment. The patient may thus feel that the referring physician has little understanding of the entire process that she or he has been through. Regular communications between the surgeon and the patient's primary care physician as well as a full discussion by the surgeon of the surgical outcome can help reduce the patient's anxiety and allow a successful conclusion of the surgeon's role in treatment.

Recent trends toward providing many patients with the option of reconstructive surgery also maintain the role of the surgeon in the follow-up period. These procedures may be requested by patients to reduce self-consciousness about a significant change in their outward appearance. Such surgery may also be a component of a planned series of surgical adjustments to the prosthesis implanted as part of a limb-salvaging procedure. In these cases, there is a preplanned sequence of visits during which the surgeon can evaluate the physical and the psychologic status of the patient.

As survival rates for patients with various tumors increase, the surgeon may have an increasing number of patients without any remaining evidence of malignant disease. These individuals may, however, find it difficult to resume their normal activities. They may experience school or job discrimination and their remission may be viewed as only temporary.[4] This attitude may prompt additional calls for reassurance to the specialist who treated them. A patient may show a heightened postoperative concern for health. Some patients may consider the slightest change in body function or pain as an ominous sign of recurrence of the tumor. These patients may benefit from the security of periodic contacts with the physician for reevaluation. Other patients may delay returning for a follow-up examination. These individuals may find it difficult to acknowledge a sign of illness recurrence because of the strong fears and memories that this recurrence causes. A system of scheduling regular follow-up visits with a thorough monitoring system for checking on cancelled or unkept appointments can help reduce this problem of noncompliance. Patients should be informed of this system at the time of the initial consultation so that they do not interpret calls for follow-up as indications that their condition has substantially deteriorated. Patients who are continuing in remission often use these follow-up visits as an opportunity to bring a sample of their achievements to their physician as a way of expressing appreciation for their ongoing care. This sharing of accomplishments is especially valuable for adolescent patients whose attainment of milestones in an orderly fashion may have been delayed by the development of cancer.

RECURRENCE AND TREATMENT

Patients who experience relapse typically repeat the pattern of shock, disbelief, and anger that they experienced at the initial diagnosis. These feelings may be accentuated and mixed with anger at the surgeon or the oncologist who did not accomplish a complete cure initially. Patients at this stage are often skeptical about what they are told regarding future therapeutic goals. They often become vulnerable to exaggerated treatment claims made by nontraditional practitioners. The cancer specialist may become an important resource for reassuring the patient that all reasonable approaches to illness have been considered.

TERMINAL PHASE

The progressive physical decline associated with many forms of cancer presents a new set of challenges to the patient, the family, and the physician. Many patients are biologically aware of the irreversible and progressive nature of their illness, even though its true nature may not have been discussed with them. At this stage, the physician must avoid either performing heroic and discomforting measures or shunning the patient to whom the physician believes she or he has nothing to contribute. Indeed, many patients in the terminal phase of their illness desire repeated reassurance that they will not be abandoned by their family or physicians. This fear is especially pronounced among children younger than 6 years, who fear the separation from their parents implied by death rather than death itself. Adolescents, on the other hand, often react with moderate to severe depression and anger. The difficult task faced by the physician at this point is to satisfy the patient's need for ongoing contact, despite the natural tendency to distance oneself when no specific diagnostic or therapeutic service can be rendered.

Areas of Intervention

PAIN

The proper management of pain requires an adequate understanding of the complex nature of this symptom. This complexity arises because the perception of pain may be modified by a number of underlying emotional and cognitive factors. Loesser and Black noted that chronic pain may be considered the outer circle of a four-part scheme.[16] At the center of this scheme is *nociception,* defined as tissue irritation at the site of the injury or illness. Nociception typically produces *pain,* which is defined as the individual's perception of the nociceptive input. However, this relationship is not inviolate, as one may experience nociceptive injury but not perceive the injury as painful. Loesser and Black noted that, when pain is perceived, the individual typically responds with emotional distress, or *suffering.* Prolonged emotional distress leads to *pain behavior,* an outward communication to the physician and significant others that the patient is in distress. Appropriate cancer pain management can occur at any level of this cycle. The orthopedist typically attempts to modify the nociceptive component of pain by surgical excision of the malignant mass. A variety of behavioral and psychotherapeutic treatments have been developed to modify the meaning of pain for the individual.[13, 22] Pain behavior can also be treated by providing important environmental supports for the person. Finally, pain perception can be modified by appropriate pharmacologic or behavioral treatments.

Pharmacologic Treatment

The overwhelming underuse of adequate narcotic analgesics for patients with acute and cancer pain and overuse of these same narcotic analgesics for patients with chronic pain of nonmalignant causes have been well documented.[1, 7, 18, 24, 31] This undertreatment of acute pain is associated with a mistaken belief that overuse of narcotic analgesics leads to respiratory depression and addiction. This myth is especially damaging because it is becoming increasingly apparent that undertreatment of acute pain itself leads to dependence, tolerance, and addiction. This phenomenon of undertreatment is especially strong when treating children. In part, this is due to mistaken ideas about children, especially that infants do not experience pain. Additionally, physicians often fear that children are more subject to respiratory depression and that they would be at higher risk for drug dependency. Finally, children with pain do not readily communicate this information to their physician, in part owing to their fear of consequences involving further painful examinations and tests. Especially with younger children, pain must be evaluated in terms of the patient's persistent crying, failure to move an extremity, abnormal gait, or changes in the patient's heart rate and blood pressure, rather than simply assessing subjective complaint or discomfort.

When treating patients with pain, nonnarcotic analgesics should first be used, the choice of drug being determined by patient's tolerance and response to the medication. The primary consideration of the clinician in this selection is the concern for gastric irritation and the decision as to whether one wants to affect platelet function. With the nonsteroidal antiinflammatory drugs (NSAIDs), there is a plateau of the analgesic effect of the medication, and further increases in dosage do not increase analgesic effectiveness but only increase adverse effects of the medication. The understood mechanism of action regarding pain is involved in the inhibition of an enzyme that ordinarily promotes the formation of prostaglandin E_2. These prostaglandins would ordinarily sensitize pain receptors to the pain-producing effects of bradykinin. These drugs work at the level of the peripheral nervous system and act synergistically with narcotic analgesics, which work on a central basis.

With the exception of choline magnesium trisalicylate (Trilisate), the NSAIDs affect platelet aggregation and are the drugs of choice if prolonged bleeding time is a concern. These drugs are particularly effective in the management of bone pain from tumor metastasis. Their use in oncology is somewhat limited if their antipyretic effects are a concern owing to their ability to mask infection. With the exception of choline magnesium trisalicylate, NSAIDs affect platelet function and promote hemorrhage in patients with thrombocytopenia and coagulation defects.

Although the NSAIDs play an important role in pain management, the narcotic analgesics are the mainstay of pain relief and are needed to manage severe cancer pain. All narcotic analgesics can be given by different routes of administration: orally, intramuscularly (IM), intraveneously (IV) either as a bolus or with a continuous infusion, rectally, epidurally, and, more recently, via transdermal patches. The onset of action and the duration of action are the important considerations. Good pain management does not involve relieving patient's pain when it becomes severe as much as preventing the patient's pain from becoming severe and distressing. Clearly, when a patient is in acute pain, IV or IM administration is most effective for bringing about quick relief. If patients are able to tolerate oral analgesics, it is much easier to maintain a steady state of pain relief by giving oral narcotic analgesics on a fixed *round-the-clock* schedule. These can be supplemented as needed if the patient experiences breakthrough pain.

All of the narcotic analgesics are equally effective in relieving pain if given in equianalgesic dosages. The clinician managing pain should have a good understanding of the equianalgesic relationships between different narcotics, their durations of action, and the different routes of administration (Table 24–1). The authors recommend that one start by giving IM injection with hydroxyzine (Vistaril) when the patient is in acute pain. The patient should be reevaluated for pain relief within about 1 hour and, if necessary, given further IM injections until he or she is comfortable. An equianalgesic dose by oral route should then be given on a continuous, round-the-clock basis. The authors' preference is for hydromorphone (Dilaudid) given every 4 hours round-the-clock, with the patient being informed that he or she will be awakened at night to be given pain medication rather than to be awakened by pain. Patients are also informed that there are escape doses available any time they should need them between the regularly scheduled doses. One can then adjust their medication dosage on a fixed schedule. Again, the advantage of round-the-clock administration of oral narcotics is that they have a much slower onset of action and a much longer period of activity; thus, with overlapping doses, one should get a relatively steady state of narcotic analgesia. The oral route is less threatening to pediatric patients than are repeated injections. With IM doses, on the other hand, there is a rapid increase and a rapid fall in the serum narcotic levels, and it is much more difficult to achieve a steady state of analgesia.

The potency of narcotic medications can be enhanced by the addition of a variety of nonnarcotic drugs that potentiate their effects. The sedating tricyclic antidepressants, such as amitriptylene and doxepin, can be used for their analgesic properties in dosages smaller than those used for the treatment of depression. This use is especially indicated when sleep disorders and anxiety are present. The authors' preference is to use doxepin (Sinequan), 25 to 75 mg orally at bedtime, for this purpose. Hydroxyzine (Vistaril), which is itself an analgesic, can also be added to this combination. In addition to its analgesic effects, hydroxyzine is helpful in controlling the nausea and vomiting that is often associated with the administration of narcotic analgesics. Finally, narcotic analgesics are constipating. Patients taking narcotics regularly should therefore be given stool softeners and laxatives routinely to counteract these effects.

It is generally recommended that children 12 years of age and older receive full adult dosages. Children 7 through 12 years generally require about 50% of the starting adult dosage, and children 2 to 6 years of age require 20 to 25% of the starting adult dosage. When dealing with infants younger than 2 years of age, the starting dosage must be calculated by weight (in milligrams per kilograms).

Behavioral Treatment

A variety of nonpharmacologic treatments can break the association between the nociceptive input from the tumor and the perception of pain and emotional suffering. These techniques emphasize training in self-regulation to produce a state of relaxation and low arousal that is incompatible with distress. They include imagery and visualization, hypnosis, autogenic training, progressive muscle relaxation, and other forms of treatment derived from cognitive behavioral approaches. These approaches share the belief that a systematic program of education, skills building, and rehearsal can help patients modify their thoughts, emotions, and behavior. They are useful for chronic pain as well as for the acute pain of invasive medical procedures such as bone marrow aspirations. A brief review of these procedures, which are probably novel to many physicians, follows.

Many patients can benefit from imagery and visualization techniques that use cognitive processes to break the linkage between nociception and pain. In imagery techniques, the patient uses imagination to create positive feelings and distance from pain. These techniques are especially suitable for children, who often have vivid imaginations. For example, these

TABLE 24–1

Narcotic Analgesics Commonly Used for Severe Pain

Name	Equianalgesic IM Dose (mg)*	PO/IM Potency	Starting Oral Dose Range (mg)	Comments	Precautions and Contraindications
Morphine-like Agonists					
Morphine	10	3**	30–60	Standard of comparison for narcotic analgesics; sustained-release preparations (MS Contin, Roxanol-SR) release drug over 8–12 hours	For all opiods, caution in patients with impaired ventilation, bronchial asthma, increased intracranial pressure, liver failure
Hydromorphone (Dilaudid)	1.5	5	4–8	Slightly shorter duration than morphine	
Methadone (Dolophine)	10	2	5–20	Good oral potency; long plasma half-life (24–36 h)	Accumulates with repetitive dosing, causing excessive sedation (on days 2–5)
Levorphanol (Levo-Dromoman)	2	2	2–4	Long plasma half-life (12–16 h)	Accumulates on days 2–3
Oxymorphone (Numorphan)		See Comments		Not available orally; 5 mg rectal suppository = 10 mg morphine IM	As for IM morphine
Meperidine (Demerol)	75	4	Not recommended	Slightly shorter acting than morphine	Normeperidine (toxic metabolite) accumulates with repetitive dosing, causing CNS excitation; avoid in patients with impaired renal function or receiving monoamine oxidase inhibitors†

Mixed Agonist-Antagonists					
Pentazocine (Talwin)	60	3	See Comments	Used orally for less severe pain; mixed agonist-antagonist; included in Schedule IV of Controlled Substances Act	May cause psychotomimetic effects; may precipitate withdrawal in narcotic-dependent patients; contraindicated in myocardial infarction†
Nalbuphine (Nubain)	10	See Comments		Not available orally; like IM pentazocine; not scheduled under Controlled Substances Act	Incidence of psychotomimetic effects lower than with pentazocine
Butorphanol (Stadol)	2	See Comments		Not available orally; action similar to that of IM nalbuphine	As for IM pentazocine
Partial Agonists					
Buprenorphine (Buprenex)	0.4	See Comments		Not available orally; sublingual preparation not yet in US; less abuse liability than morphine; does not produce psychotomimetic effects	May precipitate withdrawal in narcotic-dependent patients

For IM doses, the time to peak analgesia ranges from ½ to 1 hour and the duration from 3 to 4 hours. After oral administration, the peak analgesic effect is delayed to about 2 hours and the duration is prolonged to 3 to 6 hours.

*These doses are recommended starting IM doses from which the optimal dose for each patient is determined by titration. Equianalgesic doses are based on single-dose studies in which an IM dose of each drug listed was compared with a dose of morphine to establish relative potency.

**Although single-dose studies established the relative potency of PO/IM morphine as 6:1, in practice, repetitive dosing is the rule, and a ratio of 3:1 is more commonly used.

†Irritating to tissues with repeated IM injection.

CNS, central nervous system; IM, intramuscular; PO, oral.

From American Pain Society: Principles of Analgesic Use in the Treatment of Acute Pain and Chronic Cancer Pain: A Concise Guide to Medical Practice, 2nd ed., 1989.

children may be taught to imagine that their favorite storybook character or television hero is helping them manage their pain. Clinicians who see these techniques being practiced for the first time are often amazed at the decrease in distress experienced by responsive individuals. Simonton and others report extensive use of imagery exercises for combatting disease as adjuncts to the conventional medical and surgical management.[33, 34] Their use is indicated if they help enhance the patients' feelings of control of the disease process without placing on them the burden of guilt should their condition not improve.

Hypnosis is a particular kind of imagery-based technique that is beneficial to many patients in pain. Hypnosis can be defined as a psychophysiologic condition in which attention is focused to the point at which there is a relative reduction of peripheral awareness and critical-analytic mentation, leading to major distortions in perception, mood, and memory sufficient to produce significant behavioral and biologic changes.[41] Hypnosis uses a variety of suggestions to facilitate this shift in information processing. These strategies include (1) direct suggestions of relaxation and pain relief; (2) substitution of another sensation (e.g., pressure) for pain; (3) movement of the pain to a smaller or less important part of the body; (4) alteration of the meaning of the pain so that it becomes less frightening; and (5) dissociation or analgesia of the body part in pain.[3] Patients are often taught self-hypnosis or given an audiotape or videotape containing practice exercises. This training heightens the patients' sense of control and provides specific skills for pain management. These techniques are especially important at night and other times when hospital staff are not readily available.

Patients who desire a more structured type of therapy that shares with hypnosis a focus on suggestions may benefit from autogenic training.[17] Patients are instructed in adopting a quiet attitude and repeating to themselves phrases that are designed to relax their mind and body. Examples of such phrases are, my arms and legs are heavy and warm, and my heartbeat is calm and regular. At the other extreme are patients who benefit from relatively unstructured meditation sessions designed to bring them inner peace. These techniques are maximally beneficial when they are practiced on a regular basis and if staff and family are supportive of the patient's coping efforts.

Other techniques have more specific focuses on particular muscle areas. Progressive muscle relaxation training, for example, entails a systematic method of tensing and relaxing different muscle groups.[12] Repeated practice of this exercise helps the patient develop the skill of shifting the body from a tense reaction to stress to an overall state of relaxation. A growing body of evidence also suggests that targeted biofeedback training may be useful in the treatment of the most puzzling problem of phantom limb pain.[30] This training goes beyond general relaxation training to emphasize the attainment of specific physiologic goals like increased blood flow and decreased muscle spasm. Patients may also benefit from breathing exercises that emphasize a moderate response to environmental stimuli. The latter techniques are easy to teach to children and are useful for helping increase tolerance to the acute pain of various medical procedures.

Behavioral techniques are best taught by a specialist with training in these areas. Such consultants have the necessary expertise to match the proper nonpharmacologic techniques to the individual and to deal with any problems that interfere with the proper practice of these skills. Handing a relaxation tape to the individual with instructions to listen to it at home will probably have minimal effect on the patient's pain problem.

In this connection, one should note that patients may differ in their response to the various self-regulation techniques, depending on their beliefs and attitudes regarding the procedure being used. For example, some patients may fear that they will be "out of control" during hypnosis or perform dangerous or embarrassing acts and therefore refuse to use this type of intervention. Other patients, on the other hand, may specifically request hypnosis because of the belief that this technique is especially powerful. The experienced clinician will tailor the patient's treatment to these beliefs so that the patient can obtain maximum benefit. The consultant may also suggest specific environmental changes to be made to modify the pain behavior of the patient. These changes are helpful when analgesic intake or pain complaints appear to be intensified in association with specific environmental circumstances.[26]

Two cases in which either pharmacological management alone or pharmacological management in conjunction with behavioral techniques was used for pain management are presented.

Case Histories

A 55-year-old married man who lives with his wife had been a healthy and active man; he had been proud of maintaining himself in good physical condition and jogged regularly. Approximately 2 months prior to admission, he began experiencing pain and swelling in his right thigh; the lesion was subsequently diagnosed as sarcoma. The tumor was found to be unresectable and the patient underwent a right hip disarticulation. He had a relatively uncomplicated postoperative course but had severe phantom limb pain involving a burning sensation in his foot and ankle and a sensation of his leg's being twisted down through his bed. This was particularly distressing to the patient at night, when it would awaken him suddenly from sleep. He was treated first with supportive psychotherapy and instructed in relaxation techniques and imagery, using hypnosis to experience the amputated limb as being in a soothing, warm bath. This therapy proved to successfully manage the patient's experience of phantom pain during the day, though he continued to complain of being awakened at night with pain. He was initially given doxepin, 25 mg at bedtime, which was subsequently increased to 75 mg at bedtime. The patient soon reported good sleep through the night and an ability to control the phantom pain with imagery and self-hypnosis techniques.

A 27-year-old man was admitted to the Hospital for Joint Diseases' Orthopaedic Institute with a diagnosis of a giant cell tumor with soft tissue invasion of his right proximal femur. After radical resection of the tumor, consultation was requested for evaluation of the patient's constant complaint of inadequate pain relief. When seen, he had been receiving meperidine (Demerol), 100 mg IM every 3 hours as needed for pain, which he was requesting roughly every 3 hours. The patient reported that, although he got relief and was sedated for a while, the effects of pain medication did not last 3 hours and he was screaming and begging with nurses for pain medication for 30 to 40 minutes before his next dose was due. The meperidine IM was discontinued and patient was given hydromorphone (Dilaudid), 7 mg, with hydroxyzine (Vistaril), 25 mg, orally every 4 hours round-the-clock. He was told that the medication would be given every 4 hours, not to relieve severe pain when he was screaming, but to prevent him from ever getting to that state. In addition, he was told that, if at any time between these round-the-clock doses he should have a problem with pain, he could ask for an escape dose, which was prescribed as hydroxymorphone, 3 mg orally, to be given as needed. When seen the next day, the patient reported that he had slept well through the night without requesting any escape doses, reported his pain to be under good control, and asked that his narcotic dosage begin to be decreased.

SIDE EFFECTS OF TREATMENT

Another area of intervention concerns dysfunctional physical and behavioral responses to treatment. These side effects may include delirium as a complication of acute medical illness, treatment-induced nausea and vomiting, and anticipatory nausea and vomiting. Many patients as well as some health care professionals view the latter responses as signs of patient weakness rather than a predictable outcome of environmental conditioning that causes the previous neutral stimuli of the treatment room to elicit nausea and emesis.[6] A variety of pharmacologic and behavioral techniques can be used in the management of these conditions.

Pharmacologic Treatment

The management of treatment-induced delirium is best accomplished by using small doses of the major tranquilizers such as haloperidol (Haldol), 1 mg orally every hour until the patient is calm. This medication can be given by injection if oral administration is not possible. If more sedation is required, chlorpromazine (Thorazine), 10 mg orally or IM, can instead be given every hour until the patient is calm.

A variety of drugs can be used for the management of treatment-related side effects. The addition of hydroxyzine (Vistaril) to a narcotic analgesic often provides some relief of these symptoms. In addition, antiemetic agents such as prochlorperazine (Compazine) may be used. If the nausea and vomiting have a significant component of anxiety, antianxiety medications, including benzodiazepines, may be indicated. A common starting regimen is alprazolam (Xanax), 0.25 mg four times daily, or diazepam (Valium), 5 mg three times daily. These medications are also effective for the management of anxiety associated with an invasive medical diagnostic or treatment procedure.

Behavioral Treatment

A variety of nonpharmacologic treatments are also used for treatment-related side effects.[25] These approaches generally have the goal of teaching the patient to identify the onset of aversive sensations and to respond in a manner that is incompatible with stress. Examples are the various relaxation, imagery, and hypnotic procedures (see above).

A specific application of these techniques known as systematic desensitization has been especially useful in controlling the anticipatory side effects of chemotherapy. The patient and the therapist devise a hierarchy of anxiety-provoking stimuli relating to the feared situation, ranging from the least to the most frightening. Patients then practice relaxation while systematically visualizing the increasingly aversive scenes. This practice often helps reduce the intensity and duration of anxious responses to treatment.

A form of systematic desensitization may be especially useful for children. This technique involves the use of a child's favorite stories in conjunction with the anxiety-producing events. The therapist relates the story and introduces the feared stimuli in a hierarchic fashion from least to most distressing. The child eventually develops a feeling of self-assertion and pride, even in the previously avoided situation.

Case Histories

An 8-year-old girl had lymphoma invading the right femur. She was seen for outpatient consultation because of severe anxiety reactions to the radiotherapy treatment setting. Before treatment, she had been a good student and enjoyed reading, especially science fiction stories. She was asked to bring a favorite storybook to the treatment session and selected a story about a superheroine who used her powers to destroy enemy invaders. This image was used with the patient's first imagining the heroine destroying the negative energies around the radiotherapy machine. During each succeeding visualization, more of the negative energies were destroyed and the patient imagined herself getting closer to the machine. During the final session, the patient imagined the heroine's inviting her to receive the positive energies that had been freed. This session was followed by a brief visit to the treatment room to inspect the machine in a nonthreatening manner. The patient was able to receive subsequent treatment without experiencing any recurrence of anxiety.

A 62-year-old man was admitted to Orthopaedic Institute with a diagnosis of a tumor in his left femur. As the tumor was not thought to be resectable, he underwent a hip disarticulation. On the evening of surgery, he was found to be agitated and confused, reporting that he had seen someone standing at the window who was trying to shoot him. The patient was sedated with haloperidol (Haldol), 5 IM, and was able to fall asleep. The next morning the patient remained somewhat confused, although he no longer appeared to be agitated. Medical work-up showed no evidence of metabolic toxic causes of patient's delirium and he continued to receive haloperidol, 2 mg orally at bedtime, over the next week with no recurrence of his confusion and agitation. The medication administration was then stopped and the patient remained in remission for the remainder of his hospital course.

EMOTIONAL DISTRESS

Emotional distress can develop at any stage of diagnosis and treatment.[8, 32] Although most patients with cancer respond at some point with some anxiety and a sad and depressed mood to their diagnosis and treatment, it is important to distinguish these shifts in mood from a clinical depression that includes pervasive depressed mood lasting more than several days with the absence of normal responsiveness to usually pleasurable experiences. The latter syndrome is often associated with psychomotor agitation or retardation and necessitates treatment.

Pharmacologic Treatment

Patients often have depression as well as sleep disorders and a fair amount of agitation and often pain. The logical choice of antidepressants are therefore those that are somewhat sedating and have been shown to have associated analgesic properties. Doxepin, given at bedtime in doses of 75 to 100 mg, is especially effective when anxiety and sleep difficulties are a significant component of a patient's problem. When sedation is somewhat problematic, a tricyclic antidepressant such as nortriptylene is equally effective with somewhat less associated sedation. Therapeutic blood levels of both of these medications should be monitored. The severity of the physical illness has a direct effect on the severity of psychiatric symptoms such as anxiety and depression, and treatment dosages should be adjusted accordingly.

Behavioral Treatment

In addition to appropriate pharmacologic management, the provision of a supportive physician-patient relationship is probably the key ingredient in controlling the degree of emotional distress experienced by the patient. This support is characterized by the individualized provision of appropriate information according to the patient's needs and developmental level (see above). For example, physicians should avoid thinking that, if children do not ask questions or complain, they have low levels of emotional distress. At the other extreme, physicians should avoid fully informing children of all the risks and side effects, as the heightened suggestibility of children may intensify these effects. This information is especially crucial, as clear guidelines do not yet exist as to which children develop adjustment problems after loss of limb or other disfigurement and which do not.

The reduction of emotional distress can often be further enhanced by a routine referral to a mental health professional for evaluation of coping techniques. Cancer patients often benefit from a focused discussion of their coping skills or a course of therapy designed to help them consciously identify fears and concerns and share them with the therapist. These ventilation techniques often help sanction the expression of feelings and reactions that the patient may be too embarrassed to seek help for. These discussions frequently prevent school phobia. Therapists can also correct misperceptions by the patient and offer practical solutions to dilemmas faced by the patient.[36] These discussions are especially helpful for children whose experience of amputation may give them the false notion that their handicap will permanently prevent them from functioning at an age-appropriate level. Physicians who present the mental health referral as a routine part of the treatment protocol help ensure the acceptance of this procedure and make available to their patients a potentially useful clinical resource. Acceptance of this referral as routine is often easier when the physician's practice is based at a university-affiliated or comprehensive medical center.

Several patients may decide to enter longer-term individual psychotherapy after this evaluation. This therapy is especially useful when the diagnosis of cancer appears to activate feelings of chronic anxiety, depression, social withdrawal, or self-destructive preoccupation with the cancer diagnosis. This outcome typically occurs for patients who have experienced previous traumas. For these individuals, the diagnosis of cancer appears to reawaken a strong sense of vulnerability and fatalistic depression.[28]

Patients may also choose to enter long-term psychotherapy to help them deal with fears of dying that are posed by a disease process that has not been arrested. The purpose of these sessions is to help the person view death as part of a process rather than as a devastating insult to integrity. Kubler-Ross has identified a variety of information-processing steps with which individuals react to the threat of death.[14] These stages are (1) shock and denial at the initial phase (no, not me); (2) anger, when denial no longer works (why me?); (3) bargaining based on their religious beliefs (yes, it is me, but . . .); (4) depression and profound loss (yes, it is me); and finally (5) acceptance. Patients move through these stages at different rates, alternate between states, or develop yet other responses to the dying process. Working through these feelings can add to the patient's quality of life as well as facilitate communication among the patient, the family, and the health care professionals.

The physician may also inform the patient of the variety of community support groups that exist.[5] For example, the American Cancer Society has a wide network of peer support programs for various site-specific diagnoses. Another voluntary organization, the Candlelighters Foundation, focuses on the children and parents of children with cancer and provides an informative and supportive newsletter. Make Today Count is yet another mutual support group that focuses on emotional self-help for cancer patients and their families. These self-help groups differ from professionally led groups in that the leaders are primarily persons who have experienced the same problems as others in the group. This use of role models provides a valuable service that complements medical and surgical intervention and often facilitates postoperative rehabilitation.

Case Histories

A 17-year-old female adolescent, the oldest of three sisters, was admitted to Orthopaedic Institute with a diagnosis of osteogenic sarcoma involving her left femur. She had been a healthy and active child with a strong interest in gymnastics. The diagnosis was made after she began experiencing progressively worsening pain in her leg. Fortunately, her condition permitted salvage procedure with resection of the tumor to be followed by chemotherapy. In her postoperative course, the patient began to manifest multiple symptoms of depression. Before her surgery, she had been an outgoing young lady with several close friends. She no longer looked forward to visits with family or friends and was mostly quiet and withdrawn during their visits. Her appetite became extremely poor and she needed a great deal of coaxing to eat small amounts of food. She described her sleep as extremely poor, with difficulty in falling asleep and frequent awakening through the night, primarily with repeated concern that the cancer had spread in her body and that she was going to die. This did not seem to respond to multiple reassurances from her physicians that no evidence of cancer was found anywhere and that her prognosis was optimistic.

She was seen in consultation and started on a regimen of nortriptylene, 25 mg orally at bedtime, which over the course of the next week was gradually increased to 100 mg orally at bedtime. The patient was also seen for supportive psychotherapy and given several back issues of the Candlelighters Foundation youth newsletter that contained stories by adolescents who had responded successfully to treatment. The patient initially reported improved sleep and a gradual improvement in her appetite. Laboratory testing 5 days after patient had been receiving 100 mg at night revealed a blood level within the therapeutic range. During the course of the next few days, there was a significant return to patient's previous interest in meeting with friends, and no longer was she preoccupied with the conviction that she would die.

A 16-year-old black female adolescent had a diagnosis of osteosarcoma of the left proximal tibia. Her hospital admission was for wide resection of the left tibia after a course of outpatient chemotherapy that had been complicated by severe nausea and vomiting. The request for consultation was for treatment of the patient's severe depression and withdrawal and for training in behavioral techniques for control of nausea and vomiting.

The patient was examined and found to be withdrawn, limiting her speech to a few soft-spoken words. She was observed to be fatigued, and dietary notes indicated that she had minimal oral intake, which was considered inadequate for postoperative wound healing. The use of hypnosis was thoroughly discussed with the patient. Techniques for improving appetite and mood were used first. She responded well to the hypnotic induction using a combination of progressive relaxation and imagery suggestions. The patient was given posthypnotic suggestions for increased appetite and retention of food and improved mood. A tape was made for self-practice, and during her self-hypnosis sessions, a sign informed visitors and hospital staff that the patient was not to be disturbed. An immediate improvement was soon noted with the patient's frequent use of the tape. Instructions were given to family members and nursing staff to reinforce these improvements in mood and appetite and to encourage the use of the hypnosis tape. Additional sessions were then conducted to prepare the patient for the course of chemotherapy and to minimize her side effects. These techniques were used by the patient on an outpatient basis and helped minimize her nausea and vomiting.

Conclusions

The total care of the patient with a musculoskeletal tumor involves attention to the physical and psychologic issues. These principles should make significant contributions to the treatment and rehabilitation of the patient with cancer.

References

1. American Pain Society: Principles of Analgesic Use in the Treatment of Acute Pain and Chronic Cancer Pain: A Concise Guide to Medical Practice, 2nd ed. American Pain Society, Skokie, IL, 1989.
2. Bahnson CB: Psychologic and emotional issues in cancer: The psychotherapeutic care of the cancer patient. Semin Oncol 2:293–309, 1975.
3. Barber J, Gitelson JG: Cancer pain: Psychological management using hypnosis. CA 30:130–136, 1980.
4. Barofsky I: Job discrimination: A measure of the social death of the cancer patient. In Western States. Conference on Cancer Rehabilitation, Conference Proceedings, Bull Publishing, Palo Alto, CA, 1982.
5. Blumberg BD, Flaherty M: Services available to persons with cancer: National and regional organizations. JAMA 244:1715–1717, 1980.
6. Burish TG, Carey MI: Conditioned aversive responses in cancer chemotherapy patients: Theroretical and developmental analysis. J Consult Clin Psychol 54:593–600, 1986.
7. Chapman CR: Pain related to cancer treatment. J Pain Symptom Management 3:188–193, 1988.
8. Derogatis LR, Morrow GR, Fetting J, Penman D, Piasetsky S, Schmale AM, Hendricks M, Carnicke LM: The prevalence of psychiatric disorders among cancer patients. JAMA 249:751–757, 1983.
9. Forester BM, Kornfeld DS, Flass J: Psychiatric aspects of radiotherapy. Am J Psychiatry 135:960–963, 1978.
10. Freidenbergs I, Gordon W, Hibbard M, Levine L, Wolf C, Diller L: Psychosocial aspects of living with cancer: A review of the literature. Int J Psychiatry Med 11:303–329, 1982.
11. Goldberg RJ, Cullen LO: Factors important to psychosocial adjustment to cancer; a review of the evidence. Social Science Med 20:803–807, 1985.
12. Jacobson E: Progressive Relaxation. Chicago, University of Chicago Press, 1938.
13. Jay SM, Elliott C, Varni JW: Acute and chronic pain in adults and children with cancer. J Consult Clin Psychol 54:601–607, 1986.
14. Kubler-Ross E: On Death and Dying. New York, Macmillan, 1969.
15. Lansky SB: Impediments to treatment and rehabilitation of the childhood cancer patient. CA 35:302–306, 1985.
16. Loesser JD, Black RG: A taxonomy of pain. Pain 1:81–90, 1975.
17. Luthe W: Autogenic Therapy. New York, Grune & Stratton, 1969.
18. Marks RM, Sachar EJ: Undertreatment of medical inpatients with narcotic analgesics. Ann Intern Med 78:173–181, 1973.
19. Milano MR, Jacobs AR: The management of the surgical patient. *In* Kornfeld DS, Fickel JB (eds): Psychiatric Management for Medical Practitioners. New York, Grune & Stratton, 1982, 373–398.
20. Morthouse L: The impact of cancer on the family. An overview. Int J Psychiatry Med 13:215–240, 1983.

21. Nir Y, Maslin B: Liaison psychiatry in childhood cancer: A systems approach. Psychiatr Clin North Am 5:379–386, 1982.
22. Noyes R: Treatment of cancer pain. Psychosom Med 43:57–70, 1981.
23. Peck A, Bolard J: Emotional reactions to radiation treatment. Cancer 40:180–184, 1977.
24. Portenoy RK: Practical aspects of pain control in the patient with cancer. CA 38:327–352, 1988.
25. Redd WH: Treatment of excessive crying in a terminal cancer patient: A time series analysis. J Behav Med 5:225–235, 1982.
26. Redd WH: Behavioral approaches to treatment related distress. CA 38:138–145, 1988.
27. Redd WH, Andrykowski MA: Behavioral intervention in cancer treatment: Controlling aversion reactions to chemotherapy. Psychol Bull 50:1018–1025, 1982.
28. Sarell M, Baider L: Coping with cancer among Holocaust survivors in Israel: An exploratory study. J Hum Stress 10:121–127, 1984.
29. Schmale AH: Principles of psychosocial oncology. *In* Ruben P (ed): Clinical Oncology for Medical Students and Physicians: A Multidisciplinary Approach. New York, American Cancer Society, 1978.
30. Sherman RA, Arena JG, Sherman CJ, Ernst JL: The mystery of phantom pain: Growing evidence for psychophysiological mechanisms. Biofeedback and Self Regulation 14:267–280, 1989.
31. Short course on the management of cancer pain. J Pain Symptom Management 2 (special issue), 1987.
32. Silberfarb PM: Psychiatric treatment of the patient during cancer therapy. CA 38:133–137, 1988.
33. Simonton OC, Simonton S: Belief systems and management of the emotional aspects of malignancy. J Transpersonal Psychol 7:29–47, 1975.
34. Simonton OC, Matthews-Simonton S, Sparks TF: Psychological intervention in the treatment of cancer. Psychosomatics 21:226–233, 1980.
35. Snow BR: Compliance with therapeutic regimens. Assessment and treatment issues. *In* Finkel J (ed): Consultation/Liaison Psychiatry: Current Trends and New Perspectives. New York, Grune & Stratton, 1983, pp 97–113.
36. Stam HJ, Bultz BD, Pittman CA: Psychosocial problems and interventions in a referred sample of cancer patients. Psychosom Med 48:539–548, 1986.
37. Stam HJ, Goss C, Rosenal L, Ewens S, Urton B: Aspects of psychological distress and pain in career patients undergoing radiotherapy. Adv Pain Res Ther 9:569–573, 1985.
38. Sutherland AM, Orbach CE: Depressive reactions associated with surgery for cancer. *In* The Psychological Impact of Cancer. American Cancer Society, New York, Professional Education Publication, 1984.
39. Sutherland HJ, Llewellyn-Thomas HA, Lockwood GA, Tritchler DL, Till JE: Cancer patients: Their desire for information and participation in treatment decisions. J R Soc Med 82:260–263, 1989.
40. Weisman AD, Worden JW: The existential plight in cancer: Significance of the first 100 days. Int J Psychiatry Med 7:1–5, 1976.
41. Wickeramasekera IE: Clinical Behavioral Medicine: Some Concepts and Procedures. New York, Plenum Press, 1989.

CHAPTER 25

Psychosocial Dimensions of Bone Cancer: Social Work Services and Human Resources

GARY ROSENBERG
MICHAEL GROPPER

This chapter begins with a focus on children, not because they commonly have this disease nor because the psychosocial problems they encounter are not also experienced by adults, but because all psychosocial needs are sequenced by developmental level. To understand whatever interferes with the psychosocial tasks and achievements at any time of life, one must understand developmental tasks. Bone cancer is highly disruptive to the normal accomplishment of psychosocial development.[27] Why this is so and what the manifestations are need to be understood by personnel from every discipline involved in cancer treatment. It is a part of knowing the patient and understanding the treatment that is being given.

The emotional and social impact of any cancer on the coping mechanisms and developmental tasks of patients and those whose lives are connected with them is great because of the issues it raises. First is the possibility of death. This elicits irreversible emotional reactions. Second is the imperative of getting quality medical care, initially for diagnosis and later for sensitive, intelligent treatment. These issues entail searching for information, asking questions, and decision making for the patient and the family or friends, along with the treatment staff, oncologists, social workers, nurses, health educators, hospital administrators, and allied health care professionals. Little wonder that the state of the art approach is to include psychosocial diagnosis and treatment in the continuing care of patients with cancer and their significant others.

Thirty years ago, the treatment of cancer was mostly palliation and terminal care. Today, the importance of long-term pain and anxiety control, compliance with treatment regimens, and emotional reactions to the disease and treatment is recognized as integral to good management of the disease.[28]

The chapter considers problems relevant to developmental stages, children and adolescents with bone cancer. Parenting of children and adolescents is discussed separately because of the special problems in the coexistence of good medical treatment and good parenting. Understanding of the particular issues involved is useful both to treatment personnel and to parents. The discussion of issues facing adults with bone cancer is dependent on much of the theoretical data for children and adolescents, because each adult has a child within that becomes active under the stress of severe illness. The adult is at a different point with respect to responsibilities and concerns but may be at the child's or the adolescent's psychosocial level because of the stresses of the disease. Finally, particular interdisciplinary issues growing out of contemporary treatment methods are raised and some suggestions for resolution of problems are offered.

Children with Bone Cancer

A numerical codification of the psychosocial effects of bone cancer on children has not been done. This is because of the many social variables against which the disease and its treatment are played out. Although the struggle for precision in diagnosis and statistical data continues, treatment goes forward on the basis of the social work knowledge of the impact of bone cancer and its treatment on the child-patient and on the parents, siblings, teachers, and others on whom the child depends. Although developmental issues do not precisely follow age charts, the following discussion deals with preadolescent children.

All children are developmentally in a state of rapid change, and the interaction between them and their parents and other helpers is highly variable. Children, like most cancer patients, focus on those impairments that make them feel most abnormal at the time, and for children that signal is perceived by how caring adults see these impairments. This is one of the ways in which the development of independence is interrupted by this disease. There is not only dependence on parents, but also reliance on physicians and other treatment personnel. A fixed routine of clinic visits, hospital visits, and treatments interrupts playtime, school attendance, family activities, and friendships.[21, 22] Social work intervention is, therefore, directed toward salvaging and maintaining normal experiences for the child and those significant persons in his or her life. It is not easy for the treatment staff to normalize interventions such as surgery, chemotherapy, radiation, laboratory tests, and injections. These distract helpers from the greatest psychosocial need of a child, which is to be allowed to be a child, whether sick or well. This involves the need to play, to learn, and to be loved. The treatment staff is legitimately concerned about the debilitation of the child physically and emotionally, but may not have the knowledge or energy to identify what is most missing for the child. Each child requires, along with technical, medical excellence, attention to individual, nonmedical needs.

School is the child's workplace and that connection is crucial. Lansky and colleagues studied parents and teachers of 16 children who were survivors of cancer for 2 years or longer and were returning to school full-time.[29] They found that children who were absent at the start of the school year had the most difficult time adjusting. Given the importance of psychosocial well-being, the question must be raised whether that has been taken into account in connection with the medical treatment plan. Would it be possible for treatment to be interrupted so that a child could experience the positive value of school beginning, and then take a necessary leave, with connections having been made that would give support through the continued treatment?

Young children with cancer often experience impairment in verbal skills and academic achievement owing to high rates of absenteeism caused by their disease. This also affects the child's socialization with peers.[8, 9, 29]

Social work assessments should not interfere with treatment needs, but at the appropriate time, psychosocial elements should be introduced into the treatment-planning arena so that all staff know and take life needs into account.[23]

Closely connected with this issue is the study of fear in a child. Although bone cancer creates fear at any age, for children these fears take the shape of fear of strangers, separation anxiety, fear of loss of love and approval, fear of loss of developmental achievements, fear of loss or injury to body parts, guilt, and fear of retaliation, as well as fear of pain.[42] The use of school associates to offset some of these fears is an important resource to children and cannot be taken lightly.

Many staff members have legitimate concerns about the negative side of peer association. How will peers respond to hair loss, possible limb amputation or disfiguring surgery, weight change, and other potentially threatening side effects? In addition to the timing of school admissions, absences, and readmissions, there are several areas in which hospital-school collaboration is needed.[1]

1. Hospital staff guidance is needed by teachers. Hospital therapists know how amputation affects the child and how a prosthesis can be used. They also know how chemotherapy affects strength. These issues are easier for hospital staff than for teachers. The openness and availability of hospital staff to address questions and worries that teachers have is reassuring to teachers and is a way of giving practical treatment to the child.[6]

2. Changes in physical appearance (e.g.,

hair loss because of radiation treatment) affect children's sense of self-esteem and their peer acceptance. The child and the parent can be helped to select an attractive wig before hair loss, and plans can be made for its use. The social worker, the nurse, or another treatment person can let the teacher understand this and help the child plan how to let other children know about body changes and limitations. To help the child-patient take initiative puts him or her in a leadership position. Children have remarkable capacity to accept each other as they are, but anticipatory counseling facilitates this process.

3. The patient needs help in understanding that cancer is not a death sentence and that it is important to take responsibility for how to let friends know this. The strength of knowledge gives status. The patient can be prepared for reactions from those who are simply ignorant. To help children identify words that are clear but reassuring is important work. Teachers can be important helpers if they are also well informed.[25]

4. Medically oriented staff members can look to the social worker for initiative. The social worker consults clinical staff for particular guidance in planning and easing the transition to and from school and hospital.

Two issues with particular impact on staff are children's reactions to amputations and to fear of death. Because amputations are so visible and irreversible, they are problematic not only to children but to those who love and care for them. Social workers warn about the results of not recognizing disparate responses to this intervention. The loss of a limb may overwhelm the parent. A child may be experiencing such pain in that limb that amputation comes as a relief. Accurate empathy requires an exploration of the feelings of fear, hope, and pain of the child and the parents.

As the illness goes on, the fear of death is a part of a child's fears—differently perceived at different times. For many children with bone cancer, facing death at such a young age becomes the major problem. Transitory school phobias among fatally ill children have been reported as part of an adaptive coping mechanism, protecting children from underlying terror and overwhelming separation anxiety of death. Goldberg and Tull suggest that "it is important for staff and parents, who are struggling to make sense out of a cascade of physical and emotional stresses, to try to put a child's internal experience in some context to guide their own behaviour."[19]

Between the ages of 5 and 9 years, children are able to understand the finality of death and the seriousness of their illness and experience of separation and abandonment.[40] After age 9 years, "children perceive death as both final and inevitable."[19]

Goldberg and Tull describe the internal meaning of death for younger children.

> The child from one to five years of age perceives death as a separation, a state of being "less alive." Children in this range perceive the overall traumatic effect in terms of separation from their mothers, fathers, or individuals who have given them the most nurturing since birth.[19]

Rarely do children of this age ask directly "am I going to die?" but they can express painful feelings through drawings, cutouts, puppets, and various games. They need this opportunity for communication.

Grownups often underestimate the capacity of chronically ill younger children, especially those older than 3 years, to be aware of the painful feelings and fears associated with dying. Oncologists and persons caring for young children with cancer should remember how sensitive and how capable of expressing their fears young children are. The dying child communicates as he or she knows how. Those who care for these children need to pay close attention to the "how." These children can feel abandoned by staff if the professional caretakers withdraw during the ending stages of their lives.[16]

For some medical staff, withdrawing from a dying child serves as a protective measure against their own feelings of helplessness, defeat, and pain. Vernick warns professionals, parents, and teachers about "psychological euthanasia," which is acting on the expectation that, because a child with cancer will die, what is necessary for normal development can be withheld.[46]

Children with bone cancer are influenced by the subtle interactions of biology and treatment of the disease, family reactions and strengths, reactions of extended family and friends, community institutions' capacity and desire to accept children who look different, and a changing culture that shows signs of accepting children with cancer more easily than in the past. The professional is attentive to this environment and tries with determination and compassion to correct any imbalance that occurs between the child and those he or she knows and loves.

Adolescents with Bone Cancer

The adolescent with a malignant musculoskeletal tumor has been assaulted at a time of particular vulnerability. Normal adolescence is a period of rapid physical, psychologic, and social growth and change. Psychologically, the adolescent strives for independence and needs to begin to separate more from parents. The cancer experience is directly at odds with developmental tasks.

The adolescent with cancer is hampered in the carving out of identity through independence. The sick role is a dependent role in the hospital and even during outpatient medical treatment. Not surprisingly, power struggles with adult caretakers are common. Those treating adolescents need to be aware of their actual need to express independence and to maintain some control during the course of treatment. This is not easy for physicians or other treatment people for whom professional autonomy is the norm, but it does avert some nonproductive struggles. "Physicians were expected [by adolescents] to be open, honest, non-judgmental and respectful and to include the patient in the formulation of treatment plans."[36] If adolescent patients can be offered some options that assure them of their responsibility in the control of their disease (e.g., letting them make their own appointments, monitor their own medication dosages, and participate in the selection of their own physicians and nurses, relationships between them and their helpers will be eased. Finding options of independence without putting the patient at greater medical risk requires both imagination and patience. Only if this is seen as a pivotal factor in successful treatment does this become possible.[4]

The adolescent need for clarity has been supported by research. Adolescents reported that, on learning they had cancer, they immediately feared the worst because they did not really understand what was wrong with them.[7, 36, 40, 41] The adolescents interviewed strongly urged that full disclosure be given at the earliest possible time in clear and supportive ways. They saw the period of uncertainty after the diagnosis as the most stressful part of their experience with the disease.

Cancer treatment consists of invasive and often drastic medical procedures, which produce painful side effects and strong fears. For example, an adolescent with bone cancer may have to face an amputation of a leg. Radiation and chemotherapy produce nausea, pain, fear, and body image change.

> Chemotherapeutic and radiologic treatments sometimes make children feel as if their bodies are not their own. Their well-remembered physical responses are thrown out of kilter by the mood-changing and physique-altering effects of drugs.[7]

For adolescents, this is occurring at a time when noticeable and remarkable body changes and intensification of sexual drives and feelings are resulting from hormonal changes associated with the onset of pubescence. It is out of these conflicting realities that some young cancer patients arrive at the viewpoint of preferring death to another course of chemotherapy. To those whose mission is to save life, this attitude seems cowardly and unappreciative.

That study results and observations are often in conflict mirrors the conflictive nature of adolescence. Despite the observed examples of adolescents who express a preference for death, adolescent survivors of cancer, compared with siblings and other groups of young people of the same age, showed no higher risk for major depression and other forms of psychologic distress requiring professional help.[28, 30, 43, 44] Teta and associates studied adolescent cancer patients and 587 siblings.[44] No differences were found in the incidence of suicidal attempts, running away from home, and psychiatric hospital admissions. Does this mean that those involved in treating cancer are giving these young people needed support? Does it mean that, despite their problems or perhaps because of them, adolescent patients see life as valuable? It is an area to be further studied.

During the long ordeal of treatment, education has great importance to adolescents. Lansky and colleagues reported on the anxiety of secondary school children about educational deficits, especially losses in mathematics.[29] Their need for socialization with peers also remains strong, and Goldberg and Tull's findings that on returning to school, they feel forgotten is a sad fact.[19] Peer socialization is essential to the rehabilitative process, as a reassurance of acceptance and builder of self-esteem. Strong friendships and people with whom sadness can be shared, so that one feels comforted and less lonely, were seen as important supports to adolescents.

Adolescents are a sociable, educable, and responsive group, and these observations challenge professionals in both the classroom and the hospital to address their socialization needs. School staff members report that the most common issues facing adolescent students with cancer is teasing, the child's physical discomfort, low academic achievement, and difficulties in peer relationships.[7] Wasserman and colleagues observed that 40% of the adolescent survivors of Hodgkin's disease noted "that peers teased them about their baldness or thinness, avoided them because they might be 'contagious' or generally treated them as outcasts."[47] Because selection of suitable hair pieces is relatively simple, certainly it should be a routine part of treatment for all adolescent young men and women before hair is lost. Progress in this area is so advanced that adolescents can have any style they want.

Medical center personnel are challenged to work together with educators and parents in easing the academic reentry of the adolescent with cancer. School personnel need clear, up-to-date information about the disease, its treatment, and any physical limitations and capabilities. Teachers need help with their feelings and fears about cancer and dying to help them to respond better to the needs of the returning adolescent.[20, 24] Informed teachers and school authorities are better able to prepare schoolmates for the return of a friend, lessening the uneasiness between patient and colleagues.[25]

For patients at an age when peer support is so significant, the use of peer groups is an obvious route for intervention. Social workers can stimulate these activities, but other staff are needed as participants, as the work should be viewed as part of the treatment program.

Fears about the future are heightened for adolescent patients when their cancer goes into remission.[28, 37] The adolescent survivor of cancer is subject to particular stress. As one nurse put it, there is constant suspicion of all "lumps and bumps" and symptoms of any kind; anniversary dates for diagnosis of cancer and treatment cessation frequently trigger emotional reactions.[26]

As adolescents with bone cancer and Ewing's sarcoma survive in greater numbers, they will have to cope with the effects of chemotherapy and of bone replacement surgery. For those experiencing recurrence of cancer, amputation followed by a fitting with a prosthetic device is required. Rehabilitation becomes an important but wearisome part of therapy. Both patient and family now have added to their agenda dealing with the problems of chronic illness.

The significant help offered to adolescents by their families through the first phases of illness (diagnosis and initial treatment) can give way to discontinuities for the patient and family during the long years of chronicity. Other siblings need the parents' attention. The adolescent becomes increasingly dependent on family support at a time when separation is normal for parents as well as the child. Separating, going to college, and entering the world of later adolescence all present new psychologic problems. Adolescents also face many severe practical difficulties. For example, adolescent cancer survivors have significantly more employment, college, and health and life insurance rejections than do their siblings.[11, 45]

Like other adolescents, the adolescent with bone cancer is developmentally sometimes child and sometimes adult. Yet these young people are hampered in asserting adult freedom, to make decisions, and to defy parents and other authorities. More often, it is necessary for them to ask for help, as a child does. The struggle with the disease interferes with the struggle to break away from authority figures (represented by physicians and nurses) and parents. The usual defenses and ways of coping are interrupted.

To be a healthy adolescent is difficult. To parent a healthy adolescent is difficult. To live with adolescent bone cancer is to live with a problem that outlasts adolescence and makes adult living difficult. This is unfinished business, not only for these young people and their parents but for all of those involved in their care.

Parenting Children and Adolescents with Bone Cancer

The stresses of parenting children with bone cancer are related to the cycle of treatment, remission, and relapse. The child's condition changes, and staff expectations and reports are optimistic, guarded, or noncommittal. A parent is hopeful, in despair, grateful, reassured, discouraged, or exhausted.[13, 14] This is the content of being a parent to a child with bone cancer.

Although parents are the primary and most significant nurturers of their children, the imperatives of treatment sometimes diminish their role. Their child needs parenting, but medical matters are now critical.[5] How does the parent fit in the course of medical care and continue to reassure and comfort?

Parents are first caught up in trying to accept

the reality of the diagnosis. They must absorb an enormous amount of medical and technical information, a process whose inherent difficulties are compounded by the new language and rules of the unfamiliar medical culture. It is not easy for parents and health care professionals to adjust their styles of communication to each other.[7] When either a parent or a medical professional feels this burden, it is wise to ask a social worker to help. Not only does this facilitate understanding, but it can help the family resolve feelings about the crisis.[23]

For parents, the times of caring for a dependent patient and helping the patient with recovery or rehabilitation are painfully interlocked. They must accompany the patient to medical treatments with constant worry and uncertainty about the future. At times of remission, they may partially succeed in forgetting about the illness. Then the relapse occurs, and equilibrium is upset.

Defense Systems

Much has been written about the defense systems used by parents in their struggle to deal with the cancer of their child. Parents face the challenge of walking the narrow line between focusing on disease and its treatment, devoting time to a spouse and other children, and continuing the course of normal life. Professional staff need to know that the demand on parents is so great that they may well make use of a variety of sometimes conflicting defenses.

Denial is commonly evident early in the child's treatment. It does not mean that the parent will not move toward reality in time, but it is an appropriate defense until strength is mobilized.

Optimism, to an excessive degree and not based on reality, may also be evident as a defense. Not uncommonly, parents hang on to this as they adjust to knowledge of the child's illness. The hope fuels the strength to cope.

Search for information often helps parents to feel more in control of situations and to know which questions to ask.

Reliance on religion helps to direct emotionally painful feelings.

Search for help from others (parents, friends, and professional counselors) provides a buffer against emotional distress.

All of these mechanisms can serve usefully, and parents of children with bone cancer are likely to use all of these supports at one time or another.[11]

Because cancer is widely perceived as a synonym for death, the family confronts its basic values on life and death issues. What is the pattern for parenting a child who may die? It is, like all parenting, a day-by-day process, but feelings can overwhelm the ability to plan. The role of the social worker is to help the parents find the style and pattern that is their own.[23, 39] The disease does not proscribe this role, but will interrupt it at times. How can equilibrium be maintained so that the parent can trust his or her capacity and act spontaneously?

Support Sources

There are many ways to react to cancer, and every family member deserves appropriate guidance. Both professional counselors and self-help groups offer advice, knowledge, and emotional support and identify necessary resources for helping family members and patients cope with cancer. One of the benefits of professional guidance from a social worker is assistance with this search for sources of help.[13, 14]

To remain a healthy, helping parent requires nurturing. A group (self-help or professionally run) is a powerful resource for parents of children with cancer. Parents can meet and identify with others in a similar situation. It can offer social and emotional support as well as practical assistance with medical needs. Groups help family members with distorted perceptions about the disease and treatment. Here help is offered that improves reality testing and helps in decision making. The feelings of loneliness and alienation often associated with cancer for family members disappear as the experience is universalized. Hope is instilled in members by expressions of optimism in the group, and acceptance is provided through a feeling of mutual aid.[35, 48] One learns what other parents are saying to their children and what has helped. A group can coalesce into a remarkable support in times of crisis, when a child has a relapse, or even in the case of death.

Single-parent families are particularly in need of informal supports even if they have concerned friends who rally around. A group offers support to these mothers or fathers, whether they are faced with loneliness, lack of intimate relationships, unusual support sources, or overwhelming, unshared responsibilities. Single parents also bring a particular strength to other members.

Marital issues may be sometimes raised in a group or in individual counseling. The literature with respect to marital discord as a serious family consequence of childhood cancer is problematic. Emotional distancing, decreased frequency of sexual intimacy, sexual dysfunction, unresolved personal conflicts, disagreements, and an inability to derive personal satisfaction and comfort from the marriage were mentioned by Chesler and Barbarin.[7] They found that spouses sometimes focus on each other the pain, fear, and anger they feel because of the child's illness. They also report that the task of caring for the ill child may produce such physical and emotional fatigue that parents are unable to be physically intimate.

They also found, however, that more than 65% of spouses reported their spouse to be "very helpful" when a child had cancer. Lansky and colleagues did not find a higher divorce rate in families of children with cancer compared with families with physically healthy children.[30] Koocher and O'Malley also did not find evidence that parents of childhood cancer survivors had significantly greater marital conflicts than did other families.[28]

Whatever the meaning of these conflicting reports, awareness of the stresses that parents face causes one to take seriously Hinds' finding that the most frequently expressed unmet need perceived by families of a person with cancer was a place where they could turn to discuss their fears.[21]

Family therapy is another treatment for families who have a member with bone cancer, whether child or adult. Whether family therapy is used, or group support, or help from a social worker at particular times of crisis, some but not all of the issues discussed above are likely to surface.

The demands on parents relating to childhood cancer exceed normal capacity for coping. This is important for professional staff as well as family members to recognize. The members of such a family continue to need formal and informal ways of gathering strength for the business of living.

Each family is an individual group, each individual is unique, and parenting is a skill best understood by parents and their children.[12] Empathy and respect for this process is one of the most therapeutic contributions that people engaged in treatment can make.

Adults with Bone Cancer

The adult patient with high-grade malignant musculoskeletal tumor faces many of the problems of children and adolescent patients, because the issues of possible death, treatment, and remission are the same. A basic difference is in the impact on life goals and responsibilities, which give rise to strengths and vulnerabilities. The child and the adolescent struggle with the stigma of a diagnosis that will never go away and will hamper plans for life work, marriage, and career. The adult may have already achieved these and is concerned about how the diagnosis jeopardizes past accomplishments as well as plans for the future.

At the beginning of diagnosis and initial treatment, survival is the paramount concern. Later on, quality of life issues merit consideration and sometimes outweigh survival concerns.

Resolution of psychosocial issues for the adult patient, from the viewpoint of the social worker, begins with making a timely and skillful entrance into the work of helping both the patient and the family. The exploratory stage of treatment begins with gathering relevant information about the patient, significant others, and the family. This may entail reading the chart or talking to physicians and nurses. Staff already in contact with patient are important in this process. The social worker thinks about what kinds of issues the patient is facing—an uncertainty about the future because of a potentially terminal illness, a need to adjust to a sick role, or an attempt to absorb an enormous amount of medical and technical information about the illness within the strange and new environment of the hospital.[38] Through anticipatory empathy, the social worker knows that the patient is pressured to learn rapidly about this environment and about the biotechnical aspects of managing the bone cancer to make necessary decisions about treatment of the disease. Worries about work and financial matters are operating along with concern about the reactions of family and friends.

During the in-person interview, part of the exploratory phase, the social worker tries to understand how personal, environmental, and cultural factors are interacting; the specific problems brought on by the illness; and the patient's and the family members' perceptions of these problems. What defense mechanisms are employed to cope with the problems, and what resources does the family have to help them adapt to the demands that derive from the diagnosis of bone cancer? Setting a tone of courtesy, respect, and sincere concern facilitates communication.[17] Accurate problem definition grows out of this exploration of the stresses and coping and adaptation processes. An ecological approach to the total life space of the individual gives continuous validity to the psychosocial assessment and problem definition.

The potential for the patient or family members to experience an emotional crisis in relation to the disease is continually monitored. If a crisis occurs, clinical interventions are offered to help the patient and the family mobilize emotional resources to deal with the loss of control, hopelessness, total despair, panic, and disequilibrium that may occur.

A breakdown in family communication and connectedness can be part of the emotional fallout of this diagnosis. The social worker evaluates the change in family integration patterns and helps family members to maintain connections and openness about their fears and anxieties. If ties are maintained and strengthened, the capacity to cope with the disease and its problems is enlarged for both the patient and the family.[10]

Marital strain may result as spouse and/or children (sometimes adult children with their own set of life responsibilities and pressures) begin to manage the family's needs, coordinate financing, and provide care for the patient.[31]

The social worker helps family members to release anguish, grief, fear, pity, sadness, or resentment; encourages family discussions about the effects of cancer and changes dysfunctional communication patterns; assists in planning the patient's care; and helps the spouse maintain a healthy balance between serving the patient's and his or her own needs.

One of the most difficult roles faced by the oncology social worker, along with other members of the treatment team, is working with a dying patient and helping family members work through the emotional and practical issues surrounding this loss. Interventions are directed toward helping family members anticipate the loss of the dying person and visualize the impact that this loss will have on each of them separately as well as together as a family. The strengths and weaknesses of the patient and the family members around issues of grief and mourning are carefully evaluated in an anticipatory mourning process.[22]

Fogarty referred to an "inner pit" that therapists working with dying patients must decide to go into.

> If one decides to go into that inner pit with another person, he must do it carefully, with respect for the wishes and feelings of that person. He cannot decide how that individual should die.[15]

Knowledge and skill in helping with the psychosocial issues surrounding death and dying are crucial for oncology social workers.

Support groups for family members were discussed above. They also have value for patients. They provide a forum for the candid discussions of all concerns, including fear of the dying process, with its anticipated pain and imposed dependency; a "good" death; funeral arrangements; fantasies and beliefs about life after death; anger at various people; and thoughts about voluntarily ending one's own life.[11] Groups help cancer patients in various ways. They support hope, the fight for life, and the will to live. They help increase interpersonal skills; they also help the patient absorb the trauma of the diagnosis in small doses and protect self-esteem, narcissistic defenses, faith in religion or other powerful forces, and existential resolve. Many see this structure as an essential part of the helping process needed for patients with bone cancer. Groups provide members an opportunity to share common ideas and concerns and to evolve into a mutual aid system.[18]

Much of the of bone cancer patients' success in coping with the illness and maximizing the quality of their life during diagnosis and treatment and thereafter is related to their previous quality of life. The psychosocial support system, the nature of the work situation, and how the treatment of the disease affects and impairs major psychosocial activities are significant factors. People who are successful, particularly those with their own businesses, seem able to cope more effectively. Certainly, the financial impact of cancer on those of lower socioeconomic groups, whose ability to remain employed may be threatened by treatment, particularly by amputation, is significant. The ability to continue health insurance, to maintain economic security for their family, and to see themselves as important working and contributing members of society contrasts with the situation for children or adolescents who carry the stigma of this type of cancer in their attempts to achieve success.[34]

Despite the numerous hazards, many individuals have been able to use the cancer crisis as a way of better appreciating themselves, their families, and varied elements of their lives. They have successfully struggled and expanded their emotional, interactional, and social horizons.

Collaboration Among Disciplines

Most physicians, nurses, and social workers agree that collaboration with each other and with those from other disciplines is essential to well-balanced treatment of patients with cancer. As viewpoints, skills, and priorities are blended, quality biopsychosocial care results. Most physicians are aware that their work needs to be coordinated with that of professionals from various educational, psychologic, and social disciplines. Otherwise, the care of the related needs of both patients and families is compromised. Social workers feel the need for collegial collaborative relationships with physicians. The physicians' input is seen as an essential requirement for social work assessment in health care settings.[19, 38] Historically, social workers in hospitals relied on physicians to determine when psychosocial services were needed. As medical intervention moves more rapidly because of technological advances, and as social work increases its knowledge base, the early assessment of psychosocial needs and resources of patients has become practical and obligatory.

Martin stressed the psychosocial factors in achieving the goals of medicine, which he saw as assisting patients to achieve physical, emotional, and social well-being regardless of the presence of disease.[32] Therefore, he believed that understanding the psychosocial aspects of cancer was as important as investigating the biologic and cellular components of cancer.

Many departments of social work use independent screening mechanisms to systematically identify variables associated with high psychosocial risk.[3] These procedures enable early identification of patients at risk for psychosocial problems either at or shortly after admission to the institution.[2] Using such a device, a patient with a diagnosis of bone cancer would receive immediate attention by the social services department, because cancer is a medical problem with high psychosocial risk potential. These mechanisms enable social workers to enter a case during the preadmission phase or immediately after the patient's admission to the hospital.

When the patient is ready to leave the hospital, the fitting of the patient's limitations and abilities to the community environment requires the input of various disciplines, but always medicine, nursing, and social work are involved. Miller rated this work as having priority in the hospital social services department, noting that among the skills required were fast assessment of patient's needs, knowledge of community resources, and capacity to make a treatment plan that ensures support to the patient after the hospital stay.[33]

Guiding and connecting patients to the continuing care they need may involve obtaining financial assistance from such public sources as Social Security, Supplemental Security Income, Medicaid, Medicare, food stamps or public assistance, and arranging for needed resources such as homemaker services, or visiting nurse care. Physical therapy, transportation to and from the hospital, and referral for long-term institutional care are among the community resources that may be needed and for which careful guidance is imperative.

Hospice care is available to persons with a fatal illness and a short life expectancy. The pioneer of the hospice movement was Cicely Saunders, a British woman educated as a physician, nurse, and social worker. Saunders established St. Christopher's Hospice in London in 1967. She believed that terminal illness was a time for family members to reconcile and together face the crisis of a family member's dying. These needs were and are usually overlooked in regular hospital settings. In 1975, the hospice model arrived in the United States with the opening of the New Haven Hospice in Connecticut. In 1982, federal legislation for funding hospice care was enacted. Although a goal of hospice care is to support the patient in the home, dying patients often go in and out of the inpatient hospice setting during the final stages of life.

Important to the treatment team is the mediation function of social workers. They often help family members negotiate strains on the family system and the patient. Social workers also provide a mediating function between anxious family members and hospital treatment staff when family members have difficulties communicating questions and feelings. This role may be crucial if high-risk family factors such as cultural differences, language barriers, poverty, intellectual limitations, psychosocial family problems, and incongruent coping styles are present. Sometimes, social workers help the family maneuver a complicated medical system to be responsive to their needs.[38]

Summary

Those caring for cancer patients need to pay attention to the total needs of patients. This includes both quality medical care and quality psychosocial care and support. Although psychosocial support comes from many sources, the social worker by discipline and commitment has a responsibility to provide the oncology team with a continuing psychosocial data base. With this data, the social worker brings a quantum of empathy for the stress, excitement, and pain that constitutes the work of every colleague.

References

1. Adams D, Deveau E: Coping with Childhood Cancer. Reston, VA, Reston Publishing, 1984.
2. Berkman B, Rehr H: Early social service case finding our hospitalized patients: An experiment. Soc Service Rev 47(2), 1973.
3. Berkman B, Rehr H, Rosenberg G: A social work department creates and tests a screening mechanism to identify high social risk. Soc Work Health Care 5(4):373–385, 1980.
4. Bloctcky AD, Cohen DG, Conatser C, Klopovitch P: Psychosocial characteristics of adolescents who refuse cancer treatments. J Consult Clin Psychol 53:729–731, 1985.
5. Cassileth B, Hamilton J: The family with cancer. *In* Cassileth B (ed): The Cancer Patient: Social and Medical Aspects of Care. Philadelphia, Lea & Febiger, 1979.
6. Charlton A, Pearson D, Morris-Jones PH: Children's return to school after treatment for solid tumors. Soc Sci Med 22(12):1337–1346, 1986.
7. Chesler MA, Barbarin DA: Childhood Cancer and the Family: Meeting the Challenge of Stress and Support. New York, Brunner/Mazel Publishers, 1987, p 167.
8. Conatser C: Preparing the family for their responsibilities during treatment. Cancer 58:508–511, 1986.
9. Copeland DR, Worchel FW: Psychosocial aspects of childhood cancer. Texas Med 82:46–48, 1986.
10. Ell K: Social networks, social support and health status. Soc Service Rev 58:133–149, 1984.
11. Ell K, Northen H: Families and Health Care: Psychosocial Practice. New York, Aldine de Gruyter, 1990.
12. Ell K, Mantel J, Hamovitch M: Socioculturally sensitive intervention for patients with cancer. J Psychosoc Oncol 6:24, 1988.
13. Ell K, Nishimoto R, Mantell J, Hamovitch M: Longitudinal analysis of psychological adaptation among family members of patients with cancer. J Psychosom Res 32:429–437, 1988.
14. Ell K, Nishimoto R, Mantell J, Hamovitch M: Psychological adaptation to cancer: A comparison among patients, spouses and nonspouses. Fam Systems Med 6:335–346, 1988.
15. Fogarty TF: Chronic and life threatening illness. Family 13(2):23, 1986.
16. Futterman E, Hoffman I: Crisis and adaptation in the families of fatally ill children. *In* Anthony EJ, Koupernik C (eds): The Child in His Family: The Impact of Disease and Death (Yearbook of the International Association for Child Psychiatry and Allied Profession, Vol 2). New York, John Wiley & Sons, 1973.
17. Germain C, Gitterman A: The Life Model of Social Work Practice. New York, Columbia University Press, 1980.
18. Gitterman A: Development of group services. *In* Social Work with Groups in Maternal and Child Health. Conference proceedings, June 14 and 15, 1979. New York, Columbia University Press, 1979.
19. Goldberg RJ, Tull RM: The Psychosocial Dimensions of Cancer: A Practical Guide for Health Care Providers. New York, Free Press, 1983.
20. Green M, Solnit AJ: Reactions to the threatened loss of a child. Pediatrics 34:58–66, 1964.
21. Hinds C: The needs of families who care for patients at home: Are we meeting them? J Adv Nurs 10(6):575–581, 1985.
22. Kane R, Klein S, Bernstein L, Rothenberg R, Wales J: Hospice role in alleviating the emotional stress of terminal patients and their families. Med Care 23(3):189–197, 1985.
23. Kaplan D: Intervention strategies for families. *In* Cohen J, Cullen J, Martin LT (eds): Psychosocial Aspects of Cancer. New York, Raven Press, 1982, pp 221–233.
24. Kaplan DM, Smith A, Grobstein R, Fishman S: Family mediation of stress. Soc Work 18:60–69, 1973.
25. Katz E, Kellerman J, Rigler D, Williams K, Siegel S: School intervention with pediatric cancer patients. J Pediatr Psychol 2:72–77, 1977.
26. Koocher G: Coping with survivorship in childhood cancer: Family problems. *In* Christ A, Flomenhaft K (eds): Childhood Cancer: Impact on the Family. New York, Plenum Publishing, 1984.
27. Koocher GP: Psychosocial issues during the acute treatment of pediatric cancer. Cancer 58:468–472, 1986.
28. Koocher G, O'Malley J: The Damocles Syndrome: Psychological Consequences of Surviving Childhood Cancer. New York, McGraw-Hill, 1981.
29. Lansky S, Cairns N, Hassamien R, Wehr J, Lowman J: Childhood cancer: Parental discord and divorce. Pediatrics 62:184–188, 1978.
30. Lansky SB, Cairns NU, Lansky LL: Central nervous system prophylaxis: Studies showing impairment in verbal skills and academic achievement. Am J Pediatr Hematol Oncol 6(2):183–190, 1984.
31. Lazarus RS: Stress and coping as factors in health and illness. *In* Cohen J, Cullen JW, Martin LR (eds): Psychosocial Aspects of Cancer. New York, Raven Press, 1982, pp 163–190.
32. Martin RL: Overview of the psychosocial aspects of cancer. *In* Cohen J, Cullen JW, Martin LR (eds): Psychosocial Aspects of Cancer. New York, Raven Press, 1982, pp 1–8.
33. Miller R: Legislation and health policies. *In* Miller RS, Rehr H (eds): Social Work Issues in Health Care. Englewood Cliffs, NJ, Prentice-Hall, 1983, pp 74–120.
34. Monaco GP: Resources available to the family of the child with cancer. Cancer 58:516–521, 1986.
35. Northen H: Social work groups in health settings: Promises and problems. *In* Rosenberg G, Rehr H (eds): Advancing Social Work Practice in the Health Care Field: Emerging Issues and New Perspectives. New York, Haworth Press, 1983, pp 107–121.

36. Orr D, Hoffman M, Bennett G: Adolescents with cancer report their psychosocial needs. J Psychosoc Oncol 2(2):53, 1984.
37. Pferfferbaum B, Levenson PM: Adolescent cancer patient and physician responses to a questionnaire on patient concerns. Am J Psychiatry 139:348–351, 1982.
38. Rosenberg G: Practice roles and functions of the health social worker. *In* Miller RS, Rehr H (eds): Social Work Issues in Health Care. Englewood Cliffs, NJ, Prentice-Hall, 1983, pp 121–180.
39. Ross J: Social work intervention with families of children with cancer. Soc Work Health Care 3(3):257–282, 1978.
40. Spinetta J: The sibling of the child with cancer. *In* Spinetta J, Deasy-Spinetta P (eds): Living with Childhood Cancer. St Louis, CV Mosby, 1981.
41. Spinetta J, Deasy-Spinetta P: The patient's socialization in the community and school during therapy. Cancer 58(2 Suppl):512–515, 1986.
42. Strain J, Grossman S: Psychological Care of the Medically Ill: A Primer in Liaison Psychiatry. New York, Appleton-Century-Crofts, 1975.
43. Tarvormina J, Kastner L, Slater P, Watt S: Chronically ill children: A psychologically and emotionally deviant population? J Abnorm Child Psychol 4(2):99–110, 1976.
44. Teta MJ, Delpo M, Kasl S, Meigs JW, Meyers MH, Mulvihill J: Psychosocial consequences of pediatric cancer survival. Presented to Meeting of the Society for Epidemiologic Research, Houston, 1984.
45. Teta MJ, Delpo MC, Kasl SV, Meigs JW, Meyers MH, Mulvihill J: Psychosocial consequences of childhood and adolescent cancer survival. J Chronic Dis 39(9):751–759, 1986.
46. Vernick J: Meaningful communication with the fatally ill child. *In* Anthony EJ, Koupernik C (eds): The Child in His Family: The Impact of Disease and Death (Yearbook of the International Association for Child Psychiatry and Allied Profession, Vol 2). New York, John Wiley & Sons, 1973.
47. Wasserman AL, Thompson EI, Wilimas JA, Fairclough DL: The psychological status of survivors of childhood adolescent Hodgkin's disease. Am J Dis Child 141:627, 1987.
48. Yoak M, Chesney BK, Schwartz NH: Active Roles in Self-help Groups for Parents of Children with Cancer. Ann Arbor, University of Michigan Center for Research on Social Organization, 1983.

Suggested Readings

American Cancer Society: Cancer Facts and Figures. New York, American Cancer Society, 1984.

American Cancer Society: Cancer Facts and Figures. New York, American Cancer Society, 1985.

Aries P: The Hour of Our Death. New York, Random House, 1982.

Ashenburg NJ: Employability and insurability of the cancer patient. Paper presented at the New York State Cancer Programs Association, Inc., Rochester, NY, November 8, 1975.

Berkman BG: Innovations for social services in health care. *In* Sobey F (ed): Changing Roles in Social Work Practice. Philadelphia, Temple University Press, 1977, pp 92–126.

Berkman B, Rehr H, Rosenberg G: A social work department creates and tests a screening mechanism to identify high social risk. Soc Work Health Care 5(4):373–385, 1980.

Berkman B, Rehr H: Unanticipated consequences of the case finding system in hospital social service. Soc Work 15(2), 1970.

Black J: Practical problems: The cost of cancer. *In* Proceedings of the First National Conference for Parents of Children with Cancer: Maintaining a Normal Life. Bethesda, National Cancer Institute, 1980.

Bracht N: Health care: Issues and trends. *In* Bracht N (ed): Social Work in Health Care: A Guide to Professional Practice. New York, Haworth Press, 1978.

Caplan G: The family as a support system. *In* Caplan G, Killie M (eds): Support Systems and Mutual Help. New York, Grune & Stratton, 1976, pp 19–36.

Carpenter PT, Onufrak B: Pediatric psychiatric psychosocial oncology: A compendium of the current professional literature. J Psychosoc Oncol 2:119–136, 1984.

Cassileth B, Donovan J: Hospice: History and implications of new legislation. J Psychosoc Oncol 1:59–69, 1983.

Chesler M, Anderson B: Chronically Ill Adolescents as Health Care Consumers. Ann Arbor, MI, CRSO Working Paper 329, 1985.

Cobb S: Social support as a moderator of life stress. Psychosom Med 38:300–314, 1976.

Cohen M: Psychosocial morbidity in cancer: A clinical perspective in psychosocial aspects of cancer. *In* Cohen J, Cullen JW, Martin LR (eds): Psychosocial Aspects of Cancer. New York, Raven Press, 1982, pp 117–128.

Cohen J, Cullen JW, Martin LR: Psychosocial Aspects of Cancer. New York, Raven Press, 1982.

Cousins N: Anatomy of an Illness. New York, WW Norton, 1979.

Doremus B: The four Rs: Social diagnosis in health care. Health Soc Work 1:120–139, 1976.

Epstein L: Helping People with a Task-Centered Approach. St Louis, CV Mosby, 1980.

Erikson E: Identity, Youth, and Crisis. New York, WW Norton, 1968.

Fisher J: Effective Case Work Practice: An Eclectic Approach. New York, McGraw-Hill, 1978.

Fisher W: Hospice care of the dying and their families. *In* Lorenz K, Bonica J (eds): Pain, Discomfort and Humanitarian Care. New York, Elsevier North-Holland, 1980, pp 329–338.

Germain CB: Social Work Practice in Health Care: An Ecological Perspective. New York, Free Press, 1984.

Golan N: Treatment in Crisis Situations. New York, Free Press, 1978.

Gordon WE, Schutz ML: A natural basis for social work specializations. Soc Work 22(5):422–426, 1977.

Gottlieb F: Family force fields in health field. *In* Jacobson RC, Marton J (eds): Family Health Care: Health Promotion and Illness Care. Berkeley, University of California Press, 1976.

Harvey RF, Hollis MJ, Habeck RV: Cancer rehabilitation: An analysis of 36 program approaches. JAMA 242:2127–2131, 1982.

Hickey SS: Enabling hope. Cancer Nurs 9(3):133–137, 1986.

Hoffman AD, Becker RD: Psychotherapeutic approaches to the physically ill adolescent. Int J Child Psychother 2:492, 1973.

Kane R: The interpersonal team as a small group. Soc Work Health Care 1(1), 1975.

Kaplan D: Intervention strategies for families. *In* Cohen J, Cullen JW, Martin LR (eds): Psychosocial Aspects of Cancer. New York, Raven Press, 1982, pp 221–233.

Kirten D, Liverman M: Special educational needs of the child with cancer. J School Health 47(3):170–173, 1977.

Klein SA: Hospice care. *In* Higby DJ (ed): Issues in Supportive Care of Cancer Patients. Boston, Martinus Nijhoff Publishing, 1986, pp 173–188.

Kolodny RL: The handicapped child and his peer group: Strategy for integration. *In* Bernstein S, Daniels R, Frey LA, Garland JA, Kolodny RL, Lowy L, Paradise R (eds): Further Explorations in Group Work. Boston, Milford House, 1973.

Kremer RF: Living with childhood cancer: Healthy siblings perspective. Iss Comp Pediatr Nurs 151–181, 1981.

Kubler-Ross E: On Death and Dying. New York, Macmillan, 1969.

Kumabe K, Nishida C, O'Hara D, Woodruff C: A Handbook for Social Work Education and Practice in Community Health Settings. University of Hawaii School of Social Work, 1977.

Lansky SB, List MA, Ritter-Sterr C: Psychosocial consequences of cure. Cancer, 58(2 Suppl):529–533, 1986.

Lazarus RS, Launier R: Stress-related transactions between person and environment. *In* Pervin L, Lewis M (eds): Perspective in Interactional Psychology. New York, Plenum Press, 1978, pp 287–327.

Levy M: Behavior and Cancer: Life-style and Psychosocial Factors in the Initiation and Progression of Cancer. San Francisco, Jossey-Bass Publishers, 1985.

Letton A: The person with cancer is in the community. *In* Proceedings of the American Cancer Society. Second National Conference on Human Values and Cancer, 1977, pp 186–187.

Litman T: Family as a basic unit in health and medical care: A social behavioral overview. Soc Sci Med 8:495–519, 1974.

Lonergan EC: Humanizing the hospital experience: Report on a group program for medical patients. Health Soc Work 5(4):53–64, 1980.

McKenna RJ: Employability and Insurability of the Cancer patient. Paper presented at National Rehabilitation Conference, New York, 1974.

Mervis P: Commentary. *In* Rosenberg G, Rehr H (eds): Advancing Social Work Practice in the Health Care Field: Emerging Issues and New Perspectives. New York, Haworth Press, 1983, pp 124–128.

Miller RS, Rehr H: Health settings and health providers. *In* Miller RS, Rehr H (eds): Social Work Issues in Health Care. Englewood Cliffs, NJ, Prentice-Hall, 1983, pp 1–19.

Parry JK, Young AK: The family as a system in hospital-based social work. Health Soc Work 3(2):55–64, 1978.

Pendleton E: Too Old to Cry . . . Too Young to Die. Nashville, TN, Thomas Nelson, 1980.

Pilsecter C: Help for the dying. Soc Work 20(3):190–194, 1975.

Regensburg J: Toward education for health professions. New York, Harper & Row, 1978.

Rotman M, Rocow L, Delcon G, Heskel N: Supportive therapy in radiation oncology. Cancer 39:744–750, 1977.

Sourkes B: Siblings of the pediatric cancer patient. *In* Kellerman J (ed): Psychological Aspects of Childhood Cancer. Springfield, IL, Charles C Thomas, 1980.

Suchman EA: Stages of illness and medical care. J Health Hum Behav 6:114–128, 1965.

Van-Dongen-Melman JE, Sanders-Wouldstra JA: Psychosocial aspects of childhood cancer: A review of the literature. J Child Psychol Psychiatry 27(2):145–180, 1986.

Wellisch DJ, Jamison KR, Pasnau RO: Psychosocial aspects of mastectomy: The man's perspective. Am J Psychiatry 135:543–546, 1978.

CHAPTER 26

Nursing Considerations

DONNA M. RYNIKER
LORI STEIN FREUDMAN
DONNA M. WEINER
CARLENE CORD
HOPE A. CASTORIA
KATHRYN McLEAN

To facilitate delivery of quality nursing care to patients with high-grade malignant musculoskeletal tumors, the nurse must understand surgery, chemotherapy, and radiotherapy. The nurse's clinical knowledge should also include basic principles of the cancer disease process, the developmental process of the patient and the family, the treatment plan, the management of treatment side effects, discharge planning, and long-term follow-up. The nurse's role is instrumental in assisting the patient and the family to participate in care.

Methods in Tumor Treatment

SURGERY

Surgery is the primary and oldest treatment modality for malignant musculoskeletal tumors. Surgical excision of the tumor attempts to eradicate local disease at the primary site.[3, 49a] The early resection of a malignant tumor can reduce the risk of metastatic disease. The clinical decision about how and when to perform surgery for the malignant tumor determines the nurses' focus of care. Nursing care will include perioperative management of the patient receiving a combination of treatment modalities.

Preoperative Care

The goal of preoperative nursing care is to prepare the patient physically and psychologically for surgery and postoperative care. Preoperative preparation should include information about surgery, routine preoperative measures, anticipated postoperative care, including progression of activity level, and anticipated body image changes. The patient should be instructed in effective coughing and deep-breathing exercises, active joint range of motion exercises, and turning and positioning techniques. Turning and positioning techniques are influenced by the type of resection and the anatomic site of surgery. There must be close collaboration with the physician to clarify activity orders and to minimize immobility complications. The individualization of preoperative preparation should focus on the developmental stage of the patient and the family.

Perioperative Care

During the perioperative phase of treatment, the nurse is responsible for helping to manage the side effects of adjuvant treatments that may affect the surgical outcome and the patient's health. The nursing history and the physical examination should include an assessment of the patient's behavioral responses to cancer treatment. The assessment should include the specific adjuvant treatment received by the patient for musculoskeletal tumor management and the date of the last treatment. Preoperative chemotherapy and radiotherapy can affect the patient's physiologic response to surgery and should be scheduled 2 to 4 weeks before surgery to minimize immunosuppression and wound-healing complications.[10, 49a] A nurse should screen the following laboratory values for surgical risk factors:

1. Platelet count less than 80,000 per mm^3 indicates an alteration in physiologic hemostasis or the body's ability to control bleeding.
2. An absolute neutrophil count (ANC) less than 1000 per mm^3 is risk factor for infection.
3. Hemoglobin level less than 8.0 per g and hematocrit level less than 25 are risk factors for inadequate circulatory volume perfusion and inadequate oxygen exchange in tissues. This can precipitate hemodynamic shock and poor wound healing.
4. Serum albumin level less than 3.5 g per dL accompanied by 10% loss of body weight is a risk factor for malnutrition and potential wound-healing problems.[24, 29, 42, 45, 49a]

The nurses' paramount role during the perioperative phase of treatment is to stress the importance of surgery as a life-saving measure. The ability of the nurse to participate in this role evolves from a basic understanding of the surgical options and procedures in management of malignant musculoskeletal tumors (Table 26–1). Determination of the surgical procedure reflects the patient's age, the histologic diagnosis, associated tumor behavior, the anatomic location of the tumor, the results of staging work-up, functional goals, and patient's viewpoints in the decision-making process.[12, 24, 29, 47, 51]

TABLE 26–1

Surgical Options for Malignant Musculoskeletal Tumors

Surgical options for management of malignant musculoskeletal tumor are amputation or limb-sparing procedure. Amputation refers to excision of tumor without surgical reconstruction of anatomic site. Limb-sparing procedure refers to excision of tumor with surgical reconstructive modalities (e.g., prosthetic implant, autograft, allograft).

Surgical options can be classified according to tumor margin. Four primary procedures are

1. *Intralesional debulking,* or excision of a portion of tumor, is usually indicated in benign lesions or aggressive lesions (e.g., giant cell tumor).
2. *Marginal excision,* or shelling out of tumor with its pseudocapsule intact, is clinically indicated for benign tumor, such as lipoma. It can be called *en bloc* excision.
3. *Wide local excision* is *en bloc* excision of tumor with normal surrounding soft tissue to ensure clear surgical margins. It is clinically indicated for high-grade malignant tumors, such as osteosarcoma or Ewing's sarcoma.
4. *Radical local resection* is *en bloc* excision of tumor, including entire anatomic compartment from origin to insertion. It is also clinically indicated for high-grade malignant tumors.

Data from references 13, 16, 29, 34, 35, and 36.

SURGICAL PROCEDURES

Until the 1970s, amputation was the accepted surgical procedure for patients with malignant musculoskeletal tumors of the extremities. Limb-sparing procedure is now a surgical option as a result of advances in adjuvant treatment modalities, bioengineering designs of internal prosthetic devices, radiographic workups, and surgical techniques including tissue transfers.[12, 24, 29, 47, 51] A limb-sparing procedure involves removal of involved tissues and maintenance of vital structures (i.e., neurovascular). The goal of the limb-sparing procedure is to maintain skeletal continuity and functional use of the preserved limb. The functional expectations for the preserved limb include the ability to bear full weight in the lower extremity and use of the hand and the elbow in the upper extremity.[16, 29, 43]

High-grade malignant musculoskeletal tumors include primary bone neoplasms and soft tissue sarcomas. The surgical treatment of choice for soft tissue sarcomas is an *en bloc* resection with a surrounding cuff of normal soft tissue to prevent local recurrence and/or distant metastatic spread.[30] However, these tissues are most difficult to surgically manage because of the unpredictability of the tumor behavior. The soft tissue tumors do not have a true capsule for margin control and spread by direct local microscopic extension. Variables that affect the surgical resection include involvement of bone, lymph nodes, subcutaneous tissue, and skin.[12, 30] A wide resection of a soft tissue sarcoma could include a bone replacement, but not all soft tissue tumors involve bone.

The surgical reconstruction options in a limb-sparing procedure for primary bone neoplasms and/or soft tissue sarcomas include a resection arthrodesis, graft reconstruction (e.g., allografts and autografts), prosthetic implants, and any combination thereof (e.g., allograft and prosthesis). The surgical reconstruction method can be at the articulating surfaces or intercalary. A resection arthodesis is the resection of tumor with fusion of the joint. An allograft is a tissue transfer performed by surgically grafting cadaver bone to the host bone. An autograft is a tissue transfer performed by surgically grafting an expendable bone into a new anatomic position in the same individual (e.g., free vascularized fibula graft). The grafting of a bone is to preserve the length and function of an extremity. Stability of the graft for structure remodeling can be surgically managed by internal fixation devices or artificial ankylosis of the joint. Postoperatively, the extremity is immobilized to promote further structure remodeling and revascularization.[38, 44, 46, 47] Some surgeons prefer graft reconstruction for benign and low-grade malignant tumors. Prosthetic implants can be an alternative reconstructive choice for high-grade malignant tumors that are sensitive to chemotherapy and/or radiotherapy because there can be impaired graft bone healing at the surgical site[44, 46] with adjuvant treatment.

Tumors of the upper extremity involving the glenohumeral joint can be treated by a surgical procedure called the Tikhoff-Lindberg. This procedure involves a wide resection of the tumor with surgical reconstruction by a custom-made prosthetic implant, an allograft, an autograft, or any combination of these. The replacement for the proximal humerus stabilizes the elbow to maintain elbow-hand function. There is loss of active shoulder girdle mobility. Modification of this procedure can be done with varying degrees of functional loss determined by the anatomic location of the tumor in the shoulder girdle and soft tissue involvement. Smaller tumors of the proximal humerus can be resected alone or replaced with a metallic spacer or allograft.[12, 29] These surgical procedures can be an alternative to a forequarter amputation. A forequarter amputation is the resection of the glenohumeral joint, clavicle, scapula, and humerus without surgical reconstruction.

Tumors of the lower extremity involving the hip joint can be treated by a wide resection and surgical reconstruction with custom-made prosthesis that acts as a spacer for the proximal femur. The procedure is called a proximal femur replacement and can be an alternative to a hip disarticulation or the amputation of the limb through the hip joint. There is risk of femoral head dislocation postoperatively and the patient must be clinically managed similarly to an individual with a hip replacement to minimize this risk[36] (Table 26–2).

Tumors of the distal femur or the proximal tibia can be treated surgically by a wide resection and surgical reconstruction by a custom-made prosthesis and/or allograft. This can be an alternative to an above-knee amputation. Sometimes, there is loss of the patellar tendon function, which affects the lower extremity extensor mechanism during ambulation.[31, 51]

Tumors in the femur, the tibia, and the humerus of the growing child can be surgically managed with an internal expandable, adjustable prosthesis. This custom-made prosthesis can be lengthened to keep pace with the child's normal growth. The prosthetic adjustment is a small surgical procedure that expands this telescopic prosthesis 1 to 2 cm per surgical attempt until skeletal maturity is completed.[34, 35]

The surgical treatment of high-grade malignant musculoskeletal tumors during a limb-sparing procedure involves resection of the tumor, reconstruction of the surgical defect, and provision of adequate soft tissue coverage. The decision to initiate chemotherapy before a limb-sparing procedure is an attempt to re-

TABLE 26–2

Precautions After Total or Proximal Femur Replacement

Hip dislocation can be a complication after a total or proximal femur replacement. This type of dislocation can occur if the patient flexes the hip greater than 90 degrees or adducts the thigh. The following instructions to the patient minimize this risk:

Do not cross legs.
Do not sit in bucket seats of car.
Do not bend over or stoop to pick up things; ask for assistance or use a floor-grabbing device.
Do not lean forward to stand; slide to edge of chair and rise straight up, using armrest or crutch to help.
Do not sit on regular toilets; use an over-toilet commode or raised toilet seat.
Do not lie without pillow between the legs. Use at least one regular pillow between the knees when reclining on the back or stomach. Use at least two regular bed pillows between the knees when sleeping on the side.

duce soft tissue mass for better surgical margins and a smaller surgical defect, to allow preparation time for designing a custom-made reconstructive internal prosthesis, and to treat suspected micrometastasis.[24, 29, 47, 49a]

An extensive surgical defect can be a problem with large tumors near the knee joint. Skin coverage over the reconstructive implant must be adequate to act as a barrier against infection and to maximize functional capabilities. These extensive surgical defects can be closed by a muscle flap. The most common flaps used for this type of reconstructive surgery are the local transposition flap and the myocutaneous free flap. A local transposition flap is the rotation of muscle over the surgical defect (e.g., the gastrocnemius muscle flap). A myocutaneous free flap is the surgical transfer of muscle with attached skin from the donor site to the surgical defect (e.g., the latissimus dorsi muscle flap).[2, 41]

Postoperative Care

The goal of postoperative nursing care is to promote an optimal level of functioning by monitoring the patient's behavioral responses to the surgical outcome. Immediate physical care after a limb-sparing procedure or amputation consists of frequent monitoring of vital signs, measuring intake and output, positioning the operative extremity, and checking neurovascular circulation distal to and/or including the operative site. Postoperative monitoring of fluid and electrolyte patterns include administering replacement fluids, checking hemoglobin and hematocrit levels to measure hypovolemia, and accurately recording the color and amount of drainage to various collecting systems (e.g., Foley, Hemovac, and Jackson-Pratt drains). Recovery from the anesthesia and selected physiologic responses to surgery should be further managed on an individual basis, with special considerations given to the child and the elderly patient.

WOUND MANAGEMENT

Wound management after a reconstructive limb-sparing procedure with a flap involves measures to assess flap viability. Vascular occlusion resulting from thrombosis is the most common cause of flap failure.[18, 19] Prophylactically, patients are encouraged to minimize caffeine intake and to avoid nicotine for several months perioperatively to decrease the risk of a vascular spasm and subsequent clotting in the flap.

Flap assessment for viability includes monitoring color, capillary refill, and temperature. Temperature is the most objective assessment of flap circulation. A digital telethermometer can monitor temperature changes if one probe is attached to the flap and the second to the patient's skin distal to the flap. A difference of 2 degrees from the baseline value may indicate a vascular problem (such as interruption in the blood flow), causing heat loss and decreased flap temperature.[2, 19] These baseline norms will vary among patients. Early recognition of a postoperative complication is vital to the survival of the flap. The temperature assessment is most critical for free vascularized grafts. This graft is subcutaneous and is not visible for direct assessment of arterial and venous circulatory flow to the graft site.[20, 54]

The nurse must monitor normal body temperature and assess for deviation from the baseline norm. Loss of body temperature can cause vasoconstriction and shunting of blood to vital organs, bypassing the anastomosis site. The patient must be kept warm to promote adequate microvascular circulatory perfusion. The nurse must also initiate conservative measures to maintain the patient's anxiety at a functional level. High anxiety and pain can induce vascular spasms, causing a thrombosis at the surgical site and flap failure.

Assessments of capillary refill and color are subjective, and baseline norms must be established to minimize error in judgment. Capillary refill is assessed by pressing a finger firmly into the flap and releasing it quickly. Normal blanching occurs within 1 to 2 seconds. If the capillary refill is slow (greater than 2 seconds), arterial occlusion is suspected. If the capillary refill is rapid (less than 2 seconds), venous occlusion is suspected.[2, 30]

The color of the flap is assessed to monitor adequate arterial perfusion and adequate venous drainage from the blood vessels of the flap to the vessels in the recipient site. The color of the flap should be pink. Pale to white may indicate arterial occulsion. Cyanotic blue to purple may indicate venous occlusion.[2, 30]

All assessments should be recorded on a flowsheet every 30 minutes for the first 12 hours and hourly for the next 48 hours. The first 48 hours are most critical for flap viability, as the flap depends totally on the anastomosis of the microvessels. The anastomoses can be with blood vessels as small as 2 to 3 mm in diameter.

The postoperative neurovascular assessment of the flap is not painful because of the absence of nerve innervation to the flap. However, the donor site is painful, and analgesics should be administered every 2 to 4 hours round the clock for the first 24 to 48 hours and then as needed. The use of the patient-controlled analgesia pump or an epidural catheter can also be an effective means of postoperative pain management. As the pain decreases and the patient's activity level increases, the continuous infusion will be tapered and then discontinued. After the infusion stops, the patient may continue to experience pain. The nurse must assess the patient's pain level and medicate as necessary to promote the patient's activity. When the patient does get out of bed to a chair, the operative leg must be elevated. With ambulation, the patient's leg should be wrapped with an Ace bandage. These conservative measures are to prevent swelling and to promote venous drainage from the lower extremity.

Nursing measures to promote normal wound healing are vital to the patient's recovery. If a flap is not indicated for wound closure, healing at the incision line is by primary intention. This incision is a clean, straight line where the edges are closely approximated by sutures or staples.[45] The destruction of muscle tissue always results in scar formation. The presence of a scar is a concern to all patients, especially the adolescent. It may alleviate some of the patient's concern if the nurse gives information about surgical options for a scar revision. In many instances, a scar revision can be done after all treatment is completed.

Wound healing requires oxygen, nutrients, and adequate circulation. Factors that influence this process include the patient's age, nutritional status, circulatory status, and endocrine function; infection; fluid accumulation in dead space; and the patient's specific responses to the physiologic stressors of cancer treatment.

Dead space occurs after resection of bone and/or soft tissue, creating an empty cavity that can fill with fluid. The accumulation of excessive fluid can cause pain, dehiscence, infection, and scar tissue.[45] Postsurgical management, therefore, includes the use of low-pressure suction or drains to remove excessive fluid so healing is not delayed. The nurse is responsible for maintaining patent drainage tubes to decompress pressure build-up at the incision line and decrease risk of leakage around the tubes. The nurse should turn and position the patient so the patient is not lying on drains to prevent circulatory compromise due to tubing pressure and occlusion of the drain.[45]

The wound is covered with a dressing to prevent physical trauma, to minimize the chance of infection, and to prevent an adverse emotional reaction from the patient. The surgeon changes the dressing initially, and the nurse follows up as clinically indicated. If the wound is draining copious amounts of fluid, the physician must be notified. The dressing should be changed as often as necessary to prevent skin maceration and infection.[45] The nurse must document the color and odor of drainage and the frequency of dressing changes in the chart. Open wound dressing changes should be carried out under sterile conditions. Wound sloughing is not an uncommon complication after resection of a soft tissue sarcoma.[49a]

A potential complication that interferes with all wound healing is an infection at the surgical site. Wound infections are a primary concern for patients who receive adjuvant treatment after surgery. Chemotherapy and radiotherapy can cause poor wound healing. Chemotherapy interferes with the basic metabolic processes in cell replication, heightening the risk for neutropenia. Neutropenia is the most important factor associated with infection in the immunocompromised patient.[3, 49a] Radiotherapy causes tissue hypoxia associated with scarring and fibrosis.[10, 49a] Characteristic signs of an infection include pain in the incision area, fever after the third postoperative day, erythema, swelling, and purulent drainage. Patients experiencing neutropenia may be unable to localize pus. The nurse should suspect an infection with fever and neutropenia without the presence of purulent drainage.

The nursing assessment after surgical resection of a musculoskeletal tumor includes a heightened index of suspicion for a deep venous thrombosis (DVT). A DVT is a venous blood clot that develops from venous stasis after surgical trauma and from blood hypercoagulability, especially in the presence of a malignant tumor.[8, 21] A DVT is a clinical problem because it can be a precursor to a pulmonary embolus. A pulmonary embolus is the lodging of a venous clot in pulmonary circulation, causing sudden thoracic sharp pain and/or dyspnea. It is an important cause of postoperative mortality and is responsible for approximately 5% of postoperative deaths.[8] The elderly are at the greatest risk for a DVT.

Prophylactic measures (pharmacologic or physical) can help to reduce the incidence of

DVT. Pharmacologic measures are aimed at preventing harmful blood changes. The drugs of choice after orthopedic oncology surgery may include warfarin (Coumadin) and dextran. The nurse is involved in monitoring the blood testing for clinical response to the drugs. This assessment includes monitoring for signs of prolonged and/or increased bleeding and for an adverse reaction to the selected drug.[45]

Physical measures are aimed at assisting natural venous flow. These measures include passive leg exercises, early ambulation, use of elastic compression stockings, and active massage of the legs.[8, 21] Pain, swelling, and local tenderness in the calf are the most reliable clinical indicators of DVT in that location. Pulmonary emboli are the most common complications of a DVT in the lower extremities.[8, 21]

PAIN MANAGEMENT AND REHABILITATION

Acute postoperative pain is common after a limb-sparing procedure. It has been described as intense and sharp discomfort localized at the operative extremity, not specific to the flap. It is a most intense experience for patients with a lower extremity limb-sparing procedure. The pain usually subsides with healing and a decrease in swelling at the operative site. The most painful sensations are of limited duration, approximately 4 or 5 postoperative days. An amputation can cause acute or chronic pain. The pain after an amputation has been described as a continuous or intermittent feeling of cramping, crushing, burning, or shooting pain localized in the phantom limb, not the stump. It is called phantom pain.[6, 9] This sensation can occur immediately after surgery or have late onset. The nurse assesses the patient in pain, then schedules and administers medication in relation to the patient's needs and activities.

Special consideration should be given to the patient who must live with chronic pain. This type of pain can occur after a limb-sparing procedure or an amputation. Chronic pain from a nonmalignant cause can be a devastating, destructive experience. It has been defined as pain that is ongoing on a daily basis and is due to a non–life-threatening cause that has not responded to current available treatment methods and may continue indefinitely.[40] The patient with this type of pain could benefit from a comprehensive pain management program when the pain becomes the central feature of the individual's life. Nurses can be the primary source of referral or an integral part of the pain program in which pharmacologic modalities are used in combination with more conservative measures, including distraction, imagery, relaxation, and cutaneous stimulation.

A patient who has had a limb-sparing procedure or an amputation can experience sensory perception changes. Most common after an amputation is the sensation that the amputated limb is intact. This may diminish with time.[6, 39, 49]

Loss of nerve function during a limb-sparing procedure affects sensory and/or motor function. The anterior thigh includes structures of the quadriceps muscles and the femoral artery, vein, and nerve. Radical and wide resection of these anatomic structures affects active knee extension and decreases sensation to the anterior thigh, the knee, and the lower extremity.[16] Resection of the tibial vessels and nerves diminishes sensation to and function of the plantar surface of the foot.[16] Nurses have to instruct the patients regarding special skin care and mobility techniques. Counseling regarding the normalization of these sensations and function enables patients and their families to explore new techniques in sensitivity management. This is most helpful for patients who experience hypersensitivity at trigger points along the operative site.

In the acute postoperative period and throughout the rehabilitation process, the nurses' responsibility does include familiarity with patient's functional capabilities after a limb-sparing procedure or an amputation. The rehabilitation process assists the patient and the family to develop new independent behaviors in their environment. The possible progression of the malignant disease, additional underlying physiologic problems, side effects of adjuvant treatment modalities, and the patient's psychologic attitude affect the ongoing participation in the process of rehabilitation.

The patient's behavioral response may be impaired by weakness and fatigue from chemotherapy. The nurse should monitor hematocrit and hemoglobin levels as baseline data to develop a plan of care to increase the patient's activity level and conserve energy. The plan should include organization of activities to promote rest periods, instructions in energy-saving techniques (e.g., using a shower seat and sitting to brush one's teeth or comb one's hair), and reinforcement of the physical therapist's or the occupational therapist's instructions in exercise, transfer techniques, and ambulation strategies. The nurse should monitor the platelet count. Certain chemotherapeutic agents can cause thrombocytopenia. A platelet count less than 20,000 per mm^3 increases the patient's risk of bleeding into the joints.[3, 10, 49a] All participation in an exercise program should be discontinued until the platelet count is greater than 50,000 per mm^3.

A patient with an internal or external lower extremity prosthesis needs to participate in a program that maximizes movement and balance patterns. The exercise program focuses on standing, weight shifting, developing heel-toe balance, rocking, and stair climbing.[6, 14, 39] The strategies vary, depending on the type and location of the surgical resection: amputation or limb-sparing procedure.

Precautions on how to prevent a hip or knee joint contracture are basic components of a rehabilitation program for the patient who has had a limb-sparing procedure or an amputation. A lower extremity amputee should be instructed as follows:

Avoid sitting for long periods.
Avoid placing pillows under the residual limb.
Maintain the residual limb in proper body alignment.
Lie prone three times a day for 30 minutes to promote knee and hip extension.[6, 9, 39, 49]

An individual with a spared lower extremity will initially perform passive knee flexion and extension exercises. The exercises are organized by a physical therapist and can be facilitated by use of an assistive apparatus called a continuous passive motion machine. An individual with a transposition flap can begin passive knee motion exercises approximately 5 to 7 days postoperatively. An individual with a myocutaneous free flap can begin passive knee motion exercises approximately 10 to 14 days postoperatively. The progression to active and active-assistive knee flexion and extension exercises is determined by the recovery process, the patient's motivation, and the nature of the surgical resection.

Loss of nerve and muscle during a limb-sparing procedure does affect active motor function. Loss of the peroneal nerve results in footdrop. An orthosis that slips inside the shoe could be necessary for dorsiflexion of the foot and a smoother gait pattern. Loss of the quadriceps extensor mechanism affects stair climbing, squatting, kneeling, and rising from a chair. Compensatory mechanism are taught by the physical therapist. Loss of knee stability results from the loss of ligaments and tendons at the distal femur–proximal tibia juncture. A brace may be indicated to provide additional stability and support during ambulation.

A patient who undergoes resection of an upper extremity tumor needs to participate in a program that maximizes fine motor coordination. An individual with an internal prosthetic replacement of the humerus needs to be assessed for shoulder girdle function and taught how to maximize hand-elbow capabilities. This patient should be able to type, button a shirt, hold hands, and write. There is variable loss of active motion in the shoulder girdle secondary to the variation in the extent of the surgical resection.[16, 29] Depending on the extent of active loss of shoulder girdle motion upper extremity, an orthosis may be an option for smoother skeletal movement. An individual with a forequarter amputation is fitted with an external prosthetic replacement. New techniques for upper extremity motion after an amputation continue to be explored.

The transition from an acute care setting to ongoing rehabilitation program in the community involves comprehensive discharge planning. The educational component should focus on skin care, safety precautions, and guidelines for participation in an exercise program (Table 26–3). The follow-up component should focus on organization of the appropriate referral agencies (e.g., visiting nurse service, amputee support groups, cancer support groups, and rehabilitation programs) to maintain a supportive environment that facilitates patient compliance after discharge from the hospital. Follow-up care involves the disciplines that provide adjuvant treatment modalities. The nurses who administer adjuvant treatment continue to counsel patients and their families regarding the rehabilitation process. Ongoing nursing care incorporates careful monitoring of side effects that adversely affect the surgical outcome, such as those related to maintenance of skin integrity, participation in an exercise program, and long-term acceptance of the disability, specifically body image.

CHEMOTHERAPY

The treatment of high-grade malignant musculoskeletal tumors necessitates adjuvant chemotherapy. The goal of this therapy is to decrease the size of the primary tumor preoperatively and to prevent the progression of disease. Oncologists research the efficacy of

TABLE 26–3

Home Care Instructions for Patient After Surgery

Skin Care at Surgical Site

Skin care instructions should include measures that prevent skin breakdown and infection. The following promote healing:

1. Wash area with lukewarm water after staples or sutures are removed.
2. Keep area dry and exposed to air when possible.
3. Do not pick or scratch scabs.
4. Do not expose skin to sun. The sun will encourage scarring and may interfere with the effects of chemotherapy and/or radiation therapy. A sunscreen with a skin protection factor of 15 or greater could minimize these effects. All outdoor activities must be cleared by the physician.
5. Apply lubrication to the surgical site to prevent skin from cracking and drying. Possible lubricants are lanolin, cocoa butter, and vitamin E. Keep skin exposed to air 1–2 h after applying lubrication. Do not use products with alcohol or strong astringents.
6. Avoid exposing skin to extremes in temperature, including ice bags, heating pads, sun lamps, and hot water bottles.
7. Examine surgical site every day for signs of infection: redness, swelling, drainage, and warmth.
8. Contact physician if blisters, skin cracks, or excessive moisture appears on the surgical skin site. Radiotherapy and certain chemotherapy drugs can cause skin changes.
9. Report a fever greater than 101.2 F to the primary care physician. (If the patient has had chemotherapy, a fever may be the only sign of an infection.)

Safety Precautions

Safety precautions should focus on measures that promote mobility and independence in activities of daily living and minimize risk of infection. The following guidelines promote safety:

1. Wear shoes with nonskid soles when walking.
2. Clear environmental hazards to prevent a fall. Hazards can include scatter rugs, toys, and sports equipment.
3. Do not wear support devices too tightly (e.g., immobilizer, elastic [Ace] bandages, and slings).
4. Cut nails in a straight manner. Avoid clipping cuticles or nail corners.
5. Inform all physicians and dentists of your bone replacement. This includes for a routine dental cleaning. Antibiotics should be given as protection against infection before and after treatment.

Exercise

An organized exercise program is an excellent way to improve muscle tone, strength, and endurance after surgery. Staying active is invigorating and can be a perfect antidote for any depression or boredom that a patient may experience during treatment. It is an excellent way to reduce tension and stress. The following guidelines promote practical application of how to participate in a program. The physician and/or physical therapist may outline a more individual program.

1. Exercise is safe as long as you are able to maintain a conversation.
2. Start exercising gradually and choose a program consistent with your abilities and daily activities as guided by a physician, registered nurse, or physical therapist.
3. Have someone assist you in doing exercises for your safety and enjoyment.
4. Recognize your limitations. If you get tired or your muscles feel sore, stop and rest.[27, 53]
5. Do not participate in activities that have a "jarring" effect on internal prosthesis. Tennis, basketball, and hockey are not recommended.
6. Do participate in activities that have less of a "jarring" effect on the internal prosthesis. Hiking, swimming, and bicycling are recommended.

therapy through the development of protocols using randomized clinical trials. Clinical trials in cancer research use protocols combining surgery, radiotherapy, and chemotherapeutic drugs in an attempt to overcome tumor cell heterogeneity and drug resistance while minimizing the patient's short- and long-term side effects. Clinical trials require a follow-up period of several years to determine their outcome or cure rate. If the cure rate is better than that with the previous clinical trial, the most recent protocol becomes the standard treatment.

The nursing care involved for the patient undergoing chemotherapy entails a basic understanding of the drug's mechanism of action, safe drug administration, and the management of acute and chronic side effects.

Mechanism of Action

An understanding of the mechanism of action of chemotherapy depends on knowledge of normal cell function and division. Chemotherapeutic agents can destroy cells in several ways, including damage to the cell membrane or damage to the cellular contents (i.e., DNA responsible for cell activity and RNA responsible for protein synthesis). Some chemotherapeutic agents can affect cells during specific times in their cell cycle, whereas other agents can affect cells at any time in the cell cycle.

The cell cycle is divided into five phases: G_0, G_1, S, G_2, and M. Cells in the G_0 phase are in the resting state, and the length of this phase is variable. This includes both cells that lie dormant until activated by physiologic need and other cells that never divide.[3, 31, 32] The G_1 phase refers to cells activated into the cell cycle, and at this time, enzymes needed for DNA synthesis are produced. In the S phase, DNA is duplicated in preparation for cell replication and cells are most vulnerable. Structural damage or disarray in the DNA replication may result in cell death. The G_2 phase is characterized by hypoactivity, at which time RNA and protein synthesis occur. The M phase refers to the actual division into the daughter cells, when the cells return to G_0.[3] Neoplastic cells may divide into several new cells instead of two cells and cellular proliferation may occur without normal mechanisms of control.

The growth of malignancies depends on both the cell cycle and the growth fraction. The growth fraction refers to the ratio of the total into the number of proliferating cells.[55]

Antineoplastic agents are classified as follows:

Non–cycle-specific agents: drugs that affect both resting and proliferating cells, such as cyclophosphamide (Cytoxan), ifosfamide, doxorubicin (Adriamycin), and cisplatin.

Phase-specific agents: drugs that kill cells in a specific phase of the cell cycle, such as methotrexate (S phase), vincristine, etoposide (VP-16-213) (M phase), and bleomycin (G_2 phase).

Cycle-specific agents: drugs that damage cells in the resting and proliferating stage but are most effective with actively dividing cells, such as vincristine, etoposide, and bleomycin.[5]

Antineoplastic drugs may also be classified by their pharmacologic properties as alkylating agents, antimetabolites, antitumor antibiotics, mitotic inhibitors, hormones, plant alkaloids, and miscellaneous agents (Table 26–4).

Administration

When administering chemotherapy, the nurse must be knowledgeable regarding appropriate drug doses, correct route of administration, anticipated side effects, and necessary laboratory values. This baseline information promotes patient safety and quality care.

Safe handling and appropriate disposal of chemotherapeutic agents is necessary for the protection of all people involved with this treatment modality. In most large medical centers, chemotherapeutic agents are mixed in a central location (usually the pharmacy) by trained chemotherapy pharmacists under a biologic safety cabinet. The Occupational Safety and Health Administration (OSHA) and the National Study Commission on Cytotoxic Exposure have issued guidelines and recommendations for handling cytotoxic drugs to ensure safety during administration and handling. These include wearing disposable surgical latex unpowdered gloves, which should be changed regularly or immediately if torn or punctured, and wearing a disposable gown made of a low-permeability fabric with a closed front, long sleeves, and elastic cuffs.[42] Those precautions should also be followed while medical staff handle body secretions, such as blood, vomitus, and excreta from patients who have received antineoplastic drugs within the previous 48 hours. All equipment related to cytotoxic agents is disposed of in a puncture-resistant, leakproof container, which is handled separately from other hospital waste.

The nurse must be skilled in venous access care, including choosing appropriate vessels, monitoring the site during infusions, anticipating the possibility of extravasation and/or hypersensitivity reactions, and understanding the approved procedures for managing emergency situations. An option for patients undergoing chemotherapy is the use of subcutaneous vascular access devices. The most commonly used are the Hickman and Broviac catheters, which exit the body externally, and the implantable Port-a-Cath. These devices enable access for infusing chemotherapy, hydration, transfu-

Text continued on page 494

TABLE 26–4

Antineoplastic Drugs for High-Grade Malignant Musculoskeletal Tumors

Drug	Indication	Dosage*	Side Effects/Toxicity	Nursing Interventions
Alkylating Agents—kill cells by interfering with structure of DNA; non–cell cycle specific				
Cyclophosphamide (Cytoxan, Endoxan, Neosar)	Ewing's sarcoma, osteogenic sarcoma, other soft tissue sarcomas	500–1500 mg/m^2 IV 2–4 wk	Nausea/vomiting may occur in 3–12 h and can last up to 8–10 h.	Administer antiemetic therapy as ordered.
			Bone marrow depression 7–14 d after therapy; recovery within 7–10 d.	Instruct patient about signs and symptoms of pancytopenia and appropriate interventions. Include follow-up blood work in discharge planning.
			Inappropriate secretion of antidiuretic hormone; water intoxication, hyponatremia.	Obtain serum electrolyte values before administration, then q 12 h. Notify physician if hyponatremia develops. Institute seizure precautions. Administer appropriate fluids as ordered. Keep strict intake and output records.
			Alopecia in approximately 30% of patients (within 3 wk) with possible regrowth during treatment. Alopecia is often dose dependent.	Provide psychosocial support for patient. Provide hair loss alternatives: wigs, scarfs, and hats.
			Risk of hemorrhagic cystitis.	Vigorous hydration 3–4 L/d to maintain urine output and decrease risk of hemorrhagic cystitis. Keep strict intake and output records. Maintain urine specific gravity <1.015. For the pediatric patient IV hydration should be 2 to 2.5 times the maintenance rate for 6 h after treatment. Avoid giving drug at night.
			Potentiates the cardiotoxicites of anthracyclines.	Check patients receiving concurrent anthracyclines to ensure normal cardiac function as measured by echocardiogram and gated pool studies.
			Pneumonitis and pulmonary fibrosis have been reported with progressive respiratory insufficiency after high doses for long period of time.	Notify physician of respiratory distress. Institute appropriate measures.
			Amenorrhea and depression of sperm count with sterility may occur.	Educate patient about this potential side effect.
			Nasal stuffiness may occur when given in high doses.	Educate patient about this potential side effect.

Dacarbazine (DTIC-Dome, imidazole carboxamide)	Soft tissue sarcomas	150–250 mg/m² for 5 d IV every 3-4 wk or 800–900 mg/m² IV as a single dose every 3–4 wk	Mild bone marrow depression. May be delayed 2–3 wk.	Instruct patient about signs and symptoms of pancytopenia and measures to prevent and minimize infection and bleeding. Include follow-up blood work in discharge planning.
			Nausea and vomiting.	Administer antiemetics as ordered. When administered for 5 d, vomiting is more severe on the 1st and 2nd d.
			Influenza-like symptoms; malaise, headache, myalgia, sinus congestion.	Instruct patient that influenza-like symptoms may occur after drug administration.
			Patient may experience pain or burning at injection site and along vein.	Most patients experience burning at IV site, despite adequate blood return through IV. Ice packs may help lessen burning.
			Potent irritant, extravasation may cause thrombophlebitis with tissue damage.	Avoid extravasation. If it occurs, stop infusion and notify physician immediately. *Severe pain with infiltration.*
			Miscellaneous: metallic taste, hepatic veno-occlusive disease, photosensitivity, alopecia, facial paresthesias, and urticarial rashes have been reported.	Educate patient about potential side effects as appropriate.
Ifosfamide (Ifex, iphosphamide) (structural analogue of cyclophosphamide)	Advanced osteogenic sarcoma, relapsed Ewing's and soft tissue sarcomas	1.8–2.4 g/m² IV over 1 h for 3–5 d every 3–4 wks or 5 g/m² as single dose every 3–4 wk	Alopecia.	Instruct patient of possibility of hair loss and provide alternatives: wigs, hats, scarfs.
			Renal toxicity; problems usually more severe in patients previously treated with cisplatin.	Check serum creatinine level before administration of drug. Notify physician if not within normal range. Maintain adequate hydration for 6 h before and 12 h after ifosfamide administration, either IV or PO. Keep strict intake and output records. Notify physician if specific gravity >1.015 or if hydration cannot be maintained. Dipstick test all urines for hematuria. Administer mesna as a protection for bladder.
			Nausea and vomiting, usually more severe during first 2 d.	Administer antiemetic therapy as ordered. Assess for effectiveness and notify physician if they do not appear effective. Keep patient away from strong smells or noxious stimuli.
			Bone marrow depression.	Instruct patient about signs and symptoms of pancytopenia and measures to prevent and minimize infection and bleeding. Include follow-up blood work in discharge planning.

Table continued on following page

TABLE 26–4

Antineoplastic Drugs for High-Grade Malignant Musculoskeletal Tumors *Continued*

Drug	Indication	Dosage*	Side Effects/Toxicity	Nursing Interventions
Mesna (Mesnex)	Thiol compound with capacity of inhibiting urotoxicity of both ifosfamide and cyclophosphamide. Nontoxic addition compounds with reactive ifosfamide metabolites in urine of patients and allows regional detoxification in kidneys and urinary tract. This prevents urotoxicity associated with ifosfamide therapy.	Give 480 mg/m^2 IV just before ifosfamide and at 3, 6, 9, and 12 h after dose. Also may be mixed in ifosfamide solution. IV solution, may give orally	At dose of 60–70 mg/kg IV daily for 4 doses, abdominal pain, headache, limb and joint pain, lethargy, diarrhea, and transient hypotension have been reported.	If encountered, report to physician. *Note:* mesna is used as a rescue drug for ifosfamide. Patients should be instructed on the importance of taking all doses on schedule. Patients receiving mesna may test positive for urine ketones.
Cisplatin (CDDP, *cis*-platinum, Platinol)	Ewing's sarcoma, osteogenic sarcoma, soft tissue sarcoma	50–120 mg/m^2 IV 3–4 wk or 15–20 mg/m^2 IV every day for 5 d every 3–4 wk	Severe nausea and vomiting, usually occurring 1 h after administration and lasting 8–12 h.	Administer antiemetic therapy as ordered. Notify physician if ineffective.
			Anaphylatic reactions.	Stop infusion and administer epinephrine, antihistamine, and steroids as ordered. Notify physician.
			Mild bone marrow depression 2–4 wk after treatment.	Instruct patient about signs and symptoms of pancytopenia and measures to prevent and minimize infection and bleeding.
			Hypomagnesemia common, along with decrease in calcium, potassium, and phosphorus levels.	Monitor electrolyte levels. Assess for signs and symptoms of hypomagnesemia, hypocalcemia, hypokalemia, and hypophosphatemia. Administer supplements as ordered. Check if patient is to receive supplements after discharge and provide appropriate instructions.
			Renal toxicity.	May be avoided with adequate hydration, mannitol, furosemide, diuresis, and careful monitoring. Hydration administered to maintain urine output of 100–150 ml/h before administration and approximately 12 h after. A bolus of mannitol is often given during the infusion to maintain diuresis and decrease chances of nephrotoxicity. Damage is irreversible and results from tubular necrosis. Careful assessment of kidney function is essential before dose by checking creatinine clearance and serum blood urea nitrogen and creatinine.

			May cause thrombophlebitis with tissue damage when infiltrated.	Avoid extravasation. Notify physician if occurs.
			Ototoxic. Patients may have tinnitis and high-frequency loss. Effect may be cumulative.	Check audiogram throughout therapy. Instruct patient to notify physician of ringing in the ears or problems with hearing.
			Neurotoxicity. Uncommon, but peripheral neuropathy and seizures have been reported, including loss of taste.	Educate patient about these potential side effects. Institute seizure precautions as appropriate.
Antimetabolites—chemical analogue of an essential metabolite that is falsely substituted along metabolite pathways. Major activity is during the S phase of the cell cycle, so they can be considered cell cycle specific.				
Methotrexate (MTX, Mexate)	Osteogenic sarcomas	High-dose MTX 8–12 g/m^2 IV q 3–4 wk.* *Must be followed by folinic acid rescue.*† See Nursing Interventions.	Mild nausea and vomiting.	Administer antiemetic therapy as ordered. Notify physician if ineffective.
			Moderate bone marrow depression occurs 7–14 d after administration.	Instruct patient about signs and symptoms of pancytopenia and measures to prevent and minimize bleeding and infection.
		Allergic reactions rare; convulsions.	Stop infusion and antihistamines.	Administer epinephrine. Notify physician.
			Stomatitis with ulceration.	Notify physician if stomatitis develops. Do not administer drug until approved by physician. Instruct patient in meticulous oral hygiene and to avoid spicy and acidic foods. Administer topical preparations as ordered. Nystatin may be used to decrease risk of infection.
			Renal toxicity.	Monitor serum blood urea nitrogen and creatinine levels and creatinine clearance before administration of each dose. Notify physician if not within normal range. *Note:* renal impairment delays excretion and increases systemic toxicity. Maintain urine pH >7.0 and high urine output to prevent precipitation of MTX in renal tubules. Administer appropriate IV hydration with sodium bicarbonate. Check pH and specific gravity each void and notify physician if not in acceptable range. Patient must not be discharged until serum is obtained at 48 h after infusion and checked by physician. High MTX level may indicate delayed excretion of MTX and additional IV hydration and leucovorin may be necessary.

Table continued on following page

TABLE 26–4

Antineoplastic Drugs for High-Grade Malignant Musculoskeletal Tumors *Continued*

Drug	Indication	Dosage*	Side Effects/Toxicity	Nursing Interventions
Methotrexate (MTX, Mexate) *Continued*			Hepatic fibrosis occurs; common with long-term use.	Monitor liver function test results before each dose. Dosage may be discontinued if findings are abnormal.
			Pulmonary pneumonitis usually disappears in 1 wk. Interstitial pneumonitis may present more serious picture.	Instruct patient to notify physician of nonproductive cough, shortness of breath, and/or fever.
			Sun sensitivity.	Instruct patient to avoid exposure to sun. Sun blocks recommended.
Antitumor Antibiotics—Heterogeneous group of compounds produced by various bacterial and fungal organisms. They interfere with nuclear acid synthesis and inhibit RNA and DNA synthesis. Most are *not* cell cycle specific.				
Bleomycin (Blenoxane)	Osteogenic sarcoma	10–20 U/m^2 IV 1–2 times/wk (1 mg = 1 U). Total lifetime dose should not exceed 400 U/m^2. Many practitioners are now limiting to 300 U/m^2.	Mild nausea and vomiting.	Administer antiemetics as ordered. Notify physician if ineffective.
			Bone marrow depression is rare but can occur.	Instruct patient about signs and symptoms of pancytopenia and measures to prevent and minimize infection and bleeding.
			Fever and chills. 60% experience febrile reactions (103–105 F), which can occur 4–10 h after administration and may persist for 48 h.	Acetaminophen and antihistamines can decrease severity of febrile reactions. Administer as ordered.
			Anaphylaxis and hypotensive reactions occur rarely.	Stop infusion. Administer epinephrine and antihistamines as ordered. Notify physician at once.
			Stomatitis.	Notify physician if occurs. Administer topical lidocaine as ordered. Instruct patient on meticulous oral hygiene and avoidance of spicy or acidic foods.
			Hyperpigmentation and hyperkeratosis mainly on palms and fingertips.	Instruct patient about potential side effects and to notify physician if they occur.
			Pneumonitis with dyspnea, rales, and infiltrate that may progress to irreversible pulmonary fibrosis. Pulmonary function test results are often abnormal, usually before radiographic changes.	Patient should have routine pulmonary function tests and chest films and should be made aware of symptoms of pneumonitis. Patient should be instructed to notify physician if they occur.

Doxorubicin (Adriamycin)	Ewing's sarcoma, osteogenic sarcoma, soft tissue sarcoma	30–75 mg/m^2 IV every 3–4 wk. May also be given as a continuous infusion.	Nausea and vomiting.	Administer antiemetic therapy as ordered. Notify physician if ineffective.
			Vesicant. Severe soft tissue injury with extravasation, swelling, erythema, tenderness, and hives noted at injection site in absence of extravasation.	Avoid extravasation. Stop infusion immediately if extravasation is suspected and notify physician.
			Bone marrow depression nadir occurring 10–14 d after administration.	Instruct patient about signs and symptoms of pancytopenia and measures to prevent and minimize bleeding and infection.
			Stomatitis.	Notify physician if occurs. Instruct patient to avoid acidic and spicy food. Administer topical lidocaine. Instruct patient on meticulous oral care.
			Alopecia.	Inform patient of possibility of hair loss. Provide alternatives: hats, scarfs, and wigs.
			Arrhythmia.	When given IV push, should be given given slowly to prevent arrhythmias.
			Cardiotoxicity, occurring with high doses. Maximal cumulative doses 550 mg/m^2 (450 mg/m^2 if patient received radiotherapy to chest). Electrocardiographic changes are common but rarely permanent in absence of cardiomyopathy. Increased risk of cardiac toxicity with concomitant cyclophosphamide or previous radiation therapy.	Careful cardiac assessment is necessary. Follow protocol schedule for echocardiogram and cardiac gating testing. Young children and elderly are most susceptible to cardiotoxicity.
			Previously radiated area may experience radiation recall effect, leading to severe erythema. May be aggravated by the sun.	Instruct patient about avoidance of sun exposure and importance of using strong sunscreen.
			Discoloration of urine (red-orange-pink) for 1–48 h after infusion.	Inform patient about this potential side effect.
			Drug is metabolized by liver. In patients with elevated bilirubin levels, the dose must be reduced to avoid excessive toxicity.	Check liver function test results before administration. Notify physician if abnormal.

Table continued on following page

TABLE 26–4

Antineoplastic Drugs for High-Grade Malignant Musculoskeletal Tumors *Continued*

Drug	Indication	Dosage*	Side Effects/Toxicity	Nursing Interventions
Vincristine (Oncovin)	Soft tissue sarcoma, Ewing's sarcoma	1.5–2 mg/m^2 IV weekly to every 3 wk. Maximal dose 2 mg.	Alopecia occurs in 40–50% of cases.	Inform patient about possible hair loss and provide alternatives: wigs, hats, and scarfs.
			Neurotoxicity that can result in paresthesia of hands and feet, loss of deep tendon reflexes, footdrop, ptosis, constipation, and paralytic ileus.	Notify physician of any tingling in hands and feet and difficulty in ambulation. Symptoms may be so severe as to interfere with activities of daily living. Institute prophylactic bowel regimen as ordered by physician. Instruct patient about dietary habits to prevent constipation.
			Potent irritant and vesicant.	Avoid extravasation. Notify physician if infiltration is suspected.
			Jaw pain, metallic taste, hoarseness, and aching joint pains have been noted.	Inform patient of side effects. Administer analgesics as ordered for joint and jaw pain. Inform physician if ineffective.
			Drug is metabolized by liver. In patients with elevated bilirubin levels, the dose must be reduced to avoid excessive toxicity.	Monitor liver function test results before administration and notify physician if abnormal.
Mitotic Inhibitors—derived from the periwinkle plant; cause metaphase arrest and inhibit RNA and protein synthesis. They are cell cycle–specific agents.				
Etoposide (VP-16-213, VePesid)	Soft tissue sarcoma, Ewing's sarcoma, osteogenic sarcoma	50–100 mg/m^2 IV qd for 5 d every 2–4 wk.	Nausea and vomiting.	Administer antiemetic therapy as ordered. Notify physician if ineffective.
		125 mg/m^2 IV 3 times/wk every 4 wk. Drug is unstable in 5% dextrose in water and must be diluted in high-volume saline solution. Drug dilution must be 0.4 mg/ml.	Hypotension.	Severe hypotension with rapid infusion. Infuse over 45 min. Check blood pressure q 15 min during infusion.
			Bronchospasm.	Treat with epinephrine and antihistamines.
			Anaphylaxis.	Stop infusion immediately. Notify physician and administer epinephrine and antihistamines as ordered.
			Bone marrow depression nadir 7–14 d after infusion.	Instruct patient about signs and symptoms of pancytopenia and measures to prevent or minimize infection and bleeding.
			Alopecia.	Instruct patient about possibility of hair loss and provide alternatives: hats, scarfs, and wigs.
Actinomycin D (dactinomycin, Cosmegen)	Ewing's sarcoma, osteogenic sarcoma, and soft tissue sarcomas	15–30 μg/kg/wk IV push or 400–600 μg/m^2/d for 5 d IV.	Moderate to severe nausea and vomiting.	Administer antiemetics as ordered. Notify physician if not effective.
		Some protocols use up to 1.5 mg/m^2 IV every 3–6 wk.	Alopecia in approximately 50% of patients.	Instruct patient about hair loss and provide alternatives: wigs, scarfs, and hats.

	Bone marrow depression with nadir at 10–14 d.	Include follow-up blood work in discharge planning as ordered by physician. Instruct patient about signs and symptoms of pancytopenia and measures to prevent or minimize bleeding and infection.
	Vesicant. Infiltration causes tissue destruction.	Care must be taken to avoid extravasation. Notify physician immediately if infiltration is suspected.
	Skin reaction, characterization by acne-like rash on face. Radiation recall reaction leading to severe erythema is also possible.	Sun may aggravate skin reaction. Instruct patient to avoid sun exposure and to use strong sunscreen.
	Anorexia, stomatitis, malaise, and diarrhea.	Instruct patient about maintaining adequate hydration and nutrition. Warn about signs and symptoms of stomatitis. Notify physician if occurs.

*Dosage provided as a guide; amount and frequency may vary in different settings.

†Folinic acid (leucovorine, citrovorum factor) rescue is used following MTX to spare normal cells from the toxic effects. It allows the administration of large amounts of MTX. Folinic acid must be given exactly on schedule, as ordered. Most patients are discharged on a regimen of additional leucovorine, and adequate discharge instructions must be given regarding the importance of schedule and dosage.

sions, and hyperalimentation and for withdrawing blood for laboratory studies.[31] These devices greatly reduce the chance of extravasation of antineoplastic agents, which may cause chemical burns. They can provide psychologic comfort to patients who may otherwise require multiple attempts at peripheral venous access on their fragile veins, even by the most experienced oncology nurse.

Management of Side Effects

The ongoing assessment of these patients, and interpretation of laboratory data and diagnostic test results, combined with the precise maintenance of treatment records, is essential for the early detection and management of side effects and organ toxicities. If a patient has oral mucositis, agents such as methotrexate and doxorubicin (Adriamycin) are withheld until the lesions are healed. If a patient experiences peripheral neuropathies, decreased tendon reflexes, and motor weakness, an agent such as vincristine is withheld or the dosage is decreased until the neuropathies disappear. Laboratory data must be evaluated and should include blood counts and liver and kidney function tests. Blood counts must be at an acceptable level, with platelet levels greater than 75,000 per mm^3 and an absolute neutrophil count of greater than 500 to 1000 per mm^3, depending on which chemotherapeutic agent is to be administered and what protocol is being followed.[31] This is to minimize the risk of bleeding and infection. Liver and kidney function must be monitored to reduce the risk of organ toxicities or permanent organ damage. Table 26–4 provides a more comprehensive listing of the side effects and guidelines for administration of chemotherapeutic agents.

NAUSEA AND VOMITING

Nausea and vomiting are some of the more distressing side effects of chemotherapy experienced by the patient. It is one of the major reasons that patients dread this treatment modality. Many of the chemotherapeutic agents that are used in the treatment of high-grade malignant musculoskeletal tumors cause nausea and vomiting, which can be mild, moderate, or severe. It is important for the patient and the family to be aware of these side effects and how they will be managed to minimize their anticipated fear.

In treating nausea and vomiting, prevention is seen as a primary goal. After vomiting has occurred, it is more difficult to control. In most instances, antiemetics are administered ½ hour before the start of chemotherapy and then every 4 to 6 hours routinely for about two doses. Routine scheduling of antiemetic therapy is preferable to as-needed scheduling during the first 12 hours after treatment. However, antiemetics can produce variable results, and the nurse and the patient must work together to determine the effectiveness of these drugs. A change in antiemetic therapy or a different combination of medication may be necessary to control emesis. Some common antiemetics used are lorazepam (Ativan), diphenhydramine (Benadryl), prochlorperazine (Compazine), metoclopramide (Reglan), chlorpromazine (Thorazine), and promethazine (Phenergan) in combination with dexamethasone (Decadron) and dronabinol (Marinol). Diphenhydramine is used to control the extrapyramidal side effects that may be caused by the phenothiazides. Many patients have pronounced psychogenic vomiting and anxiety before administration of chemotherapy and may need premedication such as diazepam (Valium), diphenhydramine or prochlorperazine 12 to 24 hours before treatment. Other techniques such as hypnosis, relaxation exercises, and imagery may be helpful.[31]

Care must be taken to prevent dehydration by monitoring intake and output and adjusting the hydration as ordered by the physician. Oral intake should be controlled by the patient's desire, which is usually fairly low during this time. Most patients prefer to sleep during treatments, and interruptions should be kept to a minimum. Many patients are very sedated from the antiemetics and must have side rails up and assistance in personal hygiene.

MUCOSITIS AND STOMATITIS

Many chemotherapeutic agents can alter the oral mucosa, causing mucositis (an inflammation of the mucous membranes in general) or stomatitis (specifically, an inflammation of the mouth). This can be painful and lead to decreased nutritional health caused by poor oral intake. Good oral care is one of the major steps in preventing stomatitis; brushing gently with a soft toothbrush is recommended. However, if stomatitis develops, oral care measures must be implemented at 2- to 4-hour intervals. Using plain tooth swabs and rinsing with solutions such as normal saline with sodium bicarbonate (1 tsp of NHO_3 to 1 pint of warm water), may be helpful. Lemon and glycerin swabs are not suggested, as they can cause drying and cracking of the oral mucosa.[31]

Good oral care is essential not only in decreasing the severity of mouth sores but also in preventing infection. In many cases, nystatin suspension is given 3 or 4 times a day. Patients should be instructed to swish and swallow. This can help in preventing *Candida* infections, which commonly occur in the immunosuppressed patient.

Analgesics may sometimes be necessary in severe stomatitis. Adequate nutrition may be difficult to achieve in the patient with severe mouth sores. It is best to offer a bland diet or a soft diet that is high in protein and carbohydrates. Cold fluids are tolerated best; hot and spicy foods should be avoided. Sometimes, it is best that a patient just receive intravenous hydration for a day or two rather than attempt to eat. Solutions such as lidocaine (Xylocaine) or a combination of lidocaine, diphenhydramine, and magnesium hydroxide–aluminum hydroxide antacid (Maalox) have been used to reduce pain associated with mucositis. In addition, sodium bicarbonate solution and similar rinses have proved helpful in cleaning the oral cavity and reducing infection.[31]

NUTRITIONAL STATUS

The patient's nutritional status must be assessed on a regular basis by serial weight measurements, calorimetry, and determination of total serum protein and albumin levels.[13] The nutritionist and dietitians should be involved from the start, not only for in-hospital evaluations but also for follow-up when the patient is at home. Many patients can benefit from the use of high-calorie supplements. Many patients do better with smaller, more frequent feedings as opposed to three large meals. Owing to the nausea, vomiting, and anorexia that occur as complications of treatment, these patients are at risk for cachexia. Sometimes alternative methods, such as tube feedings or hyperalimentation, may be necessary. It is essential that the nurse assess whether the patient and/or the family are capable of handling this type of nutritional support at home, as many patients require long-term continuing nutritional support. Patients who are in adequate nutritional health tolerate chemotherapy better with less toxicity.

BONE MARROW SUPPRESSION

Bone marrow suppression is one of the most common and potentially serious side effects of chemotherapy, affecting all three cell lines: white blood cells, red blood cells, and platelets.

White Blood Cells. White blood cells are important in the patient's defense against infection. Not only is the total number of white cells important, but the percentage of granulocytes (also known as polymorphonuclear neutrophils, segmented cells, and band neutrophils) in the differential determines the patients' risk of infection. The differential is determined by multiplying the total white blood cell count by the percentage of granulocytes. This percentage is known as the absolute neutrophil count (ANC). A low granulocyte count is known as granulocytopenia or neutropenia. Less than 500 per mm^3 puts a patient at a high risk for infection.

Patients are not hospitalized for a low white blood cell count unless their temperature is 101 F, or 38.4 C, or greater. Fever with a low granulocyte count is considered to indicate an infection until proved otherwise by 72 hours of negative cultures with a rising ANC. During this time, the patient is hospitalized and antibiotic coverage is given intravenously to protect against both gram-positive and gram-negative bacteria. The work-up for infection includes cultures of blood (drawn both peripherally and centrally if a catheter is present), urine, throat, and any wound suspected of harboring infection. In addition, a chest x-ray is recommended only if the patient has signs of pulmonary infection, such as tachypnea or cough.[13] A patient who is granulocytopenic may not be able to mount the usual signs of infection, such as redness, swelling, heat, and exudate. These patients may exhibit signs such as chills, malaise, irritability, and changes in vital signs. Septic shock can occur when the body is overwhelmed by infection and may develop quite suddenly.

Strict handwashing by all those entering the patient's room is instituted as a protection for the granulocytopenic patient. Most institutions do not use reverse isolation as a protective measure because often the patient's own germs and bacteria cause an infection. A thorough examination of the patient should be done daily to check for sources of infection. Taking temperatures rectally and administering suppositories are avoided because of the possible introduction of bacteria from the rectum into the blood stream. Wound healing may be delayed in the neutropenic patient, and all wounds and suture lines should be checked daily.

The neutropenic patient is usually provided with a single room or a roommate who is noninfectious. Visitors should be instructed that the patient is more susceptible to infection. Nurses should also avoid taking care of patients with other infections so that they avoid cross contamination.

Red Blood Cells. Anemia caused by the lack of production of new red blood cells usually develops 7 to 14 days after receiving treatment. Symptoms may include weakness, lightheadedness, fatigue, orthostatic hypotension, pallor, shortness of breath, and palpitations. The patients should be aware of these symptoms because they are usually at home between treatments during the time that their blood counts are affected. Frequent rest periods may be necessary. Often, these patients adapt quite well to their anemia and may not need to undergo transfusion. Depending on the practitioner, those patients who are expected to have continuing interference with red blood cell production and/or those with a hemoglobin level of 7 to 8 g per dL are usually transfused with packed red blood cells.[13] Transfusions are used more judiciously than in the past, because of the risk of hepatitis, transfusion reactions, and concern about acquiring the human immunodeficiency virus (HIV). The use of family and friends as designated donors is a possibility at many large centers. During the administration of blood products, the nurse must be astute in observing for transfusion reactions, including hemolytic, febrile, and allergic reactions. Some centers are using irradiated blood products because of the increased risk of graft versus host disease in the immunosuppressed population.[13] In young children and elderly patients, transfusions are usually given more slowly to avoid the risk of fluid overload.

Platelets. Thrombocytopenia, a decrease in the number of platelets, is often the cause of bleeding in the patient with cancer. Signs of thrombocytopenia include petechiae, spontaneous bruises, gum bleeding, epistaxis, and blood in the urine and stool. It is uncommon for bleeding to occur with platelet levels greater than 50,000 per mm^3 and serious bleeding is unusual when the platelet count is greater than 20,000 per mm^3. The risk of bleeding tends to be greater when a fever is present, as this destroys platelets.[13] The indication for platelet transfusions is based on the total assessment of the patient. Platelets are not usually given in an attempt to maintain a specific platelet count, as any platelet transfusion may endanger the success of later transfusions. Subsequent transfusions may be less effective in achieving a significant rise in platelet levels and platelet antibodies may develop. Again, depending on the practitioner, platelets may be given prophylactically if the count is 20,000 per mm^3 or less.

Nursing care of the thrombocytopenic patient includes skin assessment for any signs of increased bruising or petechiae and testing of urine and stools for blood. Rectal treatments are usually avoided when the platelet count is low. The sites of invasive techniques such as intravenous punctures or intramuscular injection should be watched carefully for any signs of hematoma formation. Pressure and ice should be applied until signs of bleeding have stopped. Patients should be instructed that when their platelet count is low, a hard-bristled toothbrush should not be used. Instead, toothettes may be used to ensure adequate oral care. Electric razors should be used instead of straight-edged razors. Patients should also be taught to avoid strenuous activities as well as contact sports when platelet counts are low.

Renal failure may be a complication of renal damage from drugs such as cisplatin, ifosfamide, and methotrexate. Evaluation of renal function should include a 24-hour urine collection for creatinine clearance, serum creatinine, uric acid, and blood urea nitrogen determinations. Hydration is necessary during and after infusion of these medications.

Liver function tests are also monitored closely, as certain agents such as methotrexate can cause liver dysfunction. If this occurs, the drug may be withheld until the test results return to normal, the dosage may be decreased, or the medication may be discontinued.

Other toxicities include cardiomyopathy due to doxorubicin (Adriamycin). Cardiac function is monitored closely with the use of electrocardiograms, echocardiograms, and cardiac gating studies. Cisplatin is known to cause a decrease in hearing at high frequencies, and routine audiograms are necessary for these patients. Hemorrhagic cystitis is a complication of the administration of cyclophosphamide and ifosfamide, and these patients require vigorous hydration before and after therapy and the administration of mesna with the ifosfamide.[13]

The nurse is responsible for monitoring for these side effects and for implementing measures that promote the safety and health of the patient.

RADIOTHERAPY

Radiotherapy, like chemotherapy, is used to destroy primary musculoskeletal tumors and metastatic disease. Understanding some basic concepts of radiotherapy and its side effects enables the nurses caring for these patients to participate in delivery of comprehensive health care.

Mechanism of Action

Radiation destroys cells most effectively during mitosis, the time at which cells are most rapidly dividing. Cells are destroyed by damage both to the DNA and to the cell membrane.[13] The intracellular water content is also affected, and this ionization, causing further metabolic interactions, contributes to cell damage. Radiosensitivity depends on cell type, the position of the cell during the cell cycle, the extent of tumor spread, and the vascular supply and oxygenation.[51] Each treatment plan includes a carefully calculated dose of radiation, which achieves tumor control with minimal damage to normal tissue and fewer incapacitating side effects to the patient.

Osteogenic sarcoma is known as a relatively radioresistant tumor. Radioresistant indicates that the delivery of radiation doses are so high for possible tumor eradication that significant damage to the surrounding normal tissue affects structure or function. Ewing's sarcomas and many of the soft tissue sarcomas are radiosensitive. Radiosensitive indicates that the delivery of radiation doses eradicates the tumor with little damage to the normal surrounding tissue. Ewing's sarcomas and soft tissue sarcomas can be treated with concurrent radiotherapy, chemotherapy, and surgery. Radiation also can be used for palliation.

A curative course of radiotherapy is usually given in short sequential treatment sessions, 5 days a week over 4 to 6 weeks. By spreading out the treatment, healthy body tissues are less affected. The first visit to the radiation oncologist includes planning the schedule and mapping the area of tumor to be irradiated. Results of computed tomography, radiography, and/or magnetic resonance imaging are used to define the tumor margins precisely. The skin is marked with punctate indelible ink or tattoos, which remain intact until the treatment is completed. Care or maintenance of these markings is essential, as these determine the exact outline of the radiation field. The initial treatment planning session may take up to several hours or even days. For daily treatments, appointments on the average take 15 minutes, which includes appropriate positioning and the actual radiation administration, which typically lasts only 1 to 2 minutes. During this time, the patient must lie very still. Children may need sedation, such as chloral hydrate, diazepam (Valium), or sodium pentobarbital (Nembutal), or short-acting anesthesia, such as ketamine, during their treatments. Sophisticated blocks, wedges, and filters can be used to protect normal tissue and organs from scatter radiation and to improve radiation dose distribution. These are added to the machine assembly and are not applied directly over the patient.[51]

Radiation implants can be used to give a high dose of radiation to a relatively small tumor volume. Interstitial application of radiation in this manner may decrease the risk of lymphedema or other side effects, as the irradiated tissue is even more precisely defined. Radiation implants are done by a surgical procedure of needle placement under anesthesia. Needles are replaced with hollow guide tubes, which are later loaded in the patient's room with radioisotopes, such as iridium 192. Patients are then isolated, with restriction of visiting; nursing personnel are monitored with film badges; shields are placed around the bed of the patient; and pregnancy precautions are implemented. Treatment usually lasts several days. The tubes are removed in the patient's room before the patient is discharged from the hospital.[51]

Patient Education

The nurse-educator plays an important role in the patient's understanding of radiotherapy and its side effects. Useful advice in managing the local and systemic acute side effects and information on long-term effects are crucial to the comfort of the patient and include changes in skin integrity, nutrition, blood counts, and lymphedema. Additional areas to be addressed are radiation markings, scheduling of treatments, and patient comfort during treatments. Nursing care in patients undergoing palliative radiotherapy can be more difficult owing to the patients' debilitated state.

Many patients have significant fears and anxieties about radiotherapy. These concern radiation itself, machinery's falling on them, isolation and loneliness while alone in the treatment room, the noise of the machinery, and the most terrifying idea of all, developing a second tumor. Educating these patients is the single best way to allay anxiety. Other techniques involve relaxation, imagery, and self-hypnosis. These fears are greatly multiplied when the patient is a child. Children can be allowed to play with the buttons on the machinery, practice on their dolls, and bring a favorite toy into the treatment room. They may also be reassured by hearing their parents' voices via the intercom during their sessions.

Side Effects

Both local and systemic reactions are a concern to the oncologic team caring for patients with musculoskeletal tumors. Local reactions may include changes in skin integrity and lymphedema, whereas systemic reactions include nutritional changes, bone marrow depression, and growth retardation.

Changes in skin integrity are a major concern to the nurse. Local skin reactions of the irradiated areas are less severe than in the past because of advances in delivery of radiotherapy and in skin care. However, local reactions do still occur. There are four degrees of skin reactions: epilation, erythema, dry desquamation, and wet desquamation.

Epilation is loss of hair, which usually regrows 2 to 3 months after therapy is discontinued. Erythema and dry desquamation are the most common side effects to the skin. First, a redness occurs and this progresses to a dry, scaly, itchy localized reaction. Patients should be advised to keep their skin clean and dry; not to use lotions; not to expose these areas to sunlight, although fresh air is helpful; to avoid exposure of these areas to temperature extremes; and to wear 100% cotton loose-fitting clothing. Cornstarch may be useful to decrease pruritus and petrolatum (Vaseline) or vitamin A and D ointment may be useful in reducing the dryness of the skin. At this stage, there may be residual tanning, which remains on the skin after the radiotherapy is completed.

Skin reactions can progress to blistering and loss of the superficial layer of the skin, or wet desquamation. It is important to watch for signs of infection when the skin is in this condition. It may be necessary to dress the skin and use irrigations both to clean and to increase the circulation to the area.[23, 34, 51]

Actinomycin D (dactinomycin) and doxorubicin (Adriamycin) also increase skin sensitivity if given concurrently with irradiation. These drugs are usually omitted several weeks before, during, and several weeks after the radiotherapy. Occasionally, there is a late skin reaction when these drugs are reinstituted.[13, 51]

Lymphedema occurs when lymphatic vessels are damaged, causing a decrease in the drainage of the lymph fluid. Patients who have had a surgical resection of a muscloskeletal tumor need to be closely monitored for this local reaction. Lymphedema is most likely to occur in the axilla and the groin, where lymph tissue is located in large amounts. It can be an acute reaction or occur months after radiation is given. Swelling, pain, and skin breakdown may be seen in patients with lymphedema. Therapy includes use of support hosiery, exercise, and prevention of infection.

Support hosiery promotes venous and lymphatic drainage and decreases swelling in the lower extremities. The nurse must instruct the patient regarding the purpose and application and how frequently to change the support hosiery (i.e., every day after a bath or shower).

Exercise is used to maintain and build strength and to prevent joint contractures at the joints near the surgical resection of the tumor. The nurse assesses the patient's strength and mobility and encourages participation in an exercise program. Walking, leg raises, and quadricep exercises can be recommended and demonstrated to the patient by the nurse. The nurse can follow up with the appropriate referral to an organized program in close collaboration with the physician.

Infection caused by skin breakdown is always a concern to the patient receiving radiotherapy. The nurse must assess for local skin reactions and promote patient participation in maintaining skin integrity (see above).

Nutritional changes are a systemic reaction that can affect maintenance of skin integrity and participation in an exercise program. Adequate hydration and a well-balanced diet are helpful to minimize nutritional changes. Often, this is difficult because the patient experiences malaise and fatigue as a common side effect of treatment. Daily trips to the hospital are exhausting and the emotional state of the patient may also contribute to a lack of appetite. Some suggestions the nurse may offer patients are small frequent meals, high-calorie and high-carbohydrate snacks, nutritional supplements (e.g., milk shakes), and a pleasant dining atmosphere.[34]

Bone marrow depression is a reaction experienced most commonly by patients with Ewing's sarcoma and osteogenic sarcoma. The bone marrow contains lymphoid tissue that is highly sensitive to radiotherapy, therefore changes in the hematopoietic system can be expected. For soft tissue sarcomas in which there is less bone involved in the radiotherapy field, there is still some decrease in the lymphocyte count, but the other cell lines are less affected. Peripheral blood is less sensitive to treatment. The cells least affected by radiation treatment are the red blood cells and platelet precursors. Red blood cells have a much longer half-life and the threat of anemia is not as great as the risk of neutropenia. The lower limits of acceptable blood counts are set by the radiation oncologist. Patients must be aware of their need for frequent blood counts and have an understanding of the meaning of these results.[51]

Growth retardation secondary to radiation therapy can be a problem in the pediatric patient. Growing bones are highly radiosensitive. When the epiphyseal or growth plate is irradiated, cellular proliferation can be impaired or arrested altogether, depending on the dose of radiation given. This can result in a shortened standing height. Radiotherapy to the spinal axis can also result in a shortened sitting height.

Sterility and the development of secondary malignancies are a concern to all patients who receive radiotherapy. Ongoing follow-up is essential to monitor for these late effects.

Progression of Disease

Despite the advances in treatment of osteogenic sarcoma, Ewing's sarcoma, and other high-grade tumors of the musculoskeletal system, some patients develop metastasis while receiving therapy and others develop recurrent disease after therapy has been completed. The most common place for subsequent disease to occur is lung, other bones, or local sites.

The patient with progression of disease is at a cancer crisis point. The patient and the family realize that this is a setback, and hope may turn into fear and despair. The nurse's role is to help the family sort out the information and realistically discuss the alternatives and goals. Many patients may consider refusing further treatment. Clarification of the goal of therapy helps the patient and the family to make a clear decision. At this point, therapy can be to cure, to alleviate pain or symptoms, or to delay further progression of disease. The patient's and the family's trust in the medical team may be threatened. The family may feel abandoned, even though the staff appears to be available. At this time, the patient and the family may need more time and reassurance than at original diagnosis. The nurse should assess which other services need to become involved, such as rehabilitation, dietary, home care, hospice, and occupational therapy. As mentioned above, each treatment modality has specific side effects. These side effects are managed as they would be at any point throughout treatment. Patients and families require reeducation. Patients may also experience side effects from their relapse. Shortness of breath, pain, and limited mobility are a few of the symptoms that may be experienced.

The nurse's focus of care for the patient with progressive disease should be on treatment and symptom control to ensure quality of life and to help maintain the patient's and the family's optimal level of functioning.

There are a growing number of survivors with high grade musculoskeletal tumors, including patients who have experienced a relapse. Nurses are now more likely to encounter these survivors at a later stage in their lives. The nursing literature is beginning to reflect issues involved in the comprehensive rehabilitation care of these patients, including physical, psychologic, and social effects on their life style.

References

1. Baird SB: Decision Making in Oncology Nursing. Philadelphia, BC Decker, 1988.
2. Bonavita L: Free tissue transfer. Am J Nurs 85:384–387, 1985.
3. Brown J: Chemotherapy. *In* Groenwald SL (ed): Cancer Nursing: Principles and Practice. Boston, Jones & Bartlett, 1987.
4. Brown MH, Kiss ME, Gutlaw EM, Viamontes CM (eds): Standards of Oncology Nursing Practice. New York, John Wiley & Sons, 1986.
5. Bruce WR, Meeker BE, Valeriote FA: Comparison of the sensitivity of normal and hematopoietic and transplanted lymphoma colony-forming cells to chemotherapeutic agents administered *in vivo.* J Nat Cancer Inst 37:233–245, 1966.
6. Buck B, Lee AD: Amputation: Two views. Nurs Clin North Am 11:639–640, 1976.
7. Burns N: Nursing and Cancer. Philadelphia, WB Saunders Co, 1982.

7a. Consensus Conference: Perioperative red blood cell transfusion. JAMA 260:2700–2703, 1988.

8. Dalsn J: Deep vein thrombosis and pulmonary embolism developing a protocol for effective prophylaxis. Boston, Kendall Company, 1985.
9. Dittmar S: Rehabilitation Nursing. St Louis, CV Mosby, 1989.

10. Donehower MG: The behavior of malignancies. *In* Johnson BL, Gross J (eds): Handbook of Oncology Nursing. New York, John Wiley & Sons, 1985.
11. Duigon A: Anticipatory nausea and vomiting associated with cancer chemotherapy. Oncol Nurs Forum 13(1):35–40, 1986.
12. Enneking WF (ed): Limb Salvage in Musculoskeletal Oncology. New York, Churchill Livingstone, 1987.
13. Fergusson J, Fochtman D, Ford N, Pryor A: The treatment of cancer in children. *In* Fochtman D, Foley G (eds): Nursing Care of the Child with Cancer. Boston, Little, Brown, 1982.
14. Galassi AL: Cancer of the Musculoskeletal System: Osteogenic Sarcoma, Ewing's Sarcoma and Rhabdomyosarcoma. A Developmental Approach. Boston, Little, Brown, 1984.
15. Goorin AM, Dolorey MJ, et al: Prognostic significance of complete surgical resection of pulmonary metastases in patients with osteogenic sarcoma: Analysis of 32 patients. J Clin Oncol 2(5):425–431, 1989.
16. Gregorcic N: Functional abilities following limb-salvage procedures. Orthop Nurs 4(5):24–28, 1985.
17. Halperin E: Radiotherapy. *In* Hockenberry M, Coody DK (eds): Pediatric Oncology and Hematology Perspectives on Care. St Louis, CV Mosby, 1986.
18. Harii K: Microvascular free flaps for skin coverage. Clin Plast Surg 10:37–54, 1983.
19. Harrison D: Methods of assessing the viability of free flap transfer during the postoperative period. Clin Plast Surg 10:21–36, 1983.
20. Harrison DH: The osteocutaneous free fibular graft. J Bone Joint Surg 68B:804–807, 1986.
21. Hartsuck J, Greenfield LJ: Postoperative thromboembolism. Arch Surg 107:733–739, 1973.
22. Hassey KM, Rose CM: Altered skin integrity in patients receiving radiation therapy. Oncol Nurs Forum 9(4):44–50, 1982.
23. Hayes FA, Thompson EI: Metastatic Ewing's sarcoma: Remission induction and survival. J Clin Oncol 5:1199–1202, 1984.
24. Hays DM (ed): Pediatric Surgical Oncology. Orlando, FL, Grune & Stratton, 1986.
25. Hughes CB: Giving cancer drugs IV: Some guidelines. Am J Nurs 1:34–38, 1986.
26. Jaffe N, Smith E: Osteogenic sarcoma: Alternatives in the pattern of pulmonary metastases with aelyuvana chemotherapy. J Clin Oncol 1:251–253, 1983.
27. Johnson J: I Can Cope. Minneapolis, Minnesota, DLI Publishing, 1988.
28. Kaszyk LK: Cardiac toxicity associated with cancer chemotherapy. Oncol Nurs Forum 13(4):81–88, 1986.
29. Kenan S: Limb sparing reconstructive surgery in malignant and aggressive benign bone tumors of the extremities. Surgical Rounds for Orthopaedics, August 1987, pp 25–36.
30. Kenan S, Lewis M: Current concepts in the management of soft tissue sarcoma of the extremities. Bull Hosp Joint Dis Orthop Inst 46(2):108–111, 1986.
31. Knobf MK, Fischer DS, Welch-McCaffrey D: Cancer Chemotherapy: Treatment and Care. Boston, GK Hall, 1984.
32. Kupcella CE: Cellular biology of cancer. *In* Groenwald SL (ed): Cancer Nursing: Principles and Practice. Boston, Jones & Bartlett, 1987.
33. Leahy I: Nursing care of the cancer patient: Radiation therapy. *In* Bouchard-Kurtz R, Speese-Owens N (eds): Nursing Care of the Cancer Patient. St Louis, CV Mosby, 1981.
34. Lewis M: Current concept: The expandable prosthesis. Bull Hosp Joint Dis Orthop Inst 45(1):29–31, 1985.
35. Lewis M: The expandable prosthesis: An alternative to amputation for children with malignant bone tumors. AORN J 46:457–465, 1987.
35a. Lewis M: The expandable prothesis—tumor prostheses for children. Bull Hosp Joint Dis Orthop Inst 45(1):177–183, 1985.
36. Lewis M: Proximal femur replacement for neoplastic disease. Clin Orthop Rel Res 171:72–79, 1987.
37. Lydon J: Nephrotoxicity of cancer treatment. Oncol Nurs Forum 13(2):68–77, 1986.
38. Mankin HJ, Doppelt SH, Sullivan TR, Tomford WW: Osteoarticular and intercalary allograft transplantation in the management of malignant tumors of bone. Cancer 50:613–630, 1982.
39. Martin N: Comprehensive Rehabilitation Nursing. New York, McGraw-Hill, 1981.
40. McCaffery M: Pain: Clinical Management for Nursing Practice. St Louis, CV Mosby, 1989.
41. McNally JC, Stair JC, Somerville ET (eds): Guidelines for Cancer Nursing Practice. New York, Grune & Stratton, 1979.
41a. Mendenhall CM, Marcus RB Jr, Enneking WF, et al: The prognostic significance of soft tissue extension in Ewing's sarcoma. Cancer 5:913–917, 1983.
42. Oncology Nursing Society: Cancer Chemotherapy: Guidelines and Recommendations for Nursing Education and Practice. Pittsburgh, PA, Oncology Nursing Society, 1984.
43. Oster J: A cost-effectiveness analysis of prophylaxis analysis of prophylaxis against deep-vein thrombosis in major orthopaedic surgery. JAMA 257(2):203–208, 1987.
44. Parrish F: Allograft replacement of all or part of the end of a long bone following excision of a tumor. J Bone Joint Surg 55A:1–22, 1973.
45. Phipps W: Medical-Surgical Nursing: Concepts and Clinical Practice, 3rd ed. St Louis, CV Mosby, 1987.
46. Piaseck P: Bone banking: Its role in skeletal tumor reconstruction. Orthop Nurs 4(5):56–60, 1985.
47. Piasecki PA: Bone malignancies. *In* Groenwald SL (ed): Cancer Nursing: Principles and Practice. Boston, Jones & Bartlett, 1987.
48. Rhodes VA, Watson PM, Johnson MH: Association of chemotherapy and related nausea and vomiting with pretreatment and posttreatment anxiety. Oncol Nurs Forum 13(1):41–47, 1986.
49. Ritchie J: Nursing the child undergoing limb amputation. Matern Child Nurs J, 5:114–120, 1980.
49a. Rubin P (ed): Clinical Oncology: A Multidisciplinary Approach, 6th ed. Atlanta, GA, American Cancer Society, 1983.
50. Sarna LP: Concepts of nursing care for patients receiving radiation therapy. *In* Vredevoe DL, Derdiarian A, Sarna LP, Friel M, Gatan Shiplacoff JA (eds): Concepts of Oncology Nursing. Englewood Cliffs, NJ, Prentice-Hall, 1981.
51. Sim F: Reconstruction of musculoskeletal defects about the knee for tumor. Clin Orthop 221:188–200, 1987.
52. Simon R: Clinical prognostic factors in osteosarcoma. Cancer Treat Rep 62:193–196, 1978.
53. Simonton CO: Getting Well Again. New York, Bantam Books, 1981.
54. Weiland A: Vascularized bone autografts. Clin Orthop Rel Res 174:87–94, 1983.
55. Ziegfeld C (ed): Core Curriculum for Oncology Nursing. Philadelphia, WB Saunders Co, 1987.

Suggested Readings

Bender CM: Chemotherapy. *In* Ziegfeld CR (ed): Core Curriculum for Oncology Nursing. Philadelphia, WB Saunders Co, 1987.

Dudas S: Cancer rehabilitation. Oncol Nurs Forum 15(2):183–188, 1988.

Griffiths MJ, Murray KH, Russo PC: Oncology Nursing. New York, Macmillan, 1984.

Hanak M: Patient and Family Education. New York, Springer Publishing, 1986.

Hubbard SM: Cancer treatment. *In* Johnson BL, Gross J (eds): Handbook of Oncology Nursing. New York, John Wiley & Sons, 1985.

Ulrich S: Nursing Care Planning Guides: A Nursing Diagnosis Approach. Philadelphia, WB Saunders Co, 1986.

CHAPTER 27

Anesthetic Considerations in Limb Preservation Surgery for Neoplastic Disease

HATIM HYDERALLY

Currently a variety of techniques for limb preservation are available in the surgical management of patients with neoplastic disease of the musculoskeletal system. In considering the anesthetic management it is necessary to be aware of many special aspects of the medical and surgical management of these patients. In addition, with advances in modern medical management an increasing number of severely ill patients undergo surgery. Many of these patients are on concurrent complex chemotherapeutic regimens with significant life-threatening side effects that involve the respiratory, cardiovascular, and hematopoietic systems. It is therefore necessary for the anesthesiologist to be able to make a critical preoperative assessment of such patients with the understanding that complex surgical procedures now require a prolonged period of anesthesia. In addition to the usual thorough preoperative history and physical examination, the side effects and complications of chemotherapy and radiotherapy must be appreciated.

Assessment of Anesthesia Risk

Preoperative assessment is usually based on physical status, as classified by the American Society of Anesthesiologists (ASA); five classes are defined (Table 27–1).[10] This well-established classification is not intended to assess risk of anesthesia or to predict outcome but serves as a "common language" for subsequent examination of anesthetic morbidity and mortality.

In addition to the ASA classification of physical status, several other systems are available for assessment of critically ill patients in intensive care units. The Goldman multifactorial index score and the acute physiology and chronic health evaluation (APACHE) are two systems that Howland and coworkers[4] have suggested may be useful in the preoperative assessment of patients with cancer who are about to undergo major surgical procedures.

A multifactorial index score was proposed by Goldman and associates[3] for assessment of patients undergoing noncardiac surgery. This weighted system uses the following factors to assess risk and to predict outcome: jugular venous distention or S3 gallop; myocardial infarction in the preceding 6-month period; rhythm other than sinus; more than five premature ventricular beats per minute; site of operative procedure; age greater than 70 years; significant aortic valve stenosis; emergency operations; poor medical condition.

The APACHE system utilizes physiologic

TABLE 27-1

Physical Status Classification of the American Society of Anesthesiologists

Class	Disease State
ASA Class 1	No organic, physiologic, biochemical, or psychiatric disturbance.
ASA Class 2	Mild to moderate systemic disturbance that may or may not be related to the reason for surgery. Examples: Heart disease that only slightly limits physical activity, hypertension, anemia, diabetes, asthma, and chronic bronchitis.
ASA Class 3	Severe systemic disturbance that may or may not be related to the reason for surgery. Examples: Heart disease that limits physical activity, poorly controlled hypertension, diabetes with vascular complications, pulmonary disease that limits activity, history of prior myocardial infarction.
ASA Class 4	Severe systemic disease that is life-threatening with or without surgery. Examples: Congestive heart failure, persistent angina, advanced pulmonary, renal, or hepatic disease.
ASA Class 5	Moribund patients who have little chance of survival but are submitted to surgery as a last resort. Examples: Uncontrolled hemorrhage, cerebral trauma, pulmonary embolus.

and pre-admission health condition indicators and a 0 to 4 expert weighing system of several selected physiologic variables for quantification of the severity of the illness.[7] More recently, Knaus and coworkers modified the APACHE System to include only 12 routine physiologic variables and previous health conditions to assess a general measure of severity of the disease.[5] They utilize the following measurements: heart rate; mean arterial blood pressure; respiratory rate; arterial oxygen tension (PaO_2 mm Hg); arterial pH; serum sodium, potassium, and creatinine; hematocrit; white blood cell count; Glasgow coma score; and age of patient. Clearly these are complex systems applicable only to seriously and critically compromised cancer patients undergoing major surgical intervention.

Evaluation of Organ Systems

The usual patient with neoplastic musculoskeletal disease about to undergo major limb preservation surgery may not have multiorgan disease. Nevertheless, a critical evaluation of the major organ systems is required in order to plan an anesthetic technique and appropriate monitoring.

Neurologic System. Mental status must be noted, as severe preoperative anxiety may be present. Psychological reassurance and appropriate preoperative sedation with anxiolytic drugs are necessary; midazolam and diazepam are particularly useful. Brain metastases and/or raised intracranial pressure must be evaluated.

Cardiovascular System. Significant coronary artery disease and arteriosclerotic heart disease are manifested by angina, dysrhythmias, myocardial infarction, and congestive heart failure. When necessary, appropriate therapy should be instituted to optimize the medical condition of the patient preoperatively. Hypertension must be controlled adequately with appropriate therapeutic intervention. Numerous studies clearly indicate the beneficial effects of continuing hypertensive therapy up to the immediate preoperative phase of surgery.[7]

Respiratory System. Heavy smoking has several deleterious effects on the respiratory system and contributes to postoperative respiratory morbidity.[6] Patients with cancer often are elderly and occasionally are heavy smokers. Abstinence for at least 2 weeks preoperatively should be strongly encouraged.

Asthma and chronic obstructive pulmonary disease should be carefully assessed, and every attempt should be made to optimize the patient's condition with appropriate therapeutic intervention. If significant disease is present, preoperative arterial blood gas analysis is required to establish baseline guidelines for respiratory management during and after surgery.

Liver and Kidney Function. Assessment of liver and kidney function is required prior to the use of general anesthesia. Serum glutamic transaminase (SGPT) and prothrombin time (PT) are the most useful tests of liver function. PT is particularly important surgically but also as a consideration in the use of techniques such as epidural anesthesia. Serum creatinine and blood urea nitrogen levels are required for assessment of kidney function.

Hematologic System. Hemoglobin and hematocrit determinations are routine preoperatively. Anemia of a significant degree should be corrected well in advance of major orthopedic surgical intervention.

Chemotherapeutic agents have adverse effects on the hematopoietic system; therefore, a coagulation profile must be obtained and any deficiency corrected preoperatively.

Electrolyte and Acid-Base Derangements. Such abnormalities may be present in patients with cancer as a result of emesis induced by chemotherapy and radiotherapy. Serious derangements must be corrected preoperatively with the appropriate therapeutic intervention.

Chemotherapy

A variety of agents and complex regimens are currently available in the medical management of patients with musculoskeletal neoplastic disease. The adverse effects of some on these on various major organ systems are of prime importance in the anesthetic management of these patients.[9]

Chemotherapeutic agents are classified as follows: alkylating agents (nitrogen mustards, cyclophosphamide); antimetabolites (methotrexate); vinca alkaloids (vincristine); antibiotics (doxorubicin [Adriamycin], bleomycin); enzymes (asparaginase); synthetics (cisplatin); and hormones (corticosteroids).

A thorough knowledge of the adverse effects of these drugs is essential. Hemoglobin, hematocrit, platelet count, white blood cell count, coagulation profile, arterial blood gases, chest radiograph, liver and renal function tests, electrocardiogram, stress testing, and assessment of left ventricular function with echocardiography and imaging techniques may be required in the management of the cancer patient prior to surgery.

Anemia is a common side effect of several classes of chemotherapeutic agents; significant anemia must be appropriately treated prior to surgery. Oxygen transport already diminished as a result of preexisting anemia will be further reduced by blood loss during surgery. Thrombocytopenia may result in a coagulopathy. Although low levels of platelets may be acceptable during medical management of these patients, it is necessary to correct thrombocytopenia prior to major surgery.

Severe stomatitis may be aggravated by the placement of airways and endotracheal tubes. Pulmonary toxicity is a serious side effect of bleomycin therapy. Exertional dyspnea is present in mild cases, whereas arterial hypoxemia at rest and interstitial pneumonitis are seen in the more severe forms.[9]

Cardiomyopathy is dose-related and often an irreversible side effect of Adriamycin. The incidence of cardiomyopathy is negligible if the total dose is lower than 500 mg per square meter of body surface area.[9] Assessment of ventricular function with echocardiography and imaging techniques often is required to determine the degree of compromise as a result of Adriamycin-induced cardiomyopathy.

Special Considerations

The following are special considerations in the anesthetic management of patients scheduled for major limb preservation techniques with construction of free microvascular muscle flaps:

In addition to routine monitoring of the electrocardiogram, oxygen saturation (pulse oximetry), temperature, direct arterial pressure and central venous pressure, and pulmonary artery pressure monitoring with a Swan-Ganz catheter is often necessary.

Accurate measurement of fluid balance is essential. Assessment of blood loss intraoperatively and measurement of urine output are required.

Surgical procedures are often of prolonged duration, and in the cool ambient temperatures maintained in operating rooms it is not unusual for the patient to become hypothermic. Therefore, temperature must be continuously monitored and every effort should be made to maintain normothermia.

Exposed body areas are covered at all times and arms wrapped with a Kerlix bandage; the head is enclosed in a clear polyethylene bag. In addition, all intravenous fluids are warmed during intraoperative infusion. A heat and moisture exchanger filter is placed between the endotracheal tube and the breathing tube to retain heat and moisture. Pressure points are padded and protected; in lengthy procedures it is important to vary the position of the head, thereby avoiding pressure necrosis of the scalp.

Limb preservation involves not only *en-bloc*

resection and custom-built prosthetic replacement but also occasionally the preparation of free microvascular muscle flaps, often a lengthy and time-consuming procedure.

The choice of the anesthetic technique must take into account the provision of prolonged anesthesia.

Regional and general anesthetic techniques alone or in combination are suitable choices in upper and lower extremity surgery.

UPPER EXTREMITY SURGERY

Surgery of benign lesions below the elbow can be easily managed with the relatively simple technique of intravenous regional block (Bier block).[1] This simple method is not recommended for surgical excision of malignant soft tissue lesions for fear that spreading may occur during exsanguination of the arm.

This simple and reliable technique entails exsanguination of the upper extremity and subsequent injection of a measured quantity of local anesthetic that is confined to the area by use of tourniquet. A dose of 40 ml of 0.5% lidocaine provides excellent analgesia. Release of the tourniquet at the termination results in rapid disappearance of anesthesia, but with the possibility of central nervous and cardiovascular symptoms related to the entry of a bolus of local anesthetic into the systemic circulation.

Brachial plexus block can be performed by a variety of approaches. Interscalene block of the brachial plexus is achieved by injecting 20 to 40 ml of local anesthetic into the interscalene groove opposite the transverse process of the sixth cervical vertebra.[1] This block is especially effective for surgery of the shoulder or upper arm. The major complication of this block is the accidental injection of local anesthetic into the vertebral artery, resulting in convulsion. Also possible is the injection of local anesthetic solution into the epidural or subarachnoid space, resulting in central neuraxis blockade. Pneumothorax is a potential complication of interscalene block. Supraclavicular block is performed by injecting 25 to 30 ml of local anesthetic solution at the midpoint of the clavicle, where the brachial plexus crosses the first rib.[1] Paresthesia usually can be elicited with this block. This classic superclavicular block provides excellent anesthesia of the whole upper extremity from shoulder to hand. Pneumothorax, the most common complication with an incidence of about 1%, manifests initially as cough, dyspnea, and pleuritic chest pain. One advantage of this block is that a small volume of anesthetic is needed because the brachial plexus is most compact at this site. Also, the block is reliable and has a rapid onset.

Axillary block can be achieved by injecting 20 to 40 ml of local anesthetic solution into the axillary sheath in the axilla.[1] This block is most effective for surgery below the level of the elbow and is the most appropriate technique for the outpatient setting. The potential complications of pneumothorax and central neuraxis blockade are totally avoided with this approach. The most reliable technique is the transarterial approach with a ¾-inch small vein needle. The axillary artery is palpated as high up in the axilla as possible, and the needle is advanced until the neurovascular compartment is entered by piercing its sheath. In the event of definite paresthesias of the median, radial, or the ulnar nerve radiating to fingers, 20 to 40 ml of local anesthetic solution is injected. Careful repeated aspiration must be done during the injection to insure that the tip of the needle is not in the axillary artery.

LOWER EXTREMITY SURGERY

The major nerves to the lower limb are the sciatic, femoral, lateral femoral, cutaneous, and obturator; these are widely separated in the thigh. Therefore, rather than attempt multiple peripheral nerve blocks, many prefer spinal or epidural block for achieving the same degree of anesthesia.[2]

Spinal, single bolus, or continuous catheter techniques provide excellent anesthesia for surgery of the lower limb. Spinal block is usually performed with the patient in the sitting or lateral decubitus position. The needle is inserted in the midline at the most easily palpable interspace below L2, usually L3-4 or L4-5. Local anesthetic solution is injected after a clear flow of cerebrospinal fluid has been obtained. Hyperbaric, isobaric, and hypobaric solutions of local anesthetics (tetracaine, bupivacaine, and lidocaine) can be used to provide the desired duration and degree of analgesia required for surgery. Continuous lumbar epidural anesthesia is achieved by placement of a catheter in the epidural space, usually at L3-4 or L4-5. Solutions of local anesthetics such as lidocaine, mepivacaine and bupivacaine are available to provide the desired duration and degree of anesthesia.

Hypotension, a potential complication of both spinal and epidural anesthesia, is due to sympathetic nervous system blockade and consequent venous pooling, which results in decrease of preload. The hypotension is treated physiologically with administration of intravenous fluids. Occasionally sympathomimetics with positive inotropic and chronotropic effects such as ephedrine (5 to 10 mg) are administered intravenously. A distinct advantage of the continuous spinal and epidural anesthetic techniques is the ability to provide excellent postoperative analgesia with spinal or epidural narcotics.

Surgical procedures requiring the construction of free microvascular flaps may be prolonged, in which case it may be advantageous to combine regional techniques with light general anesthesia.

For general anesthesia, a variety of techniques and agents are available to produce unconsciousness, analgesia, and muscular relaxation. Loss of consciousness is usually rapidly achieved with intravenous agents such as the barbiturates (Pentothal) or the benzodiazepines (diazepam or midazolam). In small children with difficult venous access, it is possible to induce general anesthesia with the inhalational agents or ketamine given intramuscularly.

Maintenance of the state of general anesthesia is achieved with potent inhalation agents such as halothane, enflurane, and isoflurane in a mixture of nitrous oxide and oxygen. Supplementation with narcotic analgesics such as fentanyl and morphine is usually required.

Muscular relaxation for the surgical procedure is achieved with neuromuscular blocking agents such as succinylcholine, d'tubocurarine, pancuronium, vecuronium, and atracurium.

Major blood loss during limb preservation, particularly with extremely vascular lesions, is to be anticipated. Adequate supplies of blood should always be available prior to the commencement of surgery. Autologous donation before surgery should be encouraged. However, because many of these patients are anemic as a result of chemotherapy, presurgical donation is not possible. In such cases, donation from relatives should be encouraged. Acute isovolemic hemodilution techniques are currently being evaluated; with this technique the patient's own blood is salvaged for subsequent transfusion. Anesthesiologists are primarily responsible for blood transfusion intraoperatively and are aware of the possible adverse immunosuppressive effects of perioperative blood transfusion in cancer patients. In 1981 Gantt raised the possibility that patients with cancer who receive blood transfusions suppress the immune system, thereby increasing the incidence of tumor survival.[2] Rosenberg and associates noted a highly significant association between perioperative transfusion and decreased survival of patients with high-grade soft tissue sarcoma of the extremities. The risks and benefits of perioperative transfusion must therefore be carefully assessed.[8]

Absolutely meticulous attention must be paid to sterility with all anesthetic procedures and interventions. Immunosuppression is not at all uncommon in these patients, and infection may result in a poor outcome.

References

1. Dripps RD, Echenhoff JE, Vandam LD: Introduction to Anesthesia, 5th ed. Philadelphia, WB Saunders, 1977, pp 306, 292–296, 260–281.
2. Gantt CL: Red blood cells for cancer patients. Lancet 2:363, 1981.
3. Goldman L, Caldera DL, Nusbaum SR, et al: Multifactorial index of cardiac risk in non-cardiac surgical procedures. N Engl J Med 297:845, 1977.
4. Howland WS, Rooney SM, Goldiner PL: Manual of Anesthesia in Cancer Care. New York, Churchill Livingstone, 1986, p 91.
5. Knaus WA, Draper EA, Wagner DP, et al: APACHE: A severity of disease classification system. Crit Care Med 13:818, 1985.
6. Pearce AC, Jones RM: Smoking and anesthesia: Preoperative abstinence and perioperative morbidity. Anesthesiology 61:576, 1984.
7. Prys-Roberts C, Meloche R, Foex P: Studies of the anaesthesia in relation to hypertension. 1: Cardiovascular responses of treated and untreated patients. Br J Anaesth 43:122, 1971.
8. Rosenberg SA, Seipp CA, White DE, Wesley R: Perioperative blood transfusions are associated with increased risks of recurrence and decreased survival in patients with high-grade soft tissue sarcomas of the extremities. J Clin Oncol 3:698–709, 1985.
9. Stoelting RK: Chemotherapeutic drugs. *In* Pharmacology and Physiology in Anesthetic Practice. Philadelphia, JB Lippincott, 1987, pp 480–498.
10. Stoelting RK, Miller RD: Basics of Anesthesia, 2nd ed. New York, Churchill Livingstone, 1989, p 114.

Index

Note: Page numbers in *italics* indicate illustrations; those followed by t indicate tables.

B

G

H

I

M

N

P

Q

R

S

T

U

V

W

X

Z